Clinical Medical Ethics

Laura Weiss Roberts • Mark Siegler

Editors

Clinical Medical Ethics

Landmark Works of Mark Siegler, MD

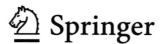 Springer

Editors
Laura Weiss Roberts
Stanford University School of Medicine
Palo Alto, CA, USA

Mark Siegler
University of Chicago
Pritzker School of Medicine
Chicago, IL, USA

ISBN 978-3-319-85262-1   ISBN 978-3-319-53875-4   (eBook)
DOI 10.1007/978-3-319-53875-4

This Springer imprint is published by Springer Nature
The registered company is Springer International Publishing AG
The registered company address is: Gewerbestrasse 11, 6330 Cham, Switzerland

Anna, this book is yours

—M.S.

For Eric, always

—L.W.R.

Preface

Throughout his career, Dr. Mark Siegler has written on topics ranging from the teaching of clinical medical ethics to end-of-life decision-making and the ethics of advances in technology. With more than 200 journal publications and 60 book chapters to choose from, the editors did their best to select representative scholarship of enduring value. We have organized our collection of 46 landmark works under the five themes of foundational scholarship, the doctor-patient relationship, education and professionalism, end-of-life care, and clinical innovation. The collected works are listed below, chronologically within the selected themes.

Reprinted works under the theme of foundational scholarship:

- Siegler M (1979) Clinical ethics and clinical medicine. Arch Intern Med 139:914–5
- Siegler M (1982) Decision-making strategy for clinical ethical problems in medicine. Arch Intern Med 142:2178–9
- La Puma J, Stocking CB, Silverstein MD, DiMartini A, Siegler M (1988) An ethics consultation service in a teaching hospital. Utilization and evaluation. JAMA 260:808–11
- Siegler M, Pellegrino ED, Singer PA (1990) Clinical medical ethics. J Clin Ethics 1:5–9
- Singer PA, Pellegrino ED, Siegler M (1990) Ethics committees and consultants. J Clin Ethics 1:263–7
- Pellegrino ED, Siegler M, Singer PA (1991) Future directions in clinical ethics. J Clin Ethics 2:5–9
- Siegler M, Singer PA (1991) Clinical ethics. In: Kelley WN (ed) Textbook of internal medicine, 2nd edn. JB Lippincott Co., Philadelphia, p 3–5
- Singer PA, Siegler M (1996) Clinical ethics in the practice of medicine. In: Wyngaarten JB, Plum F, Bennett C (eds) Cecil textbook of medicine, 20th edn. WB Saunders Co., Philadelphia, p 4–6
- Ross LF, Siegler M (1997) Five major themes in bioethics. Forum: Trends in Experimental and Clinical Medicine 7:8–17
- Siegler M (1997) The contributions of clinical ethics to patient care. Forum: Trends in Experimental and Clinical Medicine 7:244–51

Reprinted works under the theme of the doctor-patient relationship:

- Siegler M (1981) Searching for moral certainty in medicine: a proposal for a new model of the doctor-patient encounter. Bull N Y Acad Med 57:56–69
- Siegler M, Goldblatt AD (1981) Clinical intuition: a procedure for balancing the rights of patients and the responsibilities of physicians. In: Spicker SF, Healey JM, Engelhardt Jr HT (eds) The Law-Medicine Relation: A Philosophical Exploration. D. Reidel, Boston, p 5–31
- Siegler M (1981) The doctor-patient encounter and its relationship to theories of health and disease. In: Caplan AL, Engelhardt Jr HT, McCartney JJ (eds) Concepts of Health and Disease: Interdisciplinary Perspectives. Addison-Wesley, Reading, Massachusetts, p 627–44
- Siegler M (1982) The physician-patient accommodation: a central event in clinical medicine. Arch Intern Med 142:1899–1902

- Siegler M (1982) Confidentiality in medicine: a decrepit concept. N Engl J Med 307:1518–21
- Siegler M (1982) Medical consultations in the context of the physician-patient relationship. In: Agich GJ (ed) Responsibility in Health Care. D. Reidel, Boston, p 141–62
- Childress JF, Siegler M (1984) Metaphors and models of doctor-patient relationships: their implications for autonomy. Theoret Med 5:17–30
- Siegler M (1985) The progression of medicine: from physician paternalism to patient autonomy to bureaucratic parsimony. Arch Intern Med 145:713–15
- Daugherty CK, Siegler M, Ratain MJ, Zimmer G (1997) Learning from our patients: one participant's impact on clinical trial research and informed consent. Ann Intern Med 126:892–7
- Torke AM, Alexander GC, Lantos J, Siegler M (2007) The physician-surrogate relationship. Arch Intern Med 167:1117–21

Reprinted works under the theme of education and professionalism:

- Siegler M (1978) A legacy of Osler: teaching clinical ethics at the bedside. JAMA 239:951–6
- Culver C, Clouser KD, Gert B, Brody H, Fletcher J, Jonsen A, Kopelman L, Lynn J, Siegler M, Wikler D (1985) Basic curricular goals in medical ethics: the DeCamp conference on the teaching of medical ethics. N Engl J Med 312:253–56
- Lane LW, Siegler M, Miles SH, Cassel CK, Singer PA (1988) Fellowship training programs in clinical ethics. Soc Gen Intern Med Newsletter 3:4–5
- Walker RM, Lane LW, Siegler M (1989) Development of a teaching program in clinical medical ethics at the University of Chicago. Acad Med 64:723–9
- Jacobson JA, Tolle SW, Stocking C, Siegler M (1989) Internal medicine residents' preferences regarding medical ethics education. Acad Med 64:760–4
- Lane LW, Lane G, Schiedermayer DL, Spiro JH, Siegler M (1990) Caring for medical students as patients. Arch Intern Med 150:2249–53
- Pellegrino ED, Siegler M, Singer PA (1990) Teaching clinical ethics. J Clin Ethics 1:175–80
- Roberts LW, Hardee JT, Franchini G, Stidley C, Siegler M (1996) Medical students as patients: a pilot study of their health care needs, practices, and concerns. Acad Med 71:1225–32
- Roberts LW, McCarty T, Lyketsos C, Hardee JT, Jacobson J, Walker R, Hough P, Gramelspacher G, Stidley C, Arambula M, Heebink DM, Zornberg GL, Siegler M (1996) What and how psychiatry residents at ten training programs wish to learn about ethics. Acad Psychiatry 20:131–43
- Roberts LW, McCarty T, Roberts BB, Morrison N, Belitz J, Berenson C, Siegler M (1996) Clinical ethics teaching in psychiatric supervision. Acad Psychiatry 20:176–88
- Siegler M (2002) Training doctors for professionalism: some lessons from teaching clinical medical ethics. Mt. Sinai Med J 69:404–9

Reprinted works under the theme of end-of-life care:

- Siegler M (1975) Pascal's wager and the hanging of crepe. N Engl J Med 293:853–7
- Siegler M (1977) Critical illness: the limits of autonomy. Hast Cent Rep 7:12–5
- Siegler M, Wikler D (1982) Brain death and live birth. JAMA 248:1101–2
- Siegler M, Weisbard AJ (1985) Against the emerging stream: should fluids and nutritional support be discontinued? Arch Int Med 145:129–31
- Singer PA, Siegler M (1990) Euthanasia: a critique. N Engl J Med 322:1881–3
- Singer PA, Siegler M (1991) Elective use of life-sustaining treatments in internal medicine. Adv Inter Med 36:57–79

- Siegler M, Taylor RM (1993) Intimacy and caring: the legacy of Karen Ann Quinlan. Trends in Health Care Law Ethics 8:28–30, 38
- Helft P, Siegler M, Lantos J (2000) The rise and fall of the futility movement. N Engl J Med 343:293–6

Reprinted works under the theme of clinical innovation:

- Lantos JD, Siegler M, Cuttler L (1989) Ethical issues in growth hormone therapy. JAMA 261:1020–4
- Arnow P, Pottenger L, Stocking C, Siegler M, DeLeeuw H (1989) Orthopedic surgeons' attitudes and practices concerning treatment of patients with HIV infection. Public Health Reports 104:121–9
- Singer PA, Siegler M, Whitington PF, Lantos JD, Emond JC, Thistlethwaite JR, Broelsch CE (1989) Ethics of liver transplantation with living donors. N Engl J Med 321:620–2
- Kodish E, Lantos JD, Stocking CB, Singer PA, Siegler M, Johnson FL (1991) Bone marrow transplantation for sickle cell disease; a study of parents' decisions. N Eng J Med 325:1349–53
- Siegler M, Lantos JD (1992) Ethical justification for living liver donation. Camb Q Healthc Ethics 4:320–5
- Cronin D, Millis M, Siegler M (2001) Transplantation of liver grafts from living donors into adults: too much, too soon. N Eng J Med 344:1633–7
- Testa G, Angelos P, Crowley-Matoka M, Siegler M (2009) Elective surgical patients as living organ donors: a clinical and ethical innovation. Am J Transplant 9:2400–5

We express our gratitude for the permission granted to reproduce the copyrighted material in this book. Every effort has been made to trace copyright holders and to obtain their formal permission for use of copyright material. We apologize for any errors or omissions and request that we be notified of any corrections that should be incorporated in future reprints or editions of this book.

Stanford, CA, USA   Laura Weiss Roberts
Chicago, IL, USA   Mark Siegler

Acknowledgments

The editors wish to thank the contributing authors who generously shared their perspectives for *Clinical Medical Ethics: Landmark Works of Mark Siegler, M.D.* The editors sincerely thank Ann Tennier, ELS, senior managing editor, for her work in coordinating this project. We also thank Megan Cid; Katie Ryan, M.A.; Gabrielle Termuehlen; and Kevin Wright for their assistance at various stages in the preparation of this book. We thank the staff members at the MacLean Center: Kimberly Conner, office manager; research assistants Tae Yeon Kim, Christian Lowe, Mike Andersen, Wendy Tian, Cynthia J. Avila, Sarah Watanaskul, and Jasmine Solola, and Benjamin Bazin, intern. We also thank the contributors of photos for the Appendix.

The editors gratefully acknowledge the permission granted to reproduce the copyright material in this book. Every effort has been made to trace copyright holders and to obtain their permission for the use of copyright material. We apologize for any errors or omissions and would be grateful if notified of any corrections that should be incorporated in future reprints or editions of this book.

The editors also wish to thank Richard Lansing of Springer Science + Business Media, LLC, our wonderful colleague and publisher.

Contents

Contributors

Jordan J. Cohen, MD Association of American Medical Colleges, Arnold P. Gold Foundation for Humanism in Medicine, Englewood Cliffs, NJ, USA

Holly J. Humphrey, MD University of Chicago, Pritzker School of Medicine, Chicago, IL, USA

Dana Levinson, MPH University of Chicago, Pritzker School of Medicine, Chicago, IL, USA

Kenneth S. Polonsky, MD Division of the Biological Sciences, University of Chicago, Pritzker School of Medicine, Chicago, IL, USA

Laura Weiss Roberts, MD, MA Department of Psychiatry and Behavioral Sciences, Stanford University School of Medicine, Stanford, CA, USA

Mark Siegler, MD Bucksbaum Institute for Clinical Excellence, MacLean Center for Clinical Medical Ethics, University of Chicago, Pritzker School of Medicine, Chicago, IL, USA

Peter A. Singer, MD University Health Network, Grand Challenges Canada at the Sandra Rotman Centre, Toronto, ON, Canada

Daniel P. Sulmasy, MD, PhD Georgetown University, Pellegrino Center for Clinical Bioethics, Washington, DC, USA

Part I

Restoring and Transforming the Ethical Basis of Modern Clinical Medicine

An Introduction to the Work and Writings of Mark Siegler

Laura Weiss Roberts

Abstract

Dr. Mark Siegler is a founder of the interdisciplinary field of clinical medical ethics. By insisting that ethical issues in medicine could be addressed through hypothesis-driven empirical research, Siegler transformed the theoretical field of bioethics and developed an area of study that directly addressed both the everyday realities of medicine and some of the most challenging ethical questions of the past half-century. Throughout his scholarly career, Siegler has written hundreds of papers on topics ranging from the teaching of clinical medical ethics to end-of-life decision-making and the ethics of advances in technology. His work has inspired the work of many other clinician ethicists, and his innovative approaches to the physician-patient relationship and ethics consultations are widely accepted today as the premier way to provide high-level clinical care. Students and graduates from his interdisciplinary fellowship training program in clinical medical ethics have expanded on Siegler's body of work and brought his theories and teachings to every corner of the globe.

In three-piece wool suits, wire-rimmed glasses, and scuffed oxfords, Mark Siegler is not anyone's image of an innovator. With his emphasis on the doctor-patient relationship and talk of old-fashioned values in medicine, he may not sound like an innovator either. And yet, innovator he is.

1.1 Innovation

Siegler has redefined how modern clinical medicine is practiced and studied by integrating rigorous ethical decision-making into all aspects of patient care. The implications of his work are felt in every discipline of medicine, every health profession, and across society. His approach seamlessly integrates careful consideration of values, the duties of the healer, the nature of a profession, standards of care and the state of biomedical science, and novel interdisciplinary

scholarship and evidence into clinical care. "In a sense, the term 'clinical ethics' is redundant," Siegler wrote in 1979, "because good clinical medicine is necessarily ethical medicine" (p. 915 [1]). Ethics, Siegler has insisted, is not an afterthought, luxury, or secondary consideration in our care of patients — ethics is essential and necessary to excellence in clinical medicine.

Siegler has changed clinical medicine, in my view, through a number of highly innovative approaches. With colleagues and mentees, Siegler has essentially invented a new collaborative and interdisciplinary field of clinical medical ethics. As he noted, "The practice of clinical medicine has always been a unique blend of technical proficiency and ethical sensitivity, which together constitute the physician's art" (p. 914 [1]). Building upon and moving beyond this tradition in medicine, Siegler has cultivated the use of empirical inquiry and rigorous analytical scholarship from the humanities, the law, and the social and biomedical sciences to address complex issues in modern clinical medicine. This diverse interdisciplinary approach has brought wisdom and evidence forward to redefine ethical imperatives and standards in clinical care and has redesigned public policy and medical education in a lasting way.

L.W. Roberts, MD, MA (✉)
Department of Psychiatry and Behavioral Sciences,
Stanford University School of Medicine, Stanford, CA, USA
e-mail: robertsl@stanford.edu

L.W. Roberts, M. Siegler (eds.), *Clinical Medical Ethics*, DOI 10.1007/978-3-319-53875-4_1

As a natural extension of this work, Siegler championed the practice of consultation in clinical medical ethics [2], aligning the field with other consultative activities of medicine creating distinction from the work of ethics committees. Since 1985, Siegler and colleagues at the University of Chicago have performed more than many hundreds of clinical ethics consultations in diverse settings to assist physicians in their patient care decisions. Siegler articulated the view:

> Ethics case consultations, which focus on individual patient dilemmas, is a health care innovation that has been widely incorporated into many large hospitals' practices. The hope is that such consultations may help resolve dilemmas, decrease conflict, improve the decision-making process, and improve patient outcomes (p. 248 [3]).

Siegler's model of ethics consultation blended with ordinary clinical care activities for doctors — just as a primary care physician might seek counsel from a cardiologist, psychiatrist, or endocrinologist in the course of routine patient care, he or she might now also seek an ethics consultation to aid in clinical decision-making. At the time, ethics committees had only recently been adopted, largely in reaction to new regulations following the tragic case of a newborn with Down Syndrome ("Baby Doe") who died after being denied a relatively routine and life-saving surgery for esophageal atresia and a tracheoesophageal fistula specifically because of her genetically based disability [4]. With such a stormy introduction, ethics committees were perceived as serving to redirect physician behaviors and countermand their decisions. Having a clinical case "go to the ethics committee" was viewed as a vulnerability. With the innovation of routine clinical ethics consultation, Siegler changed the paradigmatic view of ethics and ethicists as "watchdogs" working against physicians in high-visibility, high-risk circumstances to a new view in which physician-ethicists, as colleagues, could enhance and strengthen the natural work of being a doctor and serving one's patients well.

In addition to clinical ethics consultation for complex patient care decisions, Siegler advanced a novel model of research ethics consultation that involved the collaboration of clinical investigators and clinical research ethicists in the review and development of a research project's design and implementation, with the goal of preemptively addressing any ethical considerations associated with the project [5]. After 1987, when Dr. Siegler and his team at the University of Chicago deemed research consultation to be a best practice in ethics [6], research ethics consultation services started to be implemented by the National Institutes of Health and dozens of universities across the United States. A casebook on research ethics consultation has recently been published, further emphasizing the value that these consultations hold in the field of human research [7].

Fighting the trend of medicine as technologically rich but interpersonally impoverished, Siegler has also elevated the therapeutic relationship. He has focused on attunement to the experience and concerns of the patient and the "accommodation" between patient and physician as central to compassionate, competent clinical care. This model resolves the tension between two dominant approaches: the traditional paternalistic relationship "premised on trust in the physician's technical competence and moral sensitivity and … characterized by patient dependency and physician control" and an emerging medical "consumerism" model in which the physician is a "passive agent, a hired technician who practices under the direction and control of his 'client'" (p. 248 [3]).

Siegler's model discards these two extreme, adversarial views of physician-patient decisions and the relationship between doctors and patients. Instead, he recommends a model of physician-patient accommodation that is "a bilateral one in which the moral and technical arrangements of a medical encounter are determined mutually, voluntarily, and autonomously by both patient and physician" (p. 60 [8]). He affirms that the "personality, character, attitude, and values" of the patient as well as of the physician, plus the physician's technical skills, the nature and gravity of the illness process, and the context of care, will each influence the accommodation that occurs between patient and physician (p. 62 [8]). Siegler characterizes the accommodation as realistic and dynamic—always changing, always in flux, and always requiring attention from the physician in order to fulfill its role in healing. In its ideal form, he suggests, this relationship will feature "mature and enduring exchanges of trust" that bring forward the patient's desired goals (p. 63 [8]).

Siegler's patient-physician accommodation model was often cited in the 1982 President's Commission for the Study of Ethical Problems in Medicine and Biomedical and Behavioral Research report on making health care decisions, which concluded that Siegler's model would "do better justice to the realities of healthcare and to the ethical values underlying the informed consent doctrine" (p. 38 [9]). The patient-physician accommodation model endures as the basis for optimal patient-centered care practices and underpins recent movements in the United States, such as current efforts toward shared decision-making elevated by the Institute of Medicine [10].

Although Siegler gravitates to everyday ethics challenges in patient care, he has taken on the most difficult and most compelling and complex issues faced in modern medicine. Highly innovative questions he has asked include the following: What is the definition of medical futility, and when should patients be allowed to die? What is the definition of death? Can physicians ethically engage in euthanasia and assisted death practices? What are the limits of patient autonomy? And what of physician autonomy? When can doctors choose not to care for certain patients? And how do physicians approach radical new interventions, such as in hand transplantations or liver transplantation with living donors?

What is the ethical justification for high-risk innovation in different areas of surgery as well as in oncology, pediatrics, internal medicine, genetics, and other medical fields? How can we ensure the highest ethical standards when performing human research? Can ethics be taught to young physicians? While other ethicists would ponder or, more cynically, pontificate on the moral complexities associated with such hard questions, Siegler has sought answers.

In advancing the field of clinical medical ethics and tackling the hardest issues encountered in modern medicine, Siegler sought answers. He acknowledges that these solutions are often imperfect and uncertain and often lead to more and equally difficult questions, but they provide clarity and possess authentic value for physicians grappling with ethical challenges in their everyday professional lives. Siegler's work, performed in collaboration with colleagues across diverse fields of medicine, has offered practical guidance for doctors, the health profession, and society as the ethical challenges of medicine have evolved with rapidity and unexpected complexity. This guidance has changed the practice of medicine and has done much to affirm the public's trust in the profession.

Finally, Siegler's innovation has extended to include a robust educational and scientific agenda over more than 40 years. For decades, every undergraduate medical student and resident at the University of Chicago's Pritzker School of Medicine has benefited from Siegler's direct teaching in the context of clinical case conferences, case consultations, seminar series, and annual conferences. Every member of the faculty and every learner, including students in the college, graduate programs, and professional schools on campus, have had the opportunity to participate in the exceptionally well-designed and rich curricular activities of the MacLean Center for Clinical Medical Ethics and, more recently, of the Bucksbaum Institute for Clinical Excellence. Literally hundreds of clinician-ethicists have trained with Mark Siegler, and his students have established ethics programs, centers, and institutes on seven continents. An outstanding educator and leader of education programs, Mark Siegler is an extraordinary and beloved mentor who has worked intensively, collaboratively, inclusively, and, many would add, relentlessly to enable the achievement and positive impact of his mentees. It is not an exaggeration to state that Siegler's educational reach is felt worldwide.

While his scholarship has been much celebrated, Siegler's scientific agenda may be underappreciated for its innovative nature and true impact. Nevertheless, it is Siegler's focus on the everyday realities of medicine and his insistence that ethics questions are amenable to empirical study, and often may be resolved through scientific inquiry, that, in my view, represents his greatest and most enduring contribution. Siegler recognized early on that hypothesis-driven empirical research was a key method for illuminating and resolving

ethical issues of genuine importance to society, including ethical issues arising in the ecology of clinical practice, clinical trials, technological innovation, "bench to bedside" translational research, and community-based participatory and population projects. While opinions — even well-informed and well-reasoned positions — are common on any number of ethics issues, they often come into conflict and do not produce actionable conclusions. Empirical study, on the other hand, can actually answer certain kinds of highly salient ethical questions and offer practicable guidance. Moreover, it is Siegler's view, and mine, that evidence drives transformational change in medicine. Seeking and applying new knowledge are central to academic medicine and these endeavors align with the practical intention of physicians.

Certainly my own ethics work on informed consent, biomedical innovation, health disparities, and special issues arising in clinical care and research involving vulnerable populations has been informed by this scientific stance. My studies funded by the National Institutes of Health have focused on ethical questions of broad importance, and our results have informed clinical, educational, and research practice and public policy. For example, with colleagues I have investigated whether people with mental illnesses may be more vulnerable to exploitation and less well protected by human research safeguards than people with other kinds of illnesses in clinical research [11]. We learned that the vulnerabilities of mentally ill individuals in the research situation, in general, do not differ in kind or seriousness than those of other human subjects and, ironically, healthy individuals may under some circumstances experience greater risk than their ill counterparts. We have learned that many people with the most serious illnesses, whether physical or mental disorders, appreciate the difference between research and usual clinical care. In addition, ill individuals express altruistic motivations far more commonly than expected. They also express their hope that doctors will do the right thing to help them, even when the interventions may differ from their expressed preferences. Such findings reinforce the value of robust safeguards in human research for all participants and also affirm the decisions made on several occasions not to create separate regulations for mental illness research.

Through science, my team and I have asked and answered several other ethically salient questions as well. Do people who live in rural and frontier areas receive a lesser standard of care due to challenges regarding not only resource availability but also special challenges for the therapeutic relationship, confidentiality, informed consent, and treatment adherence in sparsely populated community settings [12]? Do underrepresented minority individuals view genetic innovation similarly to majority individuals [13]? Do employees and employers differ in their perspectives on how personal health and genetic information should be used, or not, in the workplace [14]? How does stigma alter practices and standards in clinical care, research, and education activities in medicine [15, 16]? These questions arise from real experience in caring for patients, in engaging in clinical research, and in seeking to create health and social policies that are attuned to the needs and perspectives of all who must live them out in everyday life.

Such scientific work serves as only one example in which resolving empirical questions in medicine can bring forward new practices, standards of care, and innovation on multiple levels. Siegler, with many colleagues around the world, has engaged in robust scientific collaborations of importance and impact across medicine. He has worked to bring evidence to bear on the challenges faced by doctors and patients, leaders in medicine and government, and scholars in diverse academic disciplines. Siegler's near-Herculean efforts to advance an educational and scientific agenda at the University of Chicago have ensured that not only current medical practice but future health care practices around the world are informed by the insights and methods of clinical medical ethics.

1.2   This Book

Mark Siegler has written exceptional papers addressing both everyday and emergent ethics issues in practically every field in medicine since 1975. His scholarship is widely praised

and has been cited thousands of times. Our aim in selecting the papers for this collection of his landmark works was to include many of his best and his most highly influential publications, to include both conceptual and empirical pieces, and to show how Siegler's work changed the ethics dialogue in internal medicine, surgery, pediatrics, oncology, medical education, and other areas of medicine. Illustrations are abundant, and include early publications on controversial topics such as whether to withdraw life support from patients with terminal illness, ethics considerations in risky and innovative liver transplantation in live organ donors, futility in premature infants with low birthweight, whether surgeons could decline to operate on patients who are HIV-positive, and the "decrepit concept" of confidentiality in modern medicine. Each paper is meritorious and each paper, as the reader will recognize, was well ahead of its time.

Choosing from among more than 200 journal publications and 60 book chapters written by Siegler proved to be very difficult. We arranged our choices within the broad themes of foundational scholarship, the doctor-patient relationship, education and professionalism, end-of-life care, and clinical innovation. The end result is presented in this collection of 46 landmark works (Table 1.1). Siegler introduces this collection with his reflections, and we have invited a number of scholars to contribute perspectives to help frame the context and meaning of Siegler's work in clinical medical ethics.

Table 1.1 Mark Siegler's landmark works reprinted in this book

Foundational Scholarship
Siegler M (1979) Clinical ethics and clinical medicine. Arch Intern Med 139:914–5
Siegler M (1982) Decision-making strategy for clinical ethical problems in medicine. Arch Intern Med 142:2178–9
La Puma J, Stocking CB, Silverstein MD, DiMartini A, Siegler M (1988) An ethics consultation service in a teaching hospital. Utilization and evaluation. JAMA 260:808–11
Siegler M, Pellegrino ED, Singer PA (1990) Clinical medical ethics. J Clin Ethics 1:5–9
Singer PA, Pellegrino ED, Siegler M (1990) Ethics committees and consultants. J Clin Ethics 1:263–7
Pellegrino ED, Siegler M, Singer PA (1991) Future directions in clinical ethics. J Clin Ethics 2:5–9
Singer PA, Siegler M (1991) Clinical ethics. In: Kelley WN (ed) Textbook of internal medicine, 2nd edn. JB Lippincott Co., Philadelphia, p 3–5
Singer PA, Siegler M (1996) Clinical ethics in the practice of medicine. In: Wyngaarten JB, Plum F, Bennett C (eds) Cecil textbook of medicine, 20th edn. WB Saunders Co., Philadelphia, p 4–6
Ross LF, Siegler M (1997) Five major themes in bioethics. Forum: Trends in Experimental and Clinical Medicine 7:8–17
Siegler M (1997) The contributions of clinical ethics to patient care. Forum: Trends in Experimental and Clinical Medicine 7:244–51
The Doctor-Patient Relationship
Siegler M (1981) Searching for moral certainty in medicine: a proposal for a new model of the doctor-patient encounter. Bull N Y Acad Med 57:56–69
Siegler M, Goldblatt AD (1981) Clinical intuition: a procedure for balancing the rights of patients and the responsibilities of physicians. In: Spicker SF, Healey JM, Engelhardt Jr. HT (eds) The Law-Medicine Relation: A Philosophical Exploration. D. Reidel, Boston, p 5–31
Siegler M (1981) The doctor-patient encounter and its relationship to theories of health and disease. In: Caplan AL, Engelhardt Jr HT, McCartney JJ (eds) Concepts of Health and Disease: Interdisciplinary Perspectives. Addison-Wesley, Reading, Massachusetts, p 627–44
Siegler M (1982) The physician-patient accommodation: a central event in clinical medicine. Arch Intern Med 142:1899–1902
Siegler M (1982) Confidentiality in medicine: a decrepit concept. N Engl J Med 307:1518–21
Siegler M (1982) Medical consultations in the context of the physician-patient relationship. In: Agich GJ (ed) Responsibility in Health Care. D. Reidel, Boston, p 141–62
Childress JF, Siegler M (1984) Metaphors and models of doctor-patient relationships: their implications for autonomy. Theoret Med 5:17–30

(continued)

Table 1.1 (continued)

Siegler M (1985) The progression of medicine: from physician paternalism to patient autonomy to bureaucratic parsimony. Arch Intern Med 145:713–15

Daugherty CK, Siegler M, Ratain MJ, Zimmer G (1997) Learning from our patients: one participant's impact on clinical trial research and informed consent. Ann Intern Med 126:892–7

Torke AM, Alexander GC, Lantos J, Siegler M (2007) The physician-surrogate relationship. Arch Intern Med 167:1117–21

Education and Professionalism

Siegler M (1978) A legacy of Osler: teaching clinical ethics at the bedside. JAMA 239:951–6

Culver C, Clouser KD, Gert B, Brody H, Fletcher J, Jonsen A, Kopelman L, Lynn J, Siegler M, Wikler D (1985) Basic curricular goals in medical ethics: the DeCamp conference on the teaching of medical ethics. N Engl J Med 312:253–56

Lane LW, Siegler M, Miles SH, Cassel CK, Singer PA (1988) Fellowship training programs in clinical ethics. Soc Gen Intern Med Newsletter 3:4–5

Walker RM, Lane LW, Siegler M (1989) Development of a teaching program in clinical medical ethics at the University of Chicago. Acad Med 64:723–9

Jacobson JA, Tolle SW, Stocking C, Siegler M (1989) Internal medicine residents' preferences regarding medical ethics education. Acad Med 64:760–4

Lane LW, Lane G, Schiedermayer DL, Spiro JH, Siegler M (1990) Caring for medical students as patients. Arch Intern Med 150:2249–53

Pellegrino ED, Siegler M, Singer PA (1990) Teaching clinical ethics. J Clin Ethics 1:175–80

Roberts LW, Hardee JT, Franchini G, Stidley C, Siegler M (1996) Medical students as patients: a pilot study of their health care needs, practices, and concerns. Acad Med 71:1225–32

Roberts LW, McCarty T, Lyketsos C, Hardee JT, Jacobson J, Walker R, Hough P, Gramelspacher G, Stidley C, Arambula M, Heebink DM, Zornberg GL, Siegler M (1996) What and how psychiatry residents at ten training programs wish to learn about ethics. Acad Psychiatry 20:131–43

Roberts LW, McCarty T, Roberts BB, Morrison N, Belitz J, Berenson C, Siegler M (1996) Clinical ethics teaching in psychiatric supervision. Acad Psychiatry 20:176–88

Siegler M (2002) Training doctors for professionalism: some lessons from teaching clinical medical ethics. Mt. Sinai Med J 69:404–9

End-of-Life Care

Siegler M (1975) Pascal's wager and the hanging of crepe. N Engl J Med 293:853–7

Siegler M (1977) Critical illness: the limits of autonomy. Hast Cent Rep 7:12–15

Siegler M, Wikler D (1982) Brain death and live birth. JAMA 248:1101–2

Siegler M, Weisbard AJ (1985) Against the emerging stream: should fluids and nutritional support be discontinued? Arch Int Med 145:129–31

Singer PA, Siegler M (1990) Euthanasia: a critique. N Engl J Med 322:1881–3

Singer PA, Siegler M (1991) Elective use of life-sustaining treatments in internal medicine. Adv Inter Med 36:57–79

Siegler M, Taylor RM (1993) Intimacy and caring: the legacy of Karen Ann Quinlan. Trends in Health Care Law Ethics 8:28–30, 38

Helft P, Siegler M, Lantos J (2000) The rise and fall of the futility movement. N Engl J Med 343:293–6

Clinical Innovation

Lantos JD, Siegler M, Cuttler L (1989) Ethical issues in growth hormone therapy. JAMA 261:1020–4

Arnow P, Pottenger L, Stocking C, Siegler M., DeLeeuw H (1989) Orthopedic surgeons' attitudes and practices concerning treatment of patients with HIV infection. Public Health Reports 104:121–9

Singer PA, Siegler M, Whitington PF, Lantos JD, Emond JC, Thistlethwaite JR, Broelsch CE (1989) Ethics of liver transplantation with living donors. N Engl J Med 321:620–2

Kodish E, Lantos JD, Stocking CB, Singer PA, Siegler M, Johnson FL (1991) Bone marrow transplantation for sickle cell disease. A study of parents' decisions. N Eng J Med 325:1349–53

Siegler M, Lantos JD (1992) Ethical justification for living liver donation. Camb Q Healthc Ethics 4:320–5

Cronin D, Millis M, Siegler M (2001) Transplantation of liver grafts from living donors into adults: too much, too soon. N Eng J Med 344:1633–7

Testa G, Angelos P, Crowley-Matoka M, Siegler M (2009) Elective surgical patients as living organ donors: a clinical and ethical innovation. Am J Transplant 9:2400–5

The editors gratefully acknowledge the outstanding work of our respective teams, with heartfelt appreciation and deep respect for Ann Tennier, whose careful and tenacious efforts have brought this project to fruition. We express our gratitude for the permission granted to reproduce the copyright material in this book. Every effort has been made to trace copyright holders and to obtain their formal permission for use of copyright material. We apologize for any errors or omissions and request that we be notified of any corrections that should be incorporated in future reprints or editions of this book. We also thank Richard Lansing of Springer Publishing for his commitment to us in developing this collection, which we believe will be of value to scholars and scientists, physicians and ethicists, and especially to those of our colleagues who are all four.

References

1. Siegler M. Clinical ethics and clinical medicine. Arch Intern Med. 1979;139:914–5.
2. La Puma J, Stocking CB, Silverstein MD, DiMartini A, Siegler M. An ethics consultation service in a teaching hospital: utilization and evaluation. JAMA. 1988;260(6):808–11.
3. Siegler M. The contributions of clinical ethics to patient care. Forum: Trends in Exp Clin Med. 1997;7:244–53.
4. White M. The end at the beginning. Oschsner J. 2011;11(4): 309–16.
5. Singer PA, Siegler M, Whitington PF, et al. Ethics of liver transplantation with living donors. N Engl J Med. 1989;321:620–2.
6. The MacLean Center. Ethics consultation services [The University of Chicago Medicine website]. 2016. Accessed 1 Nov 2016 from http://macleanethics.uchicago.edu/consultation.
7. Danis M, Largent E, Grady C, et al. Research ethics consultation: a casebook. New York: Oxford University Press; 2012.
8. Siegler M. Searching for moral certainty in medicine: a proposal for a new model of the doctor-patient encounter. Bull NY Acad Med. 1981;57(1):56–69.
9. U.S. Bioethics Commission. President's commission for the study of ethical problems in medicine and biomedical and behavioral research. Making health care decisions. vol. 1. Washington, DC: US, Government Printing Office; 1982.
10. Alson C, Berger ZD, Brownlee S, et al. (2014) Shared decision-making strategies for best care: patient decision aids. Institute of Medicine. Accessed 31 Oct 2016 from https://nam.edu/wp-content/uploads/2015/06/SDMforBestCare2.pdf.
11. Roberts LW, Kim JP. Giving voice to study volunteers: comparing views of mentally ill, physically ill, and healthy protocol participants on ethical aspects of clinical research. J Psychiatr Res. 2014;56:90–7.
12. Roberts LW, Johnson ME, Brems C, Warner TD. Ethical disparities: challenges encountered by multidisciplinary providers in fulfilling ethical standards in the care of rural and minority people. J Rural Health. 2007;23:89–97.
13. Ngui EM, Warner TD, Roberts LW. Ethical responsibilities and perceptions of stakeholders of genetic research involving racial/ethnic minority participants. AJOB Empir Bioethics. 2015;6(3): 15–27.
14. Roberts LW, Barry LK, Warner TD. Potential workplace discrimination based on genetic predisposition: views of workers. AJOB Prim Res. 2011;2(3):1–12.
15. Roberts LW, Warner TD, Brody JL, et al. Stigma, ethics, and the frontier: challenges for caring for people with serious illnesses in Alaska and New Mexico. Arctic Res US. 2001;15:2–13.
16. Moutier C, Cornette M, Lehrmann J, et al. When residents need health care: stigma of the patient role. Acad Psychiatry. 2009;33(6): 431–41.

Clinical Medical Ethics

Mark Siegler

Abstract

Clinical medical ethics is a new medical field, developed and named in the 1970s, that helps patients, families, physicians, and other health professionals reach good clinical decisions by taking into account both the specific clinical situation and the patient's values and preferences. The field of clinical medical ethics is much broader and encompassing than its component of ethics consultations; it applies across the entire spectrum of routine, daily medical practice. For clinicians today, applying clinical medical ethics standards in patient care is not an elective matter but rather has become the standard of care in the United States and is mandated legally and professionally. For example, in caring for their patients, physicians must apply clinical ethics standards such as speaking truthfully to their patients, negotiating informed consent for clinical decisions, protecting patient confidentiality, assessing the patient's decisional capacity, and, when appropriate, working with surrogates or proxies to reach clinical decisions. In contrast to the 1970s, clinical medical ethics discussions have now become a part of everyday clinical discourse and are used to reach clinical decisions in outpatient and inpatient settings across the country. The goal of clinical medical ethics is to improve patient care and patient outcomes. The MacLean Center for Clinical Medical Ethics at the University of Chicago is one of the leading clinical medical ethics programs in the world and has helped to create, name, and develop this new field.

I have practiced general internal medicine for 50 years. My commitment to develop the field of clinical medical ethics derived from my primary concern of how to be a good doctor for my patients.

I have always tried to care for my patients competently and personally, the way I hoped that my family would be cared for if they were ill and needed a doctor. I never saw a tension between scientific medicine and personal care. For me, good patient care always included a high level of technical competence and clinical judgment, combined with humane, compassionate, personal relationships with patients. From my earliest medical student days, I rejected the notion that "detached concern" and "objectivity" were the optimal methods of practicing medicine. Instead, I embraced a much more social and communal view of medicine, in which patients and physicians worked together and were dedicated to the joint effort of improving the patient's symptoms and health. My ideal view of the doctor-patient relationship was when physicians worked with patients as associates, colleagues, or even, at the highest level, friends. During my years of clinical training, I was deeply influenced by the views of the great Spanish physician-humanist Dr. Pedro Laín Entralgo, who regarded medical *philia,* or friendship, as the highest form of the patient-physician relationship.

My focus on patient care has been vitally important to my development as an academic physician and clinical ethicist. I did not begin my career as a medical ethicist who felt strongly about applying medical ethics principles in the clinical setting. Rather, I started as a clinician working under the guidance of my chairman of medicine, Dr. Alvin Tarlov, in the

M. Siegler, MD (✉)
Bucksbaum Institute for Clinical Excellence, MacLean Center
for Clinical Medical Ethics, University of Chicago, Pritzker School
of Medicine, Chicago, IL, USA
e-mail: msiegler@medicine.bsd.uchicago.edu

© Springer International Publishing AG 2017
L.W. Roberts, M. Siegler (eds.), *Clinical Medical Ethics*, DOI 10.1007/978-3-319-53875-4_2

new academic fields of general internal medicine and critical care medicine. From early in my career, I recognized that a wide range of clinical ethical issues had become essential, daily concerns of clinicians. These issues had to be incorporated into medical student clinical teaching, residency, and fellowship training in order to prepare physicians who could practice competent medicine in the modern world.

2.1   Before Clinical Medical Ethics

My work in creating and developing the field of clinical medical ethics started in 1972 with my feelings of frustration and inadequacy as a medical intensive care unit (MICU) doctor.

In 1972, when I joined the University of Chicago faculty in the newly created section of general internal medicine, I was asked by Dr. Tarlov to start and direct our hospital's first MICU. In those days, there were very few MICUs, in part because there were very few effective ventilators and the specialty of critical care medicine did not exist and would not be created for another 10 years. In time, MICUs would become one of the great technological advances that saved many lives, prolonged many lives, and raised new ethical questions that clinicians had never before had to deal with.

Directing the MICU for 5 years changed my career. Our seven-bed MICU received the sickest adult patients in the hospital. Our mortality rate was over 60%. At that time, pressure ventilators rarely could support a patient for more than a few days. I daily confronted issues such as rationing beds, negotiating informed consent, deciding when we needed surrogate consent, deciding whether we could stop a treatment once we had started it, and arriving at a truthful prognostication with the patient or the family. My previous training in medicine had not prepared me for this set of problems.

Faced with these everyday questions and others like them, I soon discovered that there was no place to send my housestaff and students to find answers. The medical literature and textbooks did not discuss these matters. There was a new, emerging literature in biomedical ethics, written largely by non-clinicians—that is, philosophers, theologians, and legal scholars—but this literature rarely addressed the practical concerns raised in the MICU by medical students, residents, and physician colleagues. The language of biomedical theory was different from the language of clinicians, and bioethical theory was often not helpful in resolving the dilemmas clinicians faced while caring for sick and dying patients. Furthermore, in the early 1970s, very few clinicians were even aware of the bioethics movement, and those who were often reacted negatively and sometimes with hostility to bioethics and non-physician bioethicists.

At that time, in 1972, I first realized that if we were to improve the care of patients in the MICU and throughout the hospital, it was essential that doctors, patients, and families become more closely involved in discussions about these relatively new and difficult medical questions. Physicians and patients needed help to better understand the ethical issues in clinical practice so that they could incorporate ethical analyses into their clinical decisions. For these reasons, in 1974, with great intellectual and organizational support from Dr. Tarlov, we launched the field of clinical medical ethics in the department of medicine at the University of Chicago.

I was fortunate that in the mid-1970s four distinguished pioneering bioethicists were on the University of Chicago campus: James Gustafson (Theology), Richard McCormick (Theology), Stephen Toulmin (Philosophy and The Committee on Social Thought), and Leon Kass (The Committee on Social Thought). I found myself frequently seeking guidance about clinical dilemmas from these expert ethicists, especially from Jim Gustafson and Stephen Toulmin. I was an ethics novice, and they were wonderful teachers. I also studied with William May, a theologian from Indiana University, who introduced me to the distinguished bioethics scholars affiliated with the Hastings Center. In all of these encounters, I was struck by how important and relevant for medical practice these new bioethical insights were, while at the same time, I was acutely aware of the general absence of clinicians from these discussions and the widespread ignorance among physicians about the principles of bioethics and clinical ethics.

During those early years I realized that clinical medical ethics could not be an elective area of study for physicians. Rather, it was an essential field that was required to enable physicians to practice good medicine. I also realized that clinical medical ethics was far more closely aligned to clinical medical practice than it was to bioethical theory. The history of medicine from Hippocratic times and earlier had insisted upon the physician's beneficent commitment to the patient, the physician's obligation to minimize harm in the course of medical care, and the physician's responsibility to improve the patient's quality of life through medical interventions. The original American Medical Association Code of Ethics of 1847 reflects many of the long-standing ethical duties of physicians [1].

What had been missing for me and my students were the views of clinicians—physicians, nurses, and other health care professionals—who were responsible for caring for the critically ill patients in our MICU. While distinguished bioethicists could brilliantly teach their theoretical insights to clinicians, bioethicists could not practice medicine or provide care to patients. During those early years in the MICU, I began publishing articles on the difficult decisions we made, and colleagues would congratulate me for having written a thoughtful essay on bioethics. I then responded that I had not intended to write an ethics article but rather that my team and I had been struggling with a practical and time-sensitive clinical challenge in the MICU, one in which a clinical ethical decision had to be reached.

My central point is that intensive care medicine routinely raised many dilemmas that had ethical components and that dealing with these clinical and ethical issues became an intrinsic part of clinical decisions and clinical practice. For this reason, we needed the new medical field of clinical medical ethics, a field that assisted clinicians who were caring for patients and negotiating many decisions each day, either with the patient or with the patient's surrogate.

During my years in the MICU, I clarified my career goals: I would work to develop and expand the new field of clinical medical ethics and would train physicians and other clinicians to use the concepts of clinical ethics in their daily work while caring for patients.

2.2 Defining Clinical Medical Ethics

Alvan Feinstein, M.D., the great clinician and scholar and late Sterling Professor of Medicine at Yale University, first proposed the term *clinical medical ethics* at the annual medical meetings in Atlantic City, New Jersey, in 1974. Dr. Feinstein called his work "clinical epidemiology" because, unlike traditional studies, his epidemiology studies related closely to his clinical care of patients. Similarly, Dr. Feinstein regarded the work that I had started in the University of Chicago MICU as "clinical medical ethics," which he distinguished from "theoretical, ivory-tower, biomedical ethics." Dr. Feinstein considered our program at the University of Chicago to be the birthplace of the field of clinical medical ethics. He named the new field and the name stuck. Soon afterwards in 1974, in line with Dr. Feinstein's terminology, I renamed our ethics program at the University of Chicago as the Department of Medicine Program in Clinical Medical Ethics.

In 1975, I wrote a grant with James Gustafson and Ann Dudley Goldblatt to the former Department of Health, Education, and Welfare titled "Clinical Ethics and Human Values." The grant was approved, and we received 3 years of federal support to develop a teaching program in clinical medical ethics. In 1978, I published a paper in the *Journal of the American Medical Association* titled "A Legacy of Osler: Teaching Clinical Ethics at the Bedside" [2], which is reprinted on page 220 in this book. This article noted that the advantages of teaching clinical ethics at the bedside included dealing with actual cases to maximize the physician's personal accountability, reinforcing the relationship between clinical practice and ethical decisions, and helping to decrease the widespread resistance of the medical profession at that time to bioethics.

The following year, in 1979, I started the first section on clinical medical ethics in an American medical journal, the American Medical Association's *Archives of Internal Medicine* [3]. In 1982, Arthur Rubenstein, M.D., then chairman of medicine, and I received approval from Hanna Holborn Gray, Ph.D., the president of the University of Chicago, to establish the Center for Clinical Medical Ethics at our medical school, which is now in its 35th year. With encouragement from Dr. Gray, Dr. Rubenstein and I developed a clinical, research, and financial plan for the new center and secured initial funding for the center from several leading foundations.

I am very grateful to the Andrew W. Mellon Foundation, the Henry J. Kaiser Family Foundation, and the Pew Family Trust for their vitally important support of our center in its first decade of work. I am also deeply indebted to Dorothy Jean MacLean and Barry and Mary Ann MacLean for their early support of our program and their unwavering commitment during the past 30 years to the MacLean Center and its goals. This early support enabled us to train 15 physician-leaders in the new field of clinical medical ethics and to launch our fellowship training program. Eleven of our original trainees returned to their home institutions and became directors of clinical medical ethics programs. In 1990, I was invited along with the late Dr. Edmund Pellegrino and Dr. Peter A. Singer to describe the new field of clinical medical ethics in a series of five papers that we published in Volume I of a new journal, *The Journal of Clinical Ethics.*

In the 1970s, when my physician colleagues and I were developing clinical medical ethics, our goal was to create a new *medical* field to help patients, families, physicians, and other health professionals reach good clinical decisions by taking into account the clinical situation, the patient's values and preferences, and the ethical considerations related to the decision. Whereas theoretical bioethics looked to philosophy, theology, and law for its ethical justifications, the foundations of clinical medical ethics are grounded squarely in the practice of medicine as a profession with ancient historical roots. Clinical medical ethics is *not* a theoretical or armchair exercise. Clinical medical ethics must be practiced and applied by physicians, not ethicists, every day in the care of their patients. Vitally important, clinical medical ethics is a discipline of medicine and not a subdiscipline or subsection of biomedical ethics, philosophical ethics, theological ethics, or legal ethics. For clinicians today, applying clinical medical ethics standards in patient care is *not* an elective matter. Applying clinical ethics standards has now become the standard of care in the United States and is mandated legally and professionally.

In contrast to a narrow and mistaken view of clinical medical ethics that regards the field as focused primarily on ethics consultations, which offer expert ethics opinions about difficult clinical ethical issues, our conception of the field at the University of Chicago from the beginning in the 1970s was much broader and encompassing. We viewed clinical medical ethics as essentially a new, modern approach to medicine that seamlessly integrated ethical considerations into the entire range of medical practice. Ethics consultation is surely a component, though a relatively small component, of the larger field of clinical medical ethics. Although ethics consultations may be helpful in dealing with occasional ethical dilemmas that arise in the course of medical practice, clinical medical ethics is a much broader field that applies across the entire spectrum of routine, daily medical practice.

2.3   Changing Medicine

Clinical medical ethics has succeeded in changing medicine. In contrast to the 1970s, when physicians expressed widespread resistance to biomedical ethics, clinical medical ethics has become so well integrated into current practice that physicians often do not realize they are "practicing" or "doing" clinical medical ethics. Applying clinical ethics precepts without being aware of doing so reminds me of the character in a play by Molière who was surprised to learn that he had been speaking prose all his life. But each day physicians are practicing clinical ethics when they tell patients the truth, when they break bad news, when they maintain confidentiality, when they negotiate informed consent for a procedure or a medication, when they make decisions based on shared decision-making, or when they decide that a patient lacks decisional capacity and turn instead to surrogate decision-makers. These and other clinical ethical considerations have become so much a part of everyday medical practice that they have become widely accepted as the legal and professional standard of care. Although very few U.S. physicians today are formally trained as clinical ethicists, all physicians routinely apply clinical medical ethics approaches in their regular, daily work with patients. In fact, I would go so far as to say that today clinicians cannot practice good medicine—that is, technically competent and ethically appropriate medicine—without some knowledge of and the ability to apply the principles of clinical medicine ethics.

How has clinical medical ethics changed American medical practice? In the past 40 years, the changes have been profound and have occurred without fanfare or drama. In contrast to the 1970s, today almost every medical organization has a code of ethics and an ethics committee. Similarly, every large hospital is required by the Joint Commission to have a mechanism to resolve clinical ethical problems when they occur, usually either a hospital ethics committee or an ethics consultation service. Publications on clinical ethics issues appear regularly, both in ethics journals that clinicians infrequently read and in general and specialty medical journals that clinicians widely read. Most importantly, in contrast to the 1970s, clinical medical ethics discussions have become a part of everyday clinical discourse and clinical decisions in outpatient and inpatient settings across the United States.

2.4   Embracing Clinical Medical Ethics

Since the 1970s, physicians have changed from being unreceptive and sometimes hostile to the new bioethics that emerged in the United States in the mid-1960s to embracing and applying clinical medical ethics in their daily practice. This dramatic shift in physician attitudes occurred very swiftly, within four decades, and it would be useful to examine the factors that encouraged this rapid change.

2.4.1   Life-Saving and Life-Prolonging Medical Advances

In my view, the first key factor behind widespread acceptance of clinical medical ethics was the development of many life-saving and life-prolonging medical advances that changed medicine. These advances included intensive care units (like the MICU I started in 1972), effective ventilators, the ability to reverse end-organ failure (e.g., with organ transplantation, dialysis, or left ventricular assist devices), and the discovery of new miracle medicines including antibiotics, heart failure drugs, cancer drugs, protease inhibitors, and hepatitis C medicines. These remarkable scientific and technological advances increased the need for and the range of clinical ethics decision-making, both at the bedside and in the office.

2.4.2   Focus on Civil and Human Rights

A second key factor was a new focus on civil and human rights that led to changing the doctor-patient relationship from a paternalistic model to an autonomy model to a shared-decision making model. The latter two models required patients to be truthfully informed so that they could participate in decisions about their care. The widespread incorporation of clinical medical ethics into physician practice and patient care smoothed the transition between the earlier style of paternalistic medicine and the contemporary models of patient autonomy and shared-decision making.

2.4.3   Emergence of Bioethics

The third factor I would highlight was the emergence of bioethics in the 1960s and 1970s as a new theoretical academic discipline. As Albert Jonsen [4] wrote in his *Short History of Medical Ethics,* "Bioethicists brought to this discourse concepts and methods that had been honed in their original disciplines…. Concepts such as *autonomy* and *justice* entered the vocabulary of medical ethics…. Perhaps the most dramatic innovation was the insertion of the concept of the respect for the autonomy of the patient into the heart of the ethics of medicine" (p. 116).

In the 1960s and 1970s, the early development of biomedical ethics in the United States was led to a large degree by non-physician bioethicists—theologians, philosophers, legal scholars, and other social scientists. Physicians and other clinicians had only limited involvement in its development, and its impact on medical practice and medical education was very limited. As the historian David Rothman [5] wrote that by 1978, "Bioethics was a field, would-be ethicists had career lines to follow, and the notion that medical ethics belonged exclusively to medicine had been forgotten by most everyone, except for a cadre of older physicians and a handful of historians" (p. 189).

The development of clinical medical ethics in the late 1970s and its rapid emergence as an applied clinical skill in the 1980s and 1990s transformed the theoretical academic work of bioethicists into the new practice of clinical medical ethics by clinicians. This transition was critical in American medicine. The physician, not the bioethicist, has the special knowledge to assist patients in curing or addressing their illness or disease and to assist patients in dealing with the fear, pain, and suffering that often accompany ill health. The licensed clinician interacting with his or her patient, rather than the unlicensed bioethicist with little or no clinical experience or knowledge, is responsible for applying the following clinical ethical standards:

- speaking truthfully to the patient
- knowing when and how to break bad news
- negotiating informed consent for clinical decisions
- assessing the patient's decisional capacity
- deciding when it is appropriate to work with a surrogate to reach decisions
- assuring patients of privacy and confidentiality
- addressing and relieving patients' symptoms, including pain
- discussing with the patient end-of-life goals of care and whether aggressive or palliative care is to be pursued.

In contrast to unlicensed bioethicists, physicians are licensed by the state and are professionally, legally, and personally accountable to the patient if they fail to integrate clinical ethics into their care of patients because of lack of knowledge or skills.

2.4.4 The MacLean Center for Clinical Medical Ethics

A fourth reason for the now widespread acceptance of clinical medical ethics relates to the contributions of the MacLean Center for Clinical Medical Ethics at the University of

Table 2.1 MacLean Center for Clinical Medical Ethics

Board Co-Chairs (Immediate Past)
Barry MacLean, CEO and Chairman of MacLean-Fogg
Ann MacLean
Board Chair
Rachel Kohler, MBA, CEO of NowPow
Advisory Board Members
Duncan MacLean, MBA, MEM, President of MacLean-Fogg
Carolyn Kay Bucksbaum
Craig Duchossois, Chief Executive Office of The Duchossois Group
Nancy Foster, MBA
Dean Gestal
Anne Dudley Goldblatt, JD, LLM
Stanford J. Goldblatt, LLM
Dennis Keller, MBA
Jeff Keller, PhD
John Kinsella, MBA
Robert Murley, MBA, MS
George A. Ranny, Jr., JD, CEO of Metropolis
Carole B. Segal
Andy Silvernail, CEO, Idex Cooperation
Bryan Traubert, MD
Associate Directors
Peter Angelos, MD, PhD
Lainie Ross, MD, PhD
Daniel Sulmasy, MD, PhD
Marshall Chin, MD, MPH
Monica Peek, MD
Assistant Directors
Daniel Brauner, MD
Tracy Koogler, MD
William Meadow, MD, PhD
Emily Landon, MD
Julie Chor, MD

Chicago (Table 2.1). The MacLean Center was established at the University of Chicago in 1988 and is widely recognized as the world leader in the field of clinical medical ethics.

In the 1990s, in surveys conducted by *US News and World Report* [6], the MacLean Center for Clinical Medical Ethics was chosen by deans of American medical schools for three consecutive years as the leading medical school ethics program in the United States. In 2013, the MacLean Center became the fourth organization in the world (and only the second university program) to receive the prestigious Cornerstone Award from the American Society for Bioethics and Humanities. The award was given to the MacLean Center for "outstanding, enduring contributions by an institution that has deeply enriched and helped shape the direction of the fields of bioethics and medical humanities" [7].

The MacLean Center's contributions have changed the field of clinical medical ethics during the past 30 years. Its foremost contribution is creating, naming, developing, and continuing to lead the new field of clinical medical ethics.

Establishing clinical ethics fellowship training The MacLean Center's clinical medical ethics fellowship program is the oldest, largest, and most successful ethics fellowship program in the world. Since beginning the fellowship program in 1981, the center has trained over 440 fellows, including more than 325 physicians. Graduates of the MacLean fellowship have served as directors of more than 40 ethics programs in the United States, Canada, South America, Europe, the Middle East, Africa, Australia, and China. A former trainee, Dr. Kenneth Iserson, an emergency medicine physician, is currently the only clinical medical ethicist to have practiced in Antarctica. MacLean Center fellowship graduates have held faculty appointments at more than 60 university programs. More than 25 fellowship graduates have held endowed university professorships. Former fellows of the MacLean Center have written more than 180 books and thousands of peer-reviewed journal publications. Many of the graduates of the fellowship programs are leaders, scholars, and mentors who represent a network of expertise that advances scholarship in clinical medical ethics and works to improve patient care.

Organizing a superb leadership team The center's original associate director was Dr. Steven Miles, who was succeeded as associate director by Dr. John Lantos. Currently, the center has five outstanding associate directors: Drs. Peter Angelos, Marshall Chin, Monica Peek, Lainie Ross, and Daniel Sulmasy. Each of these leaders of the MacLean Center has made important contributions to develop the field of clinical medical ethics.

Pioneering ethics consultation services Beginning in the 1970s, the University of Chicago hospitals pioneered the development of ethics consultations to assist patients, families, physicians, and the health team. MacLean Center faculty and fellows wrote much of the early literature on ethics consultations, including the first book on the topic *Ethics Consultation*, in 1994 [8].

Introducing the concept of research ethics consultations In a landmark article in 1989 in the *New England Journal of Medicine* [9], reprinted on page 382 in this book, the MacLean Center introduced the concept of research ethics consultations, an innovative approach to the ethics of clinical and translational research. The *New England Journal of Medicine* article described research ethics consultations as follows: "Research-ethics consultation is the process in which the ethical issues raised by an innovative therapy are analyzed before a protocol is submitted to the institutional review board. This process has been an essential part of our liver-transplantation program in recent years" (p. 620). Research ethics consultations have now been widely adopted by many research groups, including the Clinical and Translational Science Award program and the National Institutes of Health [10].

Development of surgical ethics Working in close association with the American College of Surgeons, the MacLean Center has led a national effort to train surgeons in surgical ethics and to encourage research on topics related to surgical ethics. During the past 10 years, under the leadership of Dr. Peter Angelos, the MacLean Center has trained almost 50 surgeons in the new field of surgical ethics. The goal of the surgical ethics program is to prepare surgeons for academic careers that combine clinical surgery with scholarly studies in surgical ethics. Surgical ethics fellows receive training in research, teaching, and surgical ethics consultations. For the past 3 years, the MacLean Center has sponsored a joint surgical ethics fellowship program with the American College of Surgeons. Also, under the auspices of the American College of Surgeons, a new textbook on surgical ethics is being prepared, and many MacLean Center faculty and former fellows are contributing chapters.

Participating in the "empirical turn" in ethics research Beginning in the 1980s and continuing to the present, the MacLean Center and its original director of research, Carol Stocking, Ph.D., played a key role in advancing the "empirical turn" in clinical ethics scholarship. This "turn" involved the application of the techniques of clinical epidemiology, health services research, decision sciences, and evidence-based outcomes to the study of ethical matters in clinical practice. Empirical research gathers data with survey methods or clinical studies. Empirical data showing that a particular way of clinical ethical practice is better than the alternative helps develop a professional consensus that changes and improves practice. Previously, ethics research had relied primarily on non–data-based analytic scholarship done by philosophers, theologians, and legal scholars, and this scholarship had less impact on clinical practice than data-driven clinical studies.

Publishing empirical studies about the doctor-patient relationship In 1987, in an interview with James Wind for the journal *Second Opinion* [11], I stated that the most pressing future question in clinical medical ethics was related to patient decisions: Could we better understand how patients reach decisions by themselves? How do patients reach decisions working with physicians in the shared decision-making model? How were patient decisions modified or constrained by external forces such as money, available resources, family values, and so on? In the 1990s, in an effort to better understand the decision-making process of patients and physicians, I wrote a series of papers that involved what I called "disease probes," extreme illnesses that tested the decision-making process both for patients and doctors. I hoped to gain a deeper understanding by studying patients' and doctors' decision-making approaches in extreme cases that included amyotrophic lateral sclerosis, end-stage renal disease, phase

I cancer research, prostate cancer, and end-of-life issues. Many of those papers are reprinted with permission in this volume.

Defending the importance of the doctor-patient relationship The doctor-patient relationship is the central concept in clinical medical ethics. The MacLean Center is proud of its achievement in having trained hundreds of physician-ethicists and in maintaining the focus on the doctor-patient relationship. The foundation of clinical ethics is the doctor-patient encounter, an encounter that meets universal and unchanging human needs and an encounter whose central goal has changed little since the time of Hippocrates. This central goal is for the physician to meet the health needs of the person who asks for help by using scientific and personal skills to provide such help effectively.

Introducing the concept of shared decision-making Clinical medical ethics aims to improve patient outcomes by encouraging shared decision-making between patients and physicians. In a 1979 talk to the New York Academy of Medicine and a subsequent 1981 paper, "Searching for Moral Certainty in Medicine: A Proposal for a New Model of the Doctor-Patient Encounter" [12] reprinted on page 92 in this book, I introduced the concept of the doctor-patient accommodation as an alternative to either the paternalistic or the patient autonomy model. In the 1982 report "Making Health Care Decisions: A Report on the Ethical and Legal Implications of Informed Consent in the Patient-Practitioner Relationship" [13], the President's Commission for the Study of Ethical Problems in Medicine and Biomedical and Behavioral Research repeatedly cited this paper on the doctor-patient accommodation as the basis for a shared decision-making approach in medicine. The shared decision-making approach argues that neither the pure paternalism nor the pure patient autonomy model is an accurate description of the doctor-patient relationship. Both models imply an adversarial relationship between patient and physician, although the models disagree on where the ultimate power should rest, whether in the doctor's or the patient's hands. By contrast, the model of the doctor-patient accommodation and shared decision-making assumes that the physician and patient work as partners to achieve a common goal, which is to address the health care needs of the patient who has asked the doctor for help.

2.5   The Bucksbaum Institute for Clinical Excellence

In 2011, to extend our work on the central importance of the doctor-patient relationship and shared decision-making, the University of Chicago established the Bucksbaum Institute for Clinical Excellence with a transformational endowment gift from Matthew and Carolyn Bucksbaum and the

Table 2.2 Bucksbaum Institute for clinical excellence

Directors
Mark Siegler, MD, Executive Director
Matthew Sorrentino, MD, Associate Director
Angela Pace-Moody, MS, Center Director
Advisory Board
Carolyn "Kay" Bucksbaum
John Bucksbaum
Jordan J. Cohen, MD
Holly J. Humphrey, MD
Kenneth S. Polonsky, MD
Laura Roberts, MD, MA
Arthur H. Rubenstein, MBBCh

Bucksbaum Family Foundation. I was honored to be selected as the founding executive director of the new institute. The primary goal of the Bucksbaum Institute is to develop an approach for preparing and training physicians to be highly competent as well as caring and compassionate practitioners.

Initially, Bucksbaum Institute programs were designed to support the career development and activities of physicians at three career stages—as medical students, junior faculty, and master clinicians. Over time, the institute has expanded its programs to reach more trainees at multiple levels, from premedical college students to senior physicians who serve as mentors to other faculty and to residents. The program for undergraduates has now trained more than 100 undergraduate premedical students through the Clinical Excellence Scholar Track, a program that is unique among U.S. undergraduate institutions. Physicians from all 12 clinical departments at the University of Chicago Medicine now participate in the institute's programs by pursuing research and writing, by attending symposia and conferences, and by mentoring younger trainees in their clinical specialties.

Bucksbaum Institute scholars recognize and support the institute's core goals: improving doctor-patient communications and decision-making, strengthening the doctor-patient relationship, reducing health disparities, increasing faculty engagement, and creating new models for undergraduate and medical student education. In its first 5 years of operation, the Bucksbaum Institute has appointed more than 200 physicians and students at the University of Chicago who represent the ideals and goals of the institute. The advisors to the Bucksbaum Institute (Table 2.2) have demonstrated an enduring commitment to the institute that will allow it to shape medicine and medical practice for generations to come.

2.6   Conclusion

In selecting the papers that are reprinted with permission in this volume, Dr. Laura Roberts and I chose papers that reflect my career-long efforts to make clinical medical ethics an integral component of modern medical practice and to demonstrate how clinical medical ethics has improved patient care and patient outcomes. In this regard, sections of the book reprint my work on the doctor-patient relationship, medical decision-making, communication between doctor and patient, medical education, and end-of-life care. I am also proud of a section in the book describing how I helped to create the field of clinical medical ethics and how clinical medical ethics standards have become the legal and professional standards required of physicians in their daily care of patients.

References

1. American Medical Association. Code of ethics of the American Medical Association. 1847.
2. Siegler M. A legacy of osler: teaching clinical ethics at the bedside. JAMA. 1978;239(10):951–6.
3. Siegler M. Clinical ethics and clinical medicine. Arch Intern Med. 1979;139(8):914.
4. Jonsen A. A short history of medical ethics. New York: Oxford University Press; 2008.
5. Rothman D, Strangers at the bedside. New York: Basic Books; 1991.
6. Medical Ethics. US news & world report. 1993.
7. American Society for Bioethics and Humanities. Award recipients. 1998. Available from: http://asbh.org/about/awards. Last accessed 4 Oct 2016.
8. La Puma J, Schiedermayer D. Ethics consultation. Boston: Jones and Bartlett Publishers; 1994.
9. Singer P, Siegler M, Whitington P, Lantos J, Emond J, Thistlethwaite J, et al. Ethics of liver transplantation with living donors. N Engl J Med. 1989;321(9):620–2.
10. Danis M. Research ethics consultation. Oxford: Oxford University Press; 2012.
11. Siegler M. Bringing ethics to the bedside: an interview with Dr. Mark Siegler. Second Opin. 1987;3:92–107.
12. Siegler M. Searching for moral certainty in medicine: a proposal for a new model of the doctor-patient encounter. Bull N Y Acad Med. 1981;57(1):56–69.
13. U.S. Bioethics Commissions Archival Collection. Making health care decisions, a report on the ethical and legal implications of informed consent in the patient-practitioner relationship volume one: report. President's Commission for the Study of Ethical Problems in Medicine and Biomedical and Behavioral Research. Washington, DC; 1982.

Empirical Research, Consultation, and Training in Medical Ethics

Daniel P. Sulmasy

Abstract

Mark Siegler is one of the founding figures of the subfield of bioethics known as clinical medical ethics. This brief chapter outlines his contributions in developing a program of empirical research in medical ethics, an ethics consultation service, an approach to medical student ethics teaching, and a fellowship training program. These activities have become the cornerstones of clinical medical ethics.

Mark Siegler, M.D., the Lindy Bergman Distinguished Service Professor in the Departments of Medicine and Surgery and the Director of the MacLean Center for Clinical Medical Ethics at the University of Chicago, is one of the founding figures in the field of medical ethics. This volume, which collects some of his most important papers and makes them available in one place, represents an important contribution to the bioethics literature.

Siegler is most known for his contributions to a subcategory of bioethics called clinical medical ethics. Clinical medical ethics is a field that examines the practical, everyday ethical issues that arise in encounters among patients, doctors, nurses, allied health workers, and health care institutions. The goal of clinical ethics is to improve patient care and patient outcomes. Most authorities date the beginning of the contemporary era of bioethics to the 1960s. In the early days of this movement, before Siegler began his career, with the exception of the work of Edmund Pellegrino, most medical ethics was being written by philosophers and theologians. Siegler became interested in ethical questions first and foremost as a physician who was grappling with these questions at the bedside. He was an internist charged with running his hospital's new intensive care unit. He was constantly confronting ethical questions about life, death, and the proper use of new technologies such as the ventilator. He had no formal training in ethics but decided he needed to learn more. He pursued such knowledge informally through discussions and directed readings with colleagues at the University of Chicago such as James Gustafson, an ethicist and a theologian at the divinity school who had already started thinking about medical ethics. Siegler soon began sharing his own insights, publishing papers on ethics in major medical journals, beginning in 1975 with his seminal article in the *New England Journal of Medicine*, "Pascal's Wager and the Hanging of Crepe" [1], reprinted on page 308 in this book. Although it might not seem extraordinary now, it was a remarkable achievement at that time—to write an article not about medical science, diagnosis, or treatment but about ethics and the care of the dying in the world's most prestigious medical journal.

To appreciate Siegler's contributions, one must always realize that he thinks about medical ethics first and foremost as a physician. He has never been one to theorize from afar. He reflects upon his clinical experience and draws eclectically from other people's theories in order to help himself develop answers to pressing ethical questions at the bedside. This perspective has shaped his career from the beginning. He was a member of a medical school faculty in the 1970s, surrounded by basic scientists and clinical trialists, and his approach to ethics was powerfully affected by his environment. He knew that for medical ethics to survive where it counted—in medical practice—it needed a niche that would be respected in the world of academic medicine, a world dominated by science. As he worked in that world, his way of thinking almost instinctually led him to start doing for medical ethics what he saw his colleagues doing in oncology

D.P. Sulmasy, MD, PhD (✉)
Georgetown University, Pellegrino Center for Clinical Bioethics,
Washington, DC, USA
e-mail: sulmasyd@georgetown.edu

and cardiology: observing and counting. In order to do this with some measure of rigor, he turned to the methods of the recently developed field of clinical epidemiology and applied these methods to questions of medical ethics. As such, he became a pioneer in the use of empirical methods to do medical ethics research, through both his own work and the work of the fellows he trained.

Philosophers divide ethical scholarship into normative ethics, meta-ethics, and descriptive ethics. The normative questions concern how people are to act. The meta-ethical questions concern the foundational concepts, language, and logic of ethics. The descriptive ethical questions concern how people actually do think and act in normatively significant situations. One of Siegler's most important insights was that descriptive work, using the tools of other medical researchers in survey and data collection, could be of service to normative medical ethics and could also provide a vehicle for bringing medical ethics to the attention of physicians accustomed to reading empirical studies. He stands as one of the architects of the "empirical turn" in bioethics.

The first of these descriptive ethics papers was published in the *New England Journal of Medicine* in 1982, with the title "Confidentiality in Medicine: A Decrepit Concept" [2] reprinted on page 159 in this book. What Siegler did in this paper was to observe and to count. He simply asked, "How many persons have legitimate access to the chart of a patient during a hospitalization?" His answer, which was at least 25 and possibly 100, was stunning. It raised questions about how the centuries-old Hippocratic commitment to patient confidentiality could hold up in modern medicine. In the era of the electronic medical record, the challenges this paper raised have only been magnified.

Siegler was also one of the pioneers of clinical ethics consultation, establishing one of the first university hospital clinical ethics consultation services at the University of Chicago in 1983. Both courts and ethicists had already recommended consultation as a mechanism for assisting clinicians and families in resolving ethical problems encountered at the bedside for several years, but few institutions had implemented such programs. Soon after establishing their ethics consultation service, Siegler and his colleagues and former fellows began writing about their experience in doing this pioneering work. In "An Ethics Consultation Service in a Teaching Hospital: Utilization and Evaluation" [3], published in the *Journal of the American Medical Association* in 1988 and reprinted on page 40 in this book, he and his colleagues again used descriptive methods to convey their message. Eighty-one percent of consults concerned issues in care at the end of life; a third originated in the intensive care unit. Attending physicians reported that the ethics consult was "very important" in patient management. He realized that data like these could put the practice of medical ethics consultation on the mental map of physicians. He did not need to solve any dilemmas—he only needed to demonstrate that they were common and that ethics consults could help.

Siegler's method of consultation was (and remains) very much based on the medical model. Whereas other institutions relied on ethics committees, Siegler established a method by which a fellow and an attending physician would interview (and even examine!) the patient, speak with the relevant parties (family, physicians, nurses, etc.), analyze the case, and write a note in the chart reflecting that analysis and making concrete recommendations. He rejected the committee model as ethical decision-making "by bureaucracy" [4]. His alternative was the clinical ethics model—a pure consultant approach akin to consultation in nephrology, cardiology, or rheumatology. This model has been criticized as chauvinistic and exclusive, but Siegler knew that to talk to physicians effectively about ethics, it was best to talk to them as fellow physicians. He and his early fellows could speak as physicians, and they did. I have experience with both of these models and also with what is known as the mixed model of ethics consultation—a method by which a subgroup of two or three members of the ethics committee conducts the consult. Siegler's method is clearly effective. The consultant carries a beeper and can respond quickly to urgent needs, which is a distinct advantage over the pure committee model. In most cases, it seems to me that each of these three methods would arrive at the same conclusion, although I suspect that there would be differences at the margins that would depend, at least in part, upon the approach. Whether the pure consultant model is intrinsically biased toward the views of physicians remains an open question. Though difficult, it might even be a question that could be resolved using the empirical methods of clinical medical ethics that Siegler has championed.

What can be said with confidence, however, is that Siegler continues to be regarded as one of the world's experts on clinical ethical consultation. Perhaps no other individual in the world has as deep and broad an experience in this work. The MacLean Center Clinical Ethics Case Conference, at which cases from the consult service are presented and critiqued by a large and multidisciplinary group, is one of the longest running such conferences in the world. The ethics consult service still performs approximately 100 consultations per year in the 517-bed hospital of the University of Chicago Medicine.

Siegler's most salient contributions, however, have been in teaching and training. Beginning with his now classic article "A Legacy of Osler: Teaching Clinical Ethics at the Bedside," published in the *Journal of the American Medical Association* in 1978 [5] and reprinted on page 220 in this book, Siegler's greatest legacy has been in teaching clinical medical ethics to medical trainees and in teaching the teachers who would go on to impart the accumulated knowledge, experience, and wisdom of the field to other trainees. For Siegler, clinical ethics is not an optional avocation for a few interested practitioners but a set of skills integral to clinical medicine. Recalling Osler's famous epitaph "I taught medical students in the wards," Siegler has argued that ethics should also be taught on the wards and in the clinic, and not just in the lecture hall. While he has run a very successful lecture and small group discussion course for medical students at the University of Chicago for decades, he reasoned that it would only stick with students if it were related to actual cases and not merely taught in abstraction. And ethics would only be put into action by trainees if it were modeled by respected senior physicians.

Perhaps the most successful of all his endeavors in clinical ethics has been the MacLean Center fellowship, one of the world's earliest postdoctoral fellowships in bioethics, which has now trained over 440 fellows, by far the most of any clinical ethics program. Once again, he was a pioneer in this work and shared his experience by writing about it in the medical literature soon after embarking on this endeavor. He canvassed the field of ethics fellowship training in 1988 in "Fellowship Training Programs in Clinical Ethics" ([6]; reprinted on page 232 in this book), written for the newsletter of the then nascent Society of General Internal Medicine, naming only a handful of training programs. What distinguished the MacLean fellowship program from the beginning was its emphasis on clinical questions and its adaptation of well-established mechanisms of medical training to training in medical ethics. Just as there are postdoctoral fellowships in nephrology, cardiology, and rheumatology that provide further specialty training to physicians who have finished their basic residency training, so, Siegler reasoned, he could fashion a program to train young physicians in clinical medical ethics. The importance of training a cadre of physicians who could act as consultants and role models and also conduct empirical research in ethics became critical to the vision of clinical medical ethics that he, Edmund Pellegrino, and Peter Singer outlined in the inaugural issue of the *Journal of Clinical Ethics* in their 1990 contribution "Clinical Medical Ethics: The First Decade" [7], reprinted on page 45 in this book. Fellows at the MacLean Center received instruction in the rudiments of ethical theory, law, and medicine and practical training in ethics consultation and in the empirical methods pertinent to medical ethics research. These fellows have contributed enormously to the volume and quality of scholarship of the field. Further expanding the circle of his influence, a number of former MacLean Center fellows now sponsor bioethics fellowship programs of their own.

His book *Clinical Ethics* [8], co-authored with Albert Jonsen and William Winslade and first published in 1982, is now in its 8th edition. It is one of the all-time bestselling books in the field and has been widely used by clinicians. The title bespeaks, once again, Siegler's commitment to clinical ethics. The focus is on teaching medical students and house officers, and it is oriented toward bedside decision-making. It is written in clear, accessible, and straightforward prose, readily understandable by practitioners not versed in philosophy or theology. Though not theoretically oriented in its approach, it is nonetheless theoretically sound and defensible. This work expounds the "four box" approach of attending, in all medical ethics cases, to four kinds of potential moral considerations: medical indications, patient preferences, quality of life, and contextual features. To emphasize its practical focus and its targeting of physicians in training as the primary audience, the first several editions of the book were printed as small hardcover volumes and were marketed as being able to fit into the pockets of medical trainees' white coats. The book continues to stand out among introductory texts in medical ethics for clinicians and is used by a number of medical schools in their introductory courses in medical ethics.

Siegler has conducted all of his scholarship and teaching at the University of Chicago, where he founded and continues to direct the MacLean Center for Clinical Medical Ethics. The MacLean Center began in 1976 with a small 3-year grant for teaching and program development from the Department of Health, Education, and Welfare. Over the next decade, with several additional grants and a naming gift from the MacLean family, the MacLean Center became established as the first ethics program in the world to focus on clinical medical ethics. Today, the MacLean Center is seen as the birthplace of clinical ethics and remains the leading clinical ethics research and training program in the world.

In the past 30 years, clinical ethics has become one of the major components of the American bioethics movement. In contrast to 30 years ago, almost every large hospital now has an ethics committee or ethics consultation service to help resolve clinical ethical problems; almost every medical organization now has an ethics committee and code of ethics; papers on clinical ethics are published regularly, not only in ethics journals but in mainline medical journals; there is even a *Journal of Clinical Ethics;* and most significantly, clinical ethics discussions have become a part of the routine clinical discourse that occurs in outpatient and inpatient clinical settings across the country. Siegler has been an important figure in the evolution of clinical medical ethics. The papers collected in this volume help to explain why this is so.

References

1. Siegler M. Pascal's wager and the hanging of crepe. N Engl J Med. 1975;293:853–7.
2. Siegler M. Confidentiality in medicine: a decrepit concept. N Engl J Med. 1982;307:1518–21.
3. La Puma J, Stocking CB, Silverstein MD, DiMartini A, Siegler M. An ethics consultation service in a teaching hospital-utilization and evaluation. JAMA. 1988;260:808–11.
4. Siegler M. Ethics committees: decisions by bureaucracy. Hast Cent Rep. 1986;16(3):22–4.
5. Siegler M. A legacy of osler: teaching clinical ethics at the bedside. JAMA. 1978;239:951–6.
6. Lane LW, Siegler M, Miles SH, Cassel CK, Singer PA. Fellowship training programs in clinical ethics. Soc Gen Intern Med Newsl. 1988;3:4–5.
7. Siegler M, Pellegrino ED, Singer PA. Clinical medical ethics: the first decade. J Clin Ethics. 1990;1:5–9.
8. Jonsen AR, Siegler M, Winslade WJ. Clinical ethics: a practical approach to ethical decisions in clinical medicine. 8th ed. New York: McGraw-Hill; 2015.

The University of Chicago and the Work of Mark Siegler in Clinical Medical Ethics

Dana Levinson, Holly J. Humphrey, and Kenneth S. Polonsky

Abstract

In considering Dr. Mark Siegler's 50-year career on the campus of the University of Chicago, it is remarkable to appreciate the extent to which this university has molded and shaped Dr. Siegler as a teacher, physician, and scholar. In turn, it is no less true to say that Dr. Siegler's impact and contribution to the University of Chicago have been as formidable. His work in establishing a clinical medical ethics consultation service and a clinical ethics fellowship program, along with his commitment to the doctor-patient relationship, has influenced the teaching and practice of clinical medicine on our campus and throughout the world. The University of Chicago's clinical ethics consultation service was one of the first of its kind in the United States to utilize physicians as trained ethics consultants and to identify where clinical ethics needed to be taught—in true Oslerian fashion—at the bedside. Shaped as he has been by the University of Chicago, Dr. Siegler has also served as an exemplar within the specific traditions and values of the University of Chicago, and his contributions have matched those of the university's greatest faculty citizens over the many years of its history.

The University of Chicago was founded in 1890 on the basis of values and beliefs that have guided the university to the present day. The visionary ideas were due in large part to the influence of its founding president, William Rainey Harper, and the unprecedented support of its founding benefactor, John D. Rockefeller [1]. If the University of Chicago no longer seems as radically innovative as it was at its inception, it is because its system of university structure and study implemented by Harper in 1890 has been so widely imitated across the United States [1]. Chicago was "built for a long future," and its faculty and students are instilled with the commitment "to re-create that future for its successors" [1].

Those of us who have spent so much of our careers at the University of Chicago are well aware of the ongoing impact of the university's longstanding cultural and intellectual ideals on students, residents, faculty, and deans. As described in John Boyer's recently published history of the University of Chicago [1], the university's cultural and intellectual milieu was powerfully shaped and conveyed in Harper's original vision. One quality, namely his reverence for a "modern" scholarship that confronts facts courageously and thinks through complicated and controversial questions inductively, continues to be the gold standard by which our faculty and students measure themselves. As we consider Dr. Mark Siegler's long and distinguished career on the campus of the University of Chicago and his impact on our school and our students, we are reminded of how aligned he is with the value system of the University of Chicago and how himself has long served and continues to serve as one who has protected and sustained the University of Chicago's "long future." Over the 50-plus years that Mark has spent on the University of Chicago campus—as a medical student, internal medicine resident, chief resident, and faculty member—he has manifested the core values of this institution in his

D. Levinson, MPH • H.J. Humphrey, MD (✉)
University of Chicago, Pritzker School of Medicine, Chicago, IL, USA
e-mail: holly@medicine.bsd.uchicago.edu

K.S. Polonsky, MD
Division of the Biological Sciences, University of Chicago, Pritzker School of Medicine, Chicago, IL, USA

© Springer International Publishing AG 2017
L.W. Roberts, M. Siegler (eds.), *Clinical Medical Ethics*, DOI 10.1007/978-3-319-53875-4_4

dedication to innovation and scholarship in clinical medical ethics, while also maintaining a deep commitment to teaching and to providing the highest quality of clinical care for his patients.

Shaped as he has been by the University of Chicago, Dr. Siegler has also served as an exemplar within the specific traditions and values that are fundamental to the history of medical education as it unfolded at this institution. The remarks made by Richard Richter, M.D., to the graduating class of 1967—Dr. Siegler's class—and the alumni attending their reunion are very instructive in this regard. Dr. Richter, himself a 1925 graduate of the joint University of Chicago and Rush Medical School before the opening of Billings Hospital in 1927 allowed the medical school to consolidate both preclinical and clinical education on the University of Chicago campus [2], recounted the medical school's history and its unique attributes. These include the geographic and intellectual integration of the basic and clinical sciences within the division of biological sciences, a completely full-time faculty relieved of "the relentless distractions and demands of private practice and free to devote their full energies to teaching or research, or both" [3], and the commitment that all patients seen at the clinics and hospitals of the university—not just charity hospitals—be part of the teaching and research enterprise. As Dr. Richter explained to the 1967 graduates, this clinical care and educational structure, which he described as a blend of the Johns Hopkins and Mayo Clinic models, offered unique advantages for the students and patients but, most importantly, shaped the faculty in profound ways. He stated, "To make it work successfully, the modern scientific clinician must lead a double life and function also as a skillful and humane doctor, able to attract and hold patients. He must even keep in mind that old bromide, the patient-physician relationship. For the patients come not to benefit medical science after all, but because they are sick and want to be helped" [3].

This review and description of the values and traditions which animated and shaped the university in general and medical education in specific provide a crucial context for Dr. Mark Siegler's many contributions. As he has spent his entire career from medical school to the present at the University of Chicago, it is remarkable to appreciate the extent to which this university has molded and shaped Dr. Siegler as a teacher, physician, and scholar. In turn, it is no less true to say that Dr. Siegler's impact and contribution to the institution's "long future" has been no less formidable—as the "modern scientific clinician" whose work in establishing an academic clinical medical ethics program and consultation service and a clinical ethics fellowship program along with his commitment to the doctor-patient relationship has influenced the teaching and practice of clinical medicine on our campus and throughout the world.

Mark Siegler arrived in Chicago in 1963 as a young graduate of Princeton University. He joined the University of Chicago medical school class just days after meeting his future wife, Anna, on the University of Chicago's campus, thus beginning two lifelong relationships formed in Hyde Park. Dr. Siegler is proud to affirm that during his 50-plus years at the University of Chicago, he has personally known all but 3 of the 19 deans of the biological sciences division and the Pritzker School of Medicine, including our medical school's founding dean, Dr. Franklin McLean, whom Mark cared for as an internal medicine resident during Dr. McLean's hospital admissions. Mark has always honored the traditions and histories of the University of Chicago as well as its thought leaders, even going so far as to find time to pay his respects to Lowell Coggeshall, the former dean of the biological sciences division from 1947 to 1960, during his 1967 honeymoon! Amusing as an anecdote, it nonetheless says something notable about Mark and his loyalty and admiration for the history and traditions of the University of Chicago.

Following the completion of his internal medicine residency and his chief residency year, Dr. Siegler left the university for the one and only time in his career to complete training at the Hammersmith Hospital in London, England. Returning to campus as an assistant professor, Dr. Siegler met with the chairman of medicine, Alvin Tarlov, and as he is very fond of relating, took on the four jobs that comprised his first faculty role in the department of medicine. One of Dr. Tarlov's early goals as chairman of medicine was to create a strong academic section of general internal medicine to complement the strong subspecialty orientation of the department. From its inception in 1927, the department had been divided into different sections that encompassed all components of internal medicine. As explained by Dr. Franklin McLean and Ilza Veith in their history of the first 25 years of medicine at the University of Chicago [2], such a structure would leverage the benefits derived from the intense focus of specialization while limiting the dangers of limited experience by having the specialists function as generalists, practicing together in the provision of clinical care, making a separate section of general internal medicine unnecessary. However, under the leadership of the department chair George Dick, from 1933 to 1945, an "undifferentiated" clinical service grew in size such that it occupied one-third of the beds overseen by the department of medicine [4]. Following his departure, the concept of a general medicine service disappeared, until resurrected by Dr. Tarlov in 1970.

In 1973, the section of general internal medicine was formed, and Dr. Siegler became one of the first faculty members [4]. This newly constituted section was responsible for its own inpatient and outpatient services as well as a consultation service and commenced its own program of research and investigation. Mark was one of the backbones of this section as it grew—serving as inpatient director of one of the inpatient general medicine services for 8 months of the year as well as providing oversight of all medical student programs sponsored by the department of medicine, including the third year internal medicine clerkship and the fourth year electives in medicine. In addition to these two important jobs, Mark also served as the leader of the newly created general medicine consultation service to provide consultations to other departments such as surgery and obstetrics-gynecology. During this same year, Dr. Tarlov conceived of something else that was new—a medical intensive care unit. In 1972, the specialty of critical care medicine did not yet exist, but Dr. Tarlov understood that there needed to be a unit where care for the sickest patients could be monitored most closely. Dr. Siegler was to attend on the medical intensive care unit 12 months of the year!

Mark with his "four jobs" served as one of the leaders in forming this section of general internal medicine, but even more importantly, these opportunities provided an intensive "think tank" or laboratory wherein Mark found his focus and his professional direction. During the 5 years when he directed the medical intensive care unit (1972–1976) multiple important ethical issues related to medicine emerged—from end-of-life care to informed consent to surrogate decision-making to confidentiality. Mark saw students, faculty, and residents confronting ethical issues in clinical care on a daily basis without a frame of reference or background of scholarship to rely on for guidance and support. From this experience came Mark's sense of purpose for his future career and the birth of a clinical medical ethics consultation service, where the practical and difficult ethical questions arising in the care of patients could be answered with an integrated ethical analysis. This service produced two very positive outcomes: patient and family engagement increased and the confidence of clinicians in complicated ethical decision-making grew. In Mark's words, "Clinical ethics focuses on the doctor-patient relationship and helps patients, families, and physicians reach good clinical decisions, taking account of both the medical facts of the situation, as well as the patient's preferences and values" [5].

With the early support of his next department chair, Dr. Arthur Rubenstein, the Mellon Foundation, and later with the generous naming gift from the MacLean Family, Dr. Siegler founded the first Center for Clinical Medical Ethics in the department of medicine in 1984.

In 2013, in recognition of the international significance and fundamental impact of the work conducted by the MacLean Center, it became only the fourth institution (joining the Hastings Center, Kennedy Institute of Ethics at Georgetown, and the Institute for Medical Humanities at the University of Texas) to receive the Cornerstone Award from the American Society of Bioethics and Humanities for "outstanding contributions from an institution that has helped shape the direction of the field of bioethics" [6].

The MacLean Center has too many achievements and contributions to be described comprehensively, but we wish to highlight two of its most notable activities. The first is the signature program of the MacLean Center, the clinical ethics fellowship, which began in 1981. The first of its kind, this program has provided training for over 440 fellows, including more than 275 physicians. More than 40 of the fellows trained at the MacLean Center have gone on to direct university ethics programs, and more than 25 fellows now hold endowed professorships in ethics. The fellowship's impact is not only national but global—with fellows joining our campus from Argentina, Brazil, Canada, China, France, Kuwait, Russia, Spain, and Switzerland, among other countries. These individuals have published many thousands of peer-reviewed journal articles and more than 150 books advancing the field of clinical medical ethics.

A second notable achievement of the center is the creation of a unique clinical ethics consultation service in 1986 [7]. Over the prior decade, an increasing number of ethicists began focusing on issues in medicine. However, trained in the humanities and focused on theory, these scholars were not able to provide guidance on the plethora of day-to-day dilemmas encountered by the practicing physician [8]. The field of biomedical ethics' "language of theory was not helpful in resolving the dilemmas of practice" [9]. The University of Chicago's clinical ethics consultation service was, in contrast, one of the first of its kind in the United States to utilize physicians as trained ethics consultants, thereby providing, over the past 30 years, a truly unique resource for our institution's clinicians, who can rely on the body of scholarship and inductive reasoning skills of the center's faculty and fellows to help manage complex and ethically challenging clinical patient scenarios [8]. In a 1978 paper [10] reprinted in this volume on page 220, Mark was the first to use the term *clinical ethics* [8] and identify where it needed to be taught—in true Oslerian fashion—at the bedside [10]. Since the service's inception, the center's faculty and fellows have consulted on over 2500 cases at the University of Chicago. One of the papers reprinted in this collection, on page 40, assesses the preliminary impact of this ethics consultation service through a prospective study conducted in its first 2 years of operation. Even in this short time, it was eminently clear that such a consultation service had enormous value in helping physicians identify, analyze, and resolve ethical issues in patient care [7].

We have spoken of how the University of Chicago and its core values shaped Mark's work; it is equally important to note the unique opportunities that Mark found at our university as he implemented and developed the MacLean Center's programs. William Rainey Harper's original vision of the University of Chicago included a commitment to aggressive programs of original research [1], and the University of Chicago, with 89 faculty and alumni Nobel laureates, one of the highest numbers of any U.S. institution [11], is justifiably regarded as a major contributor to knowledge in multiple disciplines. Further, from its inception in 1890 the university has emphasized and encouraged interdisciplinary fields of study and cross-disciplinary collaboration [1].

In this environment, Mark Siegler enthusiastically sought out and masterfully utilized the resources and advantages of the University of Chicago, drawing on its world-renowned faculty from law, public policy, divinity, business, philosophy, and economics to contribute to the center and its work. That so many leading scholars would choose to affiliate with the MacLean Center is in fact one of the defining characteristics of the center and of its work. In 1981, Mark Siegler and Richard Epstein, then the James Parker Hall Distinguished Service Professor of Law, organized what has now become an annually offered interdisciplinary faculty seminar series, bringing together leading thinkers from across campus and throughout the world to conduct an in-depth ethical analysis of one key health issue through multiple hour-long seminars held every few weeks. This seminar series, constructed in the prototype of the university's vaunted workshop model, which was introduced in the economics department in the 1940s and has expanded across the university in the ensuing years [1], brings together faculty and students to explore multiple perspectives on complex issues affecting science and medicine. Topics have included organ transplantation, pediatric ethics, end-of-life care, global health, health care disparities, medical professionalism, confidentiality, pharmaceutical innovation and regulation, neuroethics, and reproductive ethics [12].

Mark's impact as a scholar has been felt around the world, but on our campus he is also deeply respected as a teacher and as a clinician. In 1898, William Rainey Harper stated, "I cannot conceive that a man worthy to hold the place of Dean would accept the position without the privilege of giving instruction. A man who was a Dean and who gave no instruction would merely be a clerk….So strongly do I feel this principle myself that I do the work of a professor, and shall continue to do so as long as I am President" [1]. Throughout Mark Siegler's career, while providing care to patients, developing scholarly contributions in developing a new consult service and fellowship program, creating and leading a world-renowned center, and receiving multiple honors and awards, he has followed President Harper's stricture—he has done "the work of a professor." Nor were these minimal contributions to the teaching mission. Two commitments stand out from multiple others: he was for 10 years the director of the medical school's required *Physical Diagnosis* course, and he has been for the last 16 years the director of the medical school course on the *Doctor-Patient Relationship in Clinical Practice,* required for all first-year students.

As quoted previously, Dr. Richter stated at Mark's 1967 medical school graduation that the modern scientific clinician must lead a double life and function also as a skillful and humane doctor. Mark Siegler has given an unwavering enthusiasm and commitment over 50 years to his role as clinician. He has cared for trustees and politicians and the most vulnerable patients from our South Side community with devotion and commitment. He is, for all his patients and not only for those who can afford such a privilege, a "concierge" clinician by temperament and practice. He meets his patients in the emergency department and accompanies them to the operating room. He is a role model for providing compassionate care.

It was his outstanding clinical care that served as the model on which the Bucksbaum Institute for Clinical Excellence was established in 2011, with a most generous donation by a grateful patient who admired and appreciated his collaborative relationship with patients and felt that such care should serve as an exemplar for all physicians. The central mission of the Bucksbaum Institute is to elevate the doctor-patient relationship and to make optimizing our relationship with patients a core guiding value for all our clinicians [13]. As part of the Bucksbaum Institute's support, Mark is currently co-teaching a senior medical student seminar on the doctor-patient relationship with one of us (HJH). One of his favorite teaching articles for the class is included in this book, on page 92. This paper, presented as part of a 1980 conference and published the following year, explores the tensions between the traditional paternalistic model of the doctor-patient relationship and the patient-centered, potentially consumerist model that emerged in the latter part of the twentieth century and has grown even stronger with the advent of the internet [14]. Mark's prescience in identifying this tension and his creativity in seeking a third way, which he terms "physician-patient accommodation" and which transcends the biases inherent in the competing models, is every bit as relevant today as it was 35 years ago. Dr. Mark Siegler's thoughtful consideration of the human and ethical aspects of science and medicine has made him a reference point for countless individuals. He has contributed to the intellectual life through not only the generation of new ideas but also his mentorship of students and physicians. In his history of the University of Chicago, John Boyer writes that the first faculty and leaders of the University of Chicago marveled at how our institution was created "de novo out of ambition, openness, a penchant for risk taking, and seriousness" [1]. These words and this legacy could aptly and accurately be used to describe Dr. Mark Siegler and his life's work as a physician, a teacher, and a thought leader. The essence of the University of Chicago is its faculty, and Mark's contribution to the fabric of this intellectual community enjoys a place of prominence over the many years of our institution's history.

References

1. Boyer JW. The University of Chicago: a history. Chicago: The University of Chicago Press; 2015.
2. Veith I, McLean Franklin C. The University of Chicago clinics and clinical departments: 1927 – 1952. Chicago: The University of Chicago Press; 1952.
3. Richter RB. A short history of the medical school at the University of Chicago. Chicago: Medical Alumni Bulletin; 1967.
4. Vermeulen CW. For the greatest good to the largest number: a history of the Medical Center of the University of Chicago, 1927 – 1977. Chicago: Published by The Vice President for Public Affairs, the University of Chicago; 1977.
5. Siegler M, Lowell T. Coggeshall memorial lecture: 50 extraordinary years at the University of Chicago and the development of clinical medical ethics. Lecture given on 7 Oct 2014 at the University of Chicago.
6. University of Chicago Press Release in 2013: Downloaded from http://www.uchospitals.edu/news/2013/20130924-maclean.html.
7. LaPuma J, Stocking CB, Silverstein MD, DiMartini A, Siegler M. An ethics consultation service in a teaching hospital. JAMA. 1988;260(6):808–11.
8. Tepper EB. Consults for conflict: the history of ethics consultation. Proc Bayl Univ Med Cent. 2013;26(4):417–22.
9. Siegler M. The contributions of clinical ethics to patient care. Forum Trends Exp Clin Med. 1997;7:244–53.
10. Siegler M. A legacy of Osler: teaching clinical ethics at the bedside. JAMA. 1978;239(10):951–6.
11. http://www.uchicago.edu/about/accolades/22/.
12. http://macleanethics.uchicago.edu/events/.
13. Johnson Dirk. A $42 million gift aims at improving bedside manner. The New York Times, 22 Sept 2011.
14. Siegler M. Searching for moral certainty in medicine: a proposal for doctor-patient encounter. Bull N Y Acad Med. 1981;57(1): 56–69.

Revitalizing the Field of Medical Ethics

5

Jordan J. Cohen

Abstract

Dr. Mark Siegler is a founding figure in the field of clinical medical ethics. This brief chapter discusses how he personally revitalized the field of medical ethics, which was not serving patients or physicians sufficiently when he began his work in the 1970s. Dr. Siegler's compassion, generosity, devotion to patient welfare, and attention to the doctor-patient relationship led to the founding of both the MacLean Center for Clinical Medical Ethics and the Bucksbaum Institute. Through the efforts of Dr. Siegler and these organizations, hundreds of physicians and health care professionals have been trained in the field of clinical medical ethics and the principle of caring has been embedded in the training and preparation of future physicians and clinicians.

I met Mark Siegler in 1982 when he was a rising star in the department of medicine at the University of Chicago and I had just arrived in Chicago to begin my 6-year stint as chief of medicine at Michael Reese Hospital and Medical Center. At that time, Reese was an affiliate of the University of Chicago medical school and Arthur Rubenstein was chair of medicine. Arthur and I had agreed that a closer relationship between the two departments would benefit both institutions, and we began to implement a number of changes designed to foster collaboration, especially in education and research. Mark was quick to recognize the value of combining the strengths of the University of Chicago and Reese and became a vocal advocate and close ally in these efforts. As a consequence, I had the privilege of interacting with Mark on a number of occasions. And, I am happy to say, we have remained close friends ever since.

It was clear from those early days that Mark was a physician with uncommon gifts. Not only was he a brilliant clinician and an inspiring teacher, he was most especially a mensch of the first order—kind, caring, compassionate, selfless. In all of his human interactions—whether with patients and their families, students and residents, colleagues, housekeepers, whomever—Mark's gentle and engaging manner was always evident. And it is precisely those human qualities that have been at the core of all of Mark's many seminal contributions to American medicine.

A striking example of his compelling humanity is the key role he has played in revitalizing the field of medical ethics. I believe it was his unyielding devotion to patient welfare that enabled him to recognize so early on how the fraying ethical norms in contemporary medicine was threatening the beneficent care of patients. Rather than stand by and lament the profession's ethical shortcomings, he marshaled the resources and energy to establish the MacLean Center for Clinical Medical Ethics. Moreover, it was Mark's innate reverence for the human side of medicine that has infused the center with the passion that has propelled it to worldwide preeminence. The MacLean Center has trained hundreds of physicians and other health professionals over the years, many of whom are now leading ethics centers or programs across the globe. Coupled with Mark's voluminous writings, including his widely read textbook *Clinical Ethics: A Practical Approach to Ethical Decisions in Clinical Medicine,* the MacLean Center and its staff have elevated the study and application of clinical medical ethics to a level comparable to the most relevant of clinical disciplines.

The Bucksbaum Institute for Clinical Excellence is yet another vivid example of Mark Siegler's abiding commitment

J.J. Cohen, MD (✉)
Association of American Medical Colleges, Arnold P. Gold Foundation for Humanism in Medicine, Englewood Cliffs, NJ, USA
e-mail: jjcohenmd@gmail.com

© Springer International Publishing AG 2017
L.W. Roberts, M. Siegler (eds.), *Clinical Medical Ethics*, DOI 10.1007/978-3-319-53875-4_5

to the irreducible human dimension of medicine. The emblematic doctor-patient relationship that Mark manifested in caring for the Bucksbaum family gave rise to the institute's founding. As a consequence of Mark's vision—a vision driven by his natural humanity—the Bucksbaum Institute is ensuring that the timeless principle of *caring* is embedded securely in the preparation of current and future generations of clinicians. And not just at the University of Chicago. The institute has projected its mission far beyond the University of Chicago by collaborating with other like-minded organizations, including the Arnold P. Gold Foundation and the Schwartz Center for Compassionate Healthcare.

The result, comparable to the far-reaching impact of the MacLean Center, is that Mark Siegler's menschkeit—his selfless, innate drive for doing the right and decent thing, in every possible situation—has left an enduring and immensely salutary mark on American medicine.

Study Mark Siegler and learn how one man can change the world.

6

Improving the Quality of Health Care for Patients through Clinical Medical Ethics Education

Peter A. Singer

Abstract

Dr. Mark Siegler is a founding figure in the field of clinical medical ethics. His seminal publications asserted clinical medical ethics as a worthwhile field and demonstrated its necessity within the practice of medicine. Dr. Siegler further encouraged the development of this field through the foundation of a fellowship training program in which hundreds of physician and other medical workers have learned the principles of clinical medical ethics. Through the efforts of Dr. Siegler and his many fellows, the field of clinical medical ethics is now taught, studied, and practiced internationally. By expanding the field as such, Dr. Siegler can be credited with improving the quality of health care for patients across the modern world.

Dr. Mark Siegler's seminal contribution is to have created the field of clinical medical ethics within the field of medicine.

In my career, I have had the privilege of interacting with a large number of highly distinguished physicians around the world. I trained both in clinical epidemiology with Dr. Alvan R. Feinstein at Yale and in clinical medical ethics with Dr. Siegler at the University of Chicago from 1988 to 1990. Dr. Siegler's accomplishments rise to the level of the late Dr. Alvan Feinstein, who created the field of clinical epidemiology, and the late Dr. Edmund D. Pellegrino, who was a creator of the field of medical ethics with a philosophical perspective. I knew all three of these eminent master physicians extremely well, and I can attest that they made comparable and seminal contributions in creating their respective fields.

I offer two lines of argument to support my claim: (1) Dr. Siegler's seminal papers and books, which evidence the founding of clinical medical ethics as a field within the practice of medicine and (2) how Dr. Siegler leveraged his founding of the field in the United States to make it an international movement.

Dr. Siegler created the field of clinical medical ethics in the crucible of his clinical practice and then amplified this effect through seminal publications. Dr. Siegler's very first paper, published in 1975 in the *New England Journal of Medicine*, "Pascal's Wager and the Hanging of Crepe" [1] reprinted on page 308 in this book, is a landmark article and signaled his future direction. The paper introduced and addressed the clinical phenomenon of prognostication and how clinicians would "hang crepe" to anticipate the death of a patient to the patient or loved ones. His 1978 article in the *Journal of the American Medical Association* titled "A Legacy of Osler: Teaching Clinical Ethics at the Bedside" [2], reprinted on page 220 in this book, firmly grounded his work in the Oslerian tradition, in contradistinction to prevailing approaches to medical ethics at the time, which were being pursued by philosophers and others outside the medical profession and were not grounded in the doctor-patient relationship. A similar theme was struck in his 1979 paper "Clinical Ethics and Clinical Medicine" [3], published in the *Archives of Internal Medicine* and reprinted in this book on page 34, and a bit more aggressively in "Cautionary

P.A. Singer, MD (✉)
University Health Network, Grand Challenges Canada at the Sandra Rotman Centre, Toronto, ON, Canada
e-mail: peter.singer@grandchallenges.ca

Advice for Humanists" [4], published in the *Hastings Center Report* in 1981.

These works were absolutely central to the founding of clinical medical ethics as a field within medicine that informed the care of patients and focused on strengthening the doctor-patient interaction, thus improving patient health outcomes and quality of life. The sustainability of his influence was leveraged through Dr. Siegler's more than 440 fellows in clinical medical ethics.

Dr. Siegler also internationalized the field of clinical medical ethics, which grew from its origins in the United States to a global movement. Dr. Siegler's international influence was to take the field of clinical medical ethics that he created in the United States and sow the seeds of this field in other countries. He did so in Canada, France, Spain, Switzerland, Brazil, Argentina, Australia, China, and elsewhere. Among his fellows, more than 25 now have leadership positions in clinical medical ethics in countries other than the United States. Almost all of those fellows not originating from the United States have an M.D. degree or equivalent from their nation and several, in addition to their M.D., have a Ph.D., J.D., or M.P.H. degree. Their medical specialty distribution is similar to their counterpart fellows in the United States and includes internal medicine, surgery, pediatrics, and family medicine, among other specialties. Like their counterparts in the United States, these individuals gradually work their way up a career ladder in regards to responsibility, authority, and title, often becoming program directors and establishing clinical medical ethics training programs themselves.

It appears that these former trainees are generating new clinical medical ethicists to expand the programs they direct.

One personal characteristic that drives Dr. Siegler's success is his devotion and dedication to the ongoing mentorship of trainees. One never really graduates from his training program, as the growing cohort returns en masse to Chicago annually for 2–3 days to attend a fellows conference to exchange lessons learned through practice and research, examine new formulations, and nurture collaborations for future research and writing. Dr. Siegler frequently visits his trainees' institutions to facilitate their careers and impact. Dr. Siegler also widely shares information regarding clinical medical ethics through lectures and visiting professorships, illustrating his persistence and dedication. These personal characteristics also speak to his dedication and commitment to his fellowship trainees and his patients.

I and many other trainees are in his debt. By influencing a much larger group of health care workers through his writings and teaching, Dr. Siegler has achieved what few have: improvement in patient care for a very large number of patients.

References

1. Siegler M. Pascal's wager and the hanging of crepe. New Engl J Med. 1975;293(17):853–7.
2. Siegler M. A legacy of Osler: teaching clinical ethics at the bedside. JAMA. 1978;239(10):951–6.
3. Siegler M. Clinical ethics and clinical medicine. Arch Int Med. 1979;139(8):914–5.
4. Siegler M. Cautionary advice for humanists. Hast Cent Rep. 1981; 11(2):19–20.

Part II

Landmark Works on Clinical Medical Ethics by Mark Siegler, M.D.

Foundational Scholarship

7

Laura Weiss Roberts and Mark Siegler

Abstract

This chapter contains reprinted works from Dr. Mark Siegler focusing on foundational scholarship in the field of clinical medical ethics. The earliest included works lay the foundation for the field, while later works expand on its definition and scope, anticipate future advances, and analyze the development and growth of the field through a historical lens. This selection of reprinted works specifies the improvement of patient care as the goal of clinical medical ethics and explains how the field sets itself apart from theoretical bioethics and real-life practices such as ethics consultations. The works in this chapter are reprinted with permission.

L.W. Roberts, MD, MA (✉)
Department of Psychiatry and Behavioral Sciences, Stanford
University School of Medicine, Stanford, CA, USA
e-mail: robertsl@stanford.edu

M. Siegler, MD
Bucksbaum Institute for Clinical Excellence, MacLean Center for
Clinical Medical Ethics, University of Chicago, Pritzker School of
Medicine, Chicago, IL, USA

© Springer International Publishing AG 2017
L.W. Roberts, M. Siegler (eds.), *Clinical Medical Ethics*, DOI 10.1007/978-3-319-53875-4_7

7.1   Siegler M (1979) Clinical Ethics and Clinical Medicine. Arch Intern Med 139:914–5

Clinical Ethics

Clinical Ethics and Clinical Medicine

Mark Siegler, MD

In this issue of the ARCHIVES, a new editorial department is introduced. It will appear occasionally and will present the views of practicing physicians on a broad range of clinical problems that force them to confront directly moral and ethical questions arising in their routine practice. The articles will be written by clinicians, and will be directed toward an audience of practicing physicians. This new section will be called CLINICAL ETHICS, reflecting the fact that, in the practice of medicine, clinical and ethical issues are deeply interdependent.

THE RISE OF BIOMEDICAL ETHICS

Clinical ethics, which focuses on issues that confront the physician in his daily interactions with patients, is to be contrasted with biomedical ethics (BME), which is greatly concerned with public policy issues. In the past 15 years, there has been a remarkable rise of interest in BME; it has captured the fancy of the public. The media have focused increased attention on such issues as research in human subjects, the recombinant DNA controversy, policy issues concerning national health insurance, and others; the courts have become increasingly active in the medical arena.

Biomedical ethics has become an established "field" in the United States. New scholarly journals in BME appear regularly; institutes of BME have been established; there is a proliferation of books, both academic and lay, in the field. Universities have developed graduate teaching programs in bioethics, and bioethicists testify regularly for state and federal legislative committees and the courts.

Such interdisciplinary efforts are laudable, but with some reservations. The BME establishment has been created and led to a large degree by nonphysicians, ie, theologians, philosophers, sociologists, lawyers, and historians. Physicians, scientists, and medical professionals have had only limited involvement in its development.

From the Section of General Internal Medicine, Department of Internal Medicine, University of Chicago, Pritzker School of Medicine.

Reprint requests to Box 72, University of Chicago Hospitals, 950 E 59th St, Chicago, IL 60637 (Dr Siegler).

CONCERN OVER BME

Developments in BME are disquieting and are worthy of our attention. The lack of involvement by physicians is profoundly disturbing. It has been suggested that many bioethicists have a frankly antiscientific, antimedicine bias, or at the least, that they represent interests that are quite different from those of the medical-scientific community.[1] Bioethicists who are uninvolved in the process of medical care have produced legislative, administrative, and legal changes that affect the practice of medicine, and it is clear by now that medicine has merely reacted to, rather than anticipated or participated in, most major developments in BME. Further, much of the teaching of BME to medical and other health professional students is being done by this new group of bioethicists, rather than by physicians. The proliferation of teaching medical ethicists and their virtual dominance in the teaching of medical students is another disturbing aspect in the growth of BME. It is reassuring to note that even some early leaders in the BME establishment have become concerned with this development, and have attempted to involve themselves more deeply in the realities of clinical medicine.[2]

Finally, BME is increasingly concerned with the analysis and formulation of large public policy options in medicine and science, and has not directed sufficient attention to many of the routine ethical questions that arise in the encounters between patients and physicians. Many of the leaders of the BME movement have actually expressed their disdain for traditional, Hippocratic, bedside medical ethics,[3] which, since Hippocratic times, have been overwhelmingly physician- and patient-oriented. Biomedical ethics is an intellectual movement that concerns itself with questions affecting the daily activities of medicine, but that has arisen primarily from outside the profession.

CLINICAL MEDICINE AND CLINICAL ETHICS

It is in the context of the rapid growth of BME and our concerns with that development that we encourage physicians to consider the merits of clinical ethics. The practice of clinical medicine has always been a unique blend of technical proficiency and ethical sensitivity, which together constitute the physician's art. The distinction that is too commonly made between clinical decisions and ethical decisions is an invidious, but fortunately misguided, one. In a sense, the term "clinical ethics" is redundant,[1] because good clinical medicine is necessarily ethical medicine. The reason for selecting CLINICAL ETHICS as the name of the new editorial section is that changes in modern medicine–particularly but not exclusively technological advances of the last 30 years–have created an unanticipated range of ethical dilemmas that demand creative and reflective clinical responses. We are now able to treat patients with chronic renal failure, chronic respiratory failure, and even chronic gastrointestinal failure. We have powerful antitumor drugs; the techniques of cardiopulmonary resuscitation can be used to prolong, for variable periods, the viability of every person whose heart and lungs have stopped; advances in neonatal intensive care and neonatal surgery have assured that many congenitally abnormal infants can be treated in ways that are certain to extend their existence. Each of these medical capabilities generates a range of clinical-ethical questions that must be taken into account in the course of formulating a clinical decision. These are examples of the kinds of clinical-ethical problems that increasingly test the mettle of conscientious, technically proficient, and morally scrupulous physicians.

Clinical ethics also explores the assumption that the role of the medical professional is unique. The physician's relationship to the patient is premised on specific technical training and competency. This specialized knowledge and proficiency is used to assist patients in curing or ameliorating their illness and disease, and to assist them in overcoming the fear, pain, and suffering that are often associated with ill health. Once sought out by the patient, the physician becomes involved in the patient's problem. He is never a mere observer. He cannot rely on the counterfeit courage of the noncombatant. The physician is personally accountable to the patient if he fails to perform his task adequately because of lack of skill or negligence, or because, for whatever reason, he fails to act in his patient's behalf. Søren Kierkegaard perfectly captured the distinction between the theoretician and the involved participant in his response to a question that he posed: "Is knowledge changed when it is applied?" Kierkegaard's response deserves consideration from all who would criticize medicine and physicians from a perspective removed from the actual medical setting:

Let us imagine a pilot, and assume that he had passed every examination with distinction, but that he had not as yet been at sea. Imagine him in a storm; he knows everything he ought to do, but he has not known before how terror grips the seafarer when the stars are lost in the blackness of night; he has not known the sense of impotence that comes when the pilot sees the wheel in his hand become a plaything for the waves; he has not known how the blood rushes into the head when one tries to make calculations at such a moment; in short, he has had no conception of the change that takes place in the knower when he has to apply his knowledge.[5]

A NEW EDITORIAL DEPARTMENT OF CLINICAL ETHICS

This new editorial department will be devoted to exploring issues in clinical ethics. It will be addressed to those physicians who have ". . . known how the blood rushes into the head when one tries to make calculations at such a moment. . . ." Our first symposium will serve as an example of the method we will use and it will indicate the general areas of concern to be discussed in this section in coming years. Each of the contributors to this discussion on the management of respiratory failure is a distinguished physician. Each of these contributions was unsolicited. The editors did not create a problem or a "case" and then seek out expert commentators to resolve it. This symposium should not be confused with an "ethical grand rounds." Rather, in the context of practicing clinical medicine, certain clinical quandaries appeared repeatedly. Because of the thorny nature of such problems and the lack of definitive solutions, the authors decided to struggle to articulate and defend their clinical judgment in writing.

It occurred to the editors of the ARCHIVES–themselves practicing physicians–that the types of questions that are raised by the authors of this symposium could as easily be raised about most areas of medicine. Future symposia on these pages will be devoted to similar clinical-ethical problems that arise in the practice of clinical medicine, surgery, pediatrics, obstetrics and gynecology, and psychiatry.

Our editorial plan is as follows: We will accept unsolicited articles for refereed review and will also invite distinguished clinicians to reflect on the range of clinical-ethical dilemmas that arise in their area of expertise. We will attempt to gather such articles together and publish them as symposia focusing on one clinical area. It is our hope that in time we will have generated a series of clinical reflections in most major areas of medical practice. These reflections will report ways in which physicians are dealing with these dilemmas at a time when the traditional model of the physician-patient relationship is in a state of flux, and when technological advances demand new and creative solutions. Expert clinicians will offer practical suggestions about such dilemmas from the perspective of the practicing clinician. We are hopeful that these contributions will encourage other clinicians to offer their own observations in this area, and the editors of the ARCHIVES OF INTERNAL MEDICINE have agreed to publish a substantial number of letters provoked by these articles, to indicate the range of clinical opinion on these complex and difficult subjects.

The new editorial section of the ARCHIVES OF INTERNAL MEDICINE will differ from other medical journals, such as the *New England Journal of Medicine, Clinical Research*, and the *American Journal of Medicine*, all of which increasingly publish articles that relate medicine to broad social, economic, and ethical issues. This section of the ARCHIVES will serve primarily as a forum for clinicians. We hope it will become a resource on which nonphysician-theoreticians can base their analyses and speculations.

This new section of the ARCHIVES, CLINICAL ETHICS, is certainly not intended to be reactionary. Rather, its intention is to infuse a higher degree of contact with clinical reality into the debate than has characterized BME in the past. Further, it is designed to represent more forcefully the concerns of clinicians in the councils of bioethicists. It will never be the intention of these columns to suggest that the judgment of medical professionals is correct merely because of their medical expertise. But it will be argued with vigor and fervor that the viewpoints and reflections of involved professionals, on clinical-ethical problems, merit careful consideration in the resolution of complex issues in medical ethics.

References

1. Callahan D: The ethics backlash. *Hastings Cent Rep* 5:18, 1975.
2. Jonsen AR: Books on bioethics. *Pharos* 44:39-43, 1978.
3. Veatch RM, Branson R: *Ethics and Health Policy*. Cambridge, Mass, Ballinger Publishing Co, 1976, pp xix-xx, 3-16.
4. Guttentag O: Medical humanism: A redundant phrase. *Pharos* 32:12-15, 1969.
5. Kierkegaard S: Thoughts on crucial situations in human life, in Oden TC (ed): *Parables of Kierkegaard*. Princeton, NJ, Princeton University Press, 1978, p 38.

7.2   Siegler M (1982) Decision-Making Strategy for Clinical Ethical Problems in Medicine. Arch Intern Med 142:2178–9

Reprinted with permission from the Archives of Internal Medicine, November 1982, Volume 142, Copyright 1982, American Medical Association.

Clinical Ethics

Decision-Making Strategy for Clinical-Ethical Problems in Medicine

Mark Siegler, MD

Medical education and training should prepare physicians to make decisions, because that is what they do routinely in medical practice. When physicians determine that a diagnostic procedure is warranted, or when they recommend a particular form of treatment, or even, when they assess whether and when a patient who telephones with a medical problem should be seen in the office (or in the emergency room), physicians are making decisions. None of these decisions is easy, because medicine is, as Osler described it, a science of uncertainty and an art of probability. Nevertheless, physicians generally reach clinical decisions and feel reasonably comfortable doing so.

In contrast to clinical decisions, physicians find clinical-ethical decisions of the following sort extremely difficult: Should "no-code" orders be written (for example, on a patient with irreversible senile dementia and an acute, treatable pneumonia)? Should an infant with Down's syndrome and duodenal atresia be treated with maximal aggressiveness? Should a physician accept the wishes of a young patient with bacterial meningitis who refuses to accept curative antibiotic therapy? Should the physician offer long-term renal dialysis to an overweight diabetic patient in whom renal failure develops if that patient had in the past persistently refused to take insulin or adhere to a diet? Should a physician ever violate a patient's confidentiality in the interests of third parties or in society's interest?

Clinical-ethical quandaries of these kinds provoke physician discomfort for several understandable reasons: first, these cases often involve life-and-death decisions that engage deepest human emotions and require the most delicate dealings with patients and colleagues; further, in contrast to clinical decisions, physicians rightly feel that their education and training has not prepared them to approach these problems analytically and systematically, and that they often have no basis for decision other than their common sense, intuitions, and personal value system; finally, these cases often raise the specter that the physician could be liable to civil or criminal charges *regardless* of what decision is finally made.

The question arises whether it is possible to develop a systematic approach to clinical-ethical decisions that might, to some extent, alleviate physician discomfort and that also might improve their ability to reach reasonable and legally and morally defensible decisions in these difficult situations. The method I am about to propose should help in these respects, but it is not a panacea. The method will offer a systematic approach to indicate what facts are most relevant in a case (and which are extraneous), how those facts should be organized to develop the critical considerations in a case, and how the various considerations in a case should be weighted with respect to other considerations.

Accepted for publication June 22, 1982.
From the Section of General Medicine, Department of Medicine, University of Chicago-Pritzker School of Medicine, Chicago.
Reprint requests to Box 72, University of Chicago Hospitals, 950 E 59th St, Chicago, IL 60637 (Dr Siegler).

Thus, the system should provide a checklist for physicians to guarantee that all relevant considerations are taken into account and that none is overlooked in reaching a clinical-ethical decision. It will help a clinician to clarify and consolidate the thinking about a case. However, this method will not dictate conclusions. Conclusions must be reached finally by the conscientious clinician through the application of clinical judgment.

My proposal for a systematic approach to clinical-ethical decisions involves four categories (listed in their usual order of importance) into which most considerations in a clinical case can be distributed. These categories are as follows: (1) the medical indications in a case; (2) the patient's preferences; (3) quality of life factors; and (4) factors external to the immediate physician-patient encounter (including, for example, family wishes, cost issues, societal interests, etc).

MEDICAL INDICATIONS

This is the first and most recognizable part of the decision-making scheme. It is the physician's domain. It represents the traditional clinical method of medicine and requires clinical discretion and clinical judgment. The patient is seen with a medical problem, and the physician attempts to determine what is wrong with the patient (a diagnosis); what will happen to the patient if the condition is treated or not treated (a prognosis); what the risks and benefits of various treatment programs are (therapeutic alternatives); and finally, what recommendations should be made to this particular patient in these specific circumstances (a clinical strategy). In making personal recommendations based on medical indications, the physician takes account of the nature of the disease, the risks and benefits of various courses of management, and the biologic and personal particularities (including the goals and values) of the patient. It is this action made in the interests of a particular person that transforms "medical science" into "human medicine."

PATIENT PREFERENCES

In step 1, it was the physician's obligation to recommend treatment that is medically indicated. These days, however, it is the competent adult patient's prerogative to accept or reject these recommendations in the light of personal preferences. The informed consent legal requirement reflects changes that have occurred in the physician-patient relationship. These changes emphasize the rights of patients to make decisions about their own health care. In the priority ordering of the four clinical-ethical considerations, patient preferences are probably the weightiest ethical consideration in the patient-physician encounter. However, chronologically and logically, the patient's statement of preferences must follow step 1, the physician's recommendations based on medical indications. Patients cannot express informed preferences until they are provided sufficient information about what their medical problem is and what the physician thinks should be done about it. For example, a patient who comes to the physician with a complaint of a cough of one month's duration would be unable to express any meaningful preferences regarding treatment options until the physician had determined whether the cough was caused by a viral syndrome, obstructive airway disease, tuberculosis, tumor, etc.

In most medical encounters, physicians and patients reach decisions based on steps 1 and 2 noted above. In general, the recommendations of physicians and the preferences of patients coincide. However, at times, clinical-ethical problems may arise. For example, if the medical indications in a case (say, a case of life-threatening illness) clearly point to a curative treatment that the patient refuses to authorize, the physician must determine whether the patient was expressing an *informed refusal*, ie, whether in the face of the serious illness, the patient retained the capacity to comprehend the situation and to make informed choices with irreversible (life-and-death) implications. In certain instances, the physician may decide that the patient has lost the capacity to make informed choices and that his stated preferences ought to be noted and taken into account, but that treatment should be administered anyway.

A different type of clinical-ethical dilemma may arise when physicians are confronted with situations in which the medical indications are grim (ie, no therapy offers much hope for improvement), *and* in which the patient is unable to express a preference regarding treatment or the withholding of it (eg, the patient is an infant or is an adult who is comatose or senile). If both of these conditions exist simultaneously, a clinical-ethical decision based on steps 1 and 2 of the proposed strategy becomes less likely. In these situations, physicians often take into account two additional considerations—quality of life factors and external factors—in reaching a clinical-ethical decision. If, however, only one of these conditions exist, eg, a poor medical prognosis, but the patient is capable of expressing preferences, physicians obviously would base their decisions on the stated wishes of the patient. Conversely, if the patient were unconscious, but had a treatable medical condition (eg, a ruptured spleen sustained in an automobile accident), physicians obviously would treat based on a medical indications policy, even in the absence of available statements of patient preference.

QUALITY OF LIFE CONSIDERATIONS

Although this phrase is used frequently in a variety of medical circumstances, its meaning is ambiguous. When a quality of life standard is invoked in crucial ethical deliberations about patient care, the phrase usually refers to the subjective evaluation by an onlooker about a patient's subjective experience of personal life. Usually, but not always, the phrase is used in situations where the patient is unable to make such an evaluation or is unable to express it because of mental incapacity. In a clinical setting, the phrase may be used as follows: "Is this patient's quality of life now or in the future such that it is worth treating or prolonging or preserving that life?" Quality of life considerations may operate without invoking the phrase "quality of life," as in a case where an intern asks an attending physician: "Is it *worth it* to culture that 80-year-old man's fever?" This standard, which is almost always applied by someone other than the person who is living the life that is being assessed for its "worth," represents an attempt to put a value on some collection of features of human experience. The phrase is used as if there were objective criteria, even though it rests less on facts than on one's subjective preferences about certain facts.

In the routine practice of medicine, physicians do not and

should not place much weight on quality of life considerations except those that are expressed as the patient's own preferences. However, as suggested previously, quality of life considerations (and also external considerations) will tend to be invoked in clinical circumstances in which both medical indications are limited and patient preferences are not known (and in some cases not even potentially knowable). These clinical circumstances include the following: (*a*) untreatable or terminal illnesses, (*b*) situations in which patients are permanently unconscious or brain injured or have senile dementia, (*c*) decisions regarding neonates and children, and thus, (*d*) in most no-code decisions.

EXTERNAL FACTORS

External factors refer to any consideration in a case that yields a benefit or burden to some party other than the specific patient for whom the decision is being made. External factors tend to enlarge the context in which the patient is viewed from a private physician-patient encounter (which has been the tradition of medicine since hippocratic times) to one that takes account of, for example: (*a*) the wishes and needs of the patient's family, (*b*) the costs of medical care, (*c*) the allocation of limited medical resources; (*d*) the research and teaching needs of medicine, and (*e*) the safety and well-being of society. Although almost every clinical decision will involve some external effects such as these, the question arises whether the physician should ever explicitly consider these effects and allow them to influence the clinical-ethical decision. When, if ever, is it ethically permissible to weigh the patient's interests against the interests of other persons or society? In general (except for situations already noted), external factors do not and should not be accounted great weight in routine clinical-ethical decisions.

CONCLUSION

In ordinary medical practice, physicians do and should take account of four general considerations to reach a clinical-ethical decision. Among the four factors noted, the medical indications and patient preferences, together, usually decide the case. Quality of life and external considerations are not and usually should not be important except in those specific instances noted when neither of the first two factors allows for decisive action, ie, when both medical indications are poor and patient preferences cannot be known.

Two final points should be noted. The decision-making system presented herein is one that corresponds to the way many physicians currently reach clinical-ethical decisions in practice. Thus, it represents both a description of how decisions are now being reached and an analytic prescription or a checklist to provide a model for clinical reflectiveness in the future. Lastly, although the four-part system of decision making was proposed specifically as a means for resolving clinical-ethical quandaries, it must be acknowledged that almost no medical decision is a merely technical one. All decisions are made with and for individual persons, and thus they involve human values and ethics. In this light, the decision-making proposal advanced should be applicable not only to ethical dilemmas in medicine, but to all decisions in medical practice.

This material was prepared with support from the Ethics and Values in Science and Technology program of the National Science Foundation (grant OSS-8018097) and the Humanities, Science and Technology Program of the National Endowment for the Humanities.

The views expressed herein are those of the author and do not necessarily reflect those of the National Science Foundation or the National Endowment for the Humanities.

**7.3   La Puma J, Stocking CB, Silverstein
MD, DiMartini A, Siegler M (1988)
An Ethics Consultation Service
in a Teaching Hospital. Utilization
and Evaluation. JAMA 260:808–11**

Reprinted with permission from the Journal of the American
Medical Association, August 12, 1988, Volume 260,
Copyright 1988, American Medical Association.

An Ethics Consultation Service in a Teaching Hospital

Utilization and Evaluation

John La Puma, MD; Carol B. Stocking, PhD; Marc D. Silverstein, MD; Andrea DiMartini, MD; Mark Siegler, MD

A newly established formal ethics consultation service in a university teaching hospital was prospectively evaluated. A physician-ethicist interviewed and examined patients, interviewed family and others as needed, and entered a formal consultation note in the medical record. The requesting physician and the consultant independently completed structured questionnaires. Fifty-one consultation requests were received from 45 physicians from seven departments between July 1, 1986, and June 30, 1987. Seventeen (33%) of 51 patients were in the intensive care unit, and 19 patients (37%) were fully oriented at the time of consultation. Overall, 61% of the patients survived to leave the hospital. The requesting physician sought assistance with withholding or withdrawing life-sustaining treatment in 49% of cases, with resuscitation issues in 37%, and with legal issues in 31%. Assistance with more than one issue was sought in 39 cases (76%). In 36 cases (71%), the requesting physician stated that the consultation was "very important" in patient management, in clarifying ethical issues, or in learning about medical ethics. We conclude that ethics consultation performed by physician-ethicists provides useful, clinically acceptable assistance in a teaching hospital.

(*JAMA* 1988;260:808-811)

IN A less technological, less litigious medical era, common sense and intuition were considered sufficient to resolve dilemmas of right and wrong in patient care.[1] Technological improvements in medicine and increasing legal pressure to meet a perceived standard of care[2] have highlighted the need for a systematic, rational process of ethical decision making.[3,4]

Ethics consultation services have been created to respond to this need when it arises in a particular patient's care. Few data are available about ethics consultants, their methods, or the results of their consultations. A National Institutes of Health survey of consultants attending a National Institutes of Health–University of California at San Francisco conference on ethics consultation found that each consultant received an average of nine formal requests for consultation annually.[5] One review of a pediatric institutional ethics team found that requests usually came from the attending physician.[6] Several retrospective reviews have suggested that consultations may clarify ethical issues, contribute to patient management, and teach decision-making skills to attending and house staff physicians.[7,8]

The potential clinical roles of the ethics consultant in teaching institutions recently have been discussed.[4,5,9-11] We prospectively studied the actual clinical role of a newly established clinical ethics consultation service to describe (1) the characteristics of patients for whom physicians requested ethics consultation and (2) the reasons for seeking consultation, from the viewpoints of requesting physicians and the ethics

consultant, and (3) if and how requesting physicians found ethics consultation helpful.

METHODS

Method of Consultation

A formal ethics consultation service was established on July 1, 1986, by the Center for Clinical Medical Ethics at the University of Chicago Hospitals and Clinics. Members of the ethics consultation service included three attending physicians with expertise in clinical ethics, three clinical ethics fellows (board certified in internal medicine or pediatrics), and senior medical students on monthly electives. Service resource persons included a hospital attorney and a professor of moral philosophy.

An ethics consultation format was used in performing and recording consultations.[8] When a consultation was requested by a physician, a fellow (the consultant) interviewed and examined the patient. The consultant reviewed the medical record and interviewed the requesting physician, other health care workers involved in the patient's care, family members, and, when necessary, others outside of the institution. After discussing the case with an attending physician-ethicist and one or both resource persons as needed, the consultant and the attending physician ethicist wrote an assessment and discussion of the ethical issues, as well as specific recommendations in the medical record. Patients in the hospital were followed up until their discharge or death. There was no charge for consultations.

Method of Evaluation

Consultation requests received from July 1, 1986, until June 30, 1987, were included in the evaluation. The requesting physician and the consultant independently completed parallel, structured questionnaires at the completion of the consultation. A research assistant distributed and collected the questionnaires. Responses from requesting phy-

From the Section of Clinical Ethics, Lutheran General Hospital, Park Ridge, Ill (Dr La Puma); and Center for Clinical Medical Ethics and Section of General Internal Medicine, University of Chicago Hospitals and Clinics (Drs La Puma, Stocking, Silverstein, DiMartini, and Siegler).

Presented in part at the Tenth Annual Meeting of the Society for General Internal Medicine, San Diego, May 1, 1987.

The views expressed herein are those of the authors and do not necessarily reflect the view of the supporting foundations or institutions.

Reprint requests to Section of Clinical Ethics, Lutheran General Hospital, 1775 Dempster Ave, Park Ridge, IL 60068 (Dr La Puma).

sicians were confidential and were not available to the consultant.

The consultant recorded the patient's age, sex, medical problems, mental status, and hospital location, as well as whether a do-not-resuscitate (DNR) order had been written before the consultation. The consultant also recorded the time and date of consultation request and response, the time required to complete the consultation, the identities of the persons interviewed, and the recommendations made, including whether a DNR order was recommended.

Both the requesting physician and the consultant were asked to record the reason(s) for the consultation from a list derived from the analysis of 27 formal consultations performed the previous year.[8] Both requesting physician and consultant were also asked to rate the consultation's importance in clarifying ethical issues, managing patients, and teaching the language of medical ethics.

Patients' charts were reviewed by the consultant to record whether the patient survived and, if so, whether the patient was discharged home or to a long-term care facility. One of us (J.L.) classified patients by the primary medical reason for each patient's admission. The requesting physician's participation in the evaluation was voluntary. Verbal consent to participate in the evaluation was obtained from requesting physicians after the consultant had written the recommendations. The Clinical Investigation Committee of the institution approved the evaluation protocol.

RESULTS

Forty-five physicians from seven different departments of the Hospitals and Clinics requested consultations for 51 of their patients. Twenty-one requests came from physicians in the medicine department, 13 from surgery, seven from neurology, and three from neonatology. Physicians in pediatrics, geriatrics, and dermatology all requested more than one consultation.

The patients referred for consultation ranged in age from 2 days to 93 years (average, 51 years). Thirty-one patients (61%) were in hospital rooms at the time of consultation, 17 (33%) were in an intensive care unit, and three were in other locations. Primary reasons for admission were neurologic disease (n=14), infectious disease (n=9), neoplasm (n=7), and psychiatric illness (n=4). In eight cases, other medical reasons were present.

Thirty-five patients (69%) were aware of the consultant's visit. Nineteen patients (37%) were alert and ori-

Table 1.—Requesting Physician's Reasons and Ethics Consultant's Identification of the Reasons for Consultation*

	No. (%) of Responses	
Reason	Requesting Physician (n=51)	Consulting Physician (n=51)
Withdrawing or withholding therapy	25 (49)	33 (65)
Resuscitation/DNR issues	19 (37)	19 (37)
Legal issues	16 (31)	15 (30)
Competency evaluation	12 (24)	7 (14)
Disagreement resolution	12 (24)	23 (45)
Appropriateness of current treatment	11 (22)	17 (33)
Discharge disposition	9 (18)	15 (30)
Autonomy	7 (14)	5 (10)
Cost of care	4 (8)	4 (10)
Other‡	13 (25)	20 (39)

*More than one reason for consultation could be listed for each patient. DNR indicates do not resuscitate.
†Percentage of patients for whom the reason was cited.
‡Includes assistance with advance directives, suicide attempts, and potentially rational suicide.

ented to person, place, and time at the time of consultation; another seven patients were alert and oriented to person and place. Of the 19 patients who were fully oriented, 17 (89%) survived: 15 of these patients were discharged home and two others were discharged to long-term–care facilities. Overall, 31 patients (61%) survived; 18 patients died in the hospital.

Consultant Activities

All patients were seen within a day of request by the consultation. The ethics consultation required an average of 4.8 hours (range, two to 12 hours), including team and family meetings when necessary. The consultant interviewed other physicians in 47 of 51 cases. Family members were interviewed in 35 cases, nurses in 31 cases, and social workers in 15 cases. Dietitians, clergy, and others outside the Hospitals and Clinics were consulted in 23 cases.

The consultant made specific recommendations in 48 of 51 cases. A DNR order was recommended in 13 cases and written in 12 of these cases after the completion of the consultation.

Reason for Consultation

All 51 questionnaires distributed to requesting physicians were returned (Table 1). Requesting physicians reported seeking assistance with more than one problem in 39 cases and identified an average of 2.4 reasons for consultation per case. Assistance with decisions to forego life-sustaining treatment was the most common reason for consultation.

Requesting physicians' reasons for consultation in the 19 fully alert and oriented patients were analyzed separately. Requesting physicians sought assistance with judging patient competency in nine (47%) of these patients. The cost of care was raised as a reason

by requesting physicians for four of these fully oriented patients; in three patients (16%), assistance was sought with resuscitation issues.

All 51 questionnaires distributed to the consultant were returned, and the consultant also identified reasons for consultation. The consultant responded that the requesting physician sought help with more than one reason for consultation in 46 cases (90%) and that there were an average of 3.0 reasons for consultation per case. For the 19 fully oriented patients, the consultant found the reason for consultation to concern patient competency in five cases (26%). Eight cases (42%) concerned withdrawing and withholding therapy. Four of five cost-of-care questions identified were in fully oriented patients; in four patients (21%), assistance was sought with resuscitation issues.

Evaluation of the Consultation

In 36 cases (71%), the requesting physician stated that the consultation was "very important" in patient management, in clarifying ethical issues, or in learning about medical ethics (Table 2). In 96% of cases, requesting physicians indicated that they planned to request an ethics consultation in the future. Illustrative cases are now presented.

ILLUSTRATIVE CASES

Case 1: Clarification of Ethical Issues

An unemployed, unmarried, 27-year-old man was admitted with hepatic failure. He had occasionally used intravenous cocaine and had consumed two fifths (approximately 1.5 L) of alcohol daily within seven months of admission. Vital signs were normal; results of physical examination showed an awake, alert, jaundiced man in no acute distress. The requesting physician asked,

Table 2.—Evaluation of the Ethics Consultations*

	Requesting Physician (n=51)			Consulting Physician (n=51)		
	Very Important	Somewhat Important	Not Important	Very Important	Somewhat Important	Not Important
"How important was the consultation in . . .						
. . . Clarifying ethical issues?"	51	43	6	58	42	0
. . . Patient management?"	40	48	12	61	23	2
. . . Educating the team?"	43	37	20	32	50	18

*Values are expressed as percentages of responses.

"Should this patient be a candidate for liver transplantation?"

The consultant interviewed the patient and found that the man knew the risks of transplantation and was determined to "stay off" drugs. The consultant sought to clarify three issues for the requesting physician: whether "psychosocial" criteria should be used for deciding the patient's candidacy for transplantation; whether the patient's history of substance abuse was being used to measure his individual worth and future compliance; and whether resources were available for transplantation.

The consultant presented data concerning survival and the length of abstinence required by other transplant groups (S. Iwatsuki, MD, oral communication, August 1986). The consultant outlined problems with transportation to and from the Hospitals and Clinics and with the treatment regimen's complexity, counterbalanced by the benefits of a supportive home environment and the patient's new commitment to health. Finally, the consultant discussed the clinical relevance of "dire"[12] and relative scarcity.

The consultant suggested that the patient was a transplant candidate and recommended a three-month period of medical therapy to optimize his preoperative condition. The patient was discharged home and successfully completed this three-month course. He was unable to obtain funding, however, and later filed a suit against Medicaid.[13] He won the suit but died before a liver became available for transplantation.

Case 2: Analysis of Ethical Issues

A 20-year-old woman with a history of systemic lupus erythematosus and intravenous drug use had two porcine mitral valve replacements for endocarditis in the past year. She was unemployed, uninsured, and unmarried. She was admitted with a three-week history of fever, fatigue, and weight loss; her medications included prednisone. Physical examination revealed a new systolic murmur and splenomegaly. Because the patient "had been noncompliant

regarding abstinence," the attending cardiac surgeon thought that a third valve replacement was not indicated. A house officer requested an ethics consultation, asking, "Should this patient receive a valve replacement?"

After interviewing and examining the patient, the ethics consultant found her to be competent to make her own health care decisions; to be an "undesirable patient"[14,15]; and to be in need of valve replacement and treatment of her substance dependence. Three ethical issues were identified and analyzed: the autonomy of competent, "undesirable" patients[16]; the unique ethical problems of house officers[17]; and the ethical obligations of physicians.[18] A treatment contract with the patient was recommended, involving completion of a substance dependence program after discharge. A surgeon willing to perform the operation was sought.

The patient agreed to enter a treatment program on discharge, but a surgeon was still unavailable. Her condition improved in the hospital for three weeks but she became acutely hypotensive and dyspneic. The attending internist phoned the cardiac surgeon who, because of the emergency, performed the surgery. The patient recovered, and three weeks later she left the hospital.

Case 3: Resolution of Ethical Issues

A 34-year-old woman with hypertension and renal failure had been hemodialyzed for a year. On the day of admission, she experienced a cardiopulmonary arrest at home and her husband initiated resuscitation before paramedics arrived. One week later, severe autonomic instability and anoxic encephalopathy had been diagnosed. A neurologist found that she had a "less than 1% chance of recovery." The patient's husband insisted that "everything be done," that all aggressive measures be continued, and that a miracle would occur. The physicians, who wished to withdraw life support, requested an ethics consultation, asking, "What are the roles of religion and the patient's husband in decision making?"

In this case, the ethical issues centered around the conflict between the husband's belief in miracles, the patient's terminal condition, and the obligation of the physician to continue family-requested therapies that were futile and not medically indicated. Family members may lack the legal or moral authority to make decisions for incompetent patients; physicians may not be obligated to honor these requests, even when urgent.[19]

After examining the patient and reviewing the records, the consultant agreed that she was unlikely to recover. The consultant organized a meeting of family and physicians to clarify the prognosis and the goals of treatment. All expressed hope that a miracle would occur, while acknowledging the futility of hemodialysis and mechanical ventilatory support. The consultant suggested a change in the goals of care to those of comfort instead of cure, stressing the addition of supportive and comfort-oriented care instead of the withdrawal of futile therapies. A DNR order and the discontinuation of procedures that did not contribute to patient comfort were recommended. The consultant encouraged the family to meet with their minister, but they did not wish to do so. The other suggestions were taken, and the patient died the day after the consultation.

COMMENT

A formal ethics consultation service was established in a university teaching hospital. We prospectively studied the patient population and consultation activities. We also studied the requesting physician's reasons for consultation, the consultant's perception of the reasons for consultation, and the perceived importance of the consultation in patient care. Consultations were performed in a diverse population, including critically ill, unresponsive patients and ambulatory, oriented patients. In general, the service seemed to function as an objective clinical voice in nonurgent but very difficult cases.

Requesting physicians' reasons for consultation were examined according to patient orientation at the time of consultation. For the patients who were not fully oriented, requesting physicians were most often concerned about withdrawing or withholding therapy or about DNR orders. For the patients who were fully oriented, requesting physicians still asked most often about withdrawing or withholding therapy but also asked about patient competency.

For all patients, the reasons for consultation indicated by the requesting physician and perceived by the consultant revealed the same spectrum, with a slight predominance of competency questions by the requestors, and disagreement resolution questions by the consultant.

Sixteen requesting physicians asked questions about "legal issues." These issues may have been mistaken for ethical issues or may have reflected the belief that conferring with an ethics consultant reduces potential liability. These remain untested hypotheses, but legal and ethical questions frequently overlap.

The consultation service attempted to help the requesting physician and the patient in several ways. First, the consultant facilitated patient and family participation in end-of-life care decisions by interviewing the patient or the patient's family or friends when the patient could not participate. Second, the consultant reassured physicians that patients who were dying could be allowed to die without equating this with abandonment. Third, the consultant helped physicians speak with intermittently competent patients and their families about quality of life and socioeconomic factors when the patient's wishes were unclear.

The ethics consultant did not discuss his or her recommendations with an ethics committee. A consultative function for ethics committees has been suggested,[20,21] but committees are unwieldly and may lack the clinical ethical expertise to help individual clinicians.[22-24] Until consultative committees are rigorously evaluated, their efficacy will remain unknown. A clinical ethics

consultation service may earn clinical acceptance and avoid some of the pitfalls of ethics committees that attempt to consult.[25]

A rich diversity of opinion exists about who is qualified to function as an ethics consultant. While there is certainly no currently accepted credential for ethics consultants, there is an emerging body of medical ethical knowledge. Explorations of relevant medical ethical concepts and analyses of medical ethical problems are part of a growing medical literature in medical ethics. The clinical ethics consultant's special clinical skills arise from this literature and from bedside experience with patients. The foundations of this knowledge base have been described recently.[26,27]

Physicians have previously attempted to resolve ethical dilemmas through informal discussions with colleagues, with pastoral care visits, or in ethics committee meetings. Whether ethics consultation will prove to be superior to these and other methods of resolving ethical dilemmas is unknown. Indeed, a reluctance to anger or disappoint a referring colleague with troubling advice may influence a physician-ethicist's analysis in a particular case. Like other consultants, however, physician-ethicists are bound by a standard of care[2,28] and can be held responsible for the consequences of their clinical judgment.

Our descriptive report of an ethics consultation service in a teaching hospital has limitations. Compliance with recommendations was assessed for only a single recommendation—that of writing a DNR order. Studies of medical

consultation have shown that frequent follow-up notes, fewer than five recommendations, and consultant/requestor personal contact improve compliance.[29] We chose writing a DNR order as an identifiable measure of compliance. The 92% compliance rate for writing a DNR order cannot be extrapolated to compliance with the consultant's other recommendations. Because the identification and clarification of ethical issues and the process of ethics consultation may be as important as the recommendations and references provided,[8,10,30] traditional measures such as compliance may not be the best measures of the success of an ethics consultation service. Instead, measurement of clinical expertise, communication skills, rational and humane analysis, and on-site availability may be useful.

Our findings suggest that an ethics consultation service in a university teaching hospital can help physicians identify, analyze, and resolve ethical problems in patient care. The clinical and educational value of consultation will depend on data from clinical trials of ethics consultants using diverse methods. The willingness of practicing physicians to request and consider analysis and advice may depend on the ethics consultant's credibility as a clinician, but this hypothesis has not been tested. What constitutes a "good outcome" for ethics consultation provides many opportunities for further research.

This work was supported in part by grants from the Henry J. Kaiser Family Foundation and the Andrew W. Mellon Foundation. Dr Silverstein is a Henry J. Kaiser Family Foundation Faculty Scholar in General Internal Medicine.

References

1. Jonsen AR, Siegler M, Winslade WJ: *Clinical Ethics*, ed 2. New York, Macmillan Publishing Co Inc, 1985.
2. La Puma J, Schiedermayer DL, Toulmin SE, et al: The standard of care: A case report and ethical analysis. *Ann Intern Med* 1988;108:121-124.
3. *Deciding to Forego Life Sustaining Treatment*. The President's Commission for the Study of Ethical Problems in Medicine and Biomedical and Behavioral Research, 1983, p 160.
4. Purtilo RB: Ethics consultation in the hospital. *N Engl J Med* 1984;311:983-986.
5. Bermel J: Ethics consultants: A self-portrait of decision-makers. *Hast Cent Rep* 1985;15:2.
6. Grodin MA, Markley WS, McDonald AE: Use of an institutional ethics team on a pediatric service. *QRB* 1985;11:16-19.
7. Perkins HS, Saathoff BS: How do ethics consultations benefit clinicians? abstracted. *Clin Res* 1986;34:831.
8. La Puma J: Consultations in clinical ethics: Issues and questions in 27 cases. *West J Med* 1987;146:633-637.
9. Rothenburg LS: Clinical ethicists and hospital ethics consultants: The nature and desirability of their clinical role, in Fletcher J, Jonsen AR (eds): *Proceedings of the Conference on Ethics Consultation at the National Institutes of Health*. Ann Arbor, Michigan Health Administration Press, in press.

10. Fowler MD: The role of the clinical ethicist. *Heart Lung* 1986;15:318-319.
11. Jonsen AR: Can an ethicist be a consultant? in Abernathy V (ed): *Frontiers in Medical Ethics: Applications in a Medical Setting*. Cambridge, Mass, Ballinger Publishing Co, 1980, pp 157-171.
12. Winslow GR: *Triage and Justice: The Ethics of Rationing Life-Saving Medical Resources*. Berkeley, University of California Press, 1982, pp 39-59.
13. The latest word:'In the courts.' *Hast Cent Rep* 1986;16:32.
14. Groves J: Taking care of hateful patients. *N Engl J Med* 1978;298:883-887.
15. Pepper S: The undesirable patient. *J Chronic Dis* 1970;22:777-779.
16. Outka G: Social justice and equal access to health care. *J Relig Ethics* 1974;2:11-32.
17. Winkenwerder W Jr: Ethical dilemmas for house-staff physicians: The care of critically ill and dying patients. *JAMA* 1985;254:3454-3457.
18. Zuger A, Miles SH: Physicians, AIDS, and occupational risk: Historic traditions and ethical obligations. *JAMA* 1987;258:1924-1928.
19. Brett AS, McCullough LB: When patients request specific interventions: Defining the limits of the physician's obligation. *N Engl J Med* 1986;315:1347-1351.
20. Fost N, Cranford RE: Hospital ethics committees: Administrative aspects. *JAMA* 1985;253:2687-2692.

21. Judicial Council of the American Medical Association: Guidelines for ethics committees in health care institutions. *JAMA* 1985;253:2698-2699.
22. Ahern ML: Biomedical ethics committees confront prickly issues. *Hospitals* 1984;58:66-70.
23. Siegler M: Ethics committees: Decisions by bureaucracy. *Hast Cent Rep* 1986;16:22-24.
24. La Puma J: Ethics by committee? *N Engl J Med* 1987;317:1418.
25. Lo B: Behind closed doors: Promises and pitfalls of ethics committees. *N Engl J Med* 1987;317:46-50.
26. The Ad Hoc Committee on Medical Ethics: American College of Physicians ethics manual. *Ann Intern Med* 1984;101:129-137, 263-274.
27. Siegler M, Singer P, Schiedermayer DL: *Medical Ethics: An Annotated Bibliography*. Philadelphia, The American College of Physicians, in press.
28. Robertson JA: Clinical medical ethics and the law: Rights and duties in ethics consultations, in Ackerman TF, Graber GC, Reynolds CH, et al (eds): *Clinical Medical Ethics: Exploration and Assessment*. New York, University Press of America, 1987, pp 69-81.
29. Merli GJ, Weitz HW: The medical consultant. *Med Clin North Am* 1987;71:353-355.
30. Glover JJ, Ozar DT, Thomasma DC: Teaching ethics on rounds: The ethicist as teacher, consultant and decision-maker. *Theoretical Med* 1986;7:13-32.

7.4   Siegler M, Pellegrino ED, Singer PA (1990) Clinical Medical Ethics. J Clin Ethics 1:5–9

Reprinted with permission from the Journal of Clinical Ethics, copyright 1990.

THE JOURNAL OF CLINICAL ETHICS   5

FEATURES

Clinical Medical Ethics

by Mark Siegler, Edmund D. Pellegrino, and Peter A. Singer

Introduction

Clinical medical ethics provides a special perspective on medical practice and health care. The goal of clinical ethics is to improve the quality of patient care by identifying, analyzing, and attempting to resolve the ethical problems that arise in the practice of clinical medicine. Clinical ethics emphasizes that the starting point for ethical analysis is the encounter between patient and health care provider. It stresses that the process and outcome of patient care is improved by acknowledging and respecting the importance of the patient's preferences and values and by empowering patients to make decisions based on their personal health care goals. During the past decade, clinical ethics teaching and research programs have evolved, and ethics committees and consultation services have become increasingly accessible to health professionals, patients, and families. Both physician-ethicists and professional ethicists have contributed to these developments, and continuing collaboration between these groups should be encouraged.

This first issue of *The Journal of Clinical Ethics* marks the passage of clinical ethics from childhood into adolescence and provides an appropriate forum for assessing the past and contemplating the future of the field. In describing clinical ethics more than a decade ago,[1,2] we suggested that ethics

This work was supported by the Henry J. Kaiser Family Foundation, the Andrew W. Mellon Foundation, and the Pew Charitable Trusts (M.S.) and by the Robert Wood Johnson Foundation and the Royal College of Physicians and Surgeons of Canada (P.A.S.). The opinions expressed are those of the authors and do not necessarily represent those of the foundations.

was central to clinical medicine for at least two reasons: 1) Ethical considerations cannot be avoided when physicians and patients must choose what *ought* to be done from among the many things that *can* be done for an individual patient in a particular clinical circumstance and 2) the concept of *good* clinical medicine implies that both technical and ethical considerations are taken into account. We argued that ethics informs the act of clinical decision, "the moment of clinical truth."[2] We proposed that "clinical ethics...must be taught at the bedside, in the Oslerian tradition,"[1] and, along with other colleagues, we introduced analytic systems for approaching clinical-ethical problems.[3,4]

During the past decade, many health care settings have developed clinical ethics education, research, and patient care programs. Most medical schools offer preclinical courses in medical ethics, several have vigorous teaching programs during the clinical years, and a few have established postgraduate training programs.[5,6] Published reports of both analytic or clinical research in medical ethics are increasingly common.[7,8] Many hospitals now have ethics committees[9-12] or ethics consultants[12-16] who participate directly or indirectly in patient care.

Our purpose is to assess the field of clinical ethics after its first decade and to address some fundamental questions that have arisen. What is clinical ethics? How should it be taught? What kind of research is needed in clinical ethics? What is the appropriate role for ethics committees and ethics consultants? Who should perform the teaching, research, and "patient care" functions of clinical ethics? What are

the future prospects of clinical ethics? While this paper aims to provide an overview of the field, three subsequent papers in this series will examine in greater detail how clinical ethics contributes to medical education, research, and patient care.

Clinical Ethics and Clinical Decisions

Clinical ethics is grounded in the belief that medicine is an inherently moral enterprise.[17] Medicine's moral core is found in the fact of illness and the act of profession: Sick persons ask physicians to help them get better and physicians profess to be morally committed and technically competent to help the sick.[18] This moral structure is revealed in the process of physician-patient accommodation, wherein a joint decision is reached that this patient will place his or her care in the hands of a particular physician and the physician affirms his or her ability to care for this patient.[19,20] The initial moral transaction between patient and physician creates mutual responsibilities and establishes both the goals of the clinical encounter and the process through which patient-physician decision making can occur.

The central focus of clinical ethics is individual patient-physician decision making. By contrast, biomedical ethics is a broader discipline that involves the application of ethical principles to the whole range of biomedical knowledge and extends ethical analysis from the clinical encounter to the legal and policy arenas.[21,22] The principal goal of clinical ethics is more circumscribed than that of biomedical ethics: It aims to improve the quality of patient care by identifying, analyzing, and contributing to the resolution of ethical problems that arise in the practice of clinical medicine. Clinical ethics seeks a right and good healing decision and action for a particular patient. In this respect, clinical ethics is intrinsic to the work of the physician and to the practice of medicine.

Clinical ethics is an urgent and concrete exercise enmeshed in factual uncertainty. It is often conducted in an emotionally charged atmosphere or in an emergency situation. It requires a firm grasp of clinical language and clinical knowledge. It must conclude in an action for an identifiable patient. It confronts value conflicts among physicians, patients, families, the law, social mores, and religious convictions--conflicts that must, in some way, be resolved so that a clinical decision may be made. Of course, postponing a clinical decision is itself a decision.

Clinical ethics relates as well to the standard of care.[16,23] In previous times, when a paternalistic form of medicine was condoned, the standard of care referred primarily to technical decisions that competent physicians would make for their patients. Increasingly, the standard of care has come to represent decisions reached by competent adult patients after their physicians have provided them with recommendations based on technical considerations. Thus, although ethical considerations have operated in both eras, the emphasis has shifted. In former times, the highest ethical value in medicine was physician competence and beneficence. Now this concern is coupled with a respect for patient values and self-determination.[24]

Teaching Clinical Ethics

In 1902, Sir William Osler eloquently captured the need for clinical emphasis in medical education:

In what may be called the natural method of teaching, the student begins with the patient, continues with the patient, and ends his study with the patient, using books and lectures as tools, as means to an end.... For the junior student in medicine and surgery it is a safe rule to have no teaching without a patient for a text, and the best teaching is that taught by the patient himself.[25]

Over the past decade, the teaching focus in medical ethics has moved gradually from the classroom to the bedside. Almost every US medical school has incorporated medical ethics into its undergraduate curriculum, and these courses increasingly have focused on clinical problems.[5,6] A survey of physicians' perceptions of the usefulness of medical ethics teaching concluded that "...the most effective teaching was concentrated on specific cases and was taught in the clinical years by...[physician] role models."[26] An influential consensus statement proposed that ethics teaching "should provide practicing physicians with conceptual moral-reasoning, and interactional abilities to deal successfully with most of the moral issues they confront in their daily practice."[27]

Clinical ethicists have also begun to teach medical ethics to interns and residents. In a 1983 position paper, the American Board of Internal Medicine noted that "a major responsibility of those training residents in internal medicine is to stress the importance of the humanistic qualities in the patient-physician relationship throughout the residency. The certification process must assure that this responsibility has been undertaken."[28] A response to the American Board of Internal Medicine report echoed the view that ethics "must be taught in a clinical setting, not as an academic discipline composed of theoretical concepts, but as a practical guide to action."[29] A recent survey of medical residents in six training programs indicated that almost all would like more ethics training on specific topics provided through standard clinical teaching methods.[30]

A few centers now offer specialized fellowship training in clinical ethics to prepare academic physicians.[31] Examples include the Kennedy Institute at Georgetown University, the Center for Clinical Medical Ethics at the University of Chicago, the Program in Ethics and the Professions at Harvard University, the Center for Medical Ethics at the University of Pittsburgh, and the Institute for the Study of Applied and Professional Ethics at Dartmouth.

What is the appropriate role for physicians and professional ethicists in teaching clinical ethics? The ethically sensitive physician is a superb role model. He or she can demonstrate that although the ethical and technical aspects of clinical decisions may be dissected free for pedagogic and heuristic purposes, they are ultimately inseparable in practice. It is a common observation that medical students respond better to demonstration than to rhetoric. It is essential that they see clinicians who are clinically competent and also able to engage in ethical analysis. In this way, students will learn that almost all decisions involve moral choice and that most need not be referred for ethics consultation. The physician-ethicist is well equipped to demonstrate the conscientious exercise of moral responsibility in the clinical setting. The same would be true of the nurse, the dentist, and the social worker in their own settings.

What might be the teaching role for the professional ethicist? He or she would remain the resource to convey in the preclinical years, or before medical school, the fundamental principles and theories of philosophic ethics. Professional ethicists also serve as a vital resource to introduce medical students to the broader dimensions of medical ethics in public policy and law. Finally, in undergraduate medical school courses and hospital rounds, team teaching between physicians and professional ethicists should be encouraged.

Research in Clinical Ethics

Clinical medical ethics research may be divided into two broad categories that we will call analytical and empirical. Analytical research uses the methods of logical reasoning and argument to examine the principles of philosophic and theologic ethics, law, and public policy. Analytical research aims to identify conceptual issues, structure coherent arguments, arrive at defensible recommendations for ethically acceptable practice, and justify such recommendations by appeal to normative standards. Such research may involve 1) an analysis of cases (e.g., the case of an incompetent woman who refused a brain biopsy while competent[23]); 2) an examination of conceptual and/or legal and public policy issues such as the termination of medical care,[32] active euthanasia,[33] or the concept of futility[34]; 3) an exploration of the ethical ramifications of major medical or surgical innovations (e.g., reduced-size liver transplantation[35] or liver transplantation using living donors[36]); or 4) an examination of the role of clinical

THE JOURNAL OF CLINICAL ETHICS   7

ethics itself in teaching, research, and patient care.[21]

Empirical research in clinical medical ethics involves the collection and analysis of clinical data to describe the way clinical decisions are in fact made by patients, by physicians, and within the patient-physician dyadic relationship. Empirical research examines the values that are used in clinical decision making, how they are used, by whom, and under what conditions. This type of research uses the methods of the social sciences, decision analysis, clinical epidemiology, and health services research. Examples of empirical research in medical ethics include 1) a survey of the preferences of acquired immunodeficiency syndrome patients for life-sustaining treatment[37] (social sciences), 2) an assessment of patient preferences for quality versus quantity of life in the treatment of laryngeal cancer[38] (decision analysis), 3) an examination of the prevalence of withdrawal from dialysis[39] (clinical epidemiology), and 4) evaluations of ethics consultation services[14,15] (health services research). Although empirical studies will not resolve the normative ethical question of what action is right or wrong in a particular circumstance, they can help to identify key issues, frame research questions, structure ethical analyses, and contribute to a better understanding of the normative issues that lie at the heart of clinical medical ethics.

Ideally, analytical and empirical research in ethics should be synergistic and proceed in the following way: Analyses of philosophic principles, legal requirements, and policy guidelines lead to the generation of hypotheses about ethical aspects of clinical practice. These hypotheses are tested in an empiric research project. Data are collected and analyzed, and conclusions are drawn that support, refute, or result in the modification of the original hypothesis. The empirical conclusions serve as the basis for further analysis of philosophic, legal, and policy issues affecting clinical practice. Empirical studies that point out a discrepancy between theory and practice can suggest interventions to improve clinical decision making or, on occasion, they may encourage us to rethink or refine our theories. Finally, new hypotheses are generated and the cycle begins again.

Because research in clinical ethics examines issues at the intersection of ethics, medicine, law, and public policy, interdisciplinary research is desirable and even mandatory. Health care professionals can provide practical insight into the ethical issues associated with patient care. Philosophers, theologians, lawyers, and policy experts can provide the intellectual rigor and analytic perspective of their respective disciplines. Social scientists and clinical investigators trained in decision analysis, clinical epidemiology, and health services research can provide methodologic expertise for the design of empirical research.

Clinical ethics research expands the range of issues that are addressed in traditional biomedical research by identifying and examining the ethical considerations related to the process and outcome of medical care. As in the biomedical sciences, the ultimate academic credibility of clinical ethics will depend upon its ability to develop a solid research base. More importantly, however, research in the field will further the goal of clinical ethics--to promote high-quality patient care.

Ethics Committees and Consultants

In addition to teaching and research, the clinical ethicist has service responsibilities. These are fulfilled as a consultant or member of an ethics committee.[9-16] Ethics consultations and committees can serve four functions: to educate the staff, to set institutional policy, to provide a nonjudicial mechanism for the review and resolution of cases involving conflicts, and to directly influence patient care decisions. Committees and consultants improve clinical-ethical decision making by educating the hospital staff and by developing rational and sensitive institutional policy on ethical matters, such as brain death, do not resuscitate orders, living wills, and organ transplantation. It is hoped that institutional ethics committees can assist in conflict resolution and thus spare the various parties the time, expense, and anguish of litigation and judicial intervention. A critical question still facing ethics committees and consultants, however, is whether they improve the process and outcome of clinical-ethical decision making when they become directly involved in individual patient care decisions.[16]

In theory, the difference between ethics committees and ethics consultants is analogous to the difference between a court of appeals and a lower court. Traditional ethics committees resemble the appeals court, where all the evidence has been collected, no further evidence can be entered into the record, and the decision must be based on a careful review and analysis of the established record. By contrast, ethics consultations resemble the lower court, where the record is being established and where all of the relevant evidence is entered by the parties involved in the case. Ethics consultants will evaluate a patient on request and collect much of the primary data upon which the clinical-ethical decision will be based. In practice, there are many mixed examples: an ethics committee may appoint a subcommittee of consultants or an ethics consultation service may review its conclusions with an institutional ethics committee.

Who should staff ethics committees or consultation services? The consultant clinical ethicist must be able to "do" ethics under fire in ambiguous situations. This requires not only a broad knowledge of ethics but also objectivity, compassion, and a capacity to counsel and psychologically support the participants without imposing one's own moral values upon them. The clinical ethics consultant must be available and accessible to colleagues when crucial decisions are made. He or she must be familiar with not only ethical theories and principles but also relevant policy statements, legal cases, and published research. The consultant must be knowledgeable in the clinical details of the situation and must be ready to apply clinical judgment and discernment to the case at hand.

A physician who is competent as a clinician and has been trained in medical ethics is particularly effective as a consultant. Such persons enjoy the advantages of a firm grasp of the factual tripod upon which ethical decisions must rest: diagnosis, prognosis, and therapy. They also have experience in making clinical decisions that are urgent, complex, emotionally charged, and filled with uncertainty; in addition, they are accustomed to counseling patients.

The properly trained and clinically acculturated professional ethicist should be able to meet many of these same requirements. This would, of course, mean that the professional ethicist must assimilate many elements of a medical education in order to approach the synthesis of technical and moral capability. The best professional ethicists today have done just this.

The number of ethics committees and consultants in hospitals has increased rapidly in recent years. At present, ethics committees and consultants represent promising but incompletely evaluated mechanisms of health care delivery. The degree to which committee or consultant involvement improves the process and outcome of clinical-ethical decision making is still not clear. Clinical ethicists should evaluate the impact of their ethics committees and consultation services and report their findings in the medical literature.

The Future of Clinical Medical Ethics

In this review of the first decade of clinical ethics, we have affirmed that the goal of clinical ethics is to improve the quality of patient care and that the focus of the discipline is on the process and outcome of patient-physician decision making. In particular, clinical ethics emphasizes the mutual responsibilities of physicians and patients and the view that patient attitudes, preferences, values, and aspirations are a central consideration in the decision-making process. Ethics courses in medical school, research studies in ethics, and ethics committees and consultants are means to achieve the goal of high-quality patient care. Ultimately, every physician and other health professional should feel comfortable with his or her ability to assist patients and families reaching

competent and humane clinical-ethical decisions.

Physician-ethicists and professional ethicists will continue to work side by side in the future. One is not likely to replace the other, nor is this desirable, because each brings a different perspective and different capabilities to the situation. Physician-ethicists and professional ethicists must understand each others' potential contributions. Rather than competing, they must complement and supplement each other to promote the high quality of ethical decision making now required and desired by patients.

So far as manpower and womanpower needs are concerned, the field of clinical ethics will need a variety of trained personnel. First, all physicians will have to be better educated in making the day to day clinical-ethical decisions that are an intrinsic part of every specialty of medicine. Second, to assist them with complicated cases, physicians should have available a cadre of consultants. For the foreseeable future, these consultants will be a mix of physicians trained in clinical ethics and professional medical ethicists. Third, clinical investigators and professional ethicists will be needed to pursue analytical and empirical research that will serve as the academic foundation of clinical medical ethics.

When we review the field of clinical ethics a decade from now, we hope that the focus will have shifted from ethics courses, committees, and consultants to an understanding on the part of most physicians and medical students that ethics is an inherent and inseparable part of good clinical medicine. We hope that clinical ethics will have achieved its rightful place at the interstices of relations between patients who are sick and request help and physicians who profess to be able to heal or comfort them.

NOTES

1   M. Siegler, "A Legacy of Osler: Teaching Clinical Ethics at the Bedside," *Journal of the American Medical Association* 239 (1978): 951-956.

2   E.D. Pellegrino, "Ethics and the Moment of Clinical Truth," *Journal of the American Medical Association* 239 (1978): 960-961.

3   M. Siegler, "Decision Making Strategy for Clinical-Ethical Problems in Medicine," *Archives of Internal Medicine* 142 (1982): 2178-2179.

4   A.R. Jonsen, M. Siegler, and W.J. Winslade, *Clinical Ethics: A Practical Approach to Ethical Decisions in Clinical Medicine*, New York, Macmillan, 1981.

5   E.D. Pellegrino and T.K. McElhinney, *Teaching Ethics, the Humanities and Human Values in Medical Schools: A 10 Year Overview*, Washington, DC, Institute on Human Values in Medicine, Society for Health and Human Values, 1981.

6   J. Bickel, *Integrating Human Values Teaching Programs into Medical Student's Clinical Education*, Washington, DC, Association of American Medical Colleges, 1986.

7   M. Siegler, "Recommended Reading, American College of Physicians Ethics Manual," *Annals of Internal Medicine* 101 (1984): 129-137, 263-274.

8   M. Siegler, P.A. Singer, and D.L. Schiedermayer, *Medical Ethics: An Annotated Bibliography*, Philadelphia, American College of Physicians, 1988.

9   B. Lo, "Behind Closed Doors: Promises and Pitfalls of Ethics Committees," *New England Journal of Medicine* 317 (1987): 46-50.

10   N. Fost and R.E. Cranford, "Hospital Ethics Committees: Administrative Aspects," *Journal of the American Medical Association* 253 (1985): 2687-2692.

11   F. Rosner, "Hospital Medical Ethics Committees: A Review of Their Development," *Journal of the American Medical Association* 253 (1985): 2693-2697.

12   J. La Puma and S.E. Toulmin, "Ethics Consultants and Ethics Committees," *Archives of Internal Medicine* 149 (1989): 1109-1112.

13   R.B. Purtillo, "Ethics Consultations in the Hospital," *New England Journal of Medicine* 311 (1984): 983-986.

14   J. La Puma, C.B. Stocking, M.D. Silverstein, et al., "Evaluation and Utilization of an Ethics Consultation Service in a Teaching Hospital," *Journal of the American Medical Association* 260 (1988): 808-811.

15   H.S. Perkins and B.S. Saathoff, "The Impact of Medical Ethics Consultation on Physicians: An Exploratory Study," *American Journal of Medicine* 85 (1988): 761-765.

16   M. Siegler and P.A. Singer, "Clinical Ethics Consultation: Godsend or God Squad?" *American Journal of Medicine* 85 (1988): 759-760.

17   L.R. Kass, *Toward a More Natural Science: Biology and Human Affairs*, New York, Free Press, 1985.

18   E.D. Pellegrino, "Toward a Reconstruction of Medical Morality: The Primacy of the Act of Profession and the Fact of Illness," *Journal of Medicine and Philosophy* 4 (1979): 32-56.

19   M. Siegler, "Searching for Moral Certainty in Medicine: A Proposal for a New Model of the Doctor-Patient Encounter," *Bulletin of the New York Academy of Medicine* 57 (1981): 56-69.

20   M. Siegler, "The Physician-Patient Accommodation: A Central Event in Clinical Medicine," *Archives of Internal Medicine* 142 (1982): 1899-1902.

21   E.D. Pellegrino, "Clinical Ethics: Biomedical Ethics at the Bedside," *Journal of the American Medical Association* 260 (1988): 837-839.

22   M. Siegler, "Clinical Ethics and Clinical Medicine," *Archives of Internal Medicine* 139 (1979): 914-915.

23   J. La Puma, D. Schiedermayer, S. Toulmin, *et al.*, "The Standard of Care: A Case Report and Ethical Analysis," *Annals of Internal Medicine* 108 (1988): 121-124.

24   E.D. Pellegrino and D. Thomasma, *For the Patient's Good: The Restoration of Beneficence in Health Care*, New York, Oxford University Press, 1988.

25   W. Osler, "On the Need of a Radical Reform in Our Methods of Teaching Medical Students," *Medical News* 82 (1903): 49-53.

26   E.D. Pellegrino, R.J. Hart, S.R. Henderson, *et al.*, "Relevance and Utility of Courses in Medical Ethics: A Survey of Physician's Perceptions," *Journal of the American Medical Association* 253 (1985): 49-53.

27   C.M. Culver, K.D. Clouser, B. Gert, *et al.*, "Basic Curricular Goals in Medical Ethics," *New England Journal of Medicine* 312 (1985): 253-256.

28   Subcommittee on the Evaluation of Humanistic Qualities in the Internist, American Board of Internal Medicine, "Evaluation of Humanistic Qualities in the Internist," *Annals of Internal Medicine* 99 (1983): 720-724.

29   R.M. Arnold, G.J. Povar, and J.D. Howell, "The Humanities, Humanistic Behavior, and the Humane Physician: A Cautionary Note," *Annals of Internal Medicine* 106 (1987): 313-318.

30   J.A. Jacobson, S.W. Tolle, C. Stocking, and M. Siegler, "Internal Medicine Residents' Preferences Regarding Medical Ethics Education," *Academic Medicine* 64 (1989): 760-764.

31   L.W. Lane, M. Siegler, S.H. Miles, *et al.*, "Fellowship Training Programs in Clinical Ethics, *SGIM Newsletter* 11 (1988): 4-5.

32   E.J. Emmanuel, "A Review of the Ethical and Legal Aspects of Terminating Medical Care," *American Journal of Medicine* 84 (1988): 291-301.

33   L.R. Kass, "Neither for Love Nor Money: Why Doctors Must Not Kill," *Public Interest* 14 (Winter 1989): 25-46.

34   J.D. Lantos, P.A. Singer, R.M. Walker, *et al.*, "The Illusion of Futility in Clinical Practice," *American Journal of Medicine* 87 (1989): 81-84.

35   P.A. Singer, J.D. Lantos, P.F. Whitington, *et al.*, "Equipoise and the Ethics of Segmental Liver Transplantation," *Clinical Research* 36 (1988): 539-545.

36   P.A. Singer, M. Siegler, P.F. Whitington, *et al.*, "Ethics of Liver Transplantation with Living Donors," *New England Journal of Medicine* 321 (1989): 620-622.

37   R. Steinbrook, B. Lo, J. Moulton, *et al.*, "Preferences of Homosexual Men with AIDS for Life-Sustaining Treatment," *New England Journal of Medicine* 314 (1986): 457-460.

38   B.J. McNeil, R. Weichselbaum, and S.G. Pauker, "Speech and Survival: Tradeoffs Between Quality and Quantity of Life in Laryngeal Cancer," *New England Journal of Medicine* 305 (1981): 982-987.

39   S. Neu and C.M. Kjellstrand, "Stopping Long-Term Dialysis: An Empirical Study of Withdrawal of Life-Supporting Treatment," *New England Journal of Medicine* 314 (1986): 14-20.

7.5 Singer PA, Pellegrino ED, Siegler M (1990) Ethics Committees and Consultants. J Clin Ethics 1:263–7

VOLUME 1, NUMBER 4   THE JOURNAL OF CLINICAL ETHICS   263

FEATURES

Ethics Committees and Consultants
Peter A. Singer, Edmund D. Pellegrino, and Mark Siegler

Introduction

This article is the fourth in a series on clinical ethics. The first article provided an overview of the field, the second discussed research in clinical ethics, and the third examined teaching approaches. This article focuses on ethics committees and ethics consultation services.

Ethics committees are not new.[1] The first ethics committee was formed in 1971.[2] In 1976, the Quinlan decision by the New Jersey Supreme Court encouraged health-care institutions to develop ethics committees. During the 1980s, bioethical issues increased in frequency and complexity, and in response, many health-care facilities formed ethics committees.

By contrast, formal ethics consultation services in hospitals are more recent arrivals. As early as 1982, commentators noted that psychiatric consultation often masked ethical dilemmas.[3] In 1984, one author described the operation of an ethics consultation service,[4] and in 1985, a meeting was convened at the Clinical Center of the National Institutes of Health (NIH) to hear reports about ethics consultation activity from individuals who were serving as ethics consultants.[5] However, the first clinical description of the process

Peter A. Singer, MD, MPH, FRCPC, FACP, is Assistant Professor of Medicine and Associate Director of the Centre for Bioethics at the University of Toronto.
Edmund D. Pellegrino, MD, is Director of the Center for the Advanced Study of Ethics and John Carroll Professor of Medicine and Medical Humanities at Georgetown University, Washington, DC.
Mark Siegler, MD, is Professor of Medicine and Director of the Center for Clinical Medical Ethics at the University of Chicago.

and outcome of a formal ethics consultation service was not published until 1987.[6] The precise relationship between ethics consultation services and committees still remains unclear.[7]

This article focuses on a few specific questions related to the operation of ethics committees and consultation services. What are the functions of ethics committees and consultation services? What are the dangers of ethics committees and consultations? What models exist for ethics consultation? How are committees and consultation services to be evaluated? What is the likely future of ethics committees and consultation services?

Functions of Ethics Committees and Consultants

Ethics committees and consultants represent two different approaches for achieving the essential goal of clinical medical ethics, improving patient care and patient outcomes. Both ethics committees and consultants contribute to this goal in the following three ways: by coordinating ethics education programs, by assisting in the development of institutional ethics policies, and by consulting on difficult individual cases.

Educational Programs

Ethics committees and consultation services often begin their work with efforts at self-education. This process, which may require one or two years, is highly advisable since most members of a newly-formed ethics committee have an interest, but not necessarily a significant level of expertise, in clinical ethics. The process of self-education is essential if the committee is to function

competently and establish its credibility in the institution it serves.

The second educational approach of the committee is to coordinate educational programs for all segments of the staff of a health-care facility. This includes such activities as lectures, ethics rounds, seminars, journal clubs, and "brown bag" lunches. These sessions concentrate on issues or problems of immediate clinical concern. Educational programs should be oriented not just to doctors and nurses, but also to social workers, hospital chaplains, hospital attorneys, occupational therapists, pharmacists, and health administrators. Such sessions are usually well-attended, if they are targeted to the needs and interests of the staff and are case-based. These sessions provide a valuable forum for discussion of major clinical-ethical issues or problems encountered in the day-to-day care of patients. When sessions such as these are carefully designed and competently conducted over a period of time, they can encompass most of the issues of importance in clinical bioethics.

Developing Institutional Policy

The second major function of ethics committees and consultants is to assist in the development of institutional policies related to clinical ethics. For example, many committees begin by helping to formulate the facility's brain-death policy. The policy on do-not-resuscitate orders often is the next focus of attention. Then, the committee may turn its attention to policies about the use of other life-sustaining treatments and advance directives.[8] After end-of-life concerns have been addressed, committees may turn their efforts to

264   THE JOURNAL OF CLINICAL ETHICS   WINTER 1990

such difficult ethics policy matters as informed consent, rationing, abortion, admission and discharge criteria for intensive care units, and the institution's admission policies for uninsured patients.

Policy development is an extremely important task for committees and consultants. Health-care facility policy operates at the "meso" level, filling a decision-making void between the "macro" decisions of governments and third-party payers and the "micro" decisions of individual physicians and patients. These "meso" decisions are important in a number of ways. First, by projecting a particular moral view of health care, institutional policies help to define the mission of the health-care facility.[9] Second, they help to promote the fair treatment of patients by making explicit the criteria that govern specific clinical decisions like admission to the intensive care unit, rationing of scarce resources, and the use of advance directives. Third, they foster institutional discussion about clinical situations in which appropriate management is uncertain or unclear--for example, the management of a demented, critically ill patient whose wishes regarding life-sustaining treatment are unknown and who is transferred from a nursing home to the emergency room. Institutional policies can be helpful guidelines when complex, urgent, emotionally laden clinical-ethical decisions must be made. They are preferable to ad hoc, case-by-case decisions that may be idiosyncratic and thus may not always satisfy standards of ethical propriety.

Case Consultation

The third major function of ethics committees is case consultation. Most ethics committees soon confront a pivotal operating question: should they provide consultations in the care of individual patients? Each committee must grapple with this question within the context of its own institution. In making the decision, a series of questions must be taken into account: What are the goals of an ethics case consulta-

tion? Who should be the ethics consultant, and what does he or she do? What is the nature of ethics recommendations? What are the advantages of providing consultation services? What are the potential dangers? What model of consultation should be offered?

What Are the Goals of an Ethics Consultation?

In our view, the central goal of an ethics consultation is identical to the goals of all medical and surgical consultations: to improve patient outcomes. In contrast to technical questions of what can be done for a patient (for example, *can* the patient benefit from this medication or operation?), ethical problems often raise the question of what *should* be done and often focus on the process of shared decision making that occurs between patients, health professionals, and families. Increasingly in recent years, ethics consultations also have become an important mechanism for resolving "ethical" conflicts and disagreements within the health-care institution rather than through recourse to the courts. The central goal then of ethics consultations is to assist the primary physician, the patient, and the family to reach a right and good clinical decision.[10]

Who Should Be an Ethics Consultant?

In particular, should the consultant be a physician? Although much debate has focused on this question, we believe it is misplaced. The issue is not physician versus nonphysician, but rather the essential qualifications and qualities of the individual who will perform ethics consultations. The ethics consultant will review the patient's chart; interview the patient; possibly interview family members and health-care professionals associated with the case; analyze the case from the perspective of ethics, law, and institutional policy; and make recommendations for management. These tasks require not only the skills of ethical analysis, but also a clinical orientation and sensitivity, a working knowledge of medical diagnostics, prognostics, and therapeutics,

experience in the hospital setting, good interpersonal and communication skills, and a knowledge of the relevant ethical, legal, and clinical literature. Thus, the successful ethics consultant necessarily must de facto be ethically and clinically competent, but not necessarily a physician.

What Should the Nature of the Ethics Consultant's Recommendations Be?

Ordinarily, when physicians request a consultation from colleagues, they expect recommendations. The recommendations of the ethics consultant should carry the same force as the recommendations of any other hospital or outpatient consultation. A consultant's recommendations are suggestions that the referring physician, the family, or the patient may choose to accept or reject. Well-reasoned recommendations that are supported by references to the literature, specific to the patient's actual situation, and communicated with clarity and brevity, are extremely helpful to all the participants in a clinical decision.[11] The primary clinical, moral, and legal responsibility for the care of the patient, however, remains, as always, with the attending physician.[12] Indeed, it is a serious breach of trust for the physician to follow any consultant's opinion unless convinced it is in the patient's best interest.

What Are the Advantages of Using Ethics Consultants?

There are several distinct advantages to the use of individual ethics consultants to supplement ethics committees. First, individual consultants can respond more readily in urgent clinical situations. It may take an inordinate amount of time to assemble committee members who may be otherwise engaged, traveling, or teaching. Second, it is easier for an individual consultant to review the clinical details, the points in question and disagreement among decision makers, the sources of conflict, and to see the patient about whom the decision is being made--an essential feature too often neglected by committees. Third, those who act and are accepted as consultants can be expected to possess more expertise in ethics than committee members who have an interest but do not concentrate their efforts in this field. Fourth, the ethics consultation, like any specialty consultation, should be used to educate residents and fellows in clinical ethics. Finally, a formal ethics consultation service provides the organized data collection essential to empirical research in clinical practice [13]

Dangers of Ethics Committees and Consultants

While there are clear advantages to consultations by ethics committees and consultants, there are some dangers in both. Some of these dangers are peculiar to the committee mechanism and some to the individual consultant.

Common to both processes is the temptation, already alluded to, to abrogate moral decision making and simply follow the recommendation of consultants. Given the complexity of moral decisions, the tendency to confuse legal and moral issues, the fear of legal suit, and the reality of the consultant's expertise, this is an understandable but inexcusable temptation. Physicians cannot divest themselves of their moral complicity in what happens to their patients. Theirs is the hand that writes the order.[14] They are under compulsion to weigh the consultant's advice in the light of their own covenant with the one who is ill. Neither consultants nor ethics committees can absolve physicians, nurses, or families of moral culpability, for a wrong decision.

Both individual consultants and ethics committees may, with good intention, easily overstep the fine line between clarifying the decision, raising the necessary questions, recommending courses of action, and taking over the decision-making process. If the latter occurs, one of the major benefits of any kind of consultation is lost, namely, the advantage of a more-or-less objective evaluation by persons not directly involved in the conflict or dilemma. Ideally, the ethics consultant should point out al-

ternatives, define the values involved, and negotiate conflict without apodictically deciding the issue. All of this requires not only a firm grasp of the principles and techniques of clinical ethics, but also an uncommon measure of sensitivity, counseling skill, and respect for the moral agency of those one presumes to advise.

The dangers peculiar to committees are those inherent in collective decision making. They include various combinations and possibilities, such as dominance of group dynamics by vocal or aggressive members; insufficient cultural, religious, or ethnic heterogeneity; excessive loyalty to the institution or to particularly influential or respected staff members; overemphasis on protecting against legal action; and uncritical deference to legal or ethical expertise of other committee members. Particularly disturbing, though often very subtly expressed, is the diffusion of responsibility among committee members so that the "buck" stops nowhere, but goes endlessly in a circle. Christine Cassel has emphasized this point:

> The coming together of many different perspectives and areas of expertise may provide the crucible in which the best ... decisions are made. But a committee can also provide the setting in which immoral decisions can be made for which no one has ultimate responsibility. This is most likely to occur in a setting where most persons on the committee are relatively removed from the clinical setting, where conflict of interest with administrative needs exists, and where the group dynamic is bureaucratized.[15]

Indeed, the functioning of ethics committees provides a useful model to improve our understanding of the ethics of group decision making.[16]

With individual consultants, responsibility for ethical recommendations and the decision-making process can be

localized, but this does not eliminate the dangers. Indeed, many of the dangers are similar to those noted for committees. Individual consultants may, with good intentions, intrude too far into the ethical and the clinical management of the case, especially if they are physicians. Like groups, they may subtly or overtly impose their own values onto the clinical situation. If there are repeated discussions, family and

---

Particularly disturbing is the diffusion of responsibility among committee members so that the "buck" stops nowhere, but goes endlessly in a circle.

---

friends of the patient, as well as the attending physician, may turn to the ethics consultant for a variety of evaluations. Fear of being sued, conflicts of interest pitting the patient's welfare against the hospital's, and the very fact of identifiability may make the individual consultant overly cautious.

Their dangers notwithstanding, ethics committees and ethics consultations are important mechanisms in patient care today. Like every powerful tool, they must be used with judgment, discrimination, and with clearly defined purposes. They will become even more important in the years ahead as technological progress, moral pluralism, and legal interventions further complicate the task of clinical ethical decision making. We believe ethics committees and individual consultants complement and supplement one another. They are part of a continuous spectrum of services now available to support good patient care.

Models for Ethics Case Consultation

There are four models of clinical ethical consultation in use at this time—each with its own advantages and disadvantages.

1) Pure Committee Model: In this model, the request for consultation is made to the committee as a whole. The

266   THE JOURNAL OF CLINICAL ETHICS   WINTER 1990

person originating the request (for example, a family or a physician) presents the case to the committee. The committee then discusses the case and makes its recommendations. This model is used in many hospitals as ethics committees begin to become involved in consultation.

2) Committee Member as Consultant: In this model, the request for consultation is made to the ethics committee. The committee chooses one of its members to review the patient's case. The consultant committee member then reports his or her findings to the entire committee. The committee discusses the case and makes recommendations. This is the model used at the Massachusetts General Hospital.[17]

3) Post-Facto Committee Review: In this model, the request for consultation is made directly to the individual ethics consultant. The consultant then reviews the case and makes recommendations. The case and recommendations are later reviewed by a committee. This model is used, for example, at the University of Chicago and the University of Texas at San Antonio.[18]

4) Pure Consultation Model: In this model, the request for consultation is made directly to the consultant. The consultant reviews the case and makes recommendations. The recommendations are not reviewed by a committee. This model is used, for example, at the Lutheran General Hospital in Chicago.[19]

There is, at present, insufficient evidence to establish a clear superiority for any of the models. The Pure Committee Model has the advantage of institutional consensus and support for the recommendations. The Pure Consultant Model has the advantage of a quicker response time and greater efficiency. The models that combine consultant and committee deliberation allow for access to wider discussion. Obviously, each requires individuals with extensive clinical ethics experience and expertise. The model (or models) an institution chooses will depend upon its resources, staff, and administrative preferences and the type of problems it most frequently encounters.

Evaluation of Ethics Committees and Consultants

Ethics committees and consultation services have received limited evaluation. La Puma and colleagues interviewed referring physicians of fifty-one ethics consultations at the University of Chicago.[20] In 71 percent of consultations, the referring physician stated that the consultation was very important in patient management, clarifying ethical issues, or learning about medical ethics. In 91 percent of consultations, referring physicians said they planned to request an ethics consultation in the future. Perkins and Saathoff interviewed referring physicians and reviewed medical charts of forty-four ethics consultations at the University of Texas at San Antonio.[21] According to the referring physicians, 32 percent of consultations identified ethical issues that requesters had not recognized, 89 percent clarified thinking, 41 percent changed patient management considerably, 93 percent increased requesters' confidence in final management plans, and 98 percent taught physicians. According to the chart review, 68 percent of consultations identified unrecognized issues and 66 percent changed management significantly. The most frequently overlooked issue was inappropriate family decisions for incompetent patients, and the most frequent management changes involved withholding cardiopulmonary resuscitation.

Ethics consultations, performed by committees or consultants, are difficult to evaluate because the outcomes of interest have not been sufficiently clarified. The work cited above has begun to address this deficiency. What outcome is desired? How is it to be measured? Do referring physicians learn about medical ethics through consultation? Do consultants identify unrecognized ethical issues or simply clarify issues that have been recognized? Do referring physicians perceive ethics consultations as important, helpful, or useful? Would physicians request consultation in the future? Do ethics consultations increase the confidence of referring physicians in their final management plans? Do ethics consultations change patient management, and, if so, how? Only when these questions have been addressed can the utility, effectiveness,

> ## At this time we believe it is premature to develop standards for training and certifying ethics consultants.

and optimal models of ethics consultation be fully evaluated. In 1988, two of us (Siegler and Singer) wrote:

> Ethics consultation is a promising but incompletely evaluated mechanism of health care delivery. We urge clinical ethicists to prospectively evaluate the impact of their ethics consultation services and report their findings in the medical literature.[22]

As we stated earlier in this paper, we believe the central goal of ethics case consultations is to improve patient care and patient outcomes. Patient outcomes should be measured not only in terms of mortality and morbidity, but also in terms of patient's functional status, patient satisfaction, and the cost of care. Unfortunately, since outcome data of this sort are not available for most clinical interventions (including medical and surgical consultations), we are often forced to rely on alternative and less desirable standards, such as clinical process. But again, with only a few notable exceptions,[23] the process of medical and surgical consultation has generally not been studied in detail. It therefore is not surprising that adequate outcome and process data are still unavailable for a clinical intervention as new as ethics consultations.

Thus far, we have considered the evaluation of only one of the three goals of ethics committees and consultation services--consultation in the cases of individual patients. Although arguably easier to evaluate, the other two goals of committees and consultants--education and policy development--have not been evaluated.

Future of Ethics Committees and Consultation Services

The growth and development of ethics committees and consultation services reflect the increasing attention and serious consideration given to ethical issues in health-care institutions. This larger concern promises to intensify as the medical education of the public, the use of advance directives, and the moral heterogeneity of our population expand. We believe that ethics committees and consultation services will continue to proliferate in North American health-care institutions. We hope that this proliferation will be careful and deliberate and will be studied critically by ongoing evaluative efforts.

The question has been raised whether ethics consultants (or for that matter, chairs of ethics committees) should be certified.[24] Although this issue will have to be addressed in the future, at this time we believe it is premature to develop standards for training and certifying ethics consultants. The primary reason for delay is to develop both clearer goals for ethics committees and consultants and better studies of existing committees and consultants that evaluate the efficacy of such groups in improving patient care.

The key question for ethics committees and consultation services is not whether they will exist in the future, but which functions will they perform and how will they perform them? We foresee a continuing need for education and policy development. With regard to case consultation, we are ambivalent. Ideally, we wish that ethics consultations (by committee or individual consultant) would teach clinicians how to make better ethical decisions with patients and families. As they succeed in this, the need for such ethics consultation would decrease substantially. However, given the turnover in personnel within health-care institutions and the reluctance of many physicians to learn the necessary techniques, we believe ethics consultations and ethics committees will be needed for a long time to come.

Acknowledgments

Peter A. Singer is supported by a medical scholarship from the Canadian Life and Health Insurance Association; the Centre for Bioethics is supported by a Health Systems-Linked Research Unit grant from the Ontario Ministry of Health. The Center for Clinical Medical Ethics is supported by the Henry J. Kaiser Family Foundation, the Andrew W. Mellon Foundation, and the Pew Charitable Trusts. The views expressed herein are those of the authors and may not represent those of the supporting institutions.

NOTES

1   B. Lo, "Behind Closed Doors: Promises and Pitfalls of Ethics Committees," *New England Journal of Medicine* 317 (1987): 46-50.

2   F. Rosner, "Hospital Medical Ethics Committees: A Review of Their Development," *Journal of the American Medical Association* 253 (1985): 2693-97.

3   M. Pearl and E.E. Shelps, "Psychiatric Consultation Masking Moral Dilemmas in Medicine," *New England Journal of Medicine* 307 (1982): 618-21.

4   R.B. Purtilo, "Ethics Consultation in the Hospital," *New England Journal of Medicine* 311 (1984): 983-86.

5   J. Bermel, "Ethics Consultants: A Self-Portrait of Decision Makers," *Hastings Center Report* 15 (1985): 2.

6   J. LaPuma, "Consultations in Clinical Ethics -- Issues and Questions in 27 Cases," *Western Journal of Medicine* 146 (1987): 633-37.

7   J. La Puma and S.E. Toulmin, "Ethics Consultants and Ethics Committees," *Archives of Internal Medicine* 149 (1989): 1109-12.

8   P.A. Singer and M. Siegler, "Elective Use of Life-Sustaining Treatments in Internal Medicine," in *Advances in Internal Medicine*, vol. 36, ed. G.H. Stollerman (St. Louis: Mosby, 1991), 57-79.

9   S.H. Miles, P.A. Singer, and M. Siegler, "Conflicts Between Patients' Requests to Forego Treatment and the Policies of Health Care Facilities," *New England Journal of Medicine* 321 (1989): 48-50.

10 M. Siegler, E.D. Pellegrino, and P.A. Singer, "Clinical Medical Ethics: The First Decade," *Journal of Clinical Ethics* 1 (1990): 5-9.

11 L. Goldman, T. Lee, and P. Rudd, "Ten Commandments for Effective Consultations," *Archives of Internal Medicine* 143 (1983): 1753-55.

12 M. Siegler, "Medical Consultations in the Context of the Physician-Patient Relationship," in *Responsibility in Health Care*, ed. G.J. Agich (Boston and Dordrecht, Holland: D. Reidel, 1982), 141-62.

13 P.A. Singer, M. Siegler, and E.D. Pellegrino, "Research in Clinical Medical Ethics," *Journal of Clinical Ethics* 1 (1990): 95-99.

14 E.D. Pellegrino, "Trust and Distrust in Professional Ethics," in *Ethics, Trust, and the Professions: Philosophical and Cultural Perspectives*, ed. E.D. Pellegrino, R.M. Veatch, and J.P. Langan (Washington, DC: Georgetown University Press, 1991); and M. Siegler, "Ethics Committees: Decisions by Bureaucracy," *Hastings Center Report* 16 (June 1986): 22-24.

15 C. Cassel, "Deciding to Forego Life-Sustaining Treatment: Implications for Policy in 1984," *Cardozo Law Review* 6 (May 1985): 287-302.

16 See the issue of *Journal of Medicine and Philosophy* 7 (February 1982): 1, coedited by E.D. Pellegrino and L. Newton on collective decision making.

17 T.A. Brennan, "Ethics Committees and Decisions to Limit Care: The Experience at the Massachusetts General Hospital," *Journal of the American Medical Association* 260 (1988): 803-7.

18 J. LaPuma, C.B. Stocking, M.D. Silverstein, et al., "An Ethics Consultation Service in a Teaching Hospital: Utilization and Evaluation," *Journal of the American Medical Association* 260 (1988): 808-11; and H.S. Perkins and B.S. Saathoff, "Impact of Medical Ethics Consultations on Physicians: An Exploratory Study," *American Journal of Medicine* 85 (1988): 761-65.

19 J. La Puma and D.L. Schiedermayer, "Outpatient Clinical Ethics," *Journal of General Internal Medicine* 4 (1989): 413-20.

20 J. La Puma, C.B. Stocking, M.D. Silverstein, et al., "An Ethics Consultation Service in a Teaching Hospital."

21 H.S. Perkins and B.S. Saathoff, "Impact of Medical Ethics Consultations on Physicians."

22 M. Siegler and P.A. Singer, "Clinical Ethics Consultation: Godsend or 'God Squad?' " *American Journal of Medicine* 85 (1988): 759-60.

23 M.E. Charlson, R.P. Cohen, and C.L. Sears, "General Medical Consultation: Lessons from a Clinical Service," *American Journal of Medicine* 75 (1983): 121-28; T. Lee, E.M. Pappius, and L. Goldman, "The Impact of Inter-Physician Communication on the Effectiveness of Medical Consultations," *American Journal of Medicine* 74 (1983): 106-12; and P. Rudd, M. Siegler, and R.L. Byyny, "Perioperative Diabetic Consultations: Observations and Recommendations," *Journal of Medical Education* 53 (1978): 590-96.

24 J. La Puma and D.L. Schiedermayer, "Ethics Consultation: Skills, Roles, and Training," *Annals of Internal Medicine* 114 (1991): 155-60.

7.6 Pellegrino ED, Siegler M, Singer PA (1991) Future Directions in Clinical Ethics. J Clin Ethics 2:5–9

Reprinted with permission from the Journal of Clinical Ethics, copyright 1991.

VOLUME 2, NUMBER 1   THE JOURNAL OF CLINICAL ETHICS   5

FEATURES

Future Directions in Clinical Ethics

Edmund D. Pellegrino, Mark Siegler, and Peter A. Singer

The Prologue of the Past

This article is the last in a series of articles describing the field of clinical ethics.[1] In this essay we anticipate some likely directions for clinical ethics. We have chosen to make projections for the next two decades--a period roughly equal to the entire history of the modern biomedical ethics movement in America. Over the last two decades, biomedical ethics has kept pace with revolutionary developments in biology and medicine. As a result, biomedical ethics has changed more profoundly in this period than in the whole of its previous history. Today it is of the utmost interest not just to ethicists, but to the whole of our society, including the health professions, the general public, the courts, the media, and policy makers. These developments are remarkable in a field that changed very little over 2,500 years and confined its perspective almost exclusively to the privacy of the doctor-patient relationship and to issues related to professional etiquette.

Many factors have contributed to the emergence of biomedical ethics and its new focus. We are still too close to and too much a part of these transformations to evaluate them accurately. Nevertheless, we believe the most

Edmund D. Pellegrino, MD, is Director of the Center for the Advanced Study of Ethics and John Carroll Professor of Medicine and Medical Humanities, Georgetown University, Washington, DC.
Mark Siegler, MD, is Director of the Center for Clinical Medical Ethics and Professor of Medicine, University of Chicago.
Peter A. Singer, MD, is Associate Director of the Centre for Bioethics and Assistant Professor of Medicine, University of Toronto.

important factors are the following sociocultural forces that emerged as powerful influences during the last generation: the biotechnological revolution, which presents ethical dilemmas of a kind and degree never before encountered; the rise of participatory democracy, which has shifted the locus of decision making from the doctor to the patient; the growth of moral pluralism and relativism, which place increasing emphasis on procedural rather than normative ethics; the litigious spirit of the times, which enlists the courts to settle ethical disputes; and the partial reconceptualization of medicine as a business, replete with providers and consumers and increasingly controlled by market forces or government regulation. It is our assumption that these same forces will interact in the foreseeable future to shape medical ethics. These forces provide the contextual background against which the changes we anticipate may take place.

We now offer our best guesses about six areas in which biomedical ethics is likely to play an important role in the future: 1) the impact of a continuing biomedical technical revolution; 2) the maturation of biomedical ethics as a discipline; 3) the increasing intersection of ethics and health policy; 4) the broader engagement of the public with issues in biomedical ethics; 5) changes in the conceptual foundations of bioethics; and 6) changes in the doctor-patient relationship.

The Ethics of Biomedical Technology

Despite today's truly astounding discoveries and applications of molecular

and cellular biology, we are probably only at the beginning of the biological revolution and a new era of advances in biotechnology. As our fundamental knowledge of life processes increases, our capacity to control more and more facets of human life will expand. Each new advance in reproductive biology, organ and cell culture, designer drugs, and proteins poses new questions that challenge traditional values about human life. Mapping the human genome, exploring the eugenic possibilities of somatic and gametocyte genetic engineering, and expanding the uses of artificial intelligence and artificial organs are examples of developments that surely will have profound ethical implications but whose ethical ramifications are still poorly understood.

In recent years, scientists, policy makers, and the public have come to appreciate that it is essential to develop our ethical sophistication *pari passu* with our technological know-how. This is preferable to facing the crises of knowledge application without the critical apparatus needed for intelligent ethical discussion and conflict resolution. The Human Genome Project illustrates the importance of the interrelationships of scientific advancement with law, society, politics, ethics, and economics. The genome project has the potential to radically alter the diagnosis, prevention, and treatment of many inherited disorders. Some of the ethical issues this project raises will be familiar, such as the questions of informed consent or the allocation of scarce resources. When it becomes possible to diagnose accurately such fatal, disabling diseases as Huntington's chorea or cystic fibrosis, the ethical issues will center on prenatal diagnosis, abortion, privacy, and the ownership of knowledge. Even if the ethical issues are familiar in principle, context-specific guidelines will need to be developed to regulate genetic research and practice. Our efforts in this direction can be expected to expand considerably.

On the other hand, some of the ethical issues accompanying the human genome project will be unfamiliar. One example is germ-line gene therapy--the insertion of a gene into a fertilized egg; since every cell in the body acquires the new gene, including the reproductive cells, it is passed on to succeeding generations.[2] What are our obligations to those yet to be born and yet to be conceived when we can eradicate certain diseases entirely? Which diseases do we choose? How should the needs of future generations be weighed against those of the present? Should we use somatic or germ-line gene therapy to enhance certain characteristics, such as intelligence, memory, affability, or physical abilities? Who should make such decisions for future generations? Is eugenic manipulation of the human species ever morally licit? Other kinds of questions arise if the genetic and molecular bases of Alzheimer's disease, Parkinson's disease, or aging are discovered. Should such research be undertaken, given its potential for seriously altering demographics, putting additional strains on society's resources, and limiting opportunities for the young? Whenever there are potentialities for new knowledge, there will be the need for ethical reflection. Some form of agreement on how ethical issues are to be addressed will be necessary. To its credit, the Human Genome Project has earmarked 2 percent of its budget for ethical, legal, and policy analysis. Similar provisions should be incorporated into other future research projects, genetic or otherwise. If we are to use medical knowledge wisely, humanely, and well, ethical analysis must keep pace with technological advance.

Maturation of the Discipline

It is clear that as the biological revolution continues to unfold, new ethical responses will be required. It is incumbent on the discipline and profession of bioethics to mature as well. First of all, the research base of the field must be secured, strengthened, and extended. As we pointed out earlier, there are a large number of empirical questions that must be addressed.[3] These questions are essential starting points for any serious ethical discourse. The necessary empirical data will come from a closer integration of ethical inquiry with the quantitative sciences and with traditional clinical research, since it is their methodology that is most important for descriptive ethics. Familiarity with these methods will be required for bioethicists of the future. Greater maturation will also be needed in the conceptual and foundational aspects of bioethics. This, as we will remark a little later, is a more problematic and more difficult terrain to traverse than empirical study. The second major feature of maturation will be the professionalization and perhaps regulation of clinical bioethics. This will require some standardization of educational credentials and perhaps some form of certification. As we pointed out in our previous article:

At this time we believe it is premature to develop standards for training and certifying ethics consultants. The primary reason for delay is to develop both clearer goals for ethics committees and consultants and better studies of existing committees and consultants.[4]

We should begin this work in earnest now because the trend to certification seems inevitable. "Ethicists" are being sought and employed by medical schools, hospitals, and health-care systems. They are being consulted by the media, the courts, and families. They appear on panels, symposia, and continuing education programs. They speak to and write for the general public. There is a growing need for some form of assurance that those who assume the mantle of "ethicist" do in fact bring legitimate expertise to their deliberations.

This assurance will, in our opinion, increasingly be in the form of a degree or training certificate in bioethics. For "clinical" ethics, either fellowship training or the master's degree would seem to be sufficient when combined with full qualification as a physician, nurse, social worker, or administrator. Here the emphasis is on practical decision making regarding concrete cases at the bedside, assisting others to analyze ethical issues to make their own decisions, advising ethics committees on institutional policy, and counseling families and other health professionals. Given the number of physicians who are needed to serve as clinical ethicists and the relatively few fellowship training positions available, it is likely that the combination of a degree in the health professions and either fellowship training or an advanced degree in ethics will be the standard qualification for clinical ethicists. This will not in any way diminish the need for professional ethicists who are not health professionals. Non-health professionals will, however, be much less likely in the future to do clinical ethics. They will be needed to carry out fundamental and foundational research, to teach bioethics in colleges, and to train graduate students.

A third requirement for maturation of the profession will be the acquisition of counseling and negotiation skills. When ethicists become involved in direct consultation with physicians and families, they are playing two distinct roles--one as philosopher-teacher-consultant, which is familiar, and one as counselor, which is less familiar. Counseling requires a specific set of skills. To meet the demands of both roles, the clinical ethicist needs more practical experience under supervision and perhaps even formal training in counseling and negotiation. The way information is transmitted, communication is established, and decisions are reached conjointly is of the utmost importance in an age of participatory democracy. The power of the ethics consultant is considerable, and it must be used responsibly. The ethicist's aim should be to enable, empower, and enhance the decision-making capabilities of patient, doctor, and family. The ethicist should not make the decision for them, or worse still, impose his or her ethical values or beliefs on the primary decision makers.

Intersection with Health Policy

Medical ethics has traditionally focused primarily on the interactions between individual patients and their health-care providers. During the next two decades, however, we predict that the focus will enlarge to include the ethics of health-care institutions and the health-care system as a whole. These issues of public policy are generally being recognized as ethical challenges and not simply as problems of economics or politics.

Questions of health policy, cost, access, and quality of care are, and will continue to be, major ethical issues. In 1990, the US spent $661 billion on health care (almost 12 percent of the gross national product). Health-care costs outstripped the rate of inflation, so there is danger that societal resources may be diverted away from other social goods such as education, preservation of the environment, housing, social welfare, and so on. Major policy initiatives are underway--from physician payment reform by the Medicare program, to the Oregon initiative to broaden Medicaid eligibility and to tailor the benefits package. There is also increasing emphasis on the development of clinical guidelines--a health-policy initiative focused on quality but with significant cost implications. Each of these issues--both the problems and the proposed solutions--present fundamental questions of medical ethics. We shall illustrate this point with one example, clinical guidelines.

The emergence of clinical guidelines raises at least three fundamental ethical questions. First, can ethical decision making be reduced to a paradigm and incorporated into guidelines? During the past twenty years, a crucial social, ethical, and political development in the US has been the importance of

knowing and respecting individual preferences and values. This makes it difficult to establish a single moral standard that applies to all, since the value of the individual is the key element. But what is right for a group may not be acceptable to individuals within the group. How does one balance individual preferences against group wishes? The choice will need to be made by some method of societal mediation. Ethicists should look at the criteria by which these choices are made. The "ethical fallout" of clinical guidelines can be significant in its impact on patient care, as Diagnostic Related Groups (DRGs) have been.

to incorporate such considerations into clinical guidelines. How best to do so is a subject worthy of serious scholarly attention.

These three questions are simply illustrative of the way ethical issues are embedded in policy decisions and how important it will be for bioethicists to engage the ethical implications of all major policy proposals.

Public Involvement

Biomedical ethics is now everybody's concern, not just the concern of physicians as it was in the past, or of

---

Biomedical ethics is now everybody's concern, not just the concern of physicians or professional ethicists.

A second ethical issue is the impact of clinical guidelines on physicians, the doctor-patient relationship, and the medical profession. The morale of physicians is an important element in quality health care. Physicians in the US increasingly feel demoralized, unappreciated, beleaguered, and misunderstood. Some are retiring early, others simply "go along," and others respond defensively or even vindictively. Most seem driven to justify some degree of moral compromise just to survive. This is an important matter not just for health policy, but also for medical ethics. Ethical decisions depend upon complex ethical relationships among physicians, patients, and families. The best ethical decisions depend upon the moral sensitivity of all participants.

A third ethical question about clinical guidelines is: how can patient preferences and utilities be best taken into account in the development of guidelines? To date, guidelines have focused strictly on technical issues. But medical decision making also depends upon the preferences of informed, competent, and uncoerced patients. It is important

professional ethicists as it has been in the last two decades. Sooner or later, in their own lives, or in the lives of their families or friends, every person will be called upon to make moral choices respecting medical care. This inescapable fact imposes on ethicists and health professionals the responsibility for educating the public. As never before, the public will need knowledge of how to make moral judgments in general, and specifically in their own health care.

As far as general education in making moral judgments is concerned, we are already seeing a proliferation of courses in ethics and biomedical ethics in colleges, high schools, and continuing education for the general public, as well as for health professionals. We expect this trend to continue given the ubiquity of ethical issues, not just in health care, but in matters of environment, business, politics, and virtually every facet of life. Courses in ethics should be required in any education for responsible citizenship.

In biomedical ethics specifically, there are numerous issues with which the educated public needs familiarity--

withdrawing and withholding life-sustaining treatments, organ donation, reproductive technologies, and especially advance directives. These are matters of immediate concern to clinical ethicists, who will be expected, and indeed may be required, to educate their patients in the choices available to them.

The recently passed Danforth Bill (S. 1766) is an example of governmental intervention mandating that patients, at the time of hospital admission, be informed of the use and availability of advance directives in their care. If we are not to end up with federal legislation governing every possible moral choice patients have to make, it is particularly incumbent on clinical ethicists to expand their efforts in education of the public and the health professions.

Biomedical ethics, like curative medicine, has focused largely on the individual patient in an acute clinical episode. In the future, it must also take on the perspective of preventive and public health medicine. It must develop strategies for public education, provide data and ethical analyses on which public policy can be based, and provide mechanisms for public participation. Preventing ethical conflict, confusion, and misunderstanding is analogous to preventing or containing disabling or chronic illness. Preventive ethics is less expensive, more effective, and less traumatic emotionally than litigation, bureaucratic regulation, or misunderstandings between physicians, patients, and families.

Conceptual Foundation of Bioethics

The most complex, problematic, and difficult predictions to make are related to the philosophical underpinnings of biomedical ethics. The whole structure of ethical reasoning depends upon the conceptual presuppositions and values out of which the edifice of medical ethics is built. Not to take note of the difficulties would be to ignore what is surely a major force giving shape to the future of medical ethics.

Before the entry of professional philosophers into the field, medical ethics was largely a series of statements of moral obligations. These obligations were self-imposed by physicians as a result of what they conceived medicine to be. Philosophical justification or explicit argumentation in support of those moral statements was virtually

nonexistent. Nothing like the philosophy of law, history, or politics existed.

As philosophers began to give serious attention to medical ethics, they naturally sought to link medical ethics to existing philosophical systems—mainly deontological and teleological. The philosophies of Kant and J.S. Mill, and to a lesser extent Hume and Locke, have shaped the principle-based approaches that now dominate biomedical ethical thinking.

As experience is gained in the application of these modes of thought to concrete clinical ethical decisions, some of their deficiencies are becoming apparent. Increasing numbers of thinkers consider principle-based ethics to be too abstract, too remote from the actualities of clinical decisions, too formal and stylized, and too neglectful of the character of the health professional and the affective dimensions of moral life. To remedy these shortcomings, a wide range of alternatives is being proposed, such as virtue theory, feminist psychology, experiential and essential approaches, hermeneutics, and literature. Each is seen as a way to encompass more of the multidimensional array of influences that define moral choices.

This is not the place to examine the claims of conflicting theories or models of ethics, or to confront the "foundational" issues. It is worth outlining, however, some of the foundational questions currently under discussion, the answers to which will determine what biomedical ethics will look like two decades hence.

> *Preventive ethics is less expensive, more effective, and less traumatic emotionally than litigation, bureaucratic regulation, or misunderstandings between physicians, patients, and families.*

Does the moral pluralism of world society dictate that ethics must give up its normative pretensions? Must we settle for procedural ethics only? Is there any definable foundation for ethics other than the coherence between, and consensus about, selected elements of competing theories? Are morality and ethics so culturally and historically bound that "objectivity" in ethics is an illusion? How do law, politics, ethics, and literature relate to one another? Is there some way to link the affective and cognitive components of the moral life? Is there some logically compatible way to link principle-based and alternative theories of ethics? Is medical ethics, itself, entirely encompassed within existing ethical theory, or does it have an "internal morality" of its own?

These questions are not as abstract or ephemeral as they may appear to clinicians. Ultimately, they are relevant to the most concrete dilemmas we face, and will face, in making moral choices in individual patients, in defining the obligations of health professionals, and in formulating public policy in democratic, morally heterogeneous societies.

In all likelihood, there will be some fusion of ideas drawn from a variety of ethical theories with no single theory becoming exclusively and inarguably dominant. What the resulting mosaic will look like is an open question at this time. In this case, it is clear that there is as much ferment in the foundations as there is in the applications of ethics in the clinical realm. Keeping abreast of these changes will be difficult but essential as the field of clinical ethics matures.

The Doctor-Patient Relationship

Just as the history of medical ethics was closely related to the doctor-patient relationship, so the future of medical ethics is likely to be linked to the evolution and changes that are now occurring in the doctor-patient relationship. Perhaps the most fundamental impact of the bioethics movement in America was to shift the therapeutic (and research) relationship from a traditional paternalistic model, in which the doctor knew best, to a new model in which patient rights and autonomy are acknowledged to be the most important elements in medical decisions. This evolutionary shift in authority from physician to patient has established a more equal relationship, in which therapeutic accommodations are reached based on voluntariness, mutual respect for the other party's autonomy, and negotiations.

This system of personal decisions is changing because economic, political, and structural changes in the health system have increased external control over decisions and have decreased the freedom and discretion of both patients and physicians. Essentially, we are in the midst of a new health-care revolution, in which the subjective standard of decision making is being supplanted by an externally imposed objective standard based increasingly on scientific facts, social values, and economic considerations. Among the approaches that already are being used to constrain the personal choices (and future choices) of physicians and patients are: 1) the use of probabilistic

medical outcome studies to limit physicians' discretion to offer patients choices and to respond to patients' preferences; 2) the application of statistical notions of futility, in which external authorities rather than the patient or physician define which clinical goals are legitimate to pursue and which level of probability of achieving the goals constitutes "futility"; 3) the gradual emergence of quality of life standards that may limit the pursuit of certain goals based on an external assessment that the patient's quality of life is "too poor"; and finally, 4) straightforward rationing using both medical and social utility criteria. In this new health-care environment, medical ethics will remain an essential tool for preventing morally unacceptable policies from emerging and for preserving the vital personal elements

of the doctor-patient relationship that are essential for providing excellent health care.

NOTES

1   M. Siegler, E.D. Pellegrino, and P.A. Singer, "Clinical Medical Ethics," *The Journal of Clinical Ethics* 1 (Spring 1990): 5-9; P.A. Singer, M. Siegler, and E.D. Pellegrino, "Research in Clinical Ethics," *The Journal of Clinical Ethics* 1 (Summer 1990): 95-99; E.D. Pellegrino, M. Siegler, and P.A. Singer, "Teaching Clinical Ethics," *The Journal of Clinical Ethics* 1 (Fall 1990): 175-80; P.A. Singer, E.D. Pellegrino, and M. Siegler, "Ethics Committees and Consultants," *The Journal of Clinical Ethics* 1 (Winter 1990): 263-67.
2   E.K. Nichols, *Human Gene Therapy* (Cambridge: Harvard University Press, 1988).
3   Singer, Siegler, and Pellegrino, "Research in Clinical Ethics."
4   Singer, Pellegrino, and Siegler, "Ethics Committees and Consultants," 267.

7.7 Siegler M, Singer PA (1991) Clinical Ethics. In: Kelley WN (ed) Textbook of Internal Medicine, 2nd edn. JB Lippincott Co., Philadelphia, p 3–5

Reprinted with permission from Wolters Kluwer.

C H A P T E R 2
CLINICAL ETHICS

MARK SIEGLER AND PETER A. SINGER

In the 1990s, physicians who wish to provide the high-quality personal medical care that patients have come to expect must have a working knowledge of clinical ethics, a new and practical approach to medical ethics. Patients and society now expect physicians to demonstrate not only technical proficiency but also a practical ability to respond to clinical-ethical situations. This practical working knowledge of clinical ethics should not be seen as a substitute for, but rather as an addition to, the traditional character and virtue standards expected of the good physician: integrity, compassion, and thoroughness.

The frequency, intensity, and recognition of ethical dilemmas in clinical medicine have increased in the recent past as a result of profound changes in American medicine and society. These changes have included an unprecedented growth in scientific knowledge and medical technology; a more equal relationship between patients and physicians; new organizational arrangements of medical practice and reimbursement; and a heightened sensitivity to ethical issues in medicine on the part of the public and the medical profession. Although ethical considerations are a part of every patient–physician encounter, recent clinical research suggests that physicians recognize major ethical dilemmas such as truth-telling, confidentiality, informed consent, and elective use of life-sustaining treatments in up to 17% of general internal medicine inpatient admissions and 21% of outpatient visits.

Clinical ethics emphasizes that the starting point for ethical analysis is the encounter between patient and physician, an event that both defines the goals of the patient–physician relationship and establishes mutual rights and responsibilities. Clinical ethics aims to improve decision making between patients and physicians by balancing the following three components of clinical care: (1) the medical/scientific facts; (2) the personal preferences, values, and goals of the patient; and (3) the external constraints such as cost, limited resources, and legal standards that may limit the decisional freedom of patients and physicians.

In the 1970s, clinical ethics focused on educational programs; in the 1980s, it stressed administrative approaches such as ethics committees. The additional challenge for the 1990s is to develop research in ethics that emphasizes clinical data and meets high scientific standards. The twin goals of this research are (1) to describe clinical practice to help direct ethical, legal, and policy decision making; and (2) to evaluate the use of ethical, legal, and policy standards in clinical practice. In this chapter, we begin to apply this new clinical ethics research perspective to two ethical issues that arise frequently in the practice of internal medicine: patient participation in treatment decisions and elective use of life-sustaining treatment.

PATIENT PARTICIPATION IN TREATMENT DECISIONS

In recent decades, the relationship between patients and physicians has been evolving from the traditional paternalistic relationship in which physicians made choices for patients, to a more equal relationship of shared decision making in which physicians provide information and counseling that allows competent adult patients to make their own choices. The process by which physicians and patients make decisions together, summarized in the phrase "informed consent," is based on the ethical principle of individual autonomy and the legal right of self-determination. Informed consent has three key components: *disclosure, competency,* and *voluntariness. Disclosure* means that the physician informs the patient about the medical diagnosis, prognosis, and risks and benefits of treatment options. *Competency* means that the patient is able to understand relevant information, to appreciate the situation and its consequences, to manipulate information rationally, and to communicate a treatment choice. *Voluntariness* means that the patient chooses freely, without undue coercion from the physician or anyone else. Informed consent is a process of dialogue that serves as the ethical and clinical basis for the physician–patient relationship; it is not simply an event and does not merely refer to a patient's signature on a consent form. In this process, the physician educates the patient about reasonable medical alternatives and the patient chooses treatment based on personal preferences, values, and goals.

Research studies on patient preferences, quality of life, and patient empowerment suggest important clinical reasons why physicians should involve patients in their own medical care decisions. McNeil and colleagues have shown that an individual patient's treatment preferences may not always be self-evident. For example, to avoid the risk of perioperative death, some patients with lung cancer would choose radiation therapy over surgery despite a lower 5-year survival rate. Similarly, to maintain normal voice function, some patients with laryngeal cancer would choose radiation therapy over surgery despite the lower survival rate.

When available, information about quality of life outcomes can be incorporated into the process of informing patients about treatment options. Wennberg and colleagues have evaluated patients' symptoms and quality of life after prostatectomy and incorporated functional outcome data into an experimental, interactive video-disc system that can be used to more fully inform patients with prostatism about risks and benefits as they choose between immediate transurethral resection and watchful waiting.

Empowering patients to participate in decision making appears to be associated with beneficial outcomes in several chronic diseases. In patients with diabetes, hypertension, and peptic ulcer disease, Greenfield and colleagues have shown that pilot programs aimed at increasing patient participation in medical care result in improved functional and health outcomes. In a related, long-term study (the Medical Outcomes Study), these researchers are evaluating the impact of differences in physicians' practice styles and systems of care on patient outcomes.

ELECTIVE USE OF LIFE-SUSTAINING TREATMENT

The do-not-resuscitate (DNR) order is the prototype for a clinical research approach to elective use of life-sustaining treatments. In this section, we present research data about DNR orders to illustrate how clinical research can help direct ethical, legal, and policy decision making about elective use of life-sustaining treatment.

There is a general agreement in law, public policy, and medical ethics that patients have the right to forego life-sustaining treatment, including cardiopulmonary resuscitation (CPR). In research studies, the incidence of DNR orders is 3% to 4% of hospitalized patients and 5% to 14% of patients admitted to intensive care units. Conversely, 66% to 75% of hospital deaths and 39% of deaths in intensive care units are preceded by a DNR order. Therefore, the DNR order should not be viewed as a theoretic, peripheral issue but rather as an issue in the mainstream of patient care.

According to ethical, legal, and policy guidelines, the patient's wishes should govern the use of life-sustaining treatments. In research studies, factors associated with the writing of DNR orders include older age, increased severity of illness, poor preadmission functional status, urinary incontinence, abnormal mental status or a diagnosis of dementia, residence in a nursing home, a diagnosis of cancer or the acquired immunodeficiency syndrome, and the physician's estimates of patient quality of life and prognosis (including survival and functional status). These research findings raise an important question for policymakers and ethics researchers: do the factors listed above reflect or displace patients' wishes in clinical decision making about DNR? And which of these factors should influence clinical decisions?

Advance directives (living wills or durable powers of attorney for health care) allow patients the opportunity to declare their wishes regarding DNR and other life-sustaining treatments. In surveys, 77% to 82% of elderly outpatients say they would want CPR in their current health state, but only 21% to 38% say they would want CPR if they had severe dementia, stroke, irreversible coma, or terminal cancer. In practice, however, despite evidence that advance directives are acceptable to both patients and physicians, less than 15% of patients will have left an advance directive. The infrequent use of advance directives results in part from the poor design of early versions. Emanuel and Emanuel have developed an improved advance directive that stipulates clinical scenarios and lists treatments that the patient may choose to receive or forego. Researchers are studying the reliability and validity of advance directives.

Competent patients do not require an advance directive; they can discuss the use of life-sustaining treatments directly with their physician. Studies indicate, however, that the patient is involved in only 14% to 43% of DNR decisions. Incompetency at the time of the DNR decision is a major reason for patient nonparticipation in the decision making. At the time patients are admitted to the hospital, they are often capable of making decisions, but they become incompetent in the hospital before a DNR order is discussed. Thus, policies promoting earlier discussions about DNR, when patients are still competent, may be desirable.

Relatives or friends, if available, often serve as the proxy decision maker for incompetent patients. According to recent studies, families serve as the patient's proxy in 45% to 86% of DNR decisions. The proxy decision-maker should attempt to project the patient's wishes, preferences, values, attitudes, and goals onto the current medical situation; this standard is known as *substituted judgment:* the proxy attempts to reach the decision that the incapacitated person would make if he or she were able to choose. Studies by Uhlmann and Pearlman showing poor agreement about resuscitation preferences between patients and their potential proxies raise questions about the substituted judgment standard and argue for increased use of advance directives.

Most research on elective use of life-sustaining treatment has focused on the DNR decision. Data about other life-sustaining treatments, such as mechanical ventilation, dialysis, and tube feeding, are relatively sparse. In this section, we have attempted to show how empiric data can help direct ethical, legal, and policy guidelines about DNR. We recommend that researchers evaluate the elective use of other life-sustaining treatments.

CONCLUSIONS

Research on patient participation and elective use supports the contention that ethical issues can be examined using clinical research. In the 1990s, we hope that ethicists and researchers will build on these research initiatives in clinical ethics by extending a quantitative, scientific perspective to other situations in the clinical practice of medicine. By examining the interface between clinical practice and ethics, law, and policy, clinical ethics research will help physicians provide high-quality personal care through the 1990s, an era that is likely to witness a substantial increase in the administrative regulation of medical practice.

Application of these principles in older patients is considered in chapter 513.

BIBLIOGRAPHY

Appelbaum PS, Grisso T. Assessing patients' capacities to consent to treatment. N Engl J Med 1988;319:1635

Barry MJ, Mulley AG, Fowler FJ, Wennberg JW. Watchful waiting vs immediate transurethral resection for symptomatic prostatism: the importance of patients' preferences. JAMA 1988;259:3010

Connelly JE, DalleMura S. Ethical problems in the medical office. JAMA 1988;260:812

Emanuel LL, Emanuel EJ. The medical directive: a new comprehensive advance care document. JAMA 1989;261:3288

Greenfield S, Kaplan SH, Ware JE, Yano EM, Frank HJ. Patients' participation in medical care: effects of blood sugar control and quality of life in diabetes. J Gen Intern Med 1988;3:448

Lo B, Schroeder SA. Frequency of ethical dilemmas in a medical inpatient service. Arch Intern Med 1981;141:1062

McNeil BJ, Weichselbaum R, Pauker SG. Speech and survival: tradeoffs between quality and quantity of life in laryngeal cancer. N Engl J Med 1982;305:982

Siegler M, Pellegrino ED, Singer PA. Clinical medical ethics. J Clin Ethics 1990;1:5.

Singer PA, Siegler M. Elective use of life-sustaining treatment in internal medicine. In: Stollerman GH, ed. Advances in internal medicine, vol 36. Chicago: Year Book Medical Publishers, 1991

Tarlov AL, Ware JE, Greenfield S, Nelson EC, Perrin E, Zubkoff M. The Medical Outcomes study: an application of methods for monitoring the results of medical care. JAMA 1989;262:925

Uhlmann RE, Pearlman RA, Cain KC. Physicians' and spouses' predictions of elderly patients' resuscitation preferences. J Gerontol 1988;43:M115

7.8 Singer PA, Siegler M (1996) Clinical Ethics in the Practice of Medicine. In: Wyngaarten JB, Plum F, Bennett C (eds) Cecil Textbook of Medicine, 20th edn. WB Saunders Co., Philadelphia, p 4–6

PART II

SOCIAL AND ETHICAL ISSUES IN MEDICINE

2 CLINICAL ETHICS IN THE PRACTICE OF MEDICINE

Peter A. Singer and Mark Siegler

Clinical ethics is a practical discipline that contributes to improving patient care. It focuses on the central importance of patient preferences and choices in the physician-patient relationship and on the moral obligations of physicians, such as the need for honesty, competence, compassion, and respect for the patient. Clinical ethics teaches physicians about a wide range of specifically ethical issues—informed consent, orders not to resuscitate, end-of-life decisions, advance directives, and third-party constraints on the autonomy of both patients and physicians—that arise with increasing frequency in the practice of modern medicine. Although these issues have been analyzed and seemingly resolved at a theoretical level, few physicians are comfortable with them in practice. This chapter offers guidance about the following ethical issues that arise frequently in the practice of internal medicine: (1) decision making by competent patients, (2) substitute decision making (including advance directives), (3) end-of-life decisions, (4) futility, and (5) clinical-ethical concerns in an era of health care reform.

DECISION MAKING BY COMPETENT PATIENTS

During the past generation, the relationship between patients and physicians has become more equal. Most clinical decisions are now reached by a process of shared decision making in which physicians provide information and guidance that allow competent adult patients to make their own decisions based on their personal preferences, values, and goals. Competent adult patients have an ethical and legal right to accept or refuse medical care, including life-sustaining treatments, recommended by physicians. Patients are in control of their own health care. In general, patients accept their physician's recommendations because physician and patient share the same goal—improving the patient's health status—and because patients usually trust and have confidence in both the physician's technical abilities and his/her concerns for the patient as an individual.

INFORMED CONSENT. The clinical-ethical process of shared decision making is mirrored by the legal doctrine of informed consent. Informed consent is defined as voluntary acceptance by a competent patient of a plan for medical care after the physician adequately discloses the proposed plan, its risks and benefits, and alternative approaches. The informed consent process applies not only to invasive surgical procedures but to every clinical decision. Moreover, the legal and ethical standards of informed consent are not satisfied merely by obtaining the patient's signature on a consent form but require a process of effective communication and education between the physician and patient. If the patient has decision-making capacity (see later), the physician should seek consent from the patient; if the patient lacks decision-making capacity, the physi-

cian should seek consent from the appropriate substitute decision maker. The best way for young physicians to learn how to obtain informed consent from patients is by observing a clinician who is recognized for skill in negotiating the consent process.

The patient's right to participate in treatment decisions is well recognized in law, philosophy, public policy, and clinical practice. Perhaps the clearest *legal* statement of this right was enunciated in 1914 by Justice Cardozo: "Every human being of adult years and sound mind has the right to determine what shall be done with his own body." The *philosophical* right of patients to control their own medical care is based on the principle of individual autonomy. In the 1980's, a Presidential commission clearly stated that respect for patient preferences should be the basis of *public policy* in medical ethics. Moreover, evidence from *clinical* research indicates that empowering patients to participate in their own health care may lead to improved functional outcomes in several chronic diseases.

DISCLOSURE AND TRUTH TELLING. For the purposes of informed consent, disclosure must include proposed diagnostic tests and treatments, their risks and benefits, and possible alternative approaches. Although standards for disclosure may vary from one jurisdiction to another, the physician should disclose all the information that a reasonable person in the patient's situation would want or need to know before making a decision. This usually includes information about risks that are either highly likely to occur or less likely but very serious when they do occur (e.g., death or permanent disability). Although a subjective standard of disclosure based on an individual patient's personal view is a difficult clinical standard to achieve, physicians should try to know their patients well enough to tailor disclosure to a patient's particular situation.

Another aspect of disclosure separate from the need to obtain informed consent involves telling patients the truth about unfavorable diagnoses such as metastatic cancer and their prognoses. In the United States, the current medical standard is to be honest with patients and not to conceal bad news. The patient's right to know an unfavorable diagnosis, even if no further tests or treatment is proposed, is grounded in the ethical principle of respect for persons and in the implied promise by physicians to be truthful in their relationships with a patient. Of course, the real clinical skill in "telling the truth" or delivering bad news to a patient involves determining exactly what the "truth" is in a particular case and then deciding how and when it should be imparted in a sensitive way that does not destroy the patient's hope.

COMPETENCY AND DECISION-MAKING CAPACITY. Decision-making capacity (DMC), a clinical concept, is one of the central ethical issues in clinical patient care. (Competency is the parallel legal concept.) Patients who have been determined to have DMC should make their own health care decisions (based on the principle of autonomy), whereas patients determined to lack DMC should be protected from making bad and sometimes irreversible decisions (based on the principle of beneficence). DMC is a dynamic state and may change quickly, as when a patient is admitted stuporous, hypotensive, and with sepsis, and lacks DMC, but 6 hours later, after appropriate treatment, is sitting in bed, conversing normally, and has regained DMC. Moreover, DMC is decision specific. For example, patients with substantial cognitive impairment may retain DMC to decide whether they wish to accept a recommended elective cholecystectomy.

DMC requires that a patient have the ability to communicate and understand information and appreciate the consequences of a particular decision. Unfortunately, no valid and widely accepted clinical measures exist to assess DMC. Physicians should assess DMC by asking patients if they understand and appreciate their medical problem and the risks and benefits of the proposed treatment and why they have chosen to accept or reject it. In practice, physicians often assess DMC by means of a sliding scale that varies with the likelihood and seriousness of the risks and benefits. Thus, a low level of DMC is often clinically acceptable if a patient elects a proposed life-saving treatment that has low risks and a high probability of benefit, whereas clinicians might require a higher standard of DMC if the patient refuses the same treatment.

Who should decide about DMC? In practice, the physician or health care team responsible for the patient should determine whether a patient retains or has lost DMC. When doubt exists, consulting a psychiatrist, hospital attorney, or clinical ethicist may be helpful. In cases of irremediable conflict and if clinical circumstances permit, the ultimate judge of a patient's competency is a court. Often, physicians must make decisions without the benefit of a judicial determination, relying on clinical judgment and assistance from consultants to reach the best and most ethical determination.

SUBSTITUTE DECISION MAKING

American legal theory accords incompetent patients the same rights as competent patients to consent to or refuse diagnostic tests and treatment. In practice, however, patients who lack DMC cannot exercise this right. To address this paradox and to facilitate reaching decisions for the many patients who lack DMC, substitute decision makers are permitted to make health care decisions for the patient lacking DMC. The overall goal of substitute decision making is to approximate the decisions the patient would make if he/she were still capable of making a decision. Substitute decision making policies raise two questions: Who should make decisions for the patient who lacks DMC, and by what standards should the decision be made?

The most appropriate person to make substitute decisions is someone designated by the patient while still competent, either orally or through a written proxy advance directive (see below). Other substitute decision makers, in their usual order of priority, include a spouse, adult child, parent, brother or sister, and any other relative or concerned friend. In some jurisdictions, a public official may serve as substitute decision maker for a patient who has no other decision maker available. More than 25 states have now passed health surrogate laws that permit a substitute decision maker to be appointed without going to court when a patient lacks DMC and has no formal advance directive.

The standards for making substitute decisions for patients without DMC are the following (in decreasing order of priority): explicit patient preferences, values and beliefs, and best interests. Patient preferences are prior expressions by the patient, while competent, that apply to the actual decision that needs to be made, such as whether the patient wants mechanical ventilation in the late stages of amyotrophic lateral sclerosis. Sometimes patients record their specific preferences in an instruction advance directive (see below). Values and beliefs are less specific than explicit preferences, but they allow the substitute decision maker to guess what the patient might have decided based on other past choices of the patient and his/her general approach to life. Best interests, which are "objective" estimates of the benefits and burdens of treatment to the patient, are invoked only when the patient's preferences and values are unknown.

ADVANCE DIRECTIVES. An advance directive (sometimes called a "living will") is a written document containing a person's preferences about life-sustaining treatment and about a proxy decision maker. The person completes the advance directive when competent, and the directive takes effect if the person becomes incompetent. The two types of advance directives are proxy directives, which state *whom* a person wants to make treatment decisions on his/her behalf, and instruction directives, which state *what* treatment the person would or would not want in various situations. (By far the best-studied and most widely used form of advance directive is the order not to resuscitate, i.e., DNR order, written to withhold a specific intervention, cardiopulmonary resuscitation, from a person who experiences a specific medical event, cardiorespiratory arrest.) At present, advance directives are recognized legally in every state,

and the federal Patient Self-Determination Act (PSDA) requires health care facilities to inquire whether patients have an advance directive and to inform patients of their rights under state law to complete an advance directive. Although public opinion polls indicate strong support for advance directives and although many different advance directive forms are available, relatively few Americans have filled out such directives. The development and evaluation of advance directives, including efforts to encourage their use, are areas of active empirical research.

END-OF-LIFE DECISIONS

With the possible exception of informed consent, no issue in clinical ethics has been as thoroughly analyzed as end-of-life decisions. Nevertheless, the spectrum of end-of-life decisions remains confusing for clinicians and the public. Three distinct practices can be delineated: decisions to forego life-sustaining treatment, euthanasia/physician-assisted suicide, and palliative care.

The right of patients to refuse medical interventions also applies to life-sustaining treatment such as cardiopulmonary resuscitation, mechanical ventilation, dialysis, and artificial nutrition and hydration, even if such a decision results in the patient's death. A patient's decision to not initiate (withhold) or to discontinue (withdraw) life-sustaining treatment is not considered the moral or legal equivalent of suicide, and physician participation in such an action is not the equivalent of physician-assisted suicide. These decisions may be made by the patient or substitute decision maker and are legally and ethically permissible when clinicians follow appropriate procedures, as outlined in the previous discussions of decision making by competent patients and substitute decision making. Clinicians must understand that such actions do not place them at legal risk and often reflect the best standards of clinical practice.

In contrast to foregoing life-sustaining treatment, euthanasia and assisted suicide are legally prohibited in almost every legal system in the world. Euthanasia can be defined as an action that leads directly to the death of a patient, e.g., an injection of potassium chloride. Assisted suicide can be defined as providing patients with medical means that the patient uses to commit suicide, e.g., the prescription of a large amount of barbiturates to a patient who then uses the drugs to commit suicide.

Recent cases of physician-assisted suicide reported in the medical literature and by the media and several legislative initiatives to legalize it have placed the issues of physician-assisted suicide and euthanasia high on the public policy agenda. The main arguments supporting physician-assisted suicide and euthanasia are based on respect for patient freedom of choice and the claimed right of individuals to enlist physician assistance to end their pain and suffering by either practice. The main arguments opposing these practices include respect for human life, protection of vulnerable patients, and fear of abuse. Both proponents and opponents of physician-assisted suicide and euthanasia appeal to the role-related responsibility of being a physician to support their arguments. Even if assisted suicide and euthanasia receive legal sanction in selected jurisdictions, physicians will still be confronted with the fundamental issue of whether such practices are ethical in a medical context.

A third practice in the spectrum of end-of-life decisions is the provision of palliative care. Palliative care is ethically and legally permissible, even mandatory, and is an essential component of quality clinical care of the dying. A practical problem for physicians, however, is to distinguish palliative care from euthanasia. We suggest that if a physician's actions meet all of the following three criteria, they represent appropriate palliative care: (1) subjective or objective evidence indicates that the terminally ill patient is experiencing pain; (2) the physician's therapeutic response is commensurate with the level of the patient's pain and an ongoing feedback loop between the patient's symptoms and signs and the physician's therapeutic response is evident; and (3) the physician's intention is to relieve pain and not to kill the patient (the physician's actions do not cause an immediate death, as by administering a clearly lethal dose of a drug).

FUTILITY

Futile treatments offer absolutely no possibility of changing the patient's health status or achieving any medical goals. In such cases, the physician's responsibility to the patient and substitute decision maker changes: The physician is not required to offer a futile therapy. (Of course, the physician is obligated to provide care and counseling under these circumstances.) Unfortunately, ambiguity in determining futility arises from disagreements about both the goals of therapy and the probability of attaining the goals (e.g., 0.1%, 1%, 10%) which should be considered futile. Little agreement exists currently about who has the right to decide what interventions should be called futile. Usually, a physician describes a treatment as futile either because the probability of success is very low or because the quality of life (the goal of treatment) achievable is regarded by the physician as unacceptable. The classic example of low probability of success is the use of CPR in a patient with metastatic cancer. In these cases, the core issue is usually the patient's fear of death, and this should be addressed directly. If patient and physician continue to disagree about whether CPR should be given, the physician should either provide CPR or find the patient another doctor. If the futility discussion is about quality of life, the best judge of quality of life is the patient or substitute decision maker. Sometimes physicians are uncomfortable with providing care that they describe as futile because they consider the limited benefits or low probability of success to be a waste of scarce health care resources. Such rationing decisions should not be conflated with futility but should be addressed explicitly at the level of policy guidelines. Ad hoc attempts to ration at the bedside are often clinically and ethically unsound.

CLINICAL-ETHICAL CONCERNS IN AN ERA OF HEALTH REFORM

Two forces are driving health reform: escalating and seemingly uncontrollable health costs and the substantial number of people in America who lack health insurance, limiting their access to beneficial health services. The goals of American health reform—to provide universal access to high-quality and cost-effective health care—are laudable and ethically unproblematic. The strategies for achieving these goals include reducing administrative costs, using outcome data to rationalize services and develop clinical guidelines, and encouraging patients and physicians to participate in managed care organizations, in which a primary care physician supervises the patient's overall care. Successful efforts at cost containment may also require restricting services with marginal benefits, rationing potentially beneficial services, and limiting both patient and physician freedom to make individual clinical decisions. Many of these strategies for achieving health reform will place enormous stress on the doctor-patient relationship.

Our recommendations for maintaining the ethical integrity of medical practice and for improving patient outcomes are to emphasize the following approaches: a patient-centered approach to medicine that encourages freedom of personal choice; a maximization of patient and physician autonomy even within complex bureaucratic systems like managed care organizations and health alliances; reinforcing the centrality and importance of the doctor-patient relationship; and encouraging a focus on patients' rights when developing clinical guidelines and appeal mechanisms for the large number of clinical and administrative decisions that, despite outcomes research, will continue to be made in the face of substantial uncertainty.

CONCLUSIONS

Scientific and technologic developments in medicine have created unprecedented ethical dilemmas for physicians. The coming revolution in molecular medicine will generate additional ethical problems. In the last decade, clinical ethics has emerged as a new and useful component of medical practice by emphasizing that technical and ethical concerns are inseparable in the practice of medicine. Clinical ethics focuses on the continuing centrality of the doctor-patient relationship and on how patients and physicians work within existing administrative and political structures to reach mutual agreement on clinical decisions affecting the patient. In addition, clinical ethics offers a language of discourse that broadens the medical model from one that is narrowly technical to one that takes serious account of individual patient preferences. The language and content of clinical ethics have been adopted not only by patients, physicians, nurses, other health care providers, and medical educators but also by health economists, hospital administrators, policy developers, and judges. In this regard, ethical considerations in medicine are likely to remain an important component of medical education, clinical practice, biomedical research, and the political evolution of our health care system.

Almost 2500 years ago, Plato recognized that good clinical medicine is a marriage of scientific knowledge and human care. In Book IV of *The Laws,* he described the excellent physician as one who ". . . treats disease by going into things thoroughly from the beginning in a scientific way and takes the patient and family into confidence. Thus he learns something from the sufferer . . . . He does not give prescriptions until he has won the patient's support, and when he has done so, he steadfastly aims at providing complete restoration to health by persuading the sufferer into compliance . . . ." The best clinical medicine and patient outcomes are achieved when patient and physician have established a relationship in which technical and personal aspects of care are integrated. The practice of ethical medicine in the twenty-first century will require nothing more but demand nothing less.

Appelbaum PS, Grisso T: Assessing patients' capacities to consent to treatment. N Engl J Med 319:1635, 1988. *A review of the four factors to consider in assessing patients' decision-making capacity.*

Danis M, Southerland L, Garrett JM, et al.: A prospective study of advance directives for life-sustaining care. N Engl J Med 324:882, 1991. *Empirical study examines the effect of advance directives on clinical care.*

Emanuel LL, Barry M, Stoeckle JD, et al.: Advance directives for medical care—a case for greater use. N Engl J Med 324:889, 1991. *Empirical study examines the process of completion of advance directives.*

Epstein AM: Changes in the delivery of care under comprehensive health care reform. N Engl J Med 329:1672, 1993. *An optimistic perspective that envisions that health reform will ". . . empower physicians . . . and enrich the patient relationship."*

Jonsen AR, Siegler M, Winslade WJ: Clinical Ethics: A Practical Approach to Ethical Decisions in Clinical Medicine. 3rd ed. New York, Pergamon Press, 1990. *A practical guide to help clinicians deal with ethical problems that occur frequently in medical practice.*

Menikoff JA, Sachs GA, Siegler M: Beyond advance directives: Health care surrogate laws. N Engl J Med 327:1165, 1992. *Health care surrogate laws to enable decisions to be reached for incompetent patients may meet the needs of the large majority of patients who choose not to complete advance directives.*

Paris JJ, Schreiber MD, Statter M, et al.: Beyond autonomy—physicians' refusal to use life-prolonging extracorporeal membrane oxygenation. N Engl J Med 329:354, 1993. *Patient rights are not absolute and on occasion may be overridden by clinical factors, including especially bad prognoses.*

Quill TE, Cassel CK, Meier DE: Care of the hopelessly ill. Proposed clinical criteria for physician-assisted suicide. N Engl J Med 327:1380, 1992. *Argues for legalization of physician-assisted suicide but not voluntary euthanasia; proposes clinical criteria to guide practice of assisted suicide if legalized.*

Singer PA, Siegler M: Elective use of life-sustaining treatments. *In* Stollerman GH (ed): Advances in Internal Medicine, Vol. 36. Chicago, Year Book, 1991. *Reviews empirical studies about decisions to forego life-sustaining treatment.*

**7.9   Ross LF, Siegler M (1997) Five Major
           Themes in Bioethics. Forum: Trends
           in Experimental and Clinical Medicine
           7:8–17**

Reprinted with permission from Forum Service Editore.

PROBLEMI

Five major themes in bioethics

Lainie Friedman Ross and Mark Siegler
MacLean Center for Clinical Medical Ethics, University of Chicago, Chicago

In this paper we identify five major themes in Bioethics: i. the evolving nature of the doctor-patient relationship; ii. the impact of biotechnology on birth and death; iii. the allocation of scarce resources; iv. ethical issues in human experimentation and v. the impact of genetics and the Human Genome Project on clinical medicine. These themes represent aspects of two fundamental questions in bioethics: What is the ideal relationship between physicians and patients, and what are the proper goals of medicine? These questions must be reconsidered in the light of new and rapid advances in biotechnology. Ethical reflection on these issues may help physicians focus on the primary focus of medicine: the health and well-being of individual patients and the larger community.

Key words: doctor-patient relationship, human experimentation, genetic screening

Introduction

Although the birth of modern bioethics as a formal intellectual discipline can be dated back to the mid 1960's, ethical considerations have always been an integral part of health care. The new bioethics movement is an attempt to systematically expose the ethical issues in medical practice and research, issues that have been known and debated for centuries. The Hippocratic Oath, written over 2,000 years ago, addressed the doctor-patient relationship and the proper goals of medicine, and these concerns remain at the core of bioethics. In this paper we analyse the advances in biotechnology and the changes in the health-care environment which are forcing a re-examination of the doctor-patient relationship and the goals of medicine. Specifically, we will explore: i. the evolving nature of the doctor-patient relationship; ii. the impact of biotechnology on birth and death; iii. the allocation of scarce resources; iv. ethical issues in human experimentation and v. the impact of genetics and the Human Genome Project (HGP) on clinical medicine.

The evolving nature of the doctor-patient relationship

The centre of clinical ethics is the doctor-patient relationship (DPR). The classical model was based on beneficent paternalism, physicians acted in order to maximise their "patients' best interest" as they, the physicians, perceived those interests. This model was challenged in the U.S. and in Canada in the 1960's as patients began to view health-care as a consumer good for which they, the patients, wanted to make their own decisions and choices. This movement was supported by related trends in civil rights and women's rights movements. Patient autonomy, patient self-determination, and patient rights became the major themes (1). The relationship that evolved reflected a more equal status of doctors and patients and incorporated shared decision-making by doctors and patients.

Three major forces are now modifying the DPR in the U.S. The first is the changing financial structure of health care. Managed care has placed primary care physicians in the role of gate-keepers: clinicians who must decide when, to whom, and how often to refer their patients to specialists or to use

ETICI

other medial resources (e.g., medical tests, hospital beds). This gatekeeping role is made more complex by the conflicts of interest that the various incentive plans create for physicians (2). There is also the threat to continuity of care as managed care contracts are often purchased by corporations who seek to minimise costs and not necessarily to preserve established relationships (3, 4). Patients, as consumers, also appear willing to change plans for relatively small financial benefits (5).

The second major force modifying the DPR is the growing understanding that the basis of modern medicine is population-based rather than patient-based (6). This is seen most clearly in the growing realisation of the importance of genetics for disease susceptibility, but it is also relevant in disease prevention (e.g., the need to change behaviour in order to decrease the risk of human immune deficiency virus (HIV) transmission) and in the new emphasis on cost-effective care (7, 8). This change from a concern for the health of individuals to a concern for the health of groups creates a tension between the physician's traditional obligation to benefit the patient vs the physician's obligation to use scarce health resources in the most cost-effective way to maximise the community's benefit (9).

The third major force modifying the DPR is the increasing standardisation of medical practice that is occurring because of the technological advances and the health-outcome movements which emphasise evidence-based scientific medicine derived from well-conducted clinical trials. For a treatment to be used, the evidence must show that a treatment is effective (that the benefits outweigh the harms) and that it represents a good use of limited resources. With the increasing ability to bring the newest medical advances to the most remote towns (10, 11), the "standard of care" is being set globally (12), not locally. Physicians are now expected to keep abreast of all the newest innovations or seek expert consultation (13, 14). The effort to eliminate variations in health delivery patterns change is being reflected in the development of practice guidelines (15, 16) and consensus statements (17, 18).

The impact of biotechnology on birth and death

The traditional limits to medical care were birth and death. With the advent of *in vitro* fertilisation and foetal surgery at one end and cardio-pulmonary resuscitation and prolonged mechanical ventilation at the other end, the traditional limits of birth and death are being re-defined.

Consider, first, the wide impact of the new reproductive technologies. Their use in technologically advanced medical countries is widespread since approximately 15% of married couples have infertility problems (defined as the inability to reproduce after a year of regular intercourse without contraceptives) (19). The first successful attempt at overcoming a couple's infertility was in 1790 when the surgeon John Hunter inseminated a woman using her husband's sperm (20). The first recorded case of insemination using donor sperm took place in 1884 in Philadelphia (20). Today, assisted reproductive technologies include *in vitro* fertilisation (IVF) using the couple's own gametes, aided by intracytoplasmic sperm injection (ICSI) when there are male infertility factors, or IVF with donated gametes or surrogate mothers. The two major newsworthy stories of 1997 were the birth of a healthy child to a 63 year old woman (surpassing the Italian record by eight months)[1] and the cloning of a mammal[2].

Cloning is the technique by which the nucleus of a cell from the body of an adult is transferred into an un-fertilised egg from which the nucleus has been removed. It differs from splitting embryos (blastomere separation) which occurs naturally in identical twins and can be done in a petri dish, most frequently for pre-natal diagnosis of *in vitro* embryos. What is scientifically important about cloning is that adult cells are differentiated and perform specific functions and until the report by Wilmut et al. (21), it was not believed that an adult

---

1. Kolata G. A Record and Big Questions as Woman Gives Birth at 63. New York Times April 24, 1997: A1, A12.
2. Kolata G. Scientist Reports First Cloning Ever of Adult Mammal. The New York Times. February 23, 1997: A1, A20.

PROBLEMI

cell could regain its totipotent capability which is necessary for a single cell to divide and become a full mammal.

Cloning had been raised at the beginning of the modern bioethics movement by the Nobel Laureate Joshua Lederberg in 1966 (22). His essay prompted comments from two leading bioethicists: Joseph Fletcher (23) and Paul Ramsey (24), but focus drifted away after the first successful birth of an IVF infant (25) and "the President's Commission devoted only a single footnote to cloning in its report on genetic manipulation, Splicing Life (26)". To some extent the cloning of a mammal is not very different from natural twinning and the splitting of embryos which result in two humans with identical genetic material. Actually, this is not quite accurate as a clone receives its cytoplasm from the enucleated egg which carries some genetic material. This means that the clone does not share all of its genetic material as do twins born naturally or from split embryos. Another difference is that natural twins develop simultaneously whereas clones can be born years or decades apart (the same is true with embryo splitting if one of the so-produced embryos is frozen). Clones differ from split embryos in that there is a finite number of embryos that can be created by embryo splitting because of the need for a certain amount of cytoplasmic material whereas the number of duplicated clones is theoretically infinite.

In June 1997, less than three months after Wilmut published his experiment, the U.S. National Bioethics Advisory Commission (NBAC) issued its report. NBAC concluded that creating children by nuclear transfer is unethical at this time because "it would expose the foetus and the developing child to unacceptable risks (27)". This conclusion is reminiscent of the early arguments against *in vitro* fertilisation: the uncertainty of whether conception *ex vivo* and manual implantation would have any negative impact on the developing embryo (28). All of those arguments were found, in retrospect, to be unfounded (29, 30). NBAC added that even if concerns about safety are resolved, significant concerns remain about the negative impact of the use of such a technology on both individuals and society

(27). NBAC supported continued research in cloning of animals as well as continued public debate on the ethical issues raised by the prospect of human cloning (27).

One such concern is the right of individuals to define their own personal identity. The argument is that the genetic lottery ensures the uniqueness of children so that children are free to establish their own identity. In contrast, if one clones a famous artist or scientist, the parents may only encourage particular skills so the child is not free to establish his or her own identity. The fallacy with this concern is that it ignores the fact that parents raise children with expectations and seek to develop particular traits as well as particular values and beliefs whether the child is cloned or is a product of nature's lottery. It also ignores that mating is not random: that we select our mates for particular traits and we hope to pass their desirable traits on to our children. But most importantly, it ignores the fact that an individual is defined by both his genetic make-up as well as by his environment. This is most obvious when one looks at discordance in health outcomes (31, 32), sexual identity (33), and personality and lifestyle choices between identical twins (34).

Not only have advances in biotechnology changed how and when we pro-create, they have also re-defined how and when we die. The 1960's saw the development of cardiopulmonary resuscitation (35), and the ability to reverse "death" as it was then defined. This led to the notion of "irreversible coma" and the concept of brain death (36), which was important for the emerging field of organ transplantation.

The success of the new critical care technologies were tempered by the fact that although they can restore biological function, they do not always add or restore quality to these lives. The result was that individuals began to demand the right to refuse such treatments, a right which is now generally respected in the U.S. for competent adults[3] and their proxy decision makers[4]. However, there are several studies

---

3. In re Brooks Estate, 32 Ill2d 361, 205 NE2d 435 (1965).
4. In re Quinlan 70 NJ 10, 355 A 2d 647 cert denied sub nom., Garger v. New Jersey, 429 U.S. 922 (1976).

that suggest that patient values in end-of-life decisions are often unknown, and even when known, are frequently ignored (37, 38). The right to refuse life-saving treatment has also been confused with the idea that death has somehow become elective and the 1990's have witnessed a clamour that there is or ought to be a right to die with the aid of a physician, so called physician-assisted suicide (PAS) (39). Surveys show that PAS may occur with some frequency in the U.S. (40, 41), although to date, such practices are legitimised only in the Netherlands (42). Recently, the U.S. Supreme Court denied that individuals have a right to PAS under the U.S. constitution[5].

The allocation of scarce resources

There has always been rationing of health-care, whether it come in terms of a limited number of dialysis machines or intensive care unit beds, whether it reflects the lack of access to those who do not have the ability to pay, or whether it is based on a system of queuing for a needed health resource. Yet there are still many Americans who believe that rationing of health care can be avoided[6]. They argue that if we cut waste, inefficiency and market incentives to spend more on health-care, we can have enough affordable health care for all. To some extent they are right: we can choose to allocate more and more of our gross national product (GNP) to health-care. But the need for health-care is unlimited and so at some point there will necessarily be individuals who do not get all the health care that could benefit them. In addition, the assumption that there is no need to ration only holds true if there are no resources that are scarce, irrespective of price. The paradigmatic example is organ transplantation.

Consider, then, the question of how to allocate kidneys for transplantation. In 1995, over 30,000 individuals were awaiting kidney transplant in the U.S.; but fewer than 12,000 transplants were performed[7]. Discussions of kidney organ allocation are tempered by the existence of an alternate treatment, dialysis. Long-term dialysis developed in the 1960's with the development of an artificial shunt that allowed for multiple

re-cannulations (43). Soon thereafter, the physicians at the University of Washington had to deal with the question of how to choose between the hundreds of candidates who could benefit from long-term dialysis. Their decision was to have two committees to make these decisions: i. a medical advisory committee composed of physicians interested in renal disease and a psychiatrist to choose candidates who met the medical criteria for treatment; and ii. an admissions and policy committee composed of laymen and physicians who would formulate and apply non-medical criteria. The latter committee considered the following factors in choosing patients for dialysis: "...sex of patient; marital status and number of dependents; income; net worth; emotional stability, with particular regard to the patient's capacity to accept the treatment; educational background; nature of occupation, past performance and future potential; and names of people who could serve as references[8]".

Criticisms of the Seattle program were harsh and quick. The committee was called the "God Squad," with many voicing their ethical disagreement with the criteria that were used in selecting dialysis candidates.

In response to the publicity surrounding the tragic choices that were being made by the Seattle group and other dialysis centres, Congress passed PL 92-603 in October, 1972, weeks before a major Federal election. This bill extended coverage of Medicare to greater than 90% of the U.S. population who needed kidney transplantation and dialysis as well as extending cash disability benefits. The original cost estimates in the U.S. House of Representatives for this

---

5. Washington et al. v. Glucksberg et al., U.S. Supreme Court No. 96-110. Argued January 8, 1997 - Decided June 26, 1997.

6. Lantos J. citing Magaziner I (1993) during work on the Clinton Health Care Reform Project, St Margherita di Pula, Italy 1997.

7. 1996 Annual Report of the U.S. Scientific Registry for Transplant Recipients and the Organ Procurement and Transplantation Network -Transplant Data: 1988-1995. UNOS, Richmond VA and the Division of Transplantation, Bureau of Health Resources Development, Health Resources and Services Administration, U.S. Department of Health and Human Services, Rockville, MD, 1996.

8. Alexander S. "They decide who lives, who dies: Medical miracle puts a moral burden on a small committee." Life 1962: 53 ((November 1962): 106 as cited in Fox and Swazey, op. cit.

PROBLEMI

entitlement was $35-75 million in the first year increasing to $250 million by year 4. Federal experts gave higher estimates: $135 million in the first year, $1 billion by 10 years. The actual expenses were $240 million in the first year and $1 billion in year 4 (43). By 1990, treatment for end-stage-renal-disease cost $7.3 billion[9].

Money cannot solve all scarce resource allocation issues as there are some resources which are truly scarce; e.g., organs for transplantation. Attempts to devise just criteria for the allocation of cadaveric kidneys for transplantation have met with sharp criticisms. Using histocompatibility factors alone tends to discriminate against potential minority recipients who tend to need kidneys at a disproportionate rate. As a result, the United Network of Organ Sharing (UNOS) uses a formula which gives points for length of time on the waiting-list as well as histo-compatibility criteria. Racial inequities persist despite changes in the UNOS formula (44), and they may be even greater because not all patients with end-stage kidney disease are even considered potential candidates. There are still great inequalities regarding who gets placed on the organ waiting-list in the first place and how quickly.

Recently, the Patient Care and Education Committee of the American Society of Transplant Physicians surveyed transplant centres around the country. In this survey, they found "significant heterogeneity in the approach to certain medical conditions evaluated prior to renal transplantation" from HIV to coronary-artery disease to hepatitis (45). This heterogeneity suggests the value-laden nature of what are often termed medical indications. For example, although many centres exclude all HIV-positive patients from transplant waiting-lists, there is a small but growing experience of transplantation in HIV-positive patients which show that there are cases of prolonged patient survival for up to 56 months post-transplantation[7]. Other programs exclude individuals on the basis of age alone, even though age is a poor marker for inter-individual variation of overall health, productivity, and life-expectancy.

The inequities in kidney transplantation are somewhat attenuated by the availability of dialysis, but transplantation for most other solid organs have no alternative treatment options. The criteria used in these transplant programs vary among programs (46). Transplant surgeons and ethicists argue about the appropriateness and fairness of both psycho-social as well as medical criteria. For example, liver transplant surgeons and ethicists recently decided that since livers are so scarce, that the probability of benefit should be given greater weight in the distribution of livers[10]. The public outcry regarding the new criteria is proof of the value-laden nature of these seemingly "medical criteria"[11]. Others have noted that the present criteria lead to serious gender and financial inequities in various transplant programs (47, 48).

One way to alleviate some of the stress in allocation decisions is to increase the supply of organs from both cadavers and living donors. Despite large educational campaigns (49, 50) required request laws (51), and an increased willingness to accept older and unrelated living donors (52), supply is greater than the demand and the gap continues to grow.

Despite resistance to acknowledge the need to ration in U.S. health-care debates, the criteria used in organ transplantation decisions are criteria on how to ration. Similarly, rationing occurs in triaging for intensive care unit beds and in decisions regarding access to care. The critical issue is how to develop socially and medically acceptable distribution procedures. Although ethicists have written large tomes on how scarce resources should be allocated (53, 54, 55), there is no consensus on what factors should be included and on the relative significance of these factors.

Human experimentation

The Nuremberg Code was the first code of ethics specifically written to address the

---

9. NIH Consensus Panel Report, 93: Morbidity and Mortality of Dialysis, November 1993.
10. UNOS Liver Allocation Policy Fact Sheet, 1997.
11. New Transplant Rules Upset Some. New York Times. Monday November 18, 1996: A9.

ETICI

ethics of human experimentation[12]. This code was adopted in response to the documented abuse by the Nazis of human beings as research subjects, and it was quickly followed by other national and international codes[13, 14]. Twenty years after the Nuremberg trials, Henry Beecher (56) documented the unethical research methods and practices used in many studies published in U.S. medical journals. The Tuskegee syphilis study that did not end until 1972 (57), and the more recent revelations regarding the Cold War radiation experiments performed in the U.S. in the 1940's and 1950's are proof that this topic must remain an essential focus for bioethics today[15].

The first principle in human experimentation as addressed in the Nuremberg Code was the need for informed consent: "The voluntary consent of the human subject is absolutely essential[12]. This principle has been modified to allow for proxy consent in order that some research can be done on children and other individuals who lack decision-making capacity.

One area of research that challenges the standard views of informed consent is research in the acute care setting. Often the patient-subjects are critically ill, decisionally incompetent and the experimental therapies must be given immediately. As such, there is no time to find surrogates, and even if a surrogate is present, there is no time to get full and voluntary consent. Federal Regulations were recently promulgated that allow for the waiver of informed consent requirements in certain emergency research (58).

Another controversial area of research is research in third-world countries sponsored by first-world countries. Consider, for example, a recent U.S. government-sponsored research program to test a short course of zidovudine (AZT) to prevent vertical transmission of HIV from a pregnant woman to her foetus. It is known that large doses of AZT in the last two trimesters of pregnancy, during labour and delivery, and then to the infant post-partum reduces vertical transmission from 25% to 8% (59). This regimen is too expensive for routine management of women in third-world countries. The U.S. government decided to study a short course of AZT in these countries (which would be affordable) against placebo (the present day "standard of care" in these countries). All agree that this study could not be done in the U.S. because here the short regimen would have to be tested against the longer regimen, the standard of care in the U.S. Critics contend that if the study would be unethical here, it should be unethical everywhere. The government's justification is that only if a cheap therapy can be developed will women in these countries be offered any therapy, a position supported by AIDS researchers from around the world (60).

Genetic screening and genetic therapy

The HGP was officially initiated in 1990 with a 15-year, $3 billion budget. Its goals include mapping and sequencing the human genome and developing technologies which can be transferred to medicine and industry. Three percent of the budget is allocated to considering the ethical, legal, and social implications of the HGP.

The main ethical issues raised by the new genetics are: how to procure informed consent, when to respect and when to override the principle of confidentiality, and what does justice require with respect to the new genetics. A more practical issue is that genetic testing is developing much more quickly than genetic therapy which raises the issue of what good is prediction when no treatments are presently available.

The doctrine of informed consent enables a competent adult patient to accept or refuse medical care. It is a process in which both

12. Permissible Medical Experiments. Trials of War Criminals before the Nuremberg Military Tribunals under Control Council Law No. 10: Nuremberg October 1946-April 1949. Washington: U.S. Government Printing Office (n.d.), 2: 181-182.
13. 18th World Medical Association, Declaration of Helsinki: Recommendations Guiding Medical Doctors in Biomedical Research Involving Human Subjects. Helsinki Finland, 1964 (revised most recently by the 41st World Medical Association in Hong Kong, September, 1989).
14. American Medical Association. Ethical Guidelines for Clinical Investigation (1966).
15. Faden RR et al. eds.; Advisory Committee on Human Radiation Experiments: Final Report. Washington DC: U.S. Government Printing Office, 1995.

PROBLEMI

the physician and patient play an active role. The physician discloses to the patient the prognosis, the proposed treatment and its alternatives, and the risks and benefits of the various treatments including the option of refusing treatment. The patient is free to ask questions, to consult with other health-care providers, and to discuss options with his family. The patient ultimately gives consent or refuses to give consent. Whatever decision the patient makes, the physician must respect his wishes. For adults, this same approach would apply when a physician proposes a genetic screening test.

While it is difficult to define the optimal level of disclosure, there is evidence that physicians tend to minimise uncertainty and gloss over many risks (61). This is compounded when the medical diagnosis involves genetics as there are several studies documenting physicians' misunderstanding and inability at discussing genetics (62, 63). This is due to several factors: i. the rapidly evolving nature of genetic knowledge; ii. that the same genetic condition may express at different ages and with different degrees of severity, even within one particular family; and iii. that genetic tests may only signify an increased risk rather than a pre-condition. As such, discussions regarding genetics must be explained in terms of probability and degrees of penetrance.

Informed consent for children is complicated by the need to include three parties in the DPR: the child, his or her parents and the physician. The American Academy of Pediatrics argues for a greater role for children, particularly when the decision is not life-threatening (64). If adopted this would have great implications for decisions regarding genetic testing for late-onset and/or untreatable conditions.

Confidentiality is integral to the traditional DPR, and genetic information deserves even greater protection than typical medical information because genetic information makes predictions about an individual's medical future and may have an unforeseen impact on the life of an individual and his or her family. There are, however, valid arguments against strict confidentiality of genetic information, particularly within families because genetic information applies to family members as well as to the individual. Information gleaned from testing may clearly be of vital importance to relatives, (e.g., a brother who works around environmental contaminants that may be unusually harmful due to a genetic trait) and to spouses (or potential spouses) who may desire to be informed of genetic traits prior to reproduction (65).

Given the time-consuming nature of genetic testing and genetic counselling, both will be scarce resources for the near future. This requires a public discussion of how equity can be achieved both for present day genetic testing and counselling, but also for the future when gene therapy becomes a reality (66). Major problems include; i. how to define equity in access to genetic services; ii. to what extent should access to genetic information be protected from third-parties and iii. what types of protection should be in place to guide experimentation with gene therapy.

Conclusions

Ethical considerations are integral to the clinical care of patients. Technical expertise alone does not address many of the issues raised within the DPR, a personal and moral relationship that is being challenged by interested third parties (payers, families, researchers, and health-care observers). The extraordinary technological developments of the past fifty years have revolutionised medicine. It is forcing us to reconsider what are and what ought to be the proper goals of medicine. In this paper we have addressed five areas of medicine in which the goals are being stretched or modified by new and evolving biotechnologies. We believe that medicine is, and must remain, committed primarily to the well-being of individuals while also attending to the health of the wider community, commitments which may conflict in particular cases. Ethics provides the tools to deal with such conflicts and with other challenges raised by the new technological advances in medicine.

Acknowledgements

The MacLean Center for Clinical Medical Ethics is supported by grants from The

ETICI

Andrew W. Mellon Foundation, The Pew Charitable Trusts, The Harris Foundation, and The Field Foundation of Illinois.

References

1. American Hospital Association. A *Patient's Bill of Rights*. 1973.
2. Hillman AL et al. How do financial incentives affect physicians' clinical decisions and the financial performance of health maintenance organizations? *N. Engl. J. Med.* 1989; **321**: 86-92.
3. Emanuel EJ and Brett AS. Managed Competition and the Patient-Physician Relationship. *N. Engl. J. Med.* 1993; **329**: 879-882.
4. Thomasma DC. The ethics of managed care; challenges to the principles of relationship-centered care. *J. Allied Health* 1996; **25**: 233-246.
5. Buchmueller TC and Feldstein PJ. Consumers' sensitivity to health plan premiums: evidence from a natural experiment in California. *Health Affairs* 1996; **15**: 143-151.
6. Jonsen AR. *The New Medicine and the Old Ethics*. Cambridge MA: Harvard University Press, 1990.
7. Gage BF et al. Cost-effectiveness of warfarin and aspirin for prophylaxis of stroke in patients with nonvalvular atrial fibrillation. *JAMA* 1995; **274**: 1839-1845.
8. Cronenwett JL et al. Cost-effectiveness of carotid endarterectomy in asymptomatic patients. *J. Vasc. Surg.* 1997; **25**: 298-309.
9. Jamison DT et al. Investing in health wisely. The role of needs-based technology assessment. *Int. J. Tech. Assessment in Health Care* 1995; **11**: 673-684.
10. Urban V et al. Teleconsultation: a new neurosurgical image transfer system for daily routine and emergency cases-a four-year study. *Eur. J. Emerg. Med.* 1996; **3**: 5-8.
11. Jennett PA. The use of advanced computer technology to enhance access to health care and to respond to community needs: the results of the evaluation of a technology-based clinical consultation service. *Medinfo.* 1995; **8** (part 2): 1479-1481.
12. Blonde L et al. American College of Physicians (ACP) medical informatics and telemedicine. *J. Medical Systems* 1995; **19**: 131-137.
13. Walters TJ. Deployment telemedicine: the Walter Reed Army Medical Center experience. *Military Medicine* 1996; **161**: 531-536.
14. Cheriff AD et al. Telesurgical consultation. *J. Urol.* 1996; **156**: 1391-1393.
15. Hadorn DC and Baker D. Development of the AHCPR-sponsored heart failure guideline: methodologic and procedural issues. *Joint Commission. J. Qual. Improvement* 1994; **20**: 539-547.
16. Clinton JJ et al. Enhancing clinical practice. The role of practice guidelines. *Am. Psychologist* 1994; **49**: 30-33.
17. Vanderpump MP et al. Consensus statement for good practice and audit measures in the management of hypothyroidism and hyperthyroidism. The Research Unit of the Royal College of Physicians of London, the Endocrinology and Diabetes Committee of the Royal College of Physicians of London, and the Society for Endocrinology. *Br. Med. J.* 1996; **313**: 539-544.
18. Garnick MB, Fair WR. First International Conference on Neoadjuvant Hormonal Therapy of Prostate Cancer: overview consensus statement. *Urology* 1997; **49** (Suppl. 3A): 1-4.
19. U.S. Congress, Office of Technology Assessment. *Infertility: Medical and Social Choices*. Washington DC: Government Printing Office, 1988.
20. Corea G. The Subversive Sperm: A False Strain of Blood. In: RT Hull ed.; *Ethical Issues in the New Reproductive Technologies*. Belmont CA: Wadsworth Publishing Co., 1990.
21. Wilmut I et al. Viable offspring derived from fetal and adult mammalian cells. *Nature* 1997; **385**: 810-813.
22. Lederberg J. Experimental Genetics and Human Evolution. *The American Naturalist* 1966; **100**: 519-531.
23. Fletcher J. Ethical Aspects of Genetic Controls: Designed Genetic Changes in Man. *N. Engl. J. Med.* 1971; **285**: 776-783.
24. Ramsey P. *Fabricated Man: The Ethics of Genetic Control*. New Haven CT: Yale University Press, 1970.
25. Steptoe PC and Edwards RG. Birth after the Reimplantation of a Human Embryo. *Lancet* 1978; **ii**: p. 366.
26. Annas GJ. Regulatory Models for Human Embryo Cloning: The Free Market, Professional Guidelines, and Government Restrictions. *Kennedy Institute of Ethics Journal* 1994; **4**: 235-249.
27. National Bioethics Advisory Commission. *Cloning Human Beings*. Report and Recommendations of the National Bioethics Advisory Commission. 1997.
28. Kass LR. Making Babies: The New Biology and the "Old" Morality. In: *Toward a More Natural Science*. New York: The Free Press, 1985.
29. Olivennes F et al. Follow-up of 422 children aged 6 to 13 years conceived by *in vitro* fertilization. *Fertility and Sterility* 1997; **67**: 284-289.
30. Morin NC et al. Congenital malformations

PROBLEMI

and psychosocial development in children conceived by *in vitro* fertilization. *J. Pediatr.* 1989; **115**: 222-227.

31. Smith CK et al. Life change and onset of cancer in identical twins. *J. Psychosom. Res.* 1984; **28**: 525-532.

32. Gregersen PK. Discordance for auto-immunity in monozygotic twins. Are "identical" twins really identical? *Arthritis Rheum.* 1993; **36**: 1185-1192.

33. Whitam FL et al. Homosexual orientation in twins: A report on 61 pairs and three triplet sets. *Arch. Sexual Behav.* 1993; **22**: 187-206.

34. Swan GE et al. Psychological characteristics in twins discordant for smoking behavior: A matched-twin pair analysis. *Addictive Behav.* 1988; **13**: 51-60.

35. Kouwenhoven WB et al. Closed-chest cardiac massage. JAMA 1960; **173**: 1064-1067.

36. Report of the Ad Hoc Committee of the Harvard Medical School to Examine the Definition of Brain Death. A definition of irreversible coma. JAMA 1968; **205**: 337-340.

37. A Controlled Trial to Improve Care for Seriously Ill Hospitalized Patients. The Study to Understand Prognoses and Preferences for Outcomes and Risks of Treatments (SUPPORT). JAMA 1995; **274**: 1591-1598.

38. Haas JS et al. Discussions of preferences for life-sustaining care by persons with AIDS: predictors of failure in patient-physician communication. *Arch. Intern. Med.* 1993; **153**: 1241-1248.

39. Blendon RJ et al. Should Physicians Aid Patients in Dying?: The Public Perspective. JAMA 1992; **267**: 2658-2662.

40. Back AL et al. Physician-Assisted Suicide and Euthanasia in Washington State: Patient requests and physician responses. JAMA 1996; **275**: 919-925.

41. Slome LR et al. Physician-Assisted Suicide and patients with Human Immunodeficiency Virus Disease. *N. Engl. J. Med.* 1997; **336**: 417-421.

42. van der Wal G et al. Evaluation of the notification procedure for physician-assisted death in the Netherlands. *N. Engl. J. Med.* 1996; **335**: 1706-1711.

43. Fox RC and Swazey JP. *The Courage to Fail: A Social View of Organ Transplants and Dialysis*, 2nd Edition.; revised. Chicago IL: University of Chicago Press, 1978.

44. Kasiske B et al. The effect of race on access and outcome in transplantation. *N. Engl. J. Med.* 1991; **324**: 302-307.

45. Ramos EL et al. The Evaluation of Candidates for Renal Transplantation: The Current Practice of U.S. Transplant Centers. *Transplantation* 1994; **57**: 490-497.

46. Levenson JL and Olbrisch ME. Psychosocial Evaluation of Organ Transplant Candidates: A Comparative Survey of Process, Criteria, and Outcomes in Heart, Liver, and Kidney Transplantation. *Psychosomatics* 1993; **34**: 314-323.

47. Sharples L et al. Who waits longest for heart and lung transplantation? *J. Heart and Lung Transplant.* 1994; **13**: 282-291.

48. Tuttle-Newhall JE et al. A statewide, population-based, time series analysis of access to liver transplantation. *Transplantation* 1997; **63**: 255-262.

49. Ganikos ML et al. A case study in planning for public health education: the organ and tissue donation experience. *Public Health Reports* 1994; **109**: 626-631.

50. Callender CO et al. A National Minority Organ/Tissue Transplant Education Program: The First Step in the Evolution of a National Minority Strategy and Minority Transplant Equity in the USA. *Transplant. Proc.* 1995; **27**: 1441-1443.

51. Virnig BA and Caplan AL. Required request: what difference has it made? *Transplant. Proc.* 1992; **24**: 2155-2158.

52. Spital A. Unrelated Living Kidney Donors: An Update of attitudes and use among U.S. Transplant Centers. *Transplantation* 1994; **57**: 1722-1726.

53. Kilner JF. *Who Lives? Who Dies? Ethical Criteria in Patient Selection.* New Haven CT: Yale University Press, 1990.

54. Elster J and Herpin N, eds.; *The Ethics of Medical Choice.* London UK: St Martin's Press Inc., 1994.

55. Menzel PT. *Strong Medicine: The Ethical Rationing of Health Care.* New York: Oxford University Press, 1990.

56. Beecher HK. Ethics and Clinical Research *N. Engl. J. Med.* 1966; **274**: 1354-1360.

57. Jones JH. *Bad Blood: The Tuskegee Syphilis Experiment.* New York: The Free Press, 1981.

58. National Institutes of Health, Department of Health and Human Services. Waiver of Informed Consent Requirements in Certain emergency Research. 45 CFR Part 46. *Federal Register* 1996; **61**: 51531-51533.

59. Connor EM et al. Reduction of maternal-infant transmission of human immuno-deficiency virus type 1 with zidovudine treatment. Pediatric AIDS Clinical Trials Group Protocol 076 Study Group. *N. Engl. J. Med.* 1994; **331**: 1173-1180.

60. Cohen J. Ethics of AZT Studies in Poorer Countries Attacked. *Science* 1997; **276**: p. 1022.

61. Katz J. Why Doctors Don't Disclose Uncertainty. *Hastings Center Report* 1984; **14**: 35-44.

62. Hofman K et al. Physicians Knowledge of Genetics and Genetic Tests. *Academic*

ETICI

Medicine 1993; **68**: 625-632.

63. Giardiello F et al. The Use and Interpretation of Commercial APC Gene Testing for Familial Adenomatous Polyposis. *N. Engl. J. Med.* 1997; **336**: 823-827.

64. American Academy of Pediatrics, Committee on Bioethics, Informed Consent, Parental Permission, and Assent in Pediatric Practice. *Pediatr.* 1995; **95**: 314-317.

65. Moon MR and Ross LF. Ethical Issues in the New Genetics. *FORUM Trends Exp. Clin. Med.* 1997; **3**: 295-307.

66. Murphy T and Lappe M eds.; *Justice and the human genome project.* Berkeley CA: University of California Press, 1994.

7.10 Siegler M (1997) The Contributions of Clinical Ethics to Patient Care. Forum: Trends in Experimental and Clinical Medicine 7:244–51

Reprinted with permission from Forum Service Editore.

REVIEW

The contributions of clinical ethics to patient care

Mark Siegler

MacLean Center for Clinical Medical Ethics; Department of Medicine, Section of General Internal Medicine; University of Chicago, Chicago, Illinois

This paper explores the following central questions about contemporary medical ethics: has the discipline of medical ethics improved patient care? and was improvement in clinical practice a central goal of traditional medical ethics? Although traditional medical ethics may not have improved patient care, such improvement is the principal focus of the new discpline of "clinical ethics". The paper describes the goals and methods of clinical ethics and then examines the following five specific ways in which clinical ethics improves patient care: i. by direct patient services, ii. teaching, iii. research, iv. encouraging innovations and new biotechnologies and v. by preserving the traditions of the doctor-patient relationship.
FORUM Trends in Experimental and Clinical Medicine, 7: 244-251, 1997

Key Words: clinical medical ethics, patient care, doctor-patient relationship, ethics teaching, ethics research

Introduction

For the past thirty years, the North American bioethics movement has systematically examined the moral basis of clinical and research practices and has contributed an enormously valuable perspective to medicine. Bioethics used the focus of theological ethics in the 1960's and philosophical ethics and law since the 1970's to probe and constructively criticise medicine. The bioethics movement emphasised patient autonomy, patient rights, and broad public policy concerns such as distributive justice in health care. On the whole, bioethicists have been "loving critics", of medicine but their goal has always been to improve medicine, at least in theory. But what about another goal, improving medicine in practice, that is,

improving patient care? Here, unfortunately, the contributions of bioethics are less clear. In 1978, I wrote: "Whatever else medical ethics is, it must have something to do with the practice of clinical medicine, or at least it should" (1). Others disagree, for example, Callahan (2), the former director of the Hastings Center on Bioethics, recently wrote: "While I would hardly want to overlook the needs of the [physician] practitioner, I now wonder if that is the right place to centre our attention. Does reality lie in the particularity of individual cases where most clinicians think it does or in a more general abstract and universal realm?" In this paper, I will consider the following set of questions:

i. has the discipline of medical ethics improved patient care?

ii. was improvement in patient care a central goal of medical ethics?

iii. what is clinical medical ethics?

iv. what have been the contributions of clinical medical ethics to patient care?

Correspondence should be addressed to: Mark Siegler, MacLean Center for Clinical Medical Ethics, Department of Medicine, Section of General Internal Medicine, University of Chicago, 5841 S. Maryland Avenue, MC 6098 CH, Illinois, USA

REVIEW

Has the discipline of medical ethics improved patient care?

Consider the following question: what has been the record of the North American medical ethics movement in contributing to improving the quality of patient care or improving the compassion, empathy and respect physicians have for patients, or in improving the doctor-patient relationship or the process of clinical decisions?

The short answer to these questions is "we don't know". Unfortunately, even after thirty years, there have been very few, almost no studies examining the impact of medical ethics on the quality of patient care or on patient outcomes. Eddy (3) has recently enumerated a set of principles for deciding whether to invest scarce social resources on a new treatment. I suggest the same principles could be applied to decide whether to invest in a new social or educational innovation such as medical ethics. Eddy suggests that before a new approach is adopted:

i. there must be convincing evidence that it works;
ii. that its benefits outweigh harms;
iii. that it represents good use of limited resources;
iv. that these judgments of efficiency and cost-effectiveness reflect the views not only of the community encouraging the innovation but also the preferences of those who are to receive the innovation.

Sadly, contemporary medical ethics has not met these tests. We have almost no outcome studies showing a positive benefit from the bioethics revolution.

A few years ago, Kass criticised the ethics movement for being too theoretical, philosophical, hyperrational, and ideological, while at the same time failing to examine routine practice issues and failing to consider the habits and behaviours of physicians and the profession. Kass (4) considered the issue of outcomes and wrote: "Though originally intended to improve our deeds, the practice of ethics, if truth be told, has, at best, improved our speech. The real action in practicing ethics will begin when we again see ethics as practice, as the combining of character and custom, in

conduct that both creates and manifests the human agent, negotiating the many challenges of the human condition".

There is considerable evidence to suggest that Kass is correct and that the state of medicine and of ethical medical practices is not much better in 1997 than it was at the birth of the American ethics movement thirty years ago. During that time, we have witnessed escalating health-care costs, a steady decline in access to health-care, and progressive deterioration in the doctor-patient relationship. Of course, it isn't appropriate to hold medical ethics entirely responsible for all the troubling changes in medicine that have occurred during the past thirty years. But, consider changes in one particular area, end-of-life care, a central preoccupation of American medical ethics for thirty years.

Despite hundreds of court decisions and many new laws about end-of-life care, the data from the SUPPORT study (5) is shocking on how badly we care for the dying, not only clinically, in failing to provide adequate pain medicine, but ethically, in failing to respect the wishes of dying persons. Another report from the SUPPORT investigators (6) highlights the ineffectiveness of "do not resuscitate" orders and advance directives in changing the quality of end of life care. I suspect the same findings would be uncovered if we did a SUPPORT-type study on informed consent in clinical practice or on any other ethical aspect of medicine, truth-telling, confidentiality, justice, that we believe we have resolved in theory.

Was improvement in patient care a central goal of traditional medical ethics?

During the very early years of the bioethics movement, two different kinds of clinicians, physicians such as Henry Beecher, and theologians trained in the ministry such as James Gustafsen, Paul Ramsey, Richard McCormick and Joseph Fletcher, brought a powerful clinical sense to the bioethics discipline and were dedicated to improving actual practice. In those early years, the bioethics movement focused on improving

REVIEW

clinical research, end-of-life care, and on incorporating patient values into clinical decisions.

For reasons still not entirely clear, this first wave of clinically-oriented bioethicists was soon replaced by theoreticians from non-clinical disciplines, especially philosophy, law, the humanities, and the social sciences. The new bioethicists turned away from a central focus on patient care to examine other concerns such as justice in health care, the ethics of clinical research, the definition of death, ethical issues in genetics, and the tension between patient autonomy and physician paternalism. In fact, in the 1970's, some of the non-clinician bioethicists expressed disdain for the traditional patient-physician bedside ethic that had existed in medicine from the time of Hippocrates and urged, instead, that it be replaced by a more social, political and legal perspective. In the past, I have sometimes referred to this shift from a clinical and theological perspective to a philosophical-legal-economic perspective as the secularisation of bioethics (7).

Two results of this shift in direction were that clinicians and medical students were increasingly distanced from the theoretical field of bioethics. Second, the legal reform movement, proceeding through legislation and judicial opinions, did not have as much of an impact on bedside practice and patient care as many thought or hoped it would. Again, the best evidence for this is our documented inadequacies in providing good end-of-life care despite much legislation and many judicial opinions.

These views should not be seen as an indictment of bioethicists for their failures. In fact, bioethicists and the bioethics movement did brilliantly in contributing their disciplinary insights to the task of examining and analysing medicine and, in the process, they gave clinicians and medical educators new tools to apply. Whatever failures exist in translating these insights into improving patient care should be viewed not as the responsibility of bioethicists but of clinicians and medical educators.

What is clinical medical ethics?

I will begin to answer the question from a personal perspective. In 1972, when I returned to the University of Chicago from training in England, I was given responsibility to direct our hospital's first medical intensive care unit. Of course, by modern standards, our unit was small and very primitive. Nevertheless, it was during those years that I served as director of the intensive care unit, that my students and residents began to question me about some of the practices in our unit: did we tell patients and families the truth about the patient's prognosis? Were some of our intensive care procedures experimental, and if so had the patients or their families given consent? Since we only had five beds in the unit, how did we decide which patients would be admitted to the unit and receive the benefits of a scarce resource? Once we started care with the mechanical ventilator, was it ever permissible to stop the breathing machine?

Faced with these questions and others like them, I quickly discovered that there was no place to send my housestaff and students to find answers. The medical literature and textbooks did not discuss these matters. The new literature in medical bioethics, written largely by philosophers and legal scholars, did not address the practical concerns raised by medical students and house officers. The language of theory was not helpful in resolving the dilemmas of practice. Physicians and patients needed help to better understand the ethical issues in clinical practice so they could incorporate ethical analysis into their decisions. It was essential that doctors and researchers and patients become more involved in discussions about these new questions in medical ethics. In this view, medical ethics is closer to clinical practice than it is to theoretical ethics and its main goal should be to help patients and doctors and families.

Good clinical care requires that technical and scientific considerations be integrated with personal and ethical considerations (8). Ethical concerns have always been an essential part of medical practice, from Hippocrates to James Gregory to the present day. However, the extraordinary scientific achievements of the past fifty years, achievements unparalleled in history,

REVIEW

achievements that include safe blood transfusions, antibiotics, open heart surgery, dialysis machines, transplantation, critical care units, protease inhibitors, and new reproductive technologies, with newer ones on the horizon, have increased the range, intensity and frequency of ethical issues in medicine and have contributed to the emergence of clinical ethics as an important component of medicine, not just a discipline of applied philosophy.

Goals and methods

To return to the question: what is clinical medical ethics and what are its goals? Clinical medical ethics is a practical and applied discipline that aims to improve patient care and patient outcomes (9). It focuses on the doctor-patient relationship and takes account of the ethical and legal issues that patients, doctors, and hospitals, must address to reach the best decisions for individual patients. Clinical ethics emphasises that in practising good clinical medicine, physicians must combine scientific and technical abilities with ethical concerns for the personal values of the patient who seeks their help.

Clinical ethics is more than a study of individual cases, and more than ethics consultations, and more than applied medical casuistry. Each of these, individual cases, consultations, and casuistical reasoning, is a part of clinical ethics, but the field is larger than any of these three and larger than all three together. In clinical ethics, the resolution of an individual case is a mere example, a specification, of what the goals of clinical ethics are: to improve clinical care and medical outcomes generally.

The goal of clinical ethics is to assist patients, families and health professionals to make a good health care decision for patients who come to them seeking help. In short, the goal is to improve patient care and outcome. The method used to achieve the goals of clinical medical ethics is to identify, analyse and address some specific ethical issues that arise in patient care both at the level of the patient-provider and at the level of the health system and to offer a structured approach to decision-making that can assist

patients and physicians to resolve clinical ethical problems.

Content

The content of clinical ethics includes the study of the doctor-patient relationship and of specific ethical issues. The doctor-patient relationship involves study of such issues as honesty, competence, integrity, and respect for persons. Thus clinical ethics must include a focus on the ethos of the professional and on the character and virtues of the physician, who is expected by the public to demonstrate these character qualities. In addition, clinical ethics examines specific clinical ethical issues including truth-telling, informed consent, end-of-life care, palliative care, allocation of clinical resources, and the ethics of medical research and innovations, especially how to deal in the clinical arena with new technologies.

An approach to clinical-ethical decisions

In recent decades, the relationship between patients and physicians has been evolving from that characterised by paternalism in which physicians made choices for patients based on their professional values, to a more equal relationship of shared decision-making in which physicians provide information that allows competent adult patients to make their own choices. The process by which physicians and patients make decisions together is often summarised in the phrase "informed consent". This doctrine, which is at the heart of the doctor-patient relationship, is based on the ethical principle of respect for individual autonomy and dignity and self determination.

Clinical ethics thus focuses on reaching a right and good decision in individual patient cases. Clinical ethical decisions are based primarily upon two considerations: the medical factors in the case as determined by the physician and the preferences and choices of the patient. In most cases, there is an agreement between the recommendations of the physician and the preferences of the patient because the goals of the two parties are identical. In unusual circumstances where the patient's goals may differ from the physician's, disagreements can occur and ultimately, the preferences of competent

REVIEW

adult patients should prevail. Traditionally, physicians have been reluctant to include quality of life considerations and external considerations such as economics in helping the patient to reach the best decision (10).

What have been the contributions of clinical medical ethics to patient care?

Five specific ways that clinical ethics contributes to patient care are: i. direct patient services; ii. teaching, iii. research, iv. new biotechnologies and v. preserving the traditions of the doctor-patient relationship.

Direct patient services

Clinical ethics contributes to patient care through the following kinds of direct patient services: ethics committees and ethics consultations, developing institutional policies, and by focusing on patient-centred care.

Ethics committees and ethics consultants. Clinical ethicists often serve as members of ethics committees which improve patient care by educating the staff, helping develop institutional ethics policy, providing an internal mechanism for review and resolution of cases involving conflicts, and by contributing ideas to improve patient care decisions. Ethics case consultations, which focus on individual patient dilemmas, is a health care innovation that has been widely incorporated into many large hospitals' practices. The hope is that such consultations may help resolve dilemmas, decrease conflict, improve the decision-making process, and improve patient outcomes. Our own group has provided almost two thousand ethics consultations since 1985 (11).

Institutional policies. Clinical ethics also assists hospitals to develop effective and responsive institutional ethics policies on matters such as "do not resuscitate" orders, "treatment limitation" orders, informed consent, organ transplantation, and many others.

Patient-centred care. Clinical ethics also can assist the hospital to maintain a focus on patient-centred care. Such attention can improve the atmosphere in which patient care is delivered while also providing ethical

safeguards for the rights and responsibilities of both patients and health care workers.

The teaching of clinical ethics

The teaching of clinical ethics, like any other subject in medical school, is only justified by its contribution to the care of patients (12). Therefore, the main goal in teaching clinical ethics is not to produce professional ethicists but is rather to produce ethically knowledgeable physicians and thus improve the quality of patient care. We teach clinical ethics because nowadays medical students and physicians simply must know something about ethics in order to practise competent, high quality medicine. The modern standard of care requires a practical working knowledge about such ethical subjects as informed consent, truth-telling, confidentiality, end-of-life decisions, surrogate decision-making, the use of innovative, non-standard treatments, and physicians' ethical responsibilities when working within health care bureaucracies such as managed care organisations. The modern physician is not able to practise good medicine without some working knowledge about these topics. Further, patients and society expect physicians to have not only technical proficiency but also the practical ability to recognise and respond to ethical issues such as those mentioned.

In considering when and to whom ethics should be taught, it is worth recounting the views of Osler (13) in his talk before the New York Academy of Medicine in December, 1902: "In what may be called the natural method of teaching, the student begins with the patient, continues with the patient, and ends his study with the patient, using books and lectures as tools, as means to an end. For the junior student in medicine and surgery, it is a safe rule to have no teaching without a patient for a text, and the best teaching is that taught by the patient himself". Thus, clinical ethics must be taught not only in the pre-clinical years of medical school but also during the clinical years of medical school and the crucial clinical years of training during residency. Regarding the question of how ethics should be taught, our own approach emphasises that teaching be clinically based, use real cases,

REVIEW

be continuous throughout the medical curriculum, and also be co-ordinated with students' other learning objectives. Such teaching can be provided through lectures or in practice settings such as rounds, conferences, or case conferences. The best teachers of this material are clinicians who themselves are responsible for patient care and for clinical teaching.

And how will such clinician-ethicists be prepared? Some will be trained at their own hospitals by attendance at conferences and seminars, interactions with the ethics committee and ethics consultation team, service on the ethics committee, and, perhaps, co-teaching with a trained ethicist. Some clinicians, however, may require more advanced training, for example, to become researchers in clinical ethics or to become directors in ethics programs. People seeking such training can find advanced training opportunities at a number of North American universities including Georgetown, Harvard, Pittsburgh, the University of Washington, the University of Tennessee, and at the University of Chicago. Since 1985, in our fellowship training program at the University of Chicago, we have provided a year-long training program for more than 100 clinician ethicists, of whom 80 were physicians. More than forty graduates of the University of Chicago Ethics Fellowship now serve as directors or co-directors of university ethics programs in the United States, Canada and Europe.

Research in clinical ethics

Clinical medical ethics research may be divided into two broad categories, analytical and empirical research (14). Analytical research uses the methods of legal and philosophical reasoning to examine conceptual issues and to develop defensible recommendations for ethically acceptable practice. Empirical research in clinical medical ethics involves the collection and analysis of clinical data to describe the way clinical decisions are in fact made by patients, by physicians and within the patient-physician diadic relationship. Empirical research examines the values that are used in reaching clinical decisions, how they are used, by whom and under what

conditions. This type of research uses the methods of the social sciences, decision analysis, clinical epidemiology, and health services research. This latter type of research is quite different from the legal philosophical research of analytical medical ethics. Empirical research may help to understand the ethos of professionals and the preferences and values of patients regarding a wide range of ethical issues in medicine. This type of research has helped clarify end-of-life issues and advance directives, good care of the dying, decision making in AIDS, patients' views on quality of life, and the value of ethics consultations.

Some of the most important clinical ethics research of the past fifteen years has been performed by non-ethicists who have explored aspects of the doctor-patient relationship, including communication, patient empowerment, and shared decision-making. We have learned from health service researchers that patients who have good doctor-patient relationships and who interact actively with physicians to reach a shared health care decision have greater trust in their doctor, have greater loyalty to the doctor-patient relationship, co-operate more fully to implement the shared decision, tend to make financially conservative decisions, express greater satisfaction with their health care, and have improved outcomes, at least for four chronic conditions: hypertension, *diabetes*, peptic ulcer disease, and rheumatoid arthritis.

Recently, Wennberg (15) made a statement that could serve as a future research agenda for the field of clinical ethics: "It is the job of the evaluative sciences to conduct technology assessment and outcomes research to estimate the probability for outcomes that matter to patients and to elucidate the importance of patient preferences in choosing treatment".

Biotechnology

Another important aspect of clinical ethics research deals with the ethical problems raised by new medical technologies and clinical innovations. These issues relate to but are somewhat different from standard ethical issues in clinical research. During the past ten years, our group has examined these

REVIEW

issues in our work on liver transplantation with living donors, Phase I and Phase II cancer drug studies, the ethics of doing research on critically ill patients, the ethics involved in research on patients with *dementia*, certain ethical aspects of genetic screening and testing, and most recently, ethical problems associated with a new approach to using living donors in kidney transplantation. To deal with this complex range of issues in medical and surgical innovation, our group developed an approach we have called Research Ethics Consultation. Research Ethics Consultation was first used to develop the world's first protocol study of living liver transplantation, (16) but this approach has been applied to introduce other new clinical or research innovations. Research Ethics Consultation involves open discussion and public evaluation of an innovation before it is first tried.

For example, we published our guidelines in the New England Journal of Medicine three months before performing the first living liver donor operation. We wanted to invite both public and professional comments concerning our plans. Our aim was to introduce a controversial, but innovative, surgical therapy in the most socially and ethically responsible way, and in a way that seemed most likely to decrease public attack and criticism of the sort that has occurred when other surgical innovations were introduced.

Clinical medical ethics and the doctor-patient relationship

Clinical ethics aims to re-establish the alliance between patients and physicians that traditional medical ethics may have helped weaken by artificially driving a wedge between the doctor and patient on the false dichotomy of autonomy and paternalism and by distorting the doctor-patient relationship in considering it an adversarial relationship. In the vast majority of clinical encounters, the patient and physician are not adversaries but are allies and the reason for this remarkable level of agreement is that the goals of the patient who seeks help and of the physician who offers to help coincide. The doctor-patient relationship, at the heart

of medicine and at the heart of clinical ethics, will survive for the following reasons:

i. medicine serves an unchanging human need;

ii. medicine's goals have not changed since Hippocratic times; and

iii. physicians continue to be respected and wanted by patients.

Plato's observations from 2500 years ago provide another reason why the doctor-patient relationship will survive. In a remarkable passage in book IV of "The Laws", Plato describes two different kinds of physician-patient relationships. In one type, so-called slave medicine, the physician "...never gives the patient an account of his problems nor even asks for any. The physician never gives the slave an account of his problems nor even asks for any. The physician gives an empiric treatment with an air of knowledge in the brusk fashion of a dictator, and then rushes off in haste to the next ailing slave...". Plato contrasted this inadequate relationship with what he called the physician-patient relationship for free men and women in which "...the physician treats the disease by going into things thoroughly from the beginning in a scientific way and thus takes the patient and the family into confidence. In this way, the physician learns from the patient. The physician never gives prescriptions until he has won the patient's support, and when he has done so, he aims to produce complete restoration to health by persuading the patient to comply" (17). The best clinical medicine, Plato tells us, is practised when physician and patient have concluded a fully human relationship in which the technical and scientific aspects of care are placed in the context of the doctor-patient relationship. Only in this human relationship can the benefits of modern medicine be provided in ways that patients want and in ways the physician believes to be in the patient's best interest. The contribution of clinical ethics will be to strengthen, nurture and improve this vitally important relationship.

Conclusions

Scientific and technological developments

REVIEW

in medicine and surgery have created unprecedented ethical dilemmas for physicians. The coming revolution in molecular medicine will generate additional ethical problems. In the last decade, clinical ethics has emerged as a new and useful component of medical practice by emphasising that technical and ethical concerns are inseparable in the practice of medicine. Clinical ethics focuses on the continuing centrality of the doctor-patient relationship and on how patients and physicians work within existing administrative and political structures to reach mutual agreement on clinical decisions that affect the patient. Additionally, clinical ethics offers a language of discourse that broadens the medical model from one that is narrowly technical to one that takes serious account of the preferences and needs of individual patients.

Clinical medical ethics can contribute to patient care both in general ways and also specifically in four ways: through improving direct patient care services, through teaching clinical ethics to students and physicians, through research on ethical problems in medical practice, and by helping to preserve the doctor-patient relationship. Clinical medical ethics, a new discipline, more closely aligned with medicine than ethics, can integrate valuable contributions of philosophical and legal ethics to improve the practise of clinical medicine and the care of patients. Also, clinical medical ethics, because it is firmly grounded in clinical and scientific medicine, can respond to new developments in biotechnology that will surely continue to raise challenging ethical dilemmas in the future.

References*

1. Siegler M. A Legacy of Osler: Teaching clinical ethics at the bedside. JAMA 1978;

239: 951-956.
2. Callahan D. On Living (Well) within Limits. Hastings Center Report, November-December 1996; 16-19.
3. Eddy DM. *Clinical Decision Making*. Sudbury, Mass: Jones & Bartlett, 1996, 41-48.
4. Kass LR. Practicing ethics: Where's the action? Hastings Center Report 1990; **20**: 5-12.
5. SUPPORT Principal Investigators. A controlled trial to improve care for seriously ill hospitalized patients. JAMA 1995; **274**: 1591-1598.
6. Hakim RB et al. Factors associated with do-not-resuscitate orders: Patient preferences, prognosis, and physician judgments. *Ann. Intern. Med.* 1996; **125**: 284-293.
7. Siegler M. The secularization of medical ethics. *J. Center Christian Bioethics (Loma Linda U.)* 1991; **7**: 1-8.
8. Jonsen AR et al. *Clinical Ethics: A Practical Approach to Ethical Decisions in Clinical Medicine*. 3rd Edition New York: McGraw-Hill Inc., 1992.
9. Siegler M et al. Clinical medical ethics: The first decade. *J. Clin. Ethics* 1990; **1**: 5-9.
10. Siegler M. Falling off the pedestal: What is happening to the traditional doctor-patient relationship? *Mayo Clinic Proc.* 1993; **68**: 1-7.
11. Fletcher JC et al. What are the goals of ethics consultation? A consensus statement. *J. Clin. Ethics* 1996; **7**: 122-126.
12. Pellegrino ED et al. Teaching clinical ethics. *J. Clin. Ethics* 1990; **1**: 175-180.
13. Osler W. On the need of a radical reform in our methods of teaching medical students. *Medical News* 1902; **82**: 49-53.
14. Singer PA et al. Research in clinical medical ethics. *J. Clin. Ethics* 1990; **1**: 95-99.
15. Wennberg J. Health outcomes. In: Wyngaarten JB, Plum F, and Bennett C eds.; *Cecil Textbook of Medicine*. 20th Edition Philadelphia: WB Saunders, 1996.
16. Singer PA et al. Ethics of liver transplantation with living donors. *N. Engl. J. Med.* 1989; **321**: 620-622.
17. Plato. *The Laws*. Taylor AE, translator. London: Dent, 1934, 104-105.

(The author is responsible for the accuracy of the references)

*The reference numbers written in **bold-type** indicate the selected abstracts which follow this article

Received May 13, 1997
Accepted June 16, 1997

The Doctor-Patient Relationship

Laura Weiss Roberts and Mark Siegler

Abstract

This chapter contains reprinted works from Dr. Mark Siegler focusing on the doctor-patient relationship and its connection with the field of clinical medical ethics. The works analyze the ethical issues that are often associated with the doctor-patient relationship and discuss how physicians should navigate these concerns in order to ethically provide the best patient care possible. Specific aspects of the doctor-patient relationship, such as confidentiality, patient autonomy, and informed consent, are addressed in relation to the field of clinical medical ethics. The works in this chapter are reprinted with permission.

L.W. Roberts, MD, MA (✉)
Department of Psychiatry and Behavioral Sciences,
Stanford University School of Medicine, Stanford, CA, USA
e-mail: robertsl@stanford.edu

M. Siegler, MD
Bucksbaum Institute for Clinical Excellence, MacLean Center
for Clinical Medical Ethics, University of Chicago,
Pritzker School of Medicine, Chicago, IL, USA

8.1 **Siegler M (1981) Searching for Moral**
Certainty in Medicine: A Proposal
for a New Model of the Doctor-Patient
Encounter. Bull N Y Acad Med
57:56–69

Courtesy of the New York Academy of Medicine.

56

SEARCHING FOR MORAL CERTAINTY IN MEDICINE: A PROPOSAL FOR A NEW MODEL OF THE DOCTOR-PATIENT ENCOUNTER*

MARK SIEGLER, M.D.

Section of General Internal Medicine
Department of Medicine
University of Chicago, Pritzker School of Medicine
Chicago, Illinois

PREVIOUS speakers at this conference have indicated that the physician-patient relationship is changing and remains in a state of flux. I think that assertion is incontestible, perhaps with the proviso that the relationship is changing for some patients and for some physicians, whereas others maintain more traditional notions. Despite changes in the character of the relationship, my remarks today will suggest that if moral certainty exists in medicine (that is, if it is possible to determine which actions taken in a medical context are moral and ethical, which are right and wrong), such moral certainty will be discovered not by recourse to formal laws, moral rules, or moral principles, but rather in the context of the particularities of the physician-patient relationship itself.

A problem in this line of reasoning is obvious. If the moral rightness of actions in medicine are to be discovered in the physician-patient relationship, and if the relationship is in an unstable state in which a societal consensus no longer exists regarding it, how is it possible to derive any moral guidelines from such a shifting relationship? If my thesis is correct that whatever degree of moral certainty exists in medicine is to be discovered in the physician-patient relationship, it becomes necessary then as a crucial preliminary step to develop a new and acceptable model of the doctor-patient encounter. Hence, this paper has two goals. First, the thesis will be presented and defended that if moral certainty is to be found in medicine it is to be discovered in the particularities of the physician-patient relationship, and, second, to develop a bilateral dynamic model of the doctor-patient encounter that avoids the unilateral, static notions of

*Presented in a panel. The Autonomy of the Patient and ''Consumerism,'' as part of the 1980 Annual Health Conference of the New York Academy of Medicine, *The Patient and the Health Care Professional: The Changing Pattern of Their Relations*, held April 24 and 25, 1980.

either a physician-dominated, paternalistic model or a patient-dominated, consumerist-libertarian model of medicine.

SEARCHING FOR MORAL CERTAINTY IN MEDICINE

The thesis of this paper is that moral certainty in medicine is not an entity to be discovered like a truth of nature, rather that it is defined and created in the context of a physician-patient encounter which I refer to as a physician-patient accommodation. A crucial preliminary step, then, is to understand how patients and physicians currently behave and how they describe and justify their interactions before formulating a theory for such actions. Although society's understanding of medicine is in a state of flux, the central event in medicine has not changed. This unchanging event is the clinical encounter between a person seeking help in the care of his health and the health professional—usually, the physician—whose help is sought. Although the relationship between the patient and doctor is and, frankly, always has been molded and constrained by social, political, and economic forces, there still remains enormous latitude in American medicine of 1980 for individualization of the clinical encounter and for negotiations between patient and doctor.

The approach I propose to understand moral behavior in medicine—an examination of the accommodations reached by patients and physicians in the medical encounter—must be contrasted with alternative and more traditional attempts to determine medical morality by a formulation of general moral considerations such as rules, principles, and laws. In the latter instance, one begins with such general considerations as autonomy, fidelity, and veracity, and then strives to determine whether the general consideration arises in particular cases and, if it does, how the rule or principle is to be applied to determine a proper course of action.

For example, rules concerning respect for autonomy, for truth-telling, or for fidelity to patients consistently fail to provide physicians and patients with a means of knowing what their actual duties are in particular settings and circumstances. To illustrate this point, I would like to examine briefly the concept of autonomy.

AUTONOMY

Autonomy is a form of personal liberty of action in which individuals determine their own course of action in accordance with their own life plans.[1] The principle of respect for autonomy surely recognizes that different autonomous individuals will wish to be treated in different ways by health professionals. An adequate understanding of autonomy would also include the possibility that individuals within a relationship might voluntarily and autonomously choose to relinquish or to waive a degree of independence to pursue other immediate interests. The critical question to be faced by both patient and physician is how much independence is a patient willing or eager to renounce autonomously by choosing to enter into a therapeutic relationship with a health professional. Further, if the principle of respect for autonomy applies to patients, presumably it applies with equal force to physicians. How much personal liberty of action and independence of judgment must a physician relinquish when he chooses to enter the profession of medicine? What duties, obligations, and responsibilities does the physician incur, voluntarily and autonomously, when he chooses to become a physician?

The point I am making is that the invocation of the concept of autonomy fails to provide sufficient practical guidance to morally conscientious physicians and patients to enable them to determine where on a spectrum of paternalism/consumerism or dependence/independence their professional relationship will and ought to stabilize. Invoking the principle of autonomy does not resolve the dilemma facing clinicians and patients; it merely highlights it; perhaps, at times, it even exacerbates it.

It should be noted that the principle of respect for autonomy may prove an essential regulatory component of the final arrangement between physician and patient, an arrangement that balances the respective rights and responsibilities of the two parties. But the practical clinical dilemma of how individual physicians and patients ought to establish the details of their relationship can only be understood by examining their interactions in the particularities of the clinical encounter. A clinical example may be useful to establish this point.

A Tale of Two Cities

A professional ballet dancer who suffers from moderately severe asthma moved to Chicago from New York. Upon arriving in Chicago, she became a patient of a famed specialist in asthma who is a superb clinical scientist. Within six months, the Chicago physician appeared to have managed and mastered her condition, or at least her wheezing. Despite this, she was unhappy. She called on me for another opinion and reported that she was distressed because she missed having a physician—like her New York physician—who worked with her to achieve her personal goals. She felt she now had no say in her own care. Her new doctor would not listen to her concerns or ideas. Finally, the multiple and prolonged courses of steroid drugs used to control her wheezing had caused increased muscle weakness and fluid accumulation and, as a result, the quality of her dancing had deteriorated. She didn't live just to breathe, she said; she breathed so she could dance.

I am certain that the New York doctor could have manipulated this woman's medications in the same way that the Chicago doctor did to relieve her wheezing entirely, but rather the New York physician had chosen to work with the woman to achieve alternative and important life goals which included an adequate but imperfect control of her asthma that enabled her to function effectively as a dancer. Unfortunately, the Chicago physician, although a thoroughly competent clinical scientist, could not tolerate much patient participation in medical decisions, and, more important, could not accept an alternative endpoint to that of a patient totally free of wheezes. As a result, her disease was managed, but the meaning of her life, as measured by happiness, contentment, and the ability to function as a dancer, had deteriorated.

This clinical example introduces us to three autonomous individuals, the patient and the two physicians. There is not the slightest suggestion that any of the three involved was coerced or manipulated into the two patient-physician encounters described. Each invested considerable emotional energy in developing a physician-patient bond. It must be remembered that the patient remained voluntarily in a clinical relationship with the Chicago physician for at least six months.

My concern is that the principle of respecting autonomy does not appear to resolve entirely the specification of the rights and responsibilities incurred by both patient and physician in such medical settings. Presumably, the Chicago physician believed that he acted responsibly in controlling the symptoms of the patient's disease and that she exercised her rights voluntarily and responsibly in returning for continued care and in taking her prescribed medications. The patient agreed that the Chicago physician exercised the responsibilities he believed he had assumed—to treat disease—when he became a physician. As described, the medical relationship was a failure on both a technical and a moral plane, not because it intruded on the autonomy of either patient or doctor, but because it failed to conform to the best standards of medicine.

This example reinforces my notion that if moral certainty exists in medicine, it must be explored and understood in the context of specific physician-patient encounters and cannot be deduced *a priori* from the application of general moral considerations and such principles as autonomy. This observation leads me to the second part of this paper, in which I attempt to develop a dynamic, bilateral account of the physician-patient encounter, which I refer to as the doctor-patient accommodation.

A PROPOSAL FOR A NEW MODEL OF THE PHYSICIAN-PATIENT ENCOUNTER

The traditional paternal model of medicine was premised on trust in the physician's technical competence and moral sensitivity and was characterized by patient dependency and physician control. This model is being replaced gradually by one in which patients are increasingly involved in decision-making concerning their own medical care. The rise of consumerism and the associated emergence of "rights" language in medicine has encouraged some individuals to view medicine as a "serving" profession and to regard themselves not as patients but as "medical consumers." Such "medical consumers" sometimes wish to invert the traditional model of medicine and to make the physician a passive agent, a hired technician who practices under the direction and control of his "client." However, despite these changes which affect some patients and some physicians, many patients and physicians continue to interact in a fairly traditional, paternalistic physician-patient relationship.

Both the old physician-dominated paternalism and the new patient-dominated consumerism are unilateral models in which one or the other party in the relationship is seen as dominant. By contrast, the physician-patient accommodation model I propose is a bilateral one in which the moral and technical arrangements of a medical encounter are determined mutually, voluntarily, and autonomously by both patient and physician.

In *The Methods of Ethics*, published in 1874, Henry Sidgwick considered how the moral obligations of individuals were modified when a social promise to the community (e.g., the promise of medicine) was in a state of incomplete redefinition. Sidgwick noted:

> ...The promise ought to be interpreted in the sense in which its terms are understood by the community; and, no doubt, if their usage is quite uniform and unambiguous, this role of interpretation is sufficiently obvious and simple....

> ...It seems clear that when the process [of redefinition of a community promise] is complete, we are right in adopting the new understanding as far as good faith

> is concerned....But when, as is ordinarily the case, the process is incomplete, since a portion of the community understands the engagement in the original strict sense, the obligation becomes difficult to determine, and the judgment of conscientious persons respecting it becomes divergent and perplexed.[2]

In this period of consumerism and ''rights consciousness,'' we appear to be in a phase of incomplete redefinition of a social promise, the promise of the medical profession. Possibly we have reached the stage described by Sidgwick, in which judgments of conscientious persons have become divergent and perplexed and in which a societal consensus no longer exists.

Moral dilemmas (and practical dilemmas, too) arise more frequently in periods of social uncertainty and change. The old paternalistic model of medicine held way for millenia; it was widely embraced and rarely questioned. The proper ends and limits of medicine were broadly accepted, and the determination of these ends usually was assumed to be the province of the medical practitioner. Of course, the practitioner and the patient frequently shared a common understanding in these matters. But now that a new model of medicine is evolving, one characterized by changing expectations and uncertain understandings between patient and physician, old moral quandaries again rise to the surface and some new ones seem to spring full-grown from the sea.

The central moral and practical dilemma facing concerned patients and conscientious physicians at this time is to balance the rights of patients and the responsibilities of physicians—and the rights of physicians and the responsibilities of patients—at a time when societal values and expectations are changing. This is the critical challenge facing medicine in the coming decades. This paper will suggest an approach by which the tenuous equilibrium between the rights and responsibilities of patients and physicians might be re-established on a more stable foundation. This approach will involve returning to the central event in medicine—and one which I believe remains the only possible locus of moral certainty in medicine—the physician-patient encounter.

THE PHYSICIAN-PATIENT ACCOMMODATION

The physician-patient accommodation, as I shall describe it, is both a process and an outcome. This process involves a degree of testing by both parties to decide whether this patient and this physician wish to work together. The process is one of communication and negotiation—sometimes short and to the point, sometimes extended—as to what rights and responsibilities each participant wishes to retain and which will be relinquished in the context of their medical relationship.

The accommodation process depends on all of the particularities of the medical encounter. The nature of the patient involved—his personality, character, attitude, and values—and the factors which led him to seek a medical encounter with this particular physician are central components of the process. Similarly, the personality, character, attitude, values, and technical skills of the physician affect the accommodation. Further, the quality of the interaction between patient and physician—the chemistry of the interaction—modify the process. Of course, the nature of the medical problem, including its type, acuteness, gravity, and its potential for remediation, will be a major determinant of whether a physician-patient accommodation is achieved. For example, the entire process will be modified profoundly and telescoped if the patient is acutely or critically ill and alternative medical resources are unavailable. Finally, other considerations which may affect the achievement of a physician-patient accommodation include the clinical setting, e.g., a hospital, doctor's office, or the patient's home; the organization of the medical service, Health Maintenance Organization, or fee-for-service; and also, occasionally, the claims of relevant third party interests such as those of family, insurers, or the state.

If the process of negotiation referred to as the physician-patient accommodation is concluded successfully, the result will be an outcome also called a physician-patient accommodation. In this outcome a joint decision is reached on whether this patient wishes to place his care in the hands of this physician subject to mutually agreed upon rights and responsibilities, and in which the physician also agrees to care for this particular patient. There are as many results and styles of outcome for the accommodation as there are configurations of the variables that enter into the process of negotiating the accommodation.

The physician-patient accommodation is not a permanent, stable, and unchanging relationship between a physician and a patient; it is a dyamic model and is always in flux. In one sense, the accommodation as an outcome exists only as a concept; it is always in the process either of developing or of dissolving. Patients and physicians must achieve accommodations repeatedly, even regarding the same basic conditions for which the original accommodation was concluded. For example, a patient's agreement to be cared for by a cardiologist for anginal chest pain would not commit the patient to agree with the cardiologist's recommendation to undergo coronary angiography or to accept a subsequent recommendation for cardiac surgery.

Some physician-patient accommodations are stronger than others. The resilience of an accommodation is determined largely by the extent of trust and confidence exchanged between patient and physician. However, the stability of an accommodation is constantly threatened by new circumstances because changes in the patient, the physician, or the disease all may result in a reassessment of the accommodation and perhaps a failure to reach an accommodation on the same or a new issue. If an accommodation is not achieved on an important matter (a situation roughly analogous to a prime minister who loses a vote of confidence), patient or physician legitimately could decide to dissolve their professional relationship, again with the proviso that the patient's emergency health care needs are attended to.

In contrast to previous descriptions of the physician-patient relationship which tend to regard it as an established, static arrangement between doctor and patient,[3,4] the physician-patient accommodation provides a more dynamic and more realistic model of the medical encounter. Perhaps physician-patent relationships as such rarely exist; rather, what we regard as a relationship may really be repeatedly negotiated physician-patient accommodations. More likely, a physician-patient relationship represents a specific and increasingly uncommon variant of the accommodation. It is one characterized by mature and enduring exchanges of trust between patient and physician that establish an almost insunderable bond. A decline in personal medical care and a rise in high technology and in institutional, specialized medical care probably has accelerated the decline of the traditional relationship model and has contributed to the emergence of the accomodation model.

FURTHER REFLECTIONS ON THE PHYSICIAN-PATIENT ACCOMMODATION

Either the patient or the physician may decide not to conclude an accommodation. We could surely imagine reasons for patients not wishing to enter or continue an accommodation with a particular physician. For example, if the physician had a poor bedside manner, seemed incompetent, had the wrong diplomas on the wall or none at all, maintained a shabby office, charged excessive fees, had too long a queue, didn't have the proper hospital privileges, or had a personality or value system which clashed repeatedly with the patient's, the patient might choose to go elsewhere. The patient has a choice, at least in our current medical system.

Although the physician may be less free to choose than the patient (e.g., legally a physician-patient relationship may exist from the time of a physician's first encounter with a patient), the accommodation model encourages or even obligates the physician to make a conscious decision to assume the care of the person who asks for medical assistance. A physician's decision to care for a patient is based on two determinations: his ability to help the patient, which remains a central concern in clinical medicine, and his own concept of professional standards and norms of behavior for physicians.

Therefore, a physician may be obligated not to enter a physician-patient accommodation if he believes that he is unable to help the patient or if he believes that even if he could help the patient, he could do so only by sacrificing his own conscientious standards of what it means to be a good and responsible physician and human being. Some reasons why a physician might believe himself unable to help a particular patient could include a lack of technical skills to respond to a particular problem, personality conflicts with the patient serious enough to impair the healing relationship, a profound incompatability of goals being pursued by patient and physician, or a determination that the patient was unwilling to assume responsibilities to work jointly with the physician in the care or maintenance of the patient's health. A physician might also refuse to enter an accommodation because of a belief that his involvement would violate his personal sense of responsible conduct. This might occur when the physician considers an action to be illegal or immoral or when he believes that a patient's problem is not legitimately a medical matter and could be handled more appropriately in another institutional setting.

Some of these positions may appear controversial, particularly the notion that a physician may be obligated not to enter a physician-patient accommodation if doing so would violate the physician's conscientious sense of professional and personal responsibility. One could justify the rights of both parties to refuse to enter an accommodation on the following grounds:

1) If medicine is aimed at achieving desirable ends for patients, it is to

both parties' advantage that they exhibit prudence and discretion in not entering into accommodations doomed to failure. The healing relationship is bilateral and depends on trust and confidence as much as on pills and surgery to achieve its goals.

2) The model of medicine implied by an emphasis on the need for patient and physician to achieve an accommodation is one of mutuality, voluntariness, and respect for autonomy. The freedom of both patient and physician to enter an accommodation is the core of morally acceptable medical practice.

3) The alternative, in which neither patient nor physician were free to determine these arrangements, would result in an inferior, mechanical form of medicine, such as that described by Plato (in *The Laws*) as being practiced by slave physicians on slave patients.[5]

CONCLUSION

This paper has attempted to locate the moral center of medicine in the particularities of encounters between patients and physicians. In times of social change, these encounters must develop within the context of unclear social expectations and indistinct senses of obligation. It seems necessary, under these conditions, to articulate a new and more widely acceptable model of the physician-patient encounter. This new arrangement, referred to as the physician-patient accommodation, is based upon mutuality, voluntariness, and respect for autonomy.

The physician-patient encounter is the site of human agency, the point at which individuals possessed of special needs and personal perspectives and values interact. The physician-patient accommodation model describes both the *process* of achieving a voluntary and mutually acknowledged arrangement, and the *outcome* itself, which will reflect the particular configuration of moral, medical, and personal factors which shaped the accommodation. The accommodation model focuses upon the process by which, for example, *this* physician and *this* patient under *these* circumstances negotiate *this* relationship committed towards *these* ends. By such painstaking attention to the site, conditions, and factors of human agency and medical practice, the accommodation model permits us to offer a model of medical practice which describes the processes and outcomes of physician-patient encounters and to place the locus of moral certainty in the very processes and outcomes that constitute each new arrangement. One is gradually led to the conclusion that the principles upon which the physician-patient accommodation is based may themselves be the central determinants of morally acceptable medical practice.

As a model of medical practice which describes the processes and outcomes of physician-patient encounters, the accommodation model offers unique conceptual, methodological, and clinically pragmatic insights.

By providing a powerful conceptual schema, the accommodation mode may allow us to understand better the nature and extent of the deterioration of social consensus concerning the proper limits, means, and ends of medicine. Attention to the outcome of physician-patient accommodations is likely to provide information from a plenitude of cases from which an "understanding of the community" may be derived. From the facts of a number of cases (the accommodated outcomes of which can be expected to reflect personal, medical, and moral positions) we may more readily discern the social and professional "rules of the game" as they exist in practice. At least, the general outline of procedural principles appropriate to this period of uncertainty may be made visible.

Conceptually, the accommodation model permits analysis of a critical dimension of medicine without the biases found in either the paternal or consumer/libertarian models. These other models simply do not help to predict the true sources of conflict and to prescribe remedies that can be applied broadly. Viewing the physician-patient encounter as an authoritarian intervention, adversarial conflict, or exercise in consumer choice obscures the fact that the actual character and form of medical relationships depends upon a variety of factors and varies widely for different patients and physicians.

As a methodological guide, the accommodation model encourages us to examine the influence and interaction of such diverse factors as clinical setting, the nature of the medical problem, possible third party interests, and, most important, the attitudes and values of physician and patient. And because each accommodation must take place within a social context characterized by uncertainty, and because the uncertainty concerns such issues as autonomy, responsibility, and obligation, attention to physician-patient accommodations is attention to precisely those areas of controversy which manifest themselves in practice.

Most important, the accommodation model exhibits useful features that lend themselves to the development of more humane and effective clinical practice. The model allows for maximum flexibility of decision-making for both physician and patient, while searching for that equilibrium point at which voluntary and mutual actions can be agreed upon. The patient retains the ability to claim or to relinquish various degrees of autonomy and the opportunity to inform the physician of relevant personal factors that might influence medical decisions. The discretion of physicans for entering an accommodation is limited naturally by direct patient needs; nevertheless, the physician remains an autonomous party to the accommodation. The accommodation model permits a physician better to understand a patient's expectations of him, and a patient more adequately to understand the exact nature of the commitments and expectations the physician is willing to exchange. In this way, use of the accommodation model in clinical practice encourages an ongoing, bilateral analysis of the technical, personal, and interpersonal dimensions of each case. It encourages attention to the elements of accommodation, thus acting to humanize and personalize the physician-patient encounter. Relationships based on mutually understood values and ends are those most likely to result in an exchange of trust, and trust remains an essential component of the healing relationship.

The case of the ballet dancer illustrates the conceptual, methodological, and practical usefulness of the accommodation model. Conceptually, the model enables us to analyze this case as one in which physician and patient were unable to agree upon mutual goals and interests. Methodologically, the model identifies the nature of the medical problem, the values of patient and physician, and the interaction of patient and physician as influential factors in a process which resulted in an incomplete and imperfect accommodation of goals.

In this case, attention to the principle of accommodation might have resulted in agreement upon a technical-medical endpoint which would have satisfied the physician's sense of "good medical practice" and the dancer's sense of adequate control of her condition. As it was, the dancer felt forced to choose between complete control of her asthma and retention of her skills as a dancer. And the physician could not tolerate a treatment failure narrowly construed, i.e., the persistance of wheezes which he could abolish with sufficiently potent medication.

Eventually, of course, this medical relationship dissolved. Perhaps, had physician and patient explored and negotiated together the nature of the expectations and obligations each was willing to exchange by entering a relationship, this conflict might have been avoided. If it became apparent that their conflict of purposes and interests was intractable, not resolvable even by good faith negotiations, each would have been obligated neither to accept the arrangement nor conclude an accommodation. In any event, attention to the principle of accommodation would have encouraged mutual understanding of the positions of physician and patient and prevented the needless frustration, anxiety, and confusion which characterized this case.

The physician-patient accommodation model is a useful descriptive and theoretical device. Further, an analysis of the constituents of successful, failed, and unconcluded accommodations enables us to gather information about what medical practice *is*, a necessary preparation for discussions of what medical practice *should be*.

The ingredients essential for a physician-patient accommodation—mutuality, voluntariness, respect for autonomy, and communication and negotiation between physician and patient—are surely preconditions for the practice of morally acceptable medicine. These principles of accommodation are also essential for the effective practice of the art of medicine. Thus, the circle comes full course; we find that the same principles which allow us to describe technically satisfactory physician-patient encounters are precisely those necessary for the formation of morally acceptable medical relationships.

Recognition of this fact is not a recent development. In a remarkable passage in Book IV of *The Laws*, Plato describes two different kinds of physician-patient relationships. In one type, in which slave-physicians treat slave-patients, the physician "...never gives him any account of his complaints, nor asks him for any; he gives him some empiric injunction with an air of finished knowledge in the brusque fashion of a dictator, and then is off in hot haste to the next ailing slave...."

In the physician-patient relationship befitting free men, the citizen-physician

> ...treats their disease by going into things thoroughly from the beginning in a scientific way and takes the patient and his family into confidence. Thus he learns something from the sufferers....He does not give prescriptions until he has won the patient's support, and when he has done so, he steadily aims at producing complete restoration to health by persuading the sufferer into compliance...[6]

The best clinical medicine, Plato tells us, is practiced when physician and patient have concluded a fully human relationship in which technical aspects of care are placed in the context of an appreciation for the most widely construed interests of each. It is in this regard that the principles and activity of the physician-patient accommodation establish a bond of trust between two individuals who together challenge the mutability that is the only certainty in medicine. And it is to the particularities of the physician-patient encounter that we, as healers, must turn as we seek the center of good, and therefore morally acceptable, medical practice.

ACKNOWLEDGMENTS

I gratefully acknowlege important criticism and suggestions by Professor Stephen Toulmin of the University of Chicago. I am particularly indebted to Robert T. Kinscheriff, M.A., for his valuable assistance and in particular for his help in drafting the concluding section of this paper.

REFERENCES

1. Beauchamp, T. L. and Childress, J. F.: *Principles of Biomedical Ethics*. New York and Oxford, Oxford University Press, 1979, pp. 56-96.
2. Sidgwick, H.: *The Methods of Ethics*. London, Macmillan, 1874, pp. 308-10.
3. Szasz, T. S. and Hollender, M.: The basic models of the doctor-patient rela-tionship. *Arch. Int. Med. 97:*585-92, 1956.
4. Veatch, R. M.: Models for ethical medicine in a revolutionary age. *Hast. Cent. Rep. 2:*5-7, 1972.
5. Plato: *The Laws*, Taylor, A. E., translator. London, Dent, 1934, pp. 104-05.
6. Ibid.

For more detailed discussion of some of the issues raised in the present paper and for citations of the relevant literature, see:

Siegler, M.: On the Nature and Limits of Clinical Medicine. In: *Changing Values in Medicine*, Cassell, E. J. and Siegler, M., editors. Chicago, University of Chicago Press, 1981.

Siegler, M.: The Doctor-Patient Encounter and its Relationship to Theories of Health and Disease. In: *Concepts of Health and Disease: Interdisciplinary Perspectives*, Caplan, A. L., Engelhardt, H. T., Jr., and McCartney, J. J., editors. Reading, Mass., Addison-Wesley, 1981.

Siegler, M. and Goldblatt, A. D.: Clinical Intuition: A Procedure for Balancing the Rights of Patients and the Responsibilities of Physicians. In: *The Law-Medicine Relation: A Philosophical Exploration*, Healey, J. M., Engelhardt, H. T., Jr., and Spicker, S. F., editors. Reidel, Boston, and Dordrecht, Holland, 1980.

Siegler, M.: A right to health care: Ambiguity, professional responsibility and patient liberty. *J. Med. Phil. 4(2):*148-57, 1979.

8.2 Siegler M, Goldblatt AD (1981) Clinical Intuition: A Procedure for Balancing the Rights of Patients and the Responsibilities of Physicians. In: Spicker SF, Healey JM, Engelhardt Jr HT (eds) The Law-Medicine Relation: A Philosophical Exploration. D. Reidel, Boston, p 5–31

MARK SIEGLER AND ANN DUDLEY GOLDBLATT

CLINICAL INTUITION:
A PROCEDURE FOR BALANCING THE RIGHTS OF
PATIENTS AND THE RESPONSIBILITIES OF PHYSICIANS

I. INTRODUCTION

The assumption underlying the subtitle of this paper is that medicine in the 1970's has become an adversarial practice, requiring a procedure for adjudicating between the rights of patients and the responsibilities of physicians. It is ironic that the relationship between doctor and patient — traditionally a vital element in the healing process — should deteriorate at precisely the time when medicine has become more effective. Although the doctor-patient relationship appears to be evolving in a libertarian direction, emphasizing individual autonomy, self-determination, and rights, an ambivalence remains; witness the unclarity of attitude of the courts and legislatures. Precisely because this uncertainty exists, it is not surprising that at times the practice of medicine seems to juxtapose the interests of patients and those of physicians. This essay will consider these questions by examining two very different issues in modern medicine:

(1) the rights of patients and the responsibilities of physicians in situations in which acutely, critically ill patients who have easily treatable diseases refuse life-saving therapy, and

(2) the rights of patients and the responsibilities of physicians in situations in which ambulatory patients with self-defined senses of dis-ease or illness demand specific services from physicians.

We will attempt to show by reference to these limiting cases that the libertarian model has serious weaknesses and limitations. An attempt will be made to articulate a decision-making process which we refer to as 'clinical intuition', which takes account of both patients' rights and physicians' responsibilities. We will strive to justify our conclusion with reference to legal and philosophical principles. First, we will consider the situation of the patient refusing treatment; we will subsequently examine problems posed by the demanding patient.

The central concern of this essay — balancing the general rights of patients to self-determination with the responsibility of physicians, occasionally, to override patient decisions — has been examined frequently in recent years. One aspect of this examination has been a consideration of the change in the

5

S. F. Spicker, J. M. Healey, and H. T. Engelhardt (eds.), The Law–Medicine Relation: A Philosophical Exploration, 5–31.

6   MARK SIEGLER AND ANN DUDLEY GOLDBLATT

doctor-patient relationship [DPR], a change from a paternalistic model to one that emphasizes the patient's autonomy and right of self-determination. The contributions of humanists and social scientists have been instrumental in the reassessment of the DPR. Their commentaries have structured the issues and, in general, have resolved them in accord with libertarian principles of self-determination.

Unfortunately, practicing physicians have contributed little to the analysis of this issue, although it has a direct effect on the practice of medicine and the care of patients.[1] This essay will analyze the issue of patients' rights and physicians' responsibilities from the perspective of professionals actively involved in clinical situations, rather than by conjuring hypothetical circumstances. It is not that the judgment of medical professionals is always correct merely because they are professionals or because they possess technical expertise. However, their viewpoint merits careful consideration in the resolution of these complex issues.

The role of the professional is unique. The professional's relationship to a client or patient is premised on specific technical training and on competency. This specialized knowledge and proficiency is used to assist patients in curing or ameliorating their illness and disease, and to assist them in overcoming the fear, pain and suffering that are often associated with ill health. Once sought out by the client, a professional (in this case, a medical doctor) becomes involved in the client's concerns. He is never a mere observer. He cannot rely on the counterfeit courage of the non-combatant. The physician is accountable to the patient if he fails to perform his task adequately because of lack of skill, because of negligence, or because he fails to act in the client's behalf. This special quality of the professional enterprise was described eloquently by the Roman General Lucius Aemilius Paulus in 168 B.C.

Commanders should be counselled, chiefly, by persons of known talent; by those who have made the art of war their particular study, and whose knowledge is derived from experience; from those who are present at the scene of action, who see the country, who see the enemy; who see the advantages that occasions offer, and who, like people embarked in the same ship, are sharers of the danger. If, therefore, any one thinks himself qualified to give advice respecting the war which I am to conduct, which may prove advantageous to the public, let him not refuse his assistance to the state, but let him come with me into Macedonia. He shall be furnished with a ship, a horse, a tent; even his travelling charges shall be defrayed. But if he thinks this too much trouble, and prefers the repose of a city life to the toils of war, let him not on land assume the office of a pilot. The city, in itself, furnishes abundance of topics for conversation ([13], pp. 326–327).

Although we do not endorse Paulus's concept that only professionals are

CLINICAL INTUITION   7

capable of criticizing their professional enterprise, we do endorse the principle that professionals should contribute to the analysis and criticism of their own endeavors. This essay offers and defends a position on proper actions of physicians towards acutely, critically ill patients. It is intended to complement those commentaries on this issue proffered by non-physicians.

II. THE CHANGING DOCTOR-PATIENT RELATIONSHIP [DPR]

The DPR has changed dramatically within the last sixty years. The traditional paternal model, premised on trust in the physician and characterized by the patient's dependency and the physician's control, has been replaced by a more bilateral relationship where patients are increasingly involved in decision-making which concerns their own care. In a companion essay in this volume, Professor John Ladd discusses this change and concludes that the earlier medical model has crumbled: "The ultimate authority in medical matters has shifted away from the physician. . . . The patient or administrator can now tell the doctor what he needs and what he must do . . . ". [12].

Professor Alan Donagan has arrived at a similar conclusion. He suggests that the expressed legal and moral requirements of the informed consent doctrine represent a formal recognition of today's changes in the DRP. He notes that there has been a gradual but unmistakable change from a 'physician decides' to a 'physician proposes, patient decides' model of medicine ([3], p. 313; [19]). This dramatic change in the DRP has three major causes: the successes of scientific medicine, the increase in medical research, and the public perception of health care as a 'right'.

Paradoxically, the successes of medicine have contributed to a decreased trust in physicians and a decline in the paternalistic approach to health care. The continuity of the relationship between a patient and his personal physician has been interrupted by an increased use of medical specialists and by institutional and team care.

Increased medical research has led to distrust of medical practitioners as the public has come to see physicians as applied biologists rather than as healers. Frank mistrust of physician-scientists has been augmented by documentation of various abuses in research involving human subjects. Finally, broad social changes, including a general decline in trust in public institutions and experts and the rise of the consumer movement, has encouraged the recent claim that medical care is a 'right'. This assertion has led to another: that the physician is a mere provider of a product or service — medical care — and that this product can be purchased and consumed at the will of the consumer. All

8   MARK SIEGLER AND ANN DUDLEY GOLDBLATT

these changes have occurred in a political environment that emphasizes individual rights and liberties. There is no doubt, then, that our society's understanding of medicine is unclear and the paternalistic approach to the patient is under attack.

III. SIDGWICK AND THE PUBLIC UNDERSTANDING OF INSTITUTIONAL AND SOCIETAL PROMISES

Moral dilemmas arise in any period of social uncertainty and change. The old paternalistic model of the DPR was widely embraced and rarely questioned. The proper end and limits of medicine were accepted, and the determination of these ends was assumed to be the province of the medical practitioner. Now a new model of medicine is evolving; many new questions are being asked. Eventually, the public and the medical profession will accept and articulate a new vision of the end and limits of medicine. Until this new definition of medicine emerges, however, concepts about the proper ends of medicine will differ. The public and the profession will be unsure which model of medicine — the paternal or the libertarian — is prevailing.

In the *Methods of Ethics*, published in 1874, Henry Sidgwick discussed institutional and societal promises [17]. His discussion was particularly perceptive and remains helpful in considering the problems presently faced by physicians and patients. Sidgwick noted that social promises must change when values and expectations change. But until such a change in societal values is recognized and institutionalized, different people will have conflicting understandings of the expressed and implicit promises on which certain public activities (in the present context the practice of medicine) are based. Sidgwick stated:

We have now to observe that in the cases of promises made to the community, as a condition of obtaining some office or emolument, a certain unalterable form of words has to be used if a promise is to be made at all . . . . It may be said, indeed, *that the promise ought to be interpreted in the sense in which its terms are understood by the community*; and, no doubt, if their usage is quite uniform and unambiguous, this role of interpretation is sufficiently obvious and simple . . . .

The question then arises, how far this process of gradual . . . relaxation . . . can modify the moral obligation of the promise for a thoroughly conscientious person. It seems clear that when the process is complete, we are right in adopting the new understanding as far as good faith is concerned . . . although it is always desirable in such cases that the form of the promise should be changed to correspond with the changed substance. *But when, as is ordinarily the case, the process is incomplete, since a portion of the community understands the engagement in the original strict sense, the obligation becomes difficult to determine, and the judgment of conscientious persons respecting it becomes divergent and perplexed* ([17], pp. 308–310, emphasis added).

In this period of increased 'rights consciousness' and reduced medical authority, we appear to be in a phase of incomplete redefinition of a social promise, the promise of the medical profession. Sidgwick provides a method to analyze the community's perception of the DPR. He maintains that "the promise ought to be interpreted in the sense in which its terms are understood by the community". To use this method, we must inquire how the medical relationship is understood by the public and the profession. Our answer is that we have indeed reached the stage described by Sidgwick as one in which judgments of conscientious persons have become divergent and perplexed, and in which there is no societal consensus.

IV. ACUTE CRITICAL ILLNESS: A LIMITING CASE

What is the judgment of conscientious persons on the question of how one reconciles the rights of patients and the responsibilities of physicians within a gradually evolving model of medicine? Are there limits to a patient's rights within the medical relationship? Conversely, and starkly stated, should a physician ever override the expressed wishes of a patient who has not been found legally incompetent?

We are concerned that the movement towards patients' rights and the libertarian model of medicine has gone too far. The proper end of medicine may require a shared obligation between patient and physician. The recent tendency to move toward a patient-dominated model of medicine, led by medical ethicists and philosophers, and more recently by lawyers, is probably unworkable. We suspect that the implications of this movement are unacceptable to many patients. There is little doubt that in the case of medicine when "a portion of the community understands the engagement in the original strict sense, the obligation becomes difficult to determine, and the judgements of conscientious persons regarding it become divergent and perplexed".

We think there are medical situations in which the judgment of technically competent physicians ought to dominate regardless of the patient's statements. It must be acknowledged that situations in which it is legitimate, perhaps even mandatory, to ignore the refusal of consent to treatment by a patient who has not previously been found legally incompetent are exceptional. But if these exceptional cases are shown to warrant a limited exercise of medical paternalism, it may be possible to isolate the details of such cases

10   MARK SIEGLER AND ANN DUDLEY GOLDBLATT

and to develop guidelines for an adjudication of conflicts between the patient
and the physician. For conceptual clarity we prefer to examine cases in which
third party interests – the family, the community, the state – are not used
to justify overriding the wishes of an individual. We wish to examine the
narrower issue of whether a physician is ever justified in usurping the will
of a patient in the *patient's own interest*. The two limiting cases we propose
to examine are (1) the right of an acutely, critically ill patient to refuse
simple, life-saving treatment, and (2) the right of a patient to demand specific
services from physicians. We will return to the issue of the demanding patient
in a later section of this essay. We turn now to the question of whether an
acutely, critically ill, but treatable, patient has an absolute right to refuse
treatment.

For our purposes, we define 'acute, critical, treatable illness' as an unanticipated, immediately life-threatening condition which begins acutely and
is caused by factors beyond the patient's control. The conditions we are
considering are those for which treatment is relatively easy, standardized
and conventional. Further, if treatment were withheld then the prognosis
would be very poor in terms of high mortality, and severe long-term disability
would result if spontaneous recovery occurred. Prognosis with treatment,
however, is excellent in terms of both survival and survival without long-term
disability. Indeed, we will assume that with adequate treatment these patients
can be restored to the level of health and functioning they enjoyed prior to
the onset of the acute critical illness.

Several of the terms in this definition require additional clarification.
'Acute critical illness' must be contrasted with 'chronic illness'. 'Unanticipated
illness' distinguishes these conditions from expected and predictable life-
threatening crises that inevitably occur in the course of chronic diseases or
terminal illness. Thus, we are not thinking of an episode of acute respiratory
failure that may occur once or several times during the progression of an
underlying illness such as chronic obstructive or restrictive pulmonary disease.

The term 'immediately life-threatening condition' describes a disease
process in which events unfold in minutes or hours rather than in days or
weeks. 'Cause beyond an individual's control' is used to exclude patients who
directly try to end their own lives or to injure themselves. Infectious illnesses,
traumatic injuries and myocardial infarctions are considered diseases 'beyond
an individual's control', even if certain life choices may in a statistical sense
predispose some individuals to these diseases.

The notion of treatment which is 'relatively easy, standardized and conventional' is meant to imply short-term, 'one shot' therapy such as an operation

CLINICAL INTUITION   11

or a short course of medication. This must be distinguished from high risk, experimental treatment, or long-term painful treatment such as cancer chemotherapy. The concept of 'prognosis' is of course based on probabilities, but in this context is used to refer to the outcome of diseases for which the data is relatively unambiguous, such as pneumococcal meningitis, acute respiratory failure, or exsanguinating hemorrhage, diseases in which immediate treatment has a very great probability of preventing death and disability.

Our model cases are not examples of terminal illness, chronic disease, suicidal patients, or even patients who assert a so-called 'right to die'. We wish to examine the responsibility of physicians to acutely, critically ill patients who somehow come to the attention of a physician, either by presenting voluntarily or by being admitted to hospital, and who then refuse life-saving treatment. Consider the following cases:

Case 1. The patient presents at an emergency room with high fever, headache and stiff neck. Consent is given for a spinal fluid examination to rule out meningitis. The lumbar puncture confirms non-epidemic bacterial (pneumococcal) meningitis. Pneumococcal meningitis can be treated by administering a course of antibiotics. This treatment usually will provide a total cure. If untreated, this form of meningitis is fatal in approximately 75% of its instances. Those who survive without treatment usually have severe, permanent, physical and mental impairment. The patient refuses treatment upon learning of the confirmed diagnosis.

Case 2. The patient has completed initial treatment for second and third degree burns extending over 50% of the patient's body. Therapy has entered a stage of debridement which is extremely painful, although the pain is partially palliated by analgesic and sedative medication and occasionally by anesthesia during debridement procedures. If the therapy is completed, the patient will regain nearly normal function. If treatment is terminated prior to its completion, a fatal bacteremia will probably result. The patient refuses to continue treatment.

Case 3. A patient is brought unconscious to a hospital emergency room. Initial examination reveals serious injuries including a punctured lung, a ruptured spleen and a probable concussion. While the patient is unconscious, plans are made to proceed with emergency abdominal surgery. The patient regains consciousness, refuses to consent to surgery, and demands to leave the hospital. The patient offers no specific reason for this decision.

12   MARK SIEGLER AND ANN DUDLEY GOLDBLATT

Case 4. A patient presents to an emergency room with severe crushing chest pain. An electrocardiogram reveals an acute myocardial infarction and greater than 20 multifocal, premature ventricular contractions per minute. The patient refuses to be admitted to hospital but requests analgesic medicine for use as an outpatient.

Case 5. A consenting, hospitalized patient is started on cancer chemotherapy with high dose methotrexate. Twelve hours later the patient refuses to accept oral leucovoran 'rescue' which is necessary to prevent severe and probably fatal bone marrow depression. The patient gives no reason for the refusal.

V. CLINICAL INTUITION

It is tempting to search for simple rules or principles which will enable one to resolve all cases of critically ill patients who refuse to consent to life-saving treatment. Several years ago, one of us (M.S.) published a case in which an acutely, critically ill patient's choices were respected and he died of his illness [18]. In that paper the physician adopted a basically libertarian stance and imposed a stringent burden on those who would wish to disregard a competent patient's refusal. The major issue was whether the patient understood the consequences of his refusal or whether his critical illness so impaired his thought processes that the soundness of his mentation was in question. Because of the difficulty of distinguishing competent, rational, and authentic decisions from incompetent, irrational and inauthentic judgments, there was a temptation to choose an existential position in which any decision was acceptable.

Eric Cassell, M.D., has explored the same problem and has argued the contrary position in an essay entitled "The Function of Medicine" [1]. He argued that most acutely, critically ill patients should be presumed to be devoid of autonomy. He relied on Gerald Dworkin's definition of autonomy as 'authenticity plus independence' [4]. Cassell suggested that the function of medicine was to *restore* autonomy by treating the patient, even if this meant disregarding the patient's competent, 'rational' refusal.

Cassell's justification for overriding a patient's wishes, on the grounds that illness renders individuals inauthentic, seemed excessively broad. It raised the possibility that acute, critical illness might provide grounds for a paternalistic intervention. One might consider that all critically ill patients lacked the knowledge and emotional capacity to make decisions about life and death. They would thus be like children for whom paternalistic intrusions might be

CLINICAL INTUITION   13

permissible. One could consider acutely, critically ill patients to be ignorant of the potential dangers involved in refusing the therapy (i.e., the probability of imminent death) and therefore temporarily restrain them, just as one might restrain a blind individual who wished to cross a bridge and did not realize the bridge had been washed away.

A colleague of ours, Martin Cook, pointed out that both we and Dr. Cassell were trying to stay off the slippery slope of determining what was a competent, rational, and authentic decision, although we did so with different results. Cassell argued that each patient should be presumed to be deprived of autonomy simply by virtue of his illness. We argued that almost any choice should be acceptable. All of us were looking for a conceptually neat solution. H. L. Mencken once remarked: "For every complex problem there is a solution that is simple, neat and wrong". We now believe that some patients with acute illness are, and some are not, able to make authentic choices; it is necessary, then, to formulate criteria for assessing individual judgments.

Unable to discover a single principle or a number of general rules to delimit coercive medical intervention, we have developed an approach we call 'clinical intuition'. Clinical intuition is based on a determination and a balancing of those clinical indications which should be considered by a physician when faced with an acutely, critically ill patient who declines life-saving treatment. We have constructed a list of *prima facie* considerations which should be used, and have attempted to rank them in order of importance.[2] Although this list is not exhaustive, the factors noted should always be taken into account by conscientious physicians before deciding whether to usurp the expressed will of critically ill patients who have not been found to be legally incompetent.

(1) The most important consideration is the patient's ability to choose: to understand the nature of his problem, to be able to express the medical alternatives and to understand the prognosis with and without treatment. If this ability is absent, as it is in unconscious or profoundly irrational patients, the physician's legal and moral duty to treat and to preserve life prevails. Even if the acutely, critically ill patient is able to express a choice and articulate the consequences of his choice, the physician should attempt to determine two additional things: first, whether the patient retains sufficient intellect and rationality to make this irreversible choice, and second, whether his choice reflects a 'true will' or is merely a reaction to the pain, fear, and uncertainty of his critical condition.

(2) In addition to assessing the rationality of the patient's particular choice, the physician should also ask another question: is this choice authentic? Is

14   MARK SIEGLER AND ANN DUDLEY GOLDBLATT

it consistent with the 'kind of person' this patient is? Is the choice consistent with the patient's enduring values, with his previous choices, with the convictions he has previously asserted and defended?

Authenticity may be established in several ways. It may be established by antecedent actions. The writing of a living will, the pre-existing appointment of an agent/surrogate, membership in a religious group which has a particular stance with respect to certain kinds of therapy, all support authenticity of particular choices which otherwise might be incomprehensible. The arguments of the Jehovah's Witness who refuses potentially life-saving blood transfusions are not only convincing because the courts have upheld them as expressing a free exercise of religion, but also because these convictions have been held and defended by individual Witnesses over a period of time; they have been temporally authenticated.

Authenticity, however, does not necessarily require antecedent statements or action. All people, even acutely, critically ill persons, have the right to change their minds. Thus, the quality and character of the refusal is also relevant. This is a kind of psychodynamic demonstration. It is achieved most easily when a long-standing DPR exists, but it can be accomplished when the patient is being seen for the first time. It depends upon the physician's understanding and acceptance that the patient is committed irrevocably to his determination not to be treated.

There is always a temptation to regard any choice which is not immediately comprehensible to physicians as an irrational or incompetent choice. Authentic choices are usually, but not always, understandable to others. Choosing death rather than intractable pain or financial ruin are comprehensible choices. An observer might not make the same choice, but he could perceive the factors that had been considered relevant and that had been weighed by the agent before reaching a decision. When authentic choices are based on private, secret, personal factors not easily comprehended by an observer (for example, a private religious belief against antibiotics), it is more difficult for the patient, particularly the acutely, critically ill patient being seen for the first time, to demonstrate the authenticity of his refusal.

It is true that the determination both of rationality and of authenticity is made by the physician. Many critics of medicine would prefer that the patient's condition — i.e., his rationality or competence or authenticity — rather than the physician's judgment of his condition, actually control whether the physician overrides a patient's wishes. This notion is unworkable. Rationality, competence and authenticity are not absolute standards such as 'Middle C.' Rather, they are states of mental responses that must be construed. While

CLINICAL INTUITION   15

one would hope for a rule of action that would eliminate subjectivity and avoid wrong decisions, we have seen why conceptually neat alternatives — either libertarianism or an all encompassing medical paternalism — are even more unacceptable.

(3) A third factor is the nature of the disease. Our discussion involves acute, critical illness in the hospital setting. Patients with chronic disease or even acutely, critically ill patients who present to a physician's office can more easily reject treatment. But in cases of acute, critical illness, one important fact is its prognosis if untreated and the probability of improvement if treatment is administered. Where diagnostic uncertainty is minimal, a simple treatment is curative, and the probability of death without treatment is high, the physician will be more likely to disregard the hospitalized patient's refusal. Examples would include conditions such as life-threatening but treatable, infectious illnesses (Case 1), severe hemorrhage after an injury (Case 3), or acute myocardial infarction with a life-threatening arrhythmia (Case 4).

Our decision in the three cases noted is based upon the acute, critical illness of the patient and the extremely favorable prognosis of those illnesses if treated quickly and appropriately. In contrast, if these illnesses were left untreated, the patient would almost certainly die or become permanently disabled. Our decision is also based on the uncertainty of the patient's rationality. The patient's choices appear inauthentic; no sound reasons are advanced for them. They are incomprehensible to the neutral observer. The physical pain present in each of these circumstances raises additional questions about the patient's true wishes. The probability of metabolic brain derangement from either the infectious meningitis or the impaired cardiac output associated with shock and cardiac arrhythmias would further encourage us to intervene even when these patients had not been declared legally incompetent. In these three cases, and in cases similar to them, we would tend to override the patient's expressed wishes.

(4) Several clinical variables can modify this determination, even in cases of acute, critical illness. If the patient has an underlying terminal disease or a severely disabling chronic condition, this should weigh in favor of respecting his refusal of treatment for the acute, critical condition. The same is true if an acute condition would result in permanent physical or mental disability even if treated promptly. To the contrary, if there is considerable uncertainty concerning diagnosis and prognosis, this may weigh in favor of disregarding a patient's refusal. However, if such an undiagnosed disease is unresponsive to therapy, and if the probability for successful intervention decreases, the balance can shift again.

16   MARK SIEGLER AND ANN DUDLEY GOLDBLATT

(5) Another consideration is the patient's age. Unquestionably, age influences clinical decisions involving the patient's refusals. The older the patient, the more likely his choice will be accepted.

These are considerations physicians should weigh whenever an acutely, critically ill patient refuses treatment. No formula or simple rule will resolve all clinical dilemmas, but physicians who use clinical intuition to help determine their actual decisions in individual cases have a potentially coherent procedure which can be applied, explained and subjected to public scrutiny.

VI. FURTHER THOUGHTS ON CLINICAL INTUITION

Alvan Feinstein, M.D., published his book *Clinical Judgment* in 1967 [5]. He urged clinicians to utilize the methods of scientific reasoning to improve their ability to make *therapeutic* decisions, one type of clinical decision. In contrast to therapeutic decisions, Feinstein noted that there was another type of clinical decision which he called 'environmental' and which he believed was not susceptible to scientific analysis. Feinstein writes:

... the multiple human personal attributes considered in the environmental decisions are often too complex to be catalogued, analyzed, and rationally dissected by any conventional contemporary logic. The clinician's approach to evaluating the patient exclusively as a person is still an artful aspect of care that depends on human perception and understanding. These components of clinical care are properties of heart and spirit, of instinct and psyche, and cannot be easily identified, assessed, or quantified by ordinary methods of reasoning.

He continues:

... the personal environmental management of a patient is a challenge to the clinician's judgment as a humanistic healer. The treatment of the patient is a challenge to the clinican's judgment as an experimental scientist. It is this latter aspect of clinical judgment — the performance and appraisal of therapeutic decisions — with which these essays are primarily concerned ([5], pp. 28–30).

Feinstein concludes that environmental decisions, unlike therapeutic decisions, are not easily resolvable by the application of the traditional methods of experimental science. Earlier in this essay, we concluded that certain environmental decisions, such as how to manage the acutely, critically ill patient who refuses life-saving treatment, are not easily resolvable by the application of rigid ethical principles or moral rules. Some guidelines are desirable, however, particularly when environmental decisions must be made.

Guidelines for decision-making are necessary for several reasons. The clinician must decide. He is forced to act (even inaction is an act); he must 'sin bravely'. In emergency situations there is limited time to gather information about the patient's values; the physician often must apply ethical principles to a particular clinical case without knowing his patient's true wishes. Guidelines would be desirable and helpful. If the guidelines for such decision-making were articulated, this would allow educators to teach these principles to medical students and physicians-in-training. This would also encourage intra-professional examination and criticism of the guidelines. Enunciated, published guidelines for action, as opposed to unspoken, personal clinical maxims, would permit public scrutiny of such guidelines. If some were unacceptable they could be restructured through intra-professional decisions or legislation. The point here is that it is useful to have articulated action-guiding principles which are subject to criticism.

Clinical intuition is a preliminary excursion into this domain. Clinical intuition includes both conventional scientific clinical judgment and the informed, moral intuition of physician-clinicians. These guidelines for decision-making in acute, critical illness are premised upon the traditional professional ethic of medicine. At the same time, they are, as they must be, sensitive to the changing moral understanding of patients and society. The principles of clinical intuition presented here are not absolute; it is certainly appropriate to criticize, refine, modify or abandon them if they prove inadequate or unworkable.

The process of clinical intuition is analogous to that proposed by W. D. Ross ([16], pp. 16–29) and consists of two components. First, it may be possible for physicians to elaborate a series of technical-moral guidelines which can serve as *conditional considerations* similar to Ross's *prima facie* duties. Such a conditional duty would always be a straightforward actual duty except that in certain circumstances there are other moral considerations which must also be weighed. The enumeration of a list of conditional duties for physicians — that is, principles of action which would always be binding in the absence of countervailing duties — is not an arbitrary exercise. It is based upon personal moral values, and upon those special moral guidelines which pertain to the profession of medicine. Homiletic injunctions such as: 'help and do no harm', or 'preserve life', or 'do unto others as you would have others do unto you', are all traditional moral guidelines for physicians. These general maxims probably include Ross's more clearly stated *prima facie* duties of fidelity, reparation, gratitude, justice, beneficence, non-maleficence and self-improvement. It is entirely appropriate, indeed it is essential, that society and its institutions, particularly legislatures and courts,

18   MARK SIEGLER AND ANN DUDLEY GOLDBLATT

be involved in the construction of this list of conditional considerations and in the attempt to rank and give weight to such considerations. This, then, is the first step in the process of clinical intuition.

The second stage, again analogous to Ross's, is to try to determine what our actual duty is in situations when conflicts exist among *prima facie* duties. In this process we are balancing the various *prima facie* duties in order to decide what specific action is appropriate, i.e., offers the greatest balance of positive considerations over negative ones. In this paper we have examined appropriate responses to acutely, critically ill patients who refuse therapy. Such cases seem to involve several conditional considerations which include (1) fidelity – what is the promise of the medical profession to critically ill individuals?, (2) beneficence; and (3) non-maleficence. But even if we agree that non-maleficence is the highest good, we are still left with the dilemma of whether to usurp the acutely ill patient's conscious wishes (in the context of being uncertain as to his competency) or to let him die. Which is the greater evil?

It is in situations like this, after a rational ordering of all conditional considerations, that physicians must exercise clinical intuition to decide what their actual duty is. We do not claim that physicians can⁻rely solely upon intuition to *know* with certainty what their actual duties are. Rather, we argue that the physician must utilize clinical intuition, an inductive form of reasoning, to appreciate what clinical action is suitable to the situation. Clinical intuition is fallible, but it is preferable to any existing system for making such determinations. It can be criticized and corrected. In this sense, it is similar to Rawls's concept of reflective equilibrium, a "mutual adjustment of principles and considered judgments . . . " ([15], p. 20).

We are sensitive to many of the criticisms of intuitionism, but we cannot find a better word to describe the process we are proposing. We are by no means suggesting that anyone can do what he pleases. Precisely by means of articulating our principles, we believe that we will allow for the correction of the problem. Society will have knowledge of the *prima facie* factors physicians use to reach their decisions and will be free to accept or reject these standards. Morally responsible physicians will have a rational process to employ in making these decisions. In the final decision, the moment of clinical truth, the physician must choose which of several competing duties is his actual duty. In doing so, he must employ clinical intuition.

VII. THE JUSTIFICATION OF CLINICAL INTUITION

We recognize that our proposal contradicts the conventional wisdom of those who champion 'patient rights' and argue that the physician should honor every decision of a patient who has not been found legally incompetent. Nonetheless, we believe that the application of clinical intuition is justified even in those cases where it results in disobeying a critically, acutely ill patient's stated wish not to be treated. In such cases, it is our view that over-ruling the patient's refusal may accord most closely with the requirements of the profession of medicine, the demands of the law, and the expectations of patients and their families.

When acutely, critically ill patients expressly refuse to consent to treatment, physicians are faced with an emergency situation. Particularly in the current era of the 'malpractice phenomenon' ([14], p. xv), physicians are ill at ease with simply letting patients die, especially those patients who are not terminally ill. In addition to contradicting their professional training and code, this practice makes physicians vulnerable to the criticisms of families and the threat of civil and criminal liability.[3]

Notwithstanding the celebration of unlimited patient autonomy by some commentators on the medical scene, it is usually difficult to convince those more directly involved that the curable did not want to be cured, that the decision to refuse treatment, made in the midst of extreme pain, fear and anxiety, was authentic. Physicians who acquiesce in these decisions, or who request that acutely, critically ill patients sign papers releasing the physician and hospital from liability for nontreatment, know quite well that this provides inadequate protection from the anger of families, the disbelief of juries and the dictates of their consciences.

Even if the physician could be certain he was insulated from legal liability, he could not be certain of the authenticity of the patient's decision. When a physician is faced with a patient in acute pain, who perhaps seeks death as the only escape from an overwhelming fear of death, and when there is not enough time to get a legal declaration of incompetence, the physician — who knows that treatment will almost certainly permit the patient to survive the emergency — will often decide to overrule the patient's refusal. We believe this describes the practice of many physicians in this situation.

Modifications in the doctor-patient relationship have exacerbated the physician's dilemma. Until recently, decisions concerning treatment took place within a continuing, long-standing relationship. Physician and patient were often friends and neighbors. Relations between them were based on a mutually understood medical context. Today, however, an acutely, critically ill patient is often a stranger. The physician is forced to concentrate on the choice, because he has no existing frame of reference concerning the chooser.

20   MARK SIEGLER AND ANN DUDLEY GOLDBLATT

The decision becomes not whether this choice of a particular patient is authentic, but whether a refusal itself can ever be considered an authentic decision.

Given these conditions of uncertainty and ignorance as to individual commitments and life-plans, the physician must decide whether a patient's refusal is 'authentic'. The physician must somehow determine that it is the patient who is deciding authentically, and not because of his treatable pain, anxiety, fear and confusion.

We want to emphasize that we do not rely on the common defense of medical paternalism based on the notion of role and responsibility. This defense argues that the role of the physician as defined by societal expectations generates specific obligations, such as the duty to preserve life in all circumstances, obligations that may not be applicable to other professionals. This argument seems unpersuasive when values and role responsibilities are in flux. It quickly becomes circular. The medical role is precisely what is in question. It is not helpful to argue that a particular notion of role legitimates a coercive intervention, for to do so begs the central question.

Faced with this situation, the physician must use the most general and commonly accepted rules of human behavior. Overruling the express refusal of an acutely, critically ill patient can be justified on the principle that all living things, and particularly all rational human beings, always seek to preserve their being ([9], I, 12). The physician who overrules a critically ill patient's stated refusal acts consistently with this principle of the will to survive. Even if a patient's refusal appears rational, this 'decision' is uncertain because it contradicts the 'natural law' of self-preservation. In view of this uncertainty, permitting the physician to overrule refusals made by acutely, critically ill patients with treatable illnesses constitutes a decision favoring the lesser of two potential evils. If pain and fear have led to an inauthentic refusal, the patient whose refusal is honored dies. But if a patient is treated successfully against his (authentic) will, he has at least the ability to exert legal retribution. He has regained freedom of action.

When a physician overrules the stated refusal of an acutely, critically ill patient, he does so analogically; the patient becomes similar to an unconscious patient, a patient from whom consent to life-saving treatment is *inferred* in emergency situations.[4] An assumption of implied consent in these and similar situations is based on the reigning public consensus that the *prima facie* 'best interests' of patients needing medical care are served by providing that care.[5]

This principle has been advanced, endorsed and elaborated in many states by the enactment of Good Samaritan legislation. Good Samaritan statutes permit physicians to treat critically ill or injured patients outside the hospital setting without fear of liability based on the absence of consent ([14], pp. vx–xvi). Consent is implied from the semi-conscious as well as the unconscious emergency 'patient' outside the hospital setting. Good Samaritan statutes will not meet the need they are designed to fulfill if they exclude those accident victims who, in acute pain but apparently rational, repeatedly state 'don't touch me' to the physicians who come to their aid.

We believe that the acutely, critically ill patient who refuses necessary, life-saving treatment more closely resembles the trauma victim and the profoundly irrational patient than a patient asked to consent to elective medical procedures. As we mentioned earlier, the implicit understandings of the doctor-patient relation are in a state of flux. Particularly now, when these 'social promises' of medicine are understood differently by different people, when a portion of the community remains committed to the traditional, paternal medical model, it is irresponsible for the physician always to assume that a patient means exactly what he says. A physician cannot know which mode of the patient-physician relationship this patient endorses.

This is why we advocate a public statement of the rules and application of clinical intuition. The prior acceptance of clinical intuition cannot completely protect a patient from unanticipated reactions to severe pain, fear and confusion; nor can it insulate the physician from subsequent criticism of his decision by a surviving patient or a deceased patient's immediate family. It does, however, provide better protection than the uncertain, idiosyncratic practice of the present. An announced and applied clinical intuition is far preferable to the current situation where no standards govern these decisions concerning refusals of treatment.

The position we are advocating is quite similar to the one proposed by Professor Hans Jonas. In a discussion of "The moral restraints on my freedom to decide against treatment for myself . . . ", Professor Jonas finds these restrictions essentially identical to those that ethically restrict our right to suicide. Jonas remarks:

This, admittedly, is interference with a subject's most private freedom, but only a momentary one and in the longer perspective an act in behalf of that very freedom. For it will merely restore the status quo of a free agent with the opportunity for second thoughts, in which he can revise what may have been the decision of a moment's despair – or can persist in it. Persistence will in the end succeed anyhow. The time-bound intervention treats the time-bound act like an accident from which to be saved, even against himself, can be presumed as the victim's own more enduring, if temporarily eclipsed, wish (sometimes betrayed by the very fact of imperfect secrecy that made the intervention possible) ([10], p. 32).

22   MARK SIEGLER AND ANN DUDLEY GOLDBLATT

It is evident that we do not support the principle of unfettered individual rights as a proper primary moral principle grounding the medical relation. Our defense of clinical intuition is based on a *balancing* of patient authenticity and physician responsibility — a subtle balancing which is not biased in advance in favor of the medical professional. We agree with the enthusiastic advocates of total autonomy that patients whose continuing existence depends on long-term medical treatment have both the capacity and the repose to make these decisions authentically. Patients who require renal dialysis or extensive and painful therapy, such as the severely burned patient (see Case 2), ought not to be coerced into accepting these treatments.

We hope that those who most avidly advocate patient autonomy would agree with us that a patient ought not to use a physician or medical treatment itself as a means to suicide. We believe it is clear that a patient ought not to cause his own death by withdrawing consent in the middle of certain interconnected medical or surgical treatments. For example, a patient who has consented to methotrexate chemotherapy ought not to be allowed to refuse the leucovoran rescue drug essential to neutralize the otherwise fatal toxicity of methotrexate (see Case 5). This particular concept has obvious 'slippery slope' implications and should be limited to those interconnected treatments that a physician would not begin *but for* the prior assurance that consent will not be withdrawn. The leucovoran problem is resolved by this minimal limit on patient autonomy — the more intricate considerations of clinical intuition are not required. But if it is appropriate for physicians to contradict a decision to refuse leucovoran rescue, then patient autonomy is never absolute. And if the leucovoran example reveals something unique about the medical relation, as we believe it does, it would be unfortunate if we failed to explore its implications.

Admittedly, our exploration of the best mode of the medical relation is colored by an increasing mistrust of the medical profession and the biomedical and natural sciences. Any theory that limits the decision-making rights of individuals is unpopular. An increasingly militant opposition to all forms of medical paternalism has resulted in legal decisions that have limited the authority of physicians to impose life-saving treatment on patients who expressly refuse such treatments. These decisions have been embraced by a few commentators ([20], pp. 116–163) as somehow establishing a general rule that physicians must obey any decision made by a patient, even a refusal of life-saving medical treatment. We believe these commentators have misread the legal precedents. It is our opinion that these decisions are correctly understood as specific exceptions to a general and abiding presumption in favor of

CLINICAL INTUITION   23

life-saving treatment. Like all legal decisions, they must be interpreted on the basis of their specific facts. Thus interpreted, these decisions demonstrate some limitations on a patient's right to refuse life-saving treatments. A patient's refusals of life-saving treatments have been authorized in the following situations: (1) when the treatment indicated can at best prolong the life of a terminally ill [6] or comatose patient,[7] (2) when the treatment contravenes a recognised belief,[8] and (3) when the treatment destroys physical integrity, e.g., an amputation.[9]

The most frequently discussed precedent allowing a terminally ill patient to refuse life-prolonging treatment involved a proxy refusal made on behalf of an incompetent patient. *Superintendent of Belchertown State School v Saikewicz* involved the question of whether potentially life-prolonging treatment can be withheld without the judicially reviewed consent of an incompetent patient's legal guardian.[10] *Saikewicz* concluded that the presumption in favor of preserving life may be qualified when the question is one of prolonging the life of the terminally ill. When the illness is terminal and the patient is incompetent, a *subjective* 'substitute judgment' of what the *patient, if* he *could* make a competent choice would choose for his incompetent self is permitted.[11]

Saikewicz stated that a terminally ill incompetent patient can 'refuse' treatment to the same extent as a terminally ill competent patient.[12] *Saikewicz* says nothing about the ability of any patient legally to refuse *life-saving* treatments. The decision makes a clear distinction between a palliative and life-saving treatment:

There is a substantial distinction in the State's insistence that human life be saved where the affliction is curable as opposed to the State's interest where, as here, the issue is not whether, but when, for how long, and at what cost to the individual that life may be briefly extended.[13]

And indeed, Massachusetts courts have three times prohibited the parents of a three-year old leukemia patient from refusing to submit their child to chemotherapy, a treatment that now holds out a significant chance not just of remission but of cure ([6], p. 269).

There are a number of legal decisions upholding the right of members of Jehovah's Witnesses to refuse blood transfusions. Few have involved actual refusals of life-saving treatments.[14] These decisions are distinctive because they are based on the preferred position of the First Amendment's guarantee of freedom of religion. But even this constitutional right is limited. The reliance placed on these cases by those who would use them as evidence of a

24   MARK SIEGLER AND ANN DUDLEY GOLDBLATT

general rule ignores their particular limitations and specific circumstances. These limitations include the patient's age and the existence of dependent spouse or children.[15] Circumstances that support the patient's decision include public knowledge that Witnesses believe infusions of blood and blood products result in eternal damnation.

Additional difficulties are raised by the Jehovah's Witness precedents. In some cases, the legal decision was made after the patient was successfully transfused, after the patient successfully recovered without needing the transfusion, or when the decision was rendered moot by the patient's so-called 'willingness to be coerced'.[16] This last is particularly troublesome; for if a patient has a right to refuse treatment, what right does the physician have to attempt to coerce that patient into foregoing that right? Moreover, those commentators who use the Jehovah's Witness precedents as the basis of a general right to refuse treatment attempt to extend the constitutional rights afforded religious freedom to every patient refusal, including those based on unarticulated personal beliefs.[17] For all these reasons, the physician faced with a patient who refuses life-saving treatment on grounds other than religious conviction receives no aid from the Jehovah's Witness precedents.

A third group of legal precedents permitting patients to refuse treatment is limited to unconsented destructions of physical integrity. These decisions involve the refusals of elderly patients to consent to the amputation of a limb. The need for amputation in such patients is caused either by an underlying disease or by a chronic, incurable and ultimately terminal disease.[18] Nonetheless, the degree of physical mutilation as well as the permanency of amputation do appear to provide some basis for a general rule allowing patient refusals to this kind of life-prolonging medical treatment.

Judicial precedents upholding the right of patients to refuse certain medical treatments in specific situations neither demonstrate nor provide a basis for inferring a general right to refuse life-saving medical treatment. While emphasizing that it is inappropriate to imply *any* general rule from these precedents, the very existence of these precedents reveals an underlying presumption in favor of overruling refusals of life-saving treatment. If the law favored patient autonomy in these instances, there would be no need for litigation to create specific exceptions.

The specific exceptions created by these precedents coincide with many of the considerations we propose as elements of clinical intuition, considerations such as authenticity, rationality, consistency and medical prognosis. The legal precedents are more restrictive than our principle of clinical intuition, because they impose additional conditions limiting patient refusals. These additional

CLINICAL INTUITION   25

restrictions, such as patient responsibility for dependent spouse and children, are community considerations. Such third party interests may not be appropriate elements of a patient-physician relationship. Third party rights aside, our proposal of clinical intuition coincides with the traditional legal conception of the doctor-patient relationship as well as with developing trends in the law.

VIII. THE DEMANDING PATIENT

Throughout this paper we have been concentrating on the acutely, critically ill patient who refuses life-saving treatment. We have noted that the problem of the patient who refuses treatment has been exacerbated by changes in the DPR. Our proposal of clinical intuition is offered as a mediation between the traditional paternal model and an evolving libertarian model of the DPR. It is intended also to protect both physician and patient during a time of uncertain understanding and changing expectations. But even if our proposal were to be endorsed enthusiastically, we would not have resolved our concern with the potential consequences of a libertarian medical model.

We believe that discussions of a libertarian model have failed to consider one of its most significant consequences. It encourages the demanding medical consumer, the patient who demands medical treatment based on a personal determination of his needs and desires. Clinical medicine has always encouraged patients to present with a self-defined sense of dis-ease. But the patient who presents with symptoms and also demands specific treatment based on self-prognosis poses a different problem. Such patients view clinical medicine as one of the 'serving professions' and themselves as medical consumers. When this conception of the roles of medical practitioners and medical consumers is joined with the extreme importance most citizens place on health and medical care, treatment-of-choice becomes not only a product which can be consumed at will, but a right to which one is entitled on demand.

Perhaps this 'diagnosis' is too dismal, but the 'prognosis' is based on events of the last twenty years, beginning with a coincidence concerning patients' rights too pointed to ignore. Expanded legal requirements for informed consent to medical treatment were introduced in 1960;[19] it was also the first year in which the contraceptive pill was offered as a non-experimental, pharmacologic agent. Oral contraceptive medication was the first prescription drug that was (and is) in effect, a self-prescribed 'treatment'. Patients — i.e., 'medical consumers' desiring elective medication — demanded that physicians prescribe the contraceptive pill. Other popularly self-prescribed medications soon followed: tricyclic antidepressants, mood elevators and minor tranquilizers. Here patient demands were based at least in part on a belief that these medications were appropriate for self-diagnosed 'conditions' — not precisely diseases but rather perceived disadvantageous health states. Need was based on a belief that one was not feeling one's best and that medication would cure this malaise. Medication was requested and received for non-specific anxiety, for lethargy, for nervousness, for insecurity caused by a poor self-image. Medications and surgical procedures came to be seen as appropriate solutions or treatments for problems previously considered individual or social concerns, but in any case not biological abnormalities or specific diseases: problems such as alcoholism, hyper or hypo-activity, excessive appetite, a nose too large, hips too wide, hair too sparse.

Just when patients began to protect themselves from what they feared medicine and technology could do *to* them, they became entranced with what modern medicine could do *for* them. And what medicine can do for them, they have discovered, is not limited to medication and cosmetic surgery. By the early 1970's we were hearing of intestinal bypasses for marginal obesity, an invasive procedure that contradicts normal risk-benefit analysis for elective surgery. This procedure requires a substantial allocation of medical resources for a self-perceived need, and views a surgical treatment not as a curative procedure but as a mechanism for transformation of the self.

Physicians acknowledge the practice of surgeon-shopping for this and similar surgical procedures. Some surgeon will perform cardiac bypass surgery at the request of a patient with essential chest pain; or a cholecystectomy for a patient with functional abdominal pain, even when these self-styled patients are poor risks for elective surgery. Some doctors have praised the utility of CAT Scanning to reduce anxiety in patients with non-specific headaches. Here the CAT Scan provides the service of reassurance, a function traditionally performed by the physician as doctor, as teacher. Can CAT Scanning substitute for the physician? If the patient fears, for example, a 'brain tumor', the headache will most likely return. While the doctor can assure the patient why a tumor is unlikely, the CAT Scan can only show that no tumor has been detected — at least not yet. Because the physician has transferred the service of reassurance to the scanner, and because a machine is not, as is the physician, an experienced prognosticator, repeat scans are necessary for reassurance. Are the patient's medical needs adequately served by repeated scannings? Is this kind of service a legitimate medical practice, or is it a technological gimmick, a new and more marvelous version of the X-Ray machine in use thirty years ago that demonstrated how well children's shoes fit?

Most physicians are troubled by patients who demand treatment for self-defined conditions. Nonetheless, when treatment is available and the patient believes his sense of un-ease is 'curable' by means of physician-mediated treatment or medication, a physician willing to provide the demanded service usually can be found.

We believe the demanding patient presents a serious danger to clinical medicine. A patient who refuses treatment questions the relevance and importance of the physician's professional responsibility. He may even usurp the professional ethic that traditionally obligates the physician to maintain and to restore health, and to preserve life. But the demanding patient denies that the physician's responsibilities and expertise have any relevance except insofar as this coincides with the patient's desires. The demanding patient inverts the traditional model and makes the physician a passive agent. The patient proposes; the physician provides. The physician becomes a technician, practicing under the direction and control of his 'client'. We are not arguing that a person ought to have an enforceable legal claim to the medical procedures of his choice. Unless a patient presents with a life-threatening emergency, a physician may refuse to provide any service. But an evolving libertarian model is reinforcing a public understanding that demanded treatments can be obtained from some physician, at least so long as payment is assured.

Over 70% of all hospital costs are paid by Blue Cross, Medicare and Medicaid. Blue Cross negotiates with hospitals to determine what costs are to be reimbursed. Medicaid and Medicare limit coverage by administrative regulation. In some areas of care, such as length of hospitalization, need for hospitalization for particular services, and determinations of what medical services are necessary, the practice of medicine is already a regulated industry. This solution, and particularly the rapid rate of its expansion, is unsatisfactory to many patients and physicians. While limited financial resources and the spectre of bureaucratic control may be satisfactory practical reasons for opposing the trend towards patient-controlled clinical medicine, they are not sufficient philosophical reasons. If it is only money and the end of the exalted self-image of the physician that argue against patient control, those who favor the traditional medical model are already defeated.

One of the difficulties in making a theoretical argument against patient controlled medicine is that these arguments almost always seem 'élitist'. The knowledge and training necessary to become competent in both the science and practice of medicine require extensive specialized education. The physician faced with a patient-consumer who demands a certain medication has neither the time nor the pedagogical ability to make the patient his equal in

28   MARK SIEGLER AND ANN DUDLEY GOLDBATT

knowledge concerning the specific drug and its biological potentialities. In some cases, the physician's hesitancy in prescribing medication may be based on an unarticulated clinical judgment. Moreover, the demanding patient often comes to the physician with a pre-existing distrust; he is more convinced by his perception of what the medication has done for his friends than the statistical risks, probable effects and possibly biased predictions of usefulness the physician offers.

IX. CONCLUSION

The charge of élitism may be inescapable; it is simply true that the physician is more capable than the patient of determining a specific diagnosis and prognosis, and of designing the most beneficial course of treatment. This is not to say that patients are uneducable or should be kept ignorant. The mistrust of physicians which is one of the causes of the demanding patient is in turn a result of the patient's relative lack of information about the science and practice of medicine. More than twenty years ago C. P. Snow said that the two cultures of the modern world were separated by the science of physics. A good argument can be made today that physics has been replaced by the biological sciences, particularly molecular biology and human genetics. Basic biological and medical knowledge could reduce the mistrust the public feels toward the physician, his motives and his intentions. It would also correct inappropriate, often misconceived understandings of what the wonders of modern medicine and medical technology can and should provide. Increased general biomedical knowledge could become the basis of an individual understanding and acceptance of responsibility for health maintenance and disease prevention. This would make the physician and patient partners as to goals and more nearly partners in health care procedures and curative medicine. Education would eliminate the too common belief that the 'magic bullets' of modern clinical medicine can replace or cure the medical effects of self-inflicted abuse. Patient education could also permit (and even require) the physician to start explaining why patients should do what they should do — not just telling them what they must do. Physicians are often disliked as well as mistrusted for their authoritarian approach, but so long as explanations must be exhaustive — and even then often only marginally understood — the brusque, authoritarian physician is an excusable if not sympathetic stereotype.

If the choice between the authoritarian and libertarian models of clinical medicine assumes an uneducated patient, we would propose the authoritarian model. But if this assumption is not necessary, it is possible that no such choice need be made. Clinical intuition, including most particularly the component of publicity and a before-the-fact awareness of its use, is an important step towards patient education. Another important step that need not await more comprehensive biomedical education rests within the power of the medical profession. The medical profession needs to attend to its own house: to encourage physicians not to perform unnecessary surgery; not to order or acquiesce in unnecessary diagnostic procedures; not to prescribe excessive medication. The medical profession should attempt to persuade both its members and those it serves that the ends of medicine do not include the ability to cure the human condition or to insure the physical and mental health and social and psychological well-being of any individual [11].

If patients had a more comprehensive biomedical background and physicians and patients had mutually known and consistent goals, there would be much less need for procedures such as clinical intuition. At present severe pain, fear of death and especially fear of a lingering and costly death can cause the acutely, critically ill patient to refuse to consent to treatment. Education and partnership would eliminate much of this fear and that aspect of pain that is caused by ignorance and anxiety. At present, we believe clinical intuition is the best approach to the problem of the acutely, critically ill but not profoundly irrational patient who refuses medical treatment.

University of Chicago
Chicago, Illinois

NOTES

[1] A notable exception to this is the work of Charles Culver, M.D., a psychiatrist at the Dartmouth Medical School, and Professor Bernard Gert of the Dartmouth Department of Philosophy. They have written extensively on the subject of the responsibility of physicians to patients who require but refuse psychiatric hospitalization. They have also specifically considered issues of physician paternalism and the justification of such paternalism ([7], [8]). Their work is represented in this volume by their paper, 'The Morality of Involuntary Hospitalization'.

[2] We have adapted a method that is parallel in many respect to the process described by W. D. Ross in his essay 'What Makes Right Acts Right?' ([16], pp. 16–29). Our method is described in greater detail later in this paper (see Section VI, *Further Thoughts on Clinical Intuition*). It is important to recognize that we are not merely applying Ross's principles to a medical situation. Rather, we are using his philosophical insights to develop a clinical method we refer to as clinical intuition.

[3] *Application of President and Directors of Georgetown College*, 331 F. 2d 1000 (D. C.

30   MARK SIEGLER AND ANN DUDLEY GOLDBLATT

Cir., 1964); rehearing en banc denied, 331 F. 2d 1010 (1964); *Jones v. United States*, 308 F. 2d 307 (D. C. Cir., 1962).

[4] *In re Osborne*, 294 A. 2d 371 374–5 (D. C. Cir., 1972) "Where the patient is comatose or suffering impairment of capacity for choice, it may be better to give weight to the known instinct for survival which can in a critical situation alter previously held convictions. In such cases it cannot be determined with certainty that a deliberate and intelligent choice has been made".

[5] *Petition of Nemser*, 273 N. Y. S. 2d 624, 629 (Sup. Ct., N. Y. Cty., 1966).

[6] *Superintendent of Belchertown State School v. Saikewicz*, 370 N. E. 2d 417 (Mass., 1977).

[7] *Matter of Quinlan*, 355 A. 2d 647 (N.J., 1976).

[8] See Note 5. See also *Winters v. Miller*, 446 F. 2d 65 (2d Cir., 1971).

[9] *Matter of Quackenbush*, 383 A. 2d 785 (N.J. Super. Ct., Probate Div., 1978) (amputation of both legs); see *Petition of Nemser*, Note 5.

[10] See Note 6.

[11] See Note 6 at p. 430.

[12] See Note 6 at p. 428.

[13] See Note 6 at p. 426.

[14] See Note 4.

[15] *J. F. Kennedy Hosp. v. Heston*, 279 A 2d 670 (N. J. 1971); See also *Application of President and Directors of Georgetown College*, Note 3.

[16] *In re Estate of Brooks*, 205 N. E. 2d 435 (Illinois 1965); *In re Osborne*, 294 A 2d 372 (D. C. Cir., 1972); *United States v. George*, 239 F., Supp. 752 (D. Conn. 1965).

[17] See *Collins v. Davis*, 254 N. Y. S. 2d 666 (Sup Ct., N. Y. Cty., 1964).

[18] See Note 9. See also *Lane v. Candura*, No. M78–417, Mass, C. A., Middlesex Cty, May 22, 1978.

[19] *Natanson v. Kline*, 350 P. 2d 1093 (Kansas 1960).

BIBLIOGRAPHY

1. Cassell, E. J.: 1977, 'The Function of Medicine', *Hastings Center Report* 7, 16–19.
2. Culver, C. M. and Gert, B.: 'The Morality of Involuntary Hospitalization', in this volume, pp. 159–175.
3. Donagan, A.: 1977, 'Informed Consent in Treatment and Experimentation', *Journal of Medicine and Philosophy* 2, 307–329.
4. Dworkin, G.: 'Paternalism', *The Monist* 56, 64–84.
5. Feinstein, A. R.: 1967, *Clinical Judgment*, Williams and Wilkins Company, Baltimore.
6. George, S. L. *et al.*: 1979, 'A Reappraisal of the Results of Stopping Therapy in Childhood Leukemia', *The New England Journal of Medicine* 300, 269–273.
7. Gert, B. and Culver, C. M.: 1976, 'Paternalistic Behavior', *Philosophy and Public Affairs* 6, 45–57.
8. Gert, B. and Culver, C. M.: 1979, 'The Justification of Paternalism', *Ethics* 89, 199–210.
9. Hobbes, T.: 1651, *Leviathan* I, 12.
10. Jonas, H.: 1978, 'The Right to Die', *Hastings Center Report* 8, 31–36.

CLINICAL INTUITION   31

11. Kass, L. R.: 1975, 'Regarding the End of Medicine and the Pursuit of Health', *The Public Interest* **40**, 11–42.

12. Ladd, J.: 'Physicians and Society: Tribulations of Power and Responsibility', in this volume, pp. 33–52.

13. Livy: *History of Rome*, Book XLIV, 22, 8. Transl. by George Baker, A. J. Valpy, London, 1834, pp. 326–327.

14. *Medical Malpractice*: Report of Secretary's Commission, 1973, p. xv, DHEW Publ. No. (OS) 73–88.

15. Rawls, J.: 1971, *A Theory of Justice*, Belknap Press, Harvard University Press, Cambridge, p. 20.

16. Ross, W. D.: 1930, *The Right and the Good*, Clarendon Press, Oxford, pp. 16–29.

17. Sidgwick, H.: 1874, *The Methods of Ethics*, MacMillan and Company, London, pp. 308–310.

18. Siegler, M.: 1977, 'Critical Illness: The Limits of Autonomy', *Hastings Center Report* **7**, 12–15.

19. Szasz, T. S. and Hollender, M. H.: 1956, 'The Basic Models of the Doctor-Patient Relationship', *The Archives of Internal Medicine* **97**, 585–592.

20. Veatch, R. M.: 1976, *Death, Dying, and the Biological Revolution*, Yale University Press, New Haven, pp. 116–163.

8.3   Siegler M (1981) The Doctor-Patient Encounter and Its Relationship to Theories of Health and Disease. In: Caplan AL, Engelhardt Jr HT, McCartney JJ (eds) Concepts of Health and Disease: Interdisciplinary Perspectives. Addison-Wesley, Reading, Massachusetts, p 627–44

6.2

The Doctor-Patient Encounter and Its Relationship to Theories of Health and Disease

Mark Siegler

I. INTRODUCTION

A relationship may exist between clinical medicine and theories of health and disease; if so, this relationship will likely prove to be complex and multidimensional. It must be discovered and analyzed. The practice of clinical medicine probable influences what counts as health and disease, and simultaneously theories of health and disease probably modify the nature and limits of clinical medicine. Theoretical constructs of various models of health and disease are tested ultimately in the realities of medical practice. It might be useful to explore the nature of clinical medicine in an effort to derive further insight into various models of health and disease.

The nature of clinical medicine is not an entity to be discovered like a truth of nature; rather it is defined and created in the context of a negotiated accommodation between a doctor and a patient. There is no single "nature of clinical medicine," but many such natures. What counts as a problem of clinical medicine is mutually decided in a doctor-patient accommodation which may lead to a deeper, longer lasting, doctor-patient relationship. Without such a doctor-patient accommodation problems do not exist in clinical medicine, even though there may exist health problems, or diseases, or even problems in preventive, social, community, or research medicine. Clinical medicine requires accommodations between individual patients and physicians which are designed to achieve mutually agreed on goals.

The determination that a problem falls within the boundaries of clinical medicine (rather than saying that a problem is a disease or a health problem) is an elaborate process and is usually the result of a mutually agreed on transaction between patient and physician in which the physician's eventual agreement with the patient that a problem is a medical problem (again, rather

627

than saying that a problem is a disease or a health problem) decides the case, but in which many preliminary developments have been necessary. In general, a necessary, although not a sufficient, condition for a problem to become one for clinical medicine is that the doctor and patient agree that it is one. However, when conflicts arise between patients and physicians in which either claims that a medical problem does not exist, then, with rare exceptions, for their purposes the issue is not a problem of clinical medicine. Of course, negotiations between doctors and patients are governed and partially constrained by such external forces as the availability of resources and the political demarcation of boundaries for medicine.

My contention is that these negotiations, carried on by thousands of physicians who interact with millions of patients, determine at the individual doctor-patient level the nature and limits of clinical medicine, and further, they provide valuable data from which can be inferred societally accepted norms on the nature and limits of clinical medicine and on societal attitudes towards health and disease.

Note that although an understanding of clinical medicine may illuminate our concepts of health and disease, the distinction between clinical medicine and health and disease models must be maintained. If it could be agreed that the legitimate goal of clinical medicine is the pursuit of physical and mental health, it would be crucial to indicate that clinical mdicine is merely one means by which health can be pursued or regained. Without laboring this point, it is clear that health can be maintained or regained in the absence of clinical medical intervention by improving living conditions, nutrition, sanitation, education, and by strengthening an individual's personal responsibility for the maintenance of his own health. Not all health problems are appropriately problems of or for clinical medicine. Some health problems would be entirely legitimate as problems of clinical medicine if they ever came to the attention of the traditional medical system. However, whether because of the unavailability or inaccessibility of health services, or because of an individual's failure to recognize problems as medical, or because of an individual's own decision to seek treatment of these problems in nonmedical systems, these problems never become problems for clinical medicine. For example, a patient being treated for asthma by a physician has both a health problem and a clinical medical problem. However, another person with asthma who goes to church to pray for the relief of symptoms may have a health problem, but does not have a clinical medical problem.

II. MODELS OF HEALTH AND DISEASE

Physicians and philosophers have developed many theories of health and disease. Such constructions attempt to describe the nature of health and disease and usually attempt secondarily to use such descriptions to prescribe the proper range and scope of clinical medicine. The analyses often turn on the issue of whether disease is an objective biological state, describable and verifiable by objective criteria, or alternatively whether disease is relative to social and cultural values.

As its limit, the model of disease as an objective biological state represents an analytic, scientific view in which disease and specific etiology serve as the paradigm, and in which it is argued that dysfunctional assessments involve no value judgments. In this view, sometimes referred to as the functionalist model of medicine, disease is a fact. In contrast, the extreme relativistic model of disease holds that biological derangements may not be very relevant to dysfunctional states and that all functional assessments—both somatic and psychological—involve only value judgments. An intermediate claim might hold that functional assessments frequently involve value judgments, but nevertheless it is possible to arrive at an objective assessment of dysfunction even while acknowledging the presence of a series of value judgments. Each of these three models is represented in the writings of clinicians, although the narrow, scientific model of medicine has been in the ascendancy in recent decades (or perhaps recent centuries) and has only recently been challenged again by proponents of a broader psychosocial concept of disease.

Recently a distinguished physician (Seldin, 1977) defended the traditional scientific medical model and argued that modern medicine ought to narrow and restrict its scope to those medical, surgical, and psychiatric conditions for which effective drug or surgical therapy was available. In this view, medicine is regarded as narrowly disease-oriented and is enjoined from accepting a variety of social or political missions which it is not capable of accomplishing. This functionalist model of medicine considers the maintenance or restoration of health to be the goal of medicine. Any departure from "normal" functioning is regarded as a disease, and the goal of medicine is to alleviate such dysfunctional states. Some supporters of the functional hypothesis maintain a narrow, often merely physical view of health, and do not indicate clearly how psychological well-being falls within the purview of medicine (Kass, 1975).

In contrast to these positions describing limited goals for medicine, some have defended the functionalist model, but have suggested that medicine has been far too narrow in its scope and that what medicine needs is precisely a broader model sometimes referred to as a biopsychosocial model of medicine. This view of medicine includes as disease, that is, dysfunctional states, physical-biological derangements, psychological difficulties, and even social problems. In this model, a physician would be held responsible for evaluating and managing almost any problem with which a patient presented to a medical setting. An extreme statement of this model could be referred to as "the complaint model" of medicine, in which physicians are responsible for responding to almost all patient complaints. In this view, the range of

630 Concepts of Health and Disease

medicine is defined by complaints people make in a medical setting, and the art of medicine is regarded as responding in the most effective way to treat patient complaints (Engelhardt, 1979).

I do not deny the importance of developing these kinds of conceptual models to account for actual behavior. Nor do I deny the potential usefulness of such models in modifying the behavior of physicians and patients in the future. On the one hand, such theoretical models may, if agreed upon, influence the medical profession's own sense of the range and extent of its medical obligations. For example, if an intraprofessional consensus emerged on the limits of medicine, for example, on a narrow scientific model or on a broad "complaint model," it might be reflected eventually in medical education—perhaps in the selection process of the medical students and in the curriculum for undergraduate and postgraduate medical students—and it might also be reflected eventually in the medical marketplace. Alternatively, if health planners and legislators could agree on a particular theoretical model for medicine, whether or not the profession concurred entirely with such a model, in time, practical limits could be established (perhaps through financing mechanisms) on the scope of clinical medical activities.

My concern with these theories is that none of them quite wrestles with the actualities of medical practice in an effort to describe what clinical medicine is, what its limitations are, and what the relationship is between theories of health and disease and the practice of medicine. Specifically, neither the functional model nor the complaint model provides usable guidelines that could be followed by conscientious physicians who encounter a patient in a clinical setting. Attempts to limit the scope of medicine to physical derangements fails to take into account psychological and psychosomatic illness and also founders in a more fundamental way in an inability to define adequately the concept of boundaries to healthy existence. In contrast, a broad vision of medicine, in which all patient complaints are to be counted and addressed, fails to indicate except in the most general ways how patient demands are to be restrained in such a system. It has been suggested that certain complaints transgress medical boundaries and should be seen as educational or political problems, but frequently criteria are not offered for making such a determination. One commentator notes that certain "medical" matters ought not be addressed by physicians because a physician would be involved in unethical, immoral, frivolous, or costly endeavors, but again, the question of how this conclusion is to be arrived at and who is responsible for reaching this judgment is left unanswered (Engelhardt, 1979). My essential criticism of these theoretical constructions about the nature of health and disease centers on the unclarity of how and in what circumstances such models are to be used by health planners, and more importantly, by physicians and patients.

These various theoretical models suppose that a univocal sense of health and disease appropriately describes modern medicine and captures its nuances. Proponents of such theories believe that such encompassing constructs are context-free and are beneficial to society. It should be asked, however, whether any single theory of health and disease can satisfactorily describe a system of modern medicine that includes neurosurgery, cosmetic surgery, psychoanalysis, acupuncture, and the management of aging.

I wish to suggest that a context-dependent, rather that a context-free definition of medicine would be considerably more useful for physicians and patients, and also for health planners, in determining the goals and ends of medicine. For example, in the case of emergency surgery, a narrow functional model provides a reasonably accurate description of events, whereas in other areas of medicine, such as the psychiatric management of unhappiness, alternative constructs such as a broader biopsychosocial model are needed.

An alternative approach, one that will be pursued in this chapter, is to begin not with theories of health and disease, but rather with the actuality of health and disease. If we can understand how clinical medicine works in the realities of daily practice, we may achieve a better understanding of the nature of clinical medicine and its relationship to disease and health. It seems important, even necessary as a crucial preliminary step, to understand how patients and physicians currently behave and how they describe and justify their actions before formulating any theoretical basis for such actions. It is even possible that such an approach would indicate how theories of health and disease could be applied more appropriately to resolve practical medical dilemmas. Thus, in contrast to those who propose a theoretical model of medicine and then attempt to deduce conclusions that may be useful in clinical medicine, I propose a more inductive model that moves from the actual experience of medicine, from the negotiation processes carried on by patients and doctors, to a definition of what clinical medicine is and what its goals are.

III. THE PATIENT-DOCTOR ENCOUNTER

In an effort to explore further the thesis that a problem becomes one for clinical medicine only when the patient and doctor agree that it is one, the medical encounter can be divided into four logical moments (or stages or phases): 1) the person in a pre-patient phase, 2) the physician in the context of the initial encounter with the person who now presents as a patient, 3) the negotiated accommodation between the doctor and the patient, and 4) the doctor-patient relationship. Strictly speaking, these are moments in the logical rather than in the chronological sense, because they attempt to distinguish, for purposes of analysis, elements of an interconnected process that begins when patient and physician first meet, or in fact, when they first communicate. It is important to describe accurately what occurs in such circumstances and to avoid false compartmentalization or linearization of these moments. Nevertheless, most of the pre-patient phase of this encounter is logically prior to physician involvement, and considerable action occurs in the second clinical moment, the physician phase, which is required before concluding a patient-physician accommodation. At each stage of this process, both the patient and the doctor formulate hypotheses in their minds about what kind of problem exists and what should be done about it. It is unlikely that either the doctor or the patient relies on a theoretical construction during most of the stages of their encounter.

The Pre-Patient Phase of Clinical Medicine

The pre-patient phase of clinical medicine represents the first clinical moment. An individual's decision that he has a health problem must precede the actual medical encounter. This pre-patient phase surely represents a necessary, although not a sufficient, factor to decide that the problem is appropriate to clinical medicine. The perception of a state of ill health and a decision to seek medical help is influenced by many social, cultural, political, and economic factors, in addition to the biological manifestations of the perceived state of ill health (Parsons, 1951; Merton, 1957).

Except in instances of acute medical problems where medical care is sought in an emergency, persons usually have considered their bodily sensations, that is, their symptoms, the persistence of symptoms, and the effect such symptoms have on disrupting their ordinary personal and social activities. Further, individuals will have considered their own values and beliefs, those of their immediate family and community, and the availability, cost, and quality of medical care, before determining that a particular sensation or feeling is one that should be attended to by physicians rather than, for example, by priests or teachers or social workers or by themselves.

Some commentators have suggested that medical symptoms or physiological abnormalities may be detected in as many as 90 percent of the population, but what converts such symptoms into medical problems is the failure of individuals to adapt to the stress that accompanies these symptoms. These analysts do not indicate why this failure of adaptation to stress should cause individuals to seek care from medical sources rather than from other helping professionals.

In an effort to understand the relationship of the first clinical moment—the self-definition of illness by the prospective patient—to concepts of health and disease, a case example may be useful.

A Case Example of the Pre-Patient Phase of Clinical Medicine. An eighty-one-year-old man had long-standing, moderately severe atherosclerotic coronary and cerebrovascular problems, which manifested with chronic congestive heart failure and recurrent transient ischemic attacks. Nevertheless, assisted by a devoted wife, and on medication, he had adjusted to his functional limitations and considered his lifestyle satisfactory. Three weeks before calling me, he noted the development of ankle swelling which he treated himself by increasing his dosage of diuretic medication. One week later, he noted the onset (for the first time) of fecal incontinence and began soiling his clothes and bed. He and his wife attributed this problem to advancing age. They did not seek medical assistance. His wife consulted a social worker and inquired about the possibility of obtaining the services of a nurse to assist her in caring for her husband. The social worker replied that such continuous nursing service was unavailable, but that she would submit an application for both husband and wife at a nursing home. About four days before contacting me, the patient stopped urinating. Although he and his wife were disturbed by this development, they decided that he was probably dehydrated from taking too many diuretic pills and from his repeated episodes of loose, watery bowel movements. They therefore discontinued the diuretic pills and began to push fluids. Over the course of the next four days, he experienced gradually increasing lower abdominal pains and noted the development of a large abdominal mass below the umbilicus. He also noted breathlessness on exertion. When he finally presented to my office, three weeks after the onset of his new problems, his chief complaint was severe, unremitting lower abdominal pain and an abdominal mass, and he stated: "Doc, I'm afraid I've recently developed a cancer." He and his wife mentioned the fecal incontinence and his failure to urinate only after these problems were suspected during the physical examination.

By examining the early phases of this patient's illness and his decision to seek a medical opinion, it is possible to reach some tentative conclusions concerning the relationship between clinical medicine and theories of health and disease:

1. The distinction between a problem of health and a nonhealth matter, for example, the fecal incontinence, is frequently obscure.
2. Many social, cultural, and psychological factors may influence a particular person's judgment that he has a health problem rather than a problem whose relief should be sought from other agencies, or that he has any problem at all.
3. Even if a problem is actually perceived as a "health" problem, for example, the anuria, one may choose not to make it a problem for clinical medicine by not presenting with it to physicians.
4. Some people may be entirely asymptomatic or may suppress or deny the existence of symptoms even while harboring a serious condition, such as an occult malignancy. Some individuals may define a symptomatic problem as a nonmedical problem even when severe "disease," such as cancer, exists.
5. The existence of a pre-patient phase of clinical medicine severely limits the

direct application of either a functionalist or a complaint model of medicine. Unquestionably, for three weeks this patient's usual functional capacity was severely compromised, and yet his problem was not one of clinical medicine because he chose not to make it one. Further, the complaint model of medicine is hard-pressed to explain whether this man was appropriate in seeking relief from a social service agency rather than from medicine, and whether such an individual decision would mean that he did not have a medical problem. Cases such as these indicate clearly that one can have serious dysfunctional states and diseases and still deny or misinterpret symptoms and thus delay in presenting with complaints to physicians. This man could have died from one of several possible complications of his problems before he chose to enter the medical setting.

The Initial Encounter of Patient and Physician

David Mechanic has written that "people visit the physician because they have a problem; most frequently they come because they are ill. In one sense, at least, all persons seeking advice from a physician and presenting a symptom are 'diseased.' There is something in their life condition that impels them to seek help" (Mechanic, 1978, p. 418).

From a patient's perspective the issue appears settled at the time he requests help. His problem should be counted and responded to as a medical problem. But, the question remains: do patients present to physicians based on a theory of health and disease? At some level, I suppose they do. Some patients may respond to one level of pain or discomfort or unhappiness which they consider to be disturbing, and thus may conform to the medical model theory of disease. Other patients may present with various individual dysfunctional conditions (say, a sprained ankle in a world class runner) which more closely resembles the functionalist model of health and disease. But, in general, these theoretical constructs probably exert considerably less influence on when patients come to physicians than do the social, cultural, educational, economic, and political factors noted in our consideration of the first clinical moment.

Nevertheless, I believe that in these circumstances the physician's response is guarded and reserved. Indeed, in many instances the physician is frankly suspicious of the patient and may question at least in his own mind why the patient has chosen to appear at this time and whether the patient is in ill health and has a clinical medical problem. Some might regard this suspicion as contrary to the spirit of medicine, to the physician's duty to respond to a patient's request for help. Others might regard it as an inappropriate extension of the physician's expertise. These views, which often emanate from nonphysician critics of the medical endeavor (Veatch, 1973), are naive and misguided. In fact, this stage of the physician's thinking is a crucial technical step. The physician must analyze with precision why the patient chose to present at this particular time and the physician also must elucidate the nature of the patient's symptom formation. Psychiatrists are quite adept at these analyses, particularly for psychological symptoms, but other excellent clinicians will pursue the same conceptual analysis for physical as well as for psychological complaints.

Physicians have a theoretical notion of health and disease and it is applied in these circumstances. By and large, physicians in general (excluding perhaps psychiatrists and family practitioners) are disease-oriented. This disease orientation represents the scientific model of medicine that is emphasized during medical education and postgraduate training and it also tends to be the model perpetuated by the reimbursement schemes of insurance companies and government. Physicians get paid for treating disease.

In my discussion of the first clinical moment, the individual's perspective on his illness, I indicated how a person's decision that a problem is a medical one is based on a complex interaction of biological, psychological, and social factors. These factors may culminate in a decision to seek medical care and then the person becomes a patient. Similarly, the physician now embarks on the difficult task of disentangling these multiple factors to determine whether the patient has found his way to the proper institutional setting, i.e., a medical setting, and whether the patient's problem is properly "medical" rather than being a social, religious, political, or economic problem. An essential part of this process is to determine, to borrow Alvan Feinstein's term (Feinstein, 1967, pp. 141–155), what was the iatrotropic stimulus, that is what immediate event or events convinced the patient to seek medical attention at this time.

What usually follows after the patient's initial presentation is a process which we have come to call the clinical method. Its efficacy has been established since Hippocratic times. The clinical method may appear to some to be a mechanical, stereotyped procedure, but this view is simplistic and incorrect. The clinical method as I will describe it has two central components: 1) data-gathering, and 2) data-reduction and diagnosis. Both of these features of the clinical method, but especially the data-gathering phase, require a considerable amount of personal interaction and an exchange of information about both technical and value-laden concerns between the patient and the physician.

Data-Gathering. I want to emphasize that the heart of data-gathering occurs in the verbal and paraverbal exchanges between the patient and physician. All expert clinicians agree that no laboratory tests or technological innovations in medicine can compare to the efficiency and effectiveness of the clinician's history and physical examination, which remain unrivaled tools for gathering information about patients' problems. Medical students know very well that most diagnoses, perhaps 70 to 90 percent, are made on the basis of the medical history. This stage of the clinical encounter is absolutely and critically dependent on the interaction of two persons. By contrast, a patient-computer encounter or the collection of a written medical history questionnaire are inadequate substitutes for the interaction of the patient with a sensitive and skilled physician.

The success of the data-gathering phase of the second clinical moment depends on the interaction of the patient and doctor and on their ability to communicate effectively. As Tumulty (1970) suggests, the measure of a clinician's skill is his ability to communicate successfully with a broad and diverse group of patients. It is essential to acknowledge and to appreciate that individual responses—some conscious and some subconscious—of patients to physicians and physicians to patients can modify the effectiveness of the patient-doctor interaction.

Data-Reduction and Diagnosis. The second stage of the clinical method is designed to reduce the enormous amount of information from the history, physical examination, and laboratory studies to a useful and workable amount. The data is structured and used in some taxonomic standard of classification, as the clinician engages in the process of differential diagnosis in an effort to give a disease name to the complaint with which the patient presented. Physicians will be engaged simultaneously in attempting to generate a diagnosis or a differential diagnosis and in testing the complaints of the patient to determine for themselves whether the patient legitimately falls within the clinical medical model. The second moment is not an end in itself, but is a necessary preliminary step in deciding whether to proceed to the succeeding clinical moments: the doctor-patient accommodation and the doctor-patient relationship.

The second clinical moment, the patient's encounter with the physician, has traditionally been regarded as the doctor's domain and is too often considered to be cold, analytic, objective, rational, and ultimately, that final pejorative epithet, "scientific." But even in the second clinical moment, while the physician wears his persona of objective scientist, an enormous amount of human, personal, subjective interaction is occurring between patient and doctor. The eliciting of a medical history is no job for machines and requires the profound subtlety that only trained, sensitive humans can bring to it. As Lain Entralgo (1969) has indicated in his analysis of the doctor-patient relationship, the relationship commences when patient and physician look at each other and interact for the first time, and it deepens during the physical examination phase.

Nor do I believe that the data-reduction phase which generates a diagnosis and a differential diagnosis is a mechanical process. The apparently scientific, mechanical second clinical moment—just like the first clinical moment—is full of personal drama, and it leads inexorably to the individualization of the patient which is the central event in the third clinical moment, the doctor-patient accommodation.

The case presented earlier indicates that a complete understanding of the patient's medical problem would require that the physician recollect and recount the events that unfolded over a three-week period. Only then would the physician be able to understand fully the nature of the illness and its pathophysiology and diagnosis. The historical details presented in the case example were elicited by the physician only after repeated questioning of the patient and his wife. The patient ignored certain relevant details, had forgotten them, or was sufficiently embarrassed by them (for example, the fecal incontinence) that the original history given by the patient was substantially different from the one finally described in the case report. Some physicians might not have pursued repeatedly the historical features of the case and thus might have reached an erroneous or incomplete diagnosis. This case illustrates the essential importance of subjective interaction even in the second clinical moment, which sometimes masquerades as an entirely objective, "scientific" encounter.

The second clinical moment allows the physician to answer the patient's concerns of whether he is sick and whether he has a serious disease. It permits the physician to reach a determination of whether the patient has a disease that can be named and treated. Theories of health and disease are applied at this stage, particularly by the physician. The physician's response to the patient will be modified by his beliefs concerning the kinds of problems that ought to "count" as diseases. The physician's interpretation and management of a patient's presenting complaint will depend to a large degree on whether the physician has a commitment to a narrow medical model of disease or whether he believes in a broader biopsychosocial model.

The Doctor-Patient Accommodation

The third clinical moment, the doctor-patient accommodation (DPA), is one in which a joint decision is reached relative to the specific clinical problem for which the patient presented on whether this particular doctor will agree to care for this particular patient and in which the patient also decides whether or not to place his care in the hands of this physician (Siegler, 1981). The DPA is both a process and an outcome. The participants in the DPA process have been prepared for their encounter by a complex series of preliminary experiences which have led the patient to seek counsel from the physician and which have prepared the physician to serve the patient as knowledgeable counsellor. The process is one of communication and negotiation—sometimes short and to the point, sometimes extended—on what rights and responsibilities each of the participants wishes to retain and which will be relinquished in the context of their medical relationship. From the moment the patient originally presented to the physician's attention, testing has been undertaken by both parties to decide whether this patient and this doctor wish to work together.

During the negotiations that may culminate in a DPA, the patient and the physician are each silently thinking about a series of questions, which, if answered in the affirmative, will encourage them to conclude the DPA. It may be helpful to try to make explicit what some of these questions are. The patient wishes to know: 1) Are my symptoms serious (my fear) or trivial (my hope)? 2) Is this doctor a good doctor (for me)? 3) Can he help me? Simultaneously, the physician is thinking: 1) Are the patient's symptoms "real?" 2) Does the patient have a "disease" or just a "problem of living" which may not be a matter proper for medicine? 3) Is the patient's problem serious (his fear) or trivial (his hope)? 4) Is this patient a good patient (for me)? 5) Can I help him? 6) Can I help him and still remain loyal to my obligations as a physician and as a participant in the medical enterprise?

The accommodation process depends on all of the particularities of the medical encounter. The nature of the patient involved—personality, character, attitude, and values—and the factors which led him to seek a medical encounter with this particular physician, are a central component of the process. Similarly, the personality, character, attitude, values, and technical skills of the physician affect the DPA process. Further, the quality of the interaction between patient and physician—the chemistry of the interaction—modify the process. Other considerations that may affect the achievement of a DPA include the clinical setting, for example, a hospital, doctor's office, a prepaid medical group, or the patient's home, and also, occasionally, the claims of relevant third-party interests, such as those of family, insurers, or the state. Of course, the nature of the medical problem, including its type, acuity, gravity, and its potential for remediation, will be a major determinant of whether a DPA is achieved. For example, the entire DPA process will be modified profoundly if the patient is acutely or critically ill and alternative medical resources are unavailable.

If the process of negotiation referred to as the DPA is concluded successfully, the result will be an outcome also called a DPA. This outcome is an agreement between the patient and doctor to work together on a particular problem subject to mutually acceptable specifications. There are as many results and styles of outcome for the DPA as there are configurations of the variables which enter into the process of negotiating the DPA.

The DPA is not a permanent, stable, and unchanging relationship between a doctor and a patient; it is a dynamic model and is always in flux. In one sense, the DPA as an outcome exists only as a concept; it is always in the process either of developing or of dissolving. Patients and physicians must achieve accommodations repeatedly, even regarding the same basic conditions for which the original DPA was concluded. For example, a patient's agreement to be cared for by a cardiologist for anginal chest pain would not commit the patient to agree with the cardiologist's recommendation to undergo coronary angiography or subsequently to accept a recommendation for cardiac surgery. Or, in the case example, the person's decision to be treated for congestive heart failure and transient ischemic attacks, presumably do not commit the patient to see the same physician (or any physician, for that matter) regarding his new problems of fecal incontinence and "cancer."

Some DPAs are stronger than other. The resilience of a DPA is determined largely by the extent of trust and confidence exchanged between patient and physician. However, the stability of a DPA is constantly threatened by new circumstances. For example, changes in the patient (the development of new problems, new attitudes, or new demands), changes in the physician (a change in specialization, restriction of practice, or the development of new attitudes), or changes in the disease (for example, when chronic renal disease progresses to its end stages and a new technology such as renal dialysis is needed), all may result in a reassessment of the DPA and perhaps a failure to reach an accommodation on the same or a new issue. The DPA outcome could be regarded as a dynamic equilibrium model in which medical trust tends to drive the equation toward maintaining the stability of the accommodation, but in which new circumstances constantly force patients and physicians to reassess the stability of the accommodation. If an accommodation is not achieved on an important matter (a situation roughly analogous to a prime minister who loses a vote of confidence), the patient and/or the physician legitimately could decide to dissolve their professional relationship (again with the proviso, that the patient's emergency health care needs are attended to).

In contrast to previous descriptions of the doctor-patient relationship (DPR) which tend to regard it as an established, static arrangement between doctor and patient, the DPA provides a more dynamic and more realistic model of the medical encounter. Perhaps DPRs as such rarely exist; rather, what we regard as a DPR may really be repeatedly negotiated DPAs. More likely, a DPR represents a specific, and increasingly uncommon variant of the DPA. It may be distinguished from the DPA by its duration, depth, and maturity. The DPR is characterized by mature and enduring exchanges of trust between the patient and the physician which establish an almost inseparable bond. If such an exchange of trust occurs, it serves as a stabilizer of the medical relationship even during periods of new and difficult stresses. A decline in personal medicine and a rise in high technology and in institutional, specialized medical care probably have accelerated the decline of the traditional DPR model and have contributed to the emergence of the DPA model.

The model of medicine that is implied by my emphasis on the need for physicians and patients to achieve a DPA repeatedly is one of mutuality and voluntariness. I regard such mutual consent of patient and physician to arrive at a doctor-patient accommodation to be a necessary condition for morally acceptable medical practice. Thus, the concept of accommodation is essential in defining the nature and limits of clinical medicine. From the patient's viewpoint what is sought is help in the care of a problem that he regards as a health problem. From the physician's perspective what is important is being able to help the patient while remaining loyal to the professional responsibilities to the enterprise of medicine.

Let me emphasize again my notion that the nature of clinical medicine is defined and created in the context of a DPA which must be mutually agreed on by both participants. The concept that the nature of clinical medicine can be defined with reference to the DPA required justification. I am suggesting that medicine is defined not only by its scientific knowledge base or by its technological capabilities or by theories of health and disease. Rather, in essence, my definition of clinical medicine closely parallels the definition offered by Otto Guttentag when he states that medicine "deals with the care of health of human beings by human beings" (Guttentag, 1981). This immediate and requisite involvement of two human personalities in clinical medicine distinguishes clinical medicine from other activities in which technological skills developed from basic science discoveries are applied (ultimately) for human benefit. For example, I am distinguishing medicine from such technological enterprises as bridge building, architecture, veterinary medicine, and others that are not centered in a human-to-human encounter.

Theories of health and disease partially influence whether a DPA will be concluded. How individual patients and physicians regard the medical encounter and how they conclude their negotiations leading to a particular DPA is partially affected by their individual understandings of health and disease theories. Nevertheless, I do not believe such theories provide either a general or even a societal standard to which patients and physicians can appeal to determine whether a particular problem should be addressed by clinical medicine. Thus, despite theoretical constructs, a degree of uncertainty will always prevail, and neither patient nor physician can rely on a universal, fixed standard to decide on the appropriateness of concluding a particular DPA. The enormous latitude for negotiation between the individual patient and physician, rather than theories of health and disease, is a more important determinant of whether a DPA is concluded.

Reasons Patients Choose Not to Enter a Doctor-Patient Accommodation. We could surely imagine grounds for the patient not wishing to continue with a particular doctor. For example, if the doctor had a bad bedside manner, seemed incompetent, had the wrong diplomas on the wall or none at all, maintained a shabby office, charged excessive fees, had too long a queue, or did not have the proper hospital privileges, the patient might choose to go elsewhere. The patient has a choice, at least this is so in our current medical system. The patient selected this doctor initially, but if he is now dissatisfied, he can vote with his feet. Few of us would have any difficulty accepting this position theoretically; we might differ on such empirical questions as whether our system truly provides all patients with free choices of physicians or how frequently patients as a class exercise such options to find another doctor, but we would agree that the possibility for switching from one physician to another certainly exists.

Reasons Physicians Choose Not to Enter a Doctor-Patient Accommodation. From the point of view of the physician, the decision to enter a doctor-patient accommodation is also a critical determination, although in many regards the physician is less free to choose than the patient. Legally, a doctor-patient accommodation probably exists from the first encounter with the patient, and morally, a therapeutic relationship has begun at least from the moment doctor and patient first see each other, or more likely, from the moment the patient first makes an appointment. Despite these restraints on the physician's freedom of choice, I think it is appropriate, even obligatory, for the physician to make a conscious decision to assume the care of the person who presents asking for medical assistance.

A decision to care for a patient is based on the physician's ability to help the patient (which is a central concern in clinical medicine) and his own concept of professional standards and norms of behavior for physicians. Clinical medicine is defined in this accommodation between doctor and patient. The discipline balances the need of patients (the physician's responsibility to individuals) and the science of medicine (the physician's responsibility to professional standards). In this context, the "good" physician might be viewed as one who most successfully balances responsibility to individual patients with responsibility to the medical enterprise.

One major reason why a physician might choose not to enter a doctor-patient accommodation is because he perceives that he is not able to benefit the patient. Some reasons why a physician may be unable to help a particular patient are: lack of technical skills, profound personality conflicts with the patient, or the pursuit by patient and physician of mutually incompatible medical goals.

A second general reason why a physician might choose not to enter a DPA is because he concludes that his involvement would violate his own professional standards of what it is to be a "good" physician. The physician must consider at this point his responsibilities to the art of medicine and to its standards. A physician is not required to depart from his own standards of conscientious behavior to engage in illegal or immoral practices, to act in ways contrary to his own perception of what it is to be a good physician, or to participate in practices he believes to be outside of the legitimate medical sphere. If the physician cannot help the patient, or if he can do so only by sacrificing his own conscientious standards of loyalty to the profession, I believe it is the physician's moral and medical obligation not to enter into a DPA.

The Limited Applicability of Theories of Health and Disease. A third reason why the good physician might decide not to enter a DPA would be his personal conviction, possibly based on some broad societal notion, that the patient's problems were not medical problems and ought not to be addressed by clinical medicine. I am not suggesting that we are dealing here with a radical relativism. There exist some widely shared notions of what constitute medical problems. We could probably muster a consensus that a broken leg, hemorrhagic shock, the need for open-heart surgery, acute appendicitis, and congestive heart failure were problems that were appropriately addressed by clinical medicine. However, we would likely discover that individual physicians had widely divergent views on whether the following were properly medical matters: amniocentesis for gender identification, the management of exogenous obesity, drug addiction, control of hyperactive school children, malnutrition resulting from poverty, nonspecific anxiety, elective abortions, aging, accident-proneness, unhappiness, and unattractiveness.

This situation differs from one in which the patient and the physician were each desiring different and incompatible ends from the medical encounter, but in which both participants agreed that their encounter was one that had found its way to the appropriate institutional setting, that is, the medical setting. The decision by a physician that a particular complaint is medical or not is based on the diagnosis he has reached, on his sense of the patient's motivations for coming to the doctor, and on his own attitudes and values. Some of these values may be broadly shared by society (for example, certain norms about health and disease) and some may be quite peculiar to physicians as a group or to a particular physician as an individual. Some of these values peculiar to physicians as a group may have developed in the course of training in medicine, and some of these values may have antedated professional education and, indeed, may have contributed to an individual's choosing medicine as a career.

Models of health and disease, either those articulated by philosophers or those taught to physicians in medical school, probably find their widest application at this stage of the doctor-patient encounter. I have indicated previously that some physicians have a restricted vision of medicine which views the purpose of the medical interaction as "the treatment of illness conceived as deranged biomedical function" (Seldin, 1977, p. 39). Other commentators have described a quite different medical model, a biophysiosocial model, in which almost all complaints count (Engel, 1977). I wish to emphasize that a particular physician may place a particular patient's complaints out of the sphere of clinical medicine based on the physician's own perception of what clinical medicine is about and what the standards of the profession require.

IV. CONCLUSION

In a sense, I am rejecting the proposition that any complaint that patients present to physicians counts as a medical matter. Rather, I believe that every patient presentation generates a claim to be heard by physicians. But physicians have the professional and personal responsibility, based on their training, expertise, and values, and modified by the existence of political, economic, and scientific boundaries to medicine, to weigh patient requests and to determine if they are to be managed, at least by *this* physician, as medical problems. I also reject the functionalist position which would determine what problems ought to count as medical ones based either on theoretical dysfunctional states or on narrow notions of biomedical effectiveness. I have not denied that theories of medicine, health, and disease may influence individual decision making for both patients and physicians. I have argued, however, that such theories serve only as the intellectual background of the human encounter between patient and physician. The nature of clinical medicine, at any time, is not determined by such theories, but rather is defined and discovered principally by the resolution of individual doctor-patient accommodations.

REFERENCES

Engel, G. L. 1977. The need for a new medical model: A challenge for bio-medicine. *Science* 196:129–36.

Engelhardt, H. T., Jr. 1979. Doctoring the disease, treating the complaint, helping the patient: Some of the works of Hygeia and Panacea. In *Knowing and valuing: The search for common roots*, ed. H. T. Engelhardt, Jr. and D. Callahan. Hastings on Hudson, N. Y.: The Hastings Center.

Feinstein, A. R. 1967. *Clinical Judgment*. Baltimore: Williams and Wilkins Co.

Guttentag, O. E. 1981. *The attending physician as a central figure*. In *Changing values in medicine*, ed. E. J. Cassell and M. Siegler. Chicago: Univ. of Chicago Press.

Kass, L. R. 1975. Regarding the end of medicine and the pursuit of health. *The Public Interest* 40:11–42.

Lain Entralgo, P. 1969. *Doctor and patient*. Translated by F. Partridge. New York: McGraw-Hill Book Co.

Mechanic, D. 1978. *Medical sociology*. 2d ed. New York: Free Press.

Merton, R. K. 1957. *Social theory and social structure*. Revised ed. New York: Free Press.

Parsons, T. 1951. *The social system*. New York: Free Press.

Seldin, D. W. 1977. The medical model: Bio-medical science as the basis of medicine. In *Beyond tomorrow: Trends and prospects in medical science*, ed. Helene Jordon. New York: Rockefeller University Press.

644   Concepts of Health and Disease

Siegler, M. 1981. On the nature and limits of clinical medicine. In *Changing values in medicine*, ed. E. J. Cassell and M. Siegler. Chicago: Univ. of Chicago Press.

Tumulty, P. A. 1970. What is a clinician and what does he do? *New England Journal of Medicine* 283:20–24.

Veatch, R. M. 1973. Generalization of expertise. *The Hastings Center Studies* 1:29–40.

8.4 Siegler M (1982) The Physician-Patient Accommodation: A Central Event in Clinical Medicine. Arch Intern Med 142:1899–1902

Clinical Ethics

The Physician-Patient Accommodation

A Central Event in Clinical Medicine

Mark Siegler, MD

Physicians and medical analysts have developed many theories of health and disease, and such descriptions are often used to prescribe the proper range and scope of clinical medicine. A traditional, narrow view of clinical medicine suggests that disease is an objective biologic state and that the goals of medicine should be to treat disease[1] or alternatively to restore or maintain health.[2] By contrast, a more expansive model of medicine has been proposed in which physicians would be expected to respond effectively to any type of complaint—biologic, psychologic, social, economic—with which a person approached the physician.[3,4] These theoretical models are important because they could influence the medical profession's own sense of the range and extent of its medical obligations. Furthermore, if health planners and legislators could agree on a particular theoretical model (whether or not the profession concurred entirely), practical limits could be established (primarily through financing mechanisms) on the scope of clinical medical activities. My concern is that these theoretical accounts of the purpose and limits of clinical medicine never quite come to grips with the actualities of medical practice. Before any theory of clinical medicine can be formulated, it is essential to understand how physicians currently function and how they describe and justify their actions.[5]

The thesis of this report is that there is no single, adequate, theoretical description of the nature of clinical medicine. Rather, the determination of what will be recognized as a problem for clinical medicine will depend on three separate but interdependent events: (1) the patient's decision to come to a physician with a complaint that the patient believes to be a medical one; (2) the physician's analysis of the patient's complaint, which leads to a determination that the patient does or does not have a clinical medical problem; and (3) the achievement of a negotiated physician-patient accommodation, in which a decision is reached that the patient chooses to be cared for by *this* particular physician, and the physician agrees to care for *this* particular patient.

In general, a problem becomes one for clinical medicine only when the physician and patient agree that it is one. If either the patient or the physician denies that a medical problem exists, then, with rare exceptions (medical emergencies are one), for their purposes, the issue is not a problem for clinical medicine, although there may exist health problems or diseases, or even problems in preventive, social, community, or research medicine. Although all these determinations are constrained by political, economic, and social forces, there nevertheless remains, in American medicine of the 1980s, enormous latitude for negotiated accommodations between individual patients and individual physicians. These negotiations, carried on by thousands of physicians interacting with millions of patients, determine the boundaries of clinical medicine both at the level of individual physicians and patients, and, by aggregation, at the societal level.

THE THREE CLINICAL MOMENTS IN THE PATIENT-PHYSICIAN ENCOUNTER

To explore the thesis that a problem becomes one for clinical medicine only when the patient and physician agree that it is one, the medical encounter can be divided for purposes of analysis into three conceptual moments (or stages): (1) the person in a prepatient phase; (2) the physician in the context of an initial encounter with the person who now appears as a patient; and (3) the physician-patient accommodation. These are conceptual rather than chronological moments because they attempt to distinguish, for purposes of analysis, elements of an interconnected process that begins when patient and physician first meet, or in fact, when they first communicate. Nevertheless, most of the prepatient phase of this encounter is chronologically prior to the physician's involvement, and the second clinical moment, the physician phase, is required logically before a patient-physician accommodation can be concluded.

THE FIRST CLINICAL MOMENT: THE PREPATIENT PHASE OF CLINICAL MEDICINE

The prepatient phase of clinical medicine represents the first clinical moment. In nonemergency medical situations (the focus of this report), the determination by an individual that he has a health problem necessarily must precede the actual medical encounter with a physician. The perception of a state of ill health and a decision to seek medical help are influenced by many social, cultural, political, and economic factors, in addition to the biologic manifestations of the perceived state of ill health.[6,7]

Except in instances of acute medical problems, where medical care is sought in an emergency, persons usually have considered their bodily sensations, ie, their symptoms, the persistence of symptoms, and the effect such symptoms have on disrupting the ordinary activities of the individual and the social group. Further, individuals will have considered their own values and beliefs, those of their immediate family and community, and the availability, cost, and quality of medical care, before determining that a particular sensation or feeling is one that should be attended to by physicians rather than, for example, by priests or teachers or social workers.

Accepted for publication June 17, 1982.
From the Section of General Internal Medicine, Department of Medicine, University of Chicago-Pritzker School of Medicine.
Read before the conference on Changing Values in Medicine, New York, Nov 12, 1979.
Reprint requests to Box 72, University of Chicago Hospitals, 950 E 59th St, Chicago, IL 60637 (Dr Siegler).

A CONSIDERATION OF THE PREPATIENT PHASE OF CLINICAL MEDICINE WITH REFERENCE TO TOLSTOI'S *THE DEATH OF IVAN II'ICH*

In an effort to better understand the self-definition of illness by the prospective patient, it is instructive to examine Tolstoi's short novel, *The Death of Ivan Il'ich*. In the early chapters of this work, which recount the life and particularly the death from an abdominal malignant neoplasm of Ivan Il'ich, a judge in Imperial Russia, Tolstoi depicts skillfully the unfolding of the first clinical moment, the process by which Ivan Il'ich determined he had an illness and decided to seek medical care.

In chapter 3 of the novel, Ivan Il'ich had been passed over for a promotion and was almost in despair: "Ivan Il'ich, for the first time in his life, expressed not merely ennui, but an unendurable depression, and arrived at the conclusion that to live like this was impossible, and that it was indispensable for him to adopt some decisive measure at once." It is interesting to ask whether at this stage Ivan Il'ich sought medical care for his new sensations of profound depression. He did not. Tolstoi writes: "After passing a sleepless night . . . he resolved to go to St. Petersburg, and try to get transferred into another ministry, in order to punish those persons who did not appreciate him." Thus, Ivan Il'ich defined his problem as a social problem, or in the case of one working for government, as a political problem, but he clearly did not consider that he was suffering a medical illness of depression or that he should visit a physician with his problem. Once he assigned the problem to a particular category, ie, as a social or political matter, he immediately sought to resolve it in this context.

Later in chapter 3, Ivan Il'ich unexpectedly received a promotion at work and was delightedly furnishing his new home. While climbing on a ladder to arrange some curtains, he stumbled and knocked his side against the handle of a window frame. Tolstoi writes: "The bruise hurt him a little, but the pain soon passed off. All this time, indeed, Ivan Il'ich felt particularly bright and well. He wrote his wife: 'I feel that fifteen of my years have leaped from off my shoulders.'" In this instance, Ivan Il'ich received a definite physical injury—a bruise that caused physical pain—but again, he did not seek medical attention for this problem. Perhaps, in part, the ebullient mental state associated with receiving a promotion allowed him to state forcefully, despite having suffered a new and painful injury, "I feel that fifteen years have leaped from off my shoulders."

Some weeks after he received the injury to his side, his wife inquired how he had come to fall, and he laughingly explained: "I have not been a gymnast for nothing, anyone else would have been killed, and I merely struck myself here; if you touch it, it pains, but it is passing away already, it is a simple bruise." Thus, even after discussing the injury in a social setting with his wife, Ivan Il'ich did not perceive himself as ill, nor for that matter did his wife perceive him as ill, and she concurred implicitly with his decision not to seek medical attention.

In chapter 4, we are told:

They were all well. Ivan Il'ich sometimes said indeed that he had a bad taste in his mouth, and something was not quite right, but one could hardly call that illness. But this little indisposition happened to increase, and passed, not yet into downright illness, but into a feeling of constant aching in the side, accompanied by lowness of spirits. This lowness of spirits kept on increasing and increasing, and began to destroy that easy, pleasant, and decorous manner of life which had become an institution in the family of the Golivins.

Thus, despite a bad taste in his mouth, persistent and worsening pain in his side, and a general depression and lassitude—in fact, later in the chapter we learn that he also had experienced a loss of appetite and a severe irascibility that troubled his whole family and even threatened the

stability of his marriage—he never arrived at a self-determination that he was ill.

It is fascinating to read how and why Ivan Il'ich finally decided to see a physician. He and his wife had been having unpleasant scenes at dinner when he complained of the food and refused to eat. After one of these scenes, he believed that he had been unjust to his wife and apologized saying that he was irritable "because he did not feel well. She said to him that if he were ill he ought to be cured, and insisted that he should go see a famous doctor. He went."

Thus, the decision to seek medical counsel was reached because he had a sense of not feeling well, and to this was added his wife's urging that he seek medical attention and cure. But Ivan Il'ich and his wife were not identifying the pain or bad taste or loss of appetite as the illness; rather, they were focusing on the irritability and ill temper and the impact that this was having on the family's tranquility. It appears that Ivan Il'ich sought medical attention because of the influence of his family, because of his wife's urging, and perhaps because entering the medical system offered a potential extenuating excuse for his aberrant behavior. He obviously had sensed something was not right physically, but it had required a direct challenge from his wife to force him to act on his perception.

This examination of the early chapters of Tolstoi's *Ivan Il'ich* suggests the extraordinarily complex relationship between the biologic complaints of pain in the side, loss of appetite, a bad taste in the mouth; the psychologic concomitants of these physical pains such as bad temper and irascibility; and the social effects of these problems. These three orders of experience—biologic, psychologic, and social—cumulatively led to a decision to seek medical attention. Tolstoi's description of the early phases of Ivan Il'ich's illness and his decision to seek medical help suggests that in the prepatient phase or first clinical moment (1) the distinction between a health problem and a nonhealth matter is frequently obscure; (2) social, cultural, and psychologic factors strongly influence an individual's judgment that he has a "problem," and that it is a "health problem," the treatment for which should be sought from physicians rather than a "nonmedical problem," the relief of which should be sought from other agencies; and (3) of course, individuals may incorrectly define a problem as a nonmedical one even when severe disease exists. Alternatively, even if a problem is actually perceived by an individual to be a health problem, he may choose not to make it a problem of clinical medicine simply by not going to a physician.

THE SECOND CLINICAL MOMENT: DATA GATHERING AND DATA REDUCTION

The second clinical moment represents the physician's first entry into the situation. Of this initial encounter between patients and physicians, David Mechanic[8] has written:

People visit the physician because they have a problem; most frequently they come because they believe they are ill. In one sense, at least, all persons seeking advice from a physician and presenting a symptom are "diseased." There is something in their life condition that impels them to seek help.

From a patient's perspective, the issue appears settled at the time he requests help: his problem should be counted and responded to as a medical problem. Nevertheless, in these circumstances, the physician's response often is guarded and reserved. The physician may question why the patient has chosen to appear at this specific time and whether the patient has a clinical medical problem. Some might incorrectly regard this suspicion as contrary to the medical duty to respond to a patient's request for help or even as an inappropriate extension of the physician's expertise.[9] However, this stage of the physician's thinking represents a crucial technical step. The physician must analyze with precision why the patient chose to appear at this particular time as well as the nature of the patient's symptom formation. Psychiatrists are quite adept at these analyses, particularly for psychologic symptoms, but other excellent clinicians pursue the same conceptual analysis for physical as well as for psychologic problems. It is interesting to speculate that Ivan Il'ich's medical care might have been improved greatly (even in the absence of effective cancer chemotherapy), if any of the four physicians he consulted had been sensitive to such questions as, for example,: why did Ivan Il'ich come to a physician when he did, and what factors—social, psychologic, and family—in addition to the medical, were responsible for the development and persistence of his symptoms?

If in the first clinical moment the patient's determination that a problem is medical is based on the interaction of biologic, psychologic, and cultural factors, then, in the second clinical moment, the physician must disentangle the factors that led to this visit in order to determine for himself whether the patient's problem is medical rather than some other kind and whether the patient has come to the proper (ie, to a medical) setting. An essential part of this process is to determine the iatrotropic stimulus,[10] the immediate event or events that convinced the patient to seek medical attention at this time. For example, in the case of Ivan Il'ich, the iatrotropic stimulus was family disharmony and, incidentally, an ache in his side and a strange taste in his mouth.

What usually follows after the patient's initial appearance is a process that we have come to call the clinical method. Its efficacy has been established since hippocratic times. The two central components of the clinical method are data gathering, and data reduction and diagnosis.

Data Gathering

The heart of data gathering occurs in the verbal and paraverbal exchanges between the patient and physician. Expert clinicians agree that no laboratory tests or technological innovations in medicine can compare with the efficiency and effectiveness of a skilled clinician's history and physical examination as tools for gathering information about patients' problems.

The success of the data-gathering phase of the second clinical moment depends on the interaction of the patient and physician and on their ability to communicate effectively. As Tumulty[11] suggested, the measure of a clinician's skill is his ability to communicate successfully with a broad and diverse group of patients. It is essential to acknowledge and to appreciate that individual responses of patients to physicians and physicians to patients can modify the effectiveness of the patient-physician interaction.

Data Reduction and Diagnosis

The second stage of the clinical method is designed to reduce the enormous amount of information obtained from the history, physical examination, and laboratory studies to a useful and workable amount. The data are structured and classified according to standard taxonomies as the clinician engages in the process of differential diagnosis in an effort to give a disease label to the complaint with which the patient appeared. Even while attempting to generate a diagnosis, the physician is simultaneously testing the complaints to determine whether the patient legitimately falls within the clinical medical model. The second moment is not an end in itself but is a necessary preliminary step in deciding whether to proceed to the succeeding clinical moment: the physician-patient accommodation.

THE THIRD CLINICAL MOMENT: THE PHYSICIAN-PATIENT ACCOMMODATION

The achievement of a physician-patient accommodation is the central event in contemporary American clinical medicine. My thesis is that medicine has never been defined solely by its scientific knowledge base or by its technological capabilities. Rather, the nature of clinical medicine is understood best in the context of an interpersonal accommodation that must be agreed on mutually by both participants.

The participants in a physician-patient accommodation have been prepared for their encounter by a series of preliminary experiences that have led the patient to seek counsel from the physician (the first clinical moment) and have prepared the physician to serve the patient as knowledgeable counselor. From the moment the patient originally came to the physician (the second clinical moment), testing and evaluation have been carried out by both parties. In achieving a physician-patient accommodation, a joint decision is reached on whether *this* physician will agree to care for *this* patient, and on whether *this* patient will place his care in the hands of *this* physician.

The accommodation process depends on all of the particularities of the medical encounter. The nature of the patient involved—his personality, character, attitude, and values—and the factors that led him to seek a medical encounter with this particular physician are central components of the process. Similarly, the personality, character, attitude, values, and technical skills of the physician affect the accommodation. Further, the quality of the interaction between patient and physician, the chemistry of the interaction, modify the process. Of course, the nature of the medical problem, including its type, acuteness, gravity, and its potential for remediation, will be a major determinant of whether a physician-patient accommodation is achieved. For example, the entire process will be modified profoundly and telescoped if the patient is acutely or critically ill or if alternative medical resources are unavailable. Finally, other considerations that may affect the achievement of a physician-patient accommodation include the clinical setting, eg, a hospital, physician's office, or the patient's home; the organization of the medical service, health maintenance organization, or fee-for-service; and also, occasionally, the claims of relevant third-party interests such as those of family, insurers, or the state.

During the negotiations that may culminate in a physician-patient accommodation, the patient and the physician are each thinking silently about a series of questions. The patient wonders whether his symptoms are serious or trivial and whether this physician can help him. Simultaneously, the physician is deciding whether the patient has a "disease" or just a "problem of living," and whether the problem is one that the physician can help alleviate.

The Patient's Choice

There are many reasons why a patient might decide not to continue with a particular physician. For example, if the physician had a poor bedside manner, seemed incompetent, had the wrong diplomas on the wall (or none at all), maintained a shabby office, charged excessive fees, had too long a queue, or lacked proper hospital privileges, the patient might choose to go elsewhere. At least in our current medical system, the patient has a choice. The patient selected this physician initially, but if he becomes dissatisfied, he may change to another physician.

The Physician's Choice

The physician's decision to enter a physician-patient accommodation is also critical, although in many respects, the physician is less free to choose than the patient. Legally, a physician-patient accommodation probably exists from the first encounter with the patient; morally, a therapeutic relationship has begun at the moment physician and patient first see each other, or perhaps at the moment the patient makes an appointment. Despite these constraints, it is not only appropriate but also obligatory for the physician to make a conscious decision that he will (or will not) assume the care of the person who asks for medical assistance.

One major reason why a physician should choose not to enter a physician-patient accommodation is because he perceives that he is not able to benefit the patient. Some reasons why a physician may be unable to help a particular patient are as follows: lack of the technical skills needed by a particular patient, profound personality conflicts with the patient, or the pursuit by patient and physician of mutually incompatible medical goals.

A second general reason why a physician might choose not to enter a physician-patient accommodation is because he concludes that his involvement would violate his own professional standards of what it is to be a "good" physician. The physician must consider at this point his responsibilities to the art of medicine and to its standards. A physician is not required to depart from his own standards of conscientious behavior to engage in illegal or immoral practices, to act in ways contrary to his own perception of what it is to be a good physician, or to participate in practices that he believes to be outside of the legitimate medical sphere. If the physician cannot help the patient, or if he can do so only by sacrificing his own conscientious standards of loyalty to the profession, it is the physician's moral and medical obligation not to enter into a physician-patient accommodation.

The model of medicine implied by an emphasis on the need for patient *and* physician to achieve an accommodation is one of mutuality, voluntariness, noncoercion, and respect for autonomy. This freedom of both patient and physician to enter an accommodation is the core of morally acceptable medical practice.

THE PHYSICIAN-PATIENT ACCOMMODATION CONTRASTED WITH THE PHYSICIAN-PATIENT RELATIONSHIP

The physician-patient accommodation is not a permanent, stable, and unchanging relationship between a physician and a patient; it is a dynamic model and is always in flux. In one sense, the accommodation as an outcome exists only as a concept; it is always in the process either of developing or of dissolving. Patients and physicians must achieve accommodations repeatedly, even regarding the same basic conditions for which the original accommodation was concluded. For example, a patient's agreement to be cared for by a cardiologist for anginal chest pain would not commit the patient to agree with the cardiologist's recommendation to undergo coronary angiography or to accept a subsequent recommendation for cardiac surgery.

Some physician-patient accommodations are stronger than others. The resilience of an accommodation is determined largely by the extent of trust and confidence exchanged between patient and physician. However, the stability of an accommodation is constantly threatened by new circumstances because changes in the patient, the physician, or the disease all may result in a reassessment of the accommodation and perhaps a failure to reach an accommodation on the same or a new issue. If an accommodation is not achieved on an important matter, the patient or physician legitimately could decide to dissolve their professional relationship, again with the proviso that the patient's emergency health care needs are attended to.

In contrast to previous descriptions of the physician-patient relationship that tend to regard it as an established,

static arrangement between physician and patient,[12,13] the physician-patient accommodation provides a more dynamic and more realistic model of the medical encounter. Perhaps, these days, physician-patient relationships as such rarely exist; rather, what we regard as a relationship may really be repeatedly negotiated physician-patient accommodations. More likely, a physician-patient relationship represents a specific and increasingly uncommon variant of the accommodation. It is one characterized by mature and enduring exchanges of trust between patient and physician that establish an almost insunderable bond. A decline in personal medical care and a rise in high technology and in institutional, specialized medical care probably has accelerated the decline of the traditional relationship model and has contributed to the emergence of the accommodation model.

CONCLUSION

This report has argued that an understanding of clinical medicine must be based on an analysis of how physicians and patients currently interact rather than on a theoretical analysis of the nature of health and disease. Although such theories may influence individual decision making for both patients and physicians, they serve only as the intellectual backdrop of the human encounter between patient and physician. The spectrum of clinical medicine, at any time, is not determined by such theories, but rather is created by the aggregate resolution of individual physician-patient accommodations.

It must be noted, however, that profound changes are now occurring in American medicine. Medicine is becoming increasingly bureaucratic and political. These changes may modify the patient-centered medicine that currently exists and change the delicate physician-patient encounter from a negotiated accommodation to an impersonal contract between clients and providers. If this occurs, clinical medicine will never be the same.

This material was prepared with support from the National Science Foundation (grant OSS-8018097) and the National Endowment for the Humanities. The conference before which an earlier version of this paper was read was supported by the National Science Foundation (grant OSS-78-7838) and the National Endowment for the Humanities. The views expressed herein are those of the author and do not necessarily reflect those of the National Science Foundation or the National Endowment for the Humanities.

References

1. Seldin DW: The medical model: Biomedical science as the basis of medicine, in Jordan, H (ed): *Beyond Tomorrow: Trends and Prospects in Medical Science*. New York, Rockefeller University Press, 1977.
2. Kass LR: Regarding the end of machine and the pursuit of health. *Public Interest* 1975;40:11-42.
3. Engel GL: The need for a new medical model: A challenge for biomedicine. *Science* 1977;196:129-136.
4. Engelhardt HT Jr: Doctoring the disease, treating the complaint, helping the patient: Some of the works of Hygeia and Panacea, in Engelhardt HT Jr, Callahan D (eds): *Knowing and Valuing: The Search for Common Roots*. Hastings-on-Hudson, NY, Hastings Center, 1979, pp 225-249.
5. Siegler M: The doctor-patient encounter and its relationship to theories of health and disease, in Caplan AL, Engelhardt HT Jr, McCartney JJ (eds): *Concepts of Health and Disease: Interdisciplinary Perspectives*. Reading, Mass, Addison-Wesley, 1981, pp 627-644.
6. Parsons T: *The Social System*. New York, Free Press, 1951.
7. Merton RK: *Social Theory and Social Structure*. New York, Free Press, 1957.
8. Mechanic D: *Medical Sociology*. New York, Free Press, 1978.
9. Veatch RM: Generalization of expertise. *Hastings Center Studies* 1973;1:29-40.
10. Feinstein AR: *Clinical Judgment*. Baltimore, Williams & Wilkins Co, 1967.
11. Tumulty PA: What is a clinician and what does he do? *N Engl J Med* 1970;283:20-24.
12. Szasz TS, Hollender M: The basic models of the doctor-patient relationship. *Arch Intern Med* 1956;97:585-592.
13. Veatch RM: Models for ethical medicine in a revolutionary age. *Hastings Center Report* 1972;2:5-7.

8.5   Siegler M (1982) Confidentiality in Medicine: A Decrepit Concept. N Engl J Med 307:1518–21

1518   THE NEW ENGLAND JOURNAL OF MEDICINE   Dec. 9, 1982

CONFIDENTIALITY IN MEDICINE —
A DECREPIT CONCEPT

MEDICAL confidentiality, as it has traditionally been understood by patients and doctors, no longer exists. This ancient medical principle, which has been included in every physician's oath and code of ethics since Hippocratic times, has become old, worn-out, and useless; it is a decrepit concept. Efforts to preserve it appear doomed to failure and often give rise to more problems than solutions. Psychiatrists have tacitly acknowledged the impossibility of ensuring the confidentiality of medical records by choosing to establish a separate, more secret record. The following case illustrates how the confidentiality principle is compromised systematically in the course of routine medical care.

Vol. 307   No. 24   SOUNDING BOARDS   1519

A patient of mine with mild chronic obstructive pulmonary disease was transferred from the surgical intensive-care unit to a surgical nursing floor two days after an elective cholecystectomy. On the day of transfer, the patient saw a respiratory therapist writing in his medical chart (the therapist was recording the results of an arterial blood gas analysis) and became concerned about the confidentiality of his hospital records. The patient threatened to leave the hospital prematurely unless I could guarantee that the confidentiality of his hospital record would be respected.

This patient's complaint prompted me to enumerate the number of persons who had both access to his hospital record and a reason to examine it. I was amazed to learn that at least 25 and possibly as many as 100 health professionals and administrative personnel at our university hospital had access to the patient's record and that all of them had a legitimate need, indeed a professional responsibility, to open and use that chart. These persons included 6 attending physicians (the primary physician, the surgeon, the pulmonary consultant, and others); 12 house officers (medical, surgical, intensive-care unit, and "covering" house staff); 20 nursing personnel (on three shifts); 6 respiratory therapists; 3 nutritionists; 2 clinical pharmacists; 15 students (from medicine, nursing, respiratory therapy, and clinical pharmacy); 4 unit secretaries; 4 hospital financial officers; and 4 chart reviewers (utilization review, quality assurance review, tissue review, and insurance auditor). It is of interest that this patient's problem was straightforward, and he therefore did not require many other technical and support services that the modern hospital provides. For example, he did not need multiple consultants and fellows, such specialized procedures as dialysis, or social workers, chaplains, physical therapists, occupational therapists, and the like.

Upon completing my survey I reported to the patient that I estimated that at least 75 health professionals and hospital personnel had access to his medical record. I suggested to the patient that these people were all involved in providing or supporting his health-care services. They were, I assured him, working for him. Despite my reassurances the patient was obviously distressed and retorted, "I always believed that medical confidentiality was part of a doctor's code of ethics. Perhaps you should tell me just what you people mean by 'confidentiality'!"

TWO ASPECTS OF MEDICAL CONFIDENTIALITY

Confidentiality and Third-Party Interests

Previous discussions of medical confidentiality usually have focused on the tension between a physician's responsibility to keep information divulged by patients secret and a physician's legal and moral duty, on occasion, to reveal such confidences to third parties, such as families, employers, public-health authorities, or police authorities. In all these instances, the central question relates to the stringency of the physician's obligation to maintain patient confidentiality when the health, well-being, and safety of identifiable others or of society in general would be threatened by a failure to reveal information about the patient. The tension in such cases is between the good of the patient and the good of others.

Confidentiality and the Patient's Interest

As the example above illustrates, further challenges to confidentiality arise because the patient's personal interest in maintaining confidentiality comes into conflict with his personal interest in receiving the best possible health care. Modern high-technology health care is available principally in hospitals (often, teaching hospitals), requires many trained and specialized workers (a "health-care team"), and is very costly. The existence of such teams means that information that previously had been held in confidence by an individual physician will now necessarily be disseminated to many members of the team. Furthermore, since health-care teams are expensive and few patients can afford to pay such costs directly, it becomes essential to grant access to the patient's medical record to persons who are responsible for obtaining third-party payment. These persons include chart reviewers, financial officers, insurance auditors, and quality-of-care assessors. Finally, as medicine expands from a narrow, disease-based model to a model that encompasses psychological, social, and economic problems, not only will the size of the health-care team and medical costs increase, but more sensitive information (such as one's personal habits and financial condition) will now be included in the medical record and will no longer be confidential.

The point I wish to establish is that hospital medicine, the rise of health-care teams, the existence of third-party insurance programs, and the expanding limits of medicine all appear to be responses to the wishes of people for better and more comprehensive medical care. But each of these developments necessarily modifies our traditional understanding of medical confidentiality.

THE ROLE OF CONFIDENTIALITY IN MEDICINE

Confidentiality serves a dual purpose in medicine. In the first place, it acknowledges respect for the patient's sense of individuality and privacy. The patient's most personal physical and psychological secrets are kept confidential in order to decrease a sense of shame and vulnerability. Secondly, confidentiality is important in improving the patient's health care — a basic goal of medicine. The promise of confidentiality permits people to trust (i.e., have confidence) that information revealed to a physician in the course of a medical encounter will not be disseminated further. In this way patients are encouraged to communicate honestly and forthrightly with their doctors. This bond of trust between patient and doctor is vitally important both in the diagnostic process (which relies on an accurate history) and subsequently in the treatment phase,

1520   THE NEW ENGLAND JOURNAL OF MEDICINE   Dec. 9, 1982

which often depends as much on the patient's trust in the physician as its does on medications and surgery. These two important functions of confidentiality are as important now as they were in the past. They will not be supplanted entirely either by improvements in medical technology or by recent changes in relations between some patients and doctors toward a rights-based, consumerist model.

POSSIBLE SOLUTIONS TO THE CONFIDENTIALITY PROBLEM

First of all, in all nonbureaucratic, noninstitutional medical encounters — that is, in the millions of doctor–patient encounters that take place in physicians' offices, where more privacy can be preserved — meticulous care should be taken to guarantee that patients' medical and personal information will be kept confidential.

Secondly, in such settings as hospitals or large-scale group practices, where many persons have opportunities to examine the medical record, we should aim to provide access only to those who have "a need to know." This could be accomplished through such administrative changes as dividing the entire record into several sections — for example, a medical and financial section — and permitting only health professionals access to the medical information.

The approach favored by many psychiatrists — that of keeping a psychiatric record separate from the general medical record — is an understandable strategy but one that is not entirely satisfactory and that should not be generalized. The keeping of separate psychiatric records implies that psychiatry and medicine are different undertakings and thus drives deeper the wedge between them and between physical and psychological illness. Furthermore, it is often vitally important for internists or surgeons to know that a patient is being seen by a psychiatrist or is taking a particular medication. When separate records are kept, this information may not be available. Finally, if generalized, the practice of keeping a separate psychiatric record could lead to the unacceptable consequence of having a separate record for each type of medical problem.

Patients should be informed about what is meant by "medical confidentiality." We should establish the distinction between information about the patient that generally will be kept confidential regardless of the interest of third parties and information that will be exchanged among members of the health-care team in order to provide care for the patient. Patients should be made aware of the large number of persons in the modern hospital who require access to the medical record in order to serve the patient's medical and financial interests.

Finally, at some point most patients should have an opportunity to review their medical record and to make informed choices about whether their entire record is to be available to everyone or whether certain portions of the record are privileged and should be accessible only to their principal physician or to others designated explicitly by the patient. This approach would rely on traditional informed-consent procedural standards and might permit the patient to balance the personal value of medical confidentiality against the personal value of high-technology, team health care. There is no reason that the same procedure should not be used with psychiatric records instead of the arbitrary system now employed, in which everything related to psychiatry is kept secret.

AFTERTHOUGHT: CONFIDENTIALITY AND INDISCRETION

There is one additional aspect of confidentiality that is rarely included in discussions of the subject. I am referring here to the wanton, often inadvertent, but avoidable exchanges of confidential information that occur frequently in hospital rooms, elevators, cafeterias, doctors' offices, and at cocktail parties. Of course, as more people have access to medical information about the patient the potential for this irresponsible abuse of confidentiality increases geometrically.

Such mundane breaches of confidentiality are probably of greater concern to most patients than the broader issue of whether their medical records may be entered into a computerized data bank or whether a respiratory therapist is reviewing the results of an arterial blood gas determination. Somehow, privacy is violated and a sense of shame is heightened when intimate secrets are revealed to people one knows or is close to — friends, neighbors, acquaintances, or hospital roommates — rather than when they are disclosed to an anonymous bureaucrat sitting at a computer terminal in a distant city or to a health professional who is acting in an official capacity.

I suspect that the principles of medical confidentiality, particularly those reflected in most medical codes of ethics, were designed principally to prevent just this sort of embarrassing personal indiscretion rather than to maintain (for social, political, or economic reasons) the absolute secrecy of doctor–patient communications. In this regard, it is worth noting that Percival's Code of Medical Ethics (1803) includes the following admonition: "Patients should be interrogated concerning their complaint in a tone of voice which cannot be overheard." * We in the medical profession frequently neglect these simple courtesies.

CONCLUSION

The principle of medical confidentiality described in medical codes of ethics and still believed in by patients no longer exists. In this respect, it is a decrepit concept. Rather than perpetuate the myth of confidentiality and invest energy vainly to preserve it, the public and the profession would be better served if they devoted their

---

*Leake CD, ed. Percival's medical ethics. Baltimore: Williams & Wilkins, 1927.

Vol. 307   No. 24

CORRESPONDENCE

1521

attention to determining which aspects of the original principle of confidentiality are worth retaining. Efforts could then be directed to salvaging those.

University of Chicago–
  Pritzker School of Medicine
Chicago, IL 60637   MARK SIEGLER, M.D.

Supported by a grant (OSS-8018097) from the National Science Foundation and by the National Endowment for the Humanities. The views expressed are those of the author and do not necessarily reflect those of the National Science Foundation or the National Endowment for the Humanities.

8.6 Siegler M (1982) Medical Consultations in the Context of the Physician-Patient Relationship. In: Agich GJ (ed) Responsibility in Health Care. D. Reidel, Boston, p 141–62

MARK SIEGLER

MEDICAL CONSULTATIONS IN THE CONTEXT OF THE PHYSICIAN-PATIENT RELATIONSHIP*

There is widespread agreement that the physician-patient relationship is changing and remains in a state of flux. This assertion is incontestable with the proviso that the physician-patient relationship is changing more for some patients and physicians than for others. The traditional paternalistic medical model, characterized by the patient's trust in and dependency on the physician, has been replaced in many cases by a more equal relationship in which patient autonomy and self-determination is emphasized. While this newer model certainly has many advantages, there are times when patients' rights and physicians' responsibilities conflict. When this happens, an adversarial relationship may develop between physician and patient which could negate the cooperative, reciprocal, mutual, voluntary, and goal-oriented engagement essential for both parties.

An analysis of the rights of patients and the responsibilities of physicians may be beneficial in understanding why these conflicts arise and how they may be prevented. For this reason I have chosen to examine the physician-patient relationship in the complex but fascinating setting of medical consultations.[1] (The complexity may be partly responsible for the paucity of either medical or ethical literature on the subject of medical consultations.) An attempt will be made to describe medical consultations as they currently operate in medicine, to distinguish them from other forms of physician-patient encounters, and to indicate the remarkable spectrum of possible interactions that can be described properly as medical consultations.[2]

An understanding of the rights and responsibilities of individuals within the arrangement referred to as medical consultation requires a preliminary understanding of what medical encounters qualify as consultations. The term *medical consultation* as it is used here and in contemporary American medicine is defined as the evaluation of a patient by a physician-consultant for the purpose of providing the primary care physician with additional information which will assist him in the care of the patient.[3] The situation described is one in which Dr. A requests that Dr. B evaluate Patient C and render an opinion or perform a diagnostic or therapeutic procedure on Patient C. As used here the term consultation involves three persons — two physicians and a patient — and thus differs in profound ways from the

141

George J. Agich (ed.), Responsibility in Health Care, 141–162.
Copyright © 1982 by D. Reidel Publishing Company, Dordrecht, Holland.

standard two-person physician-patient encounter that characterizes much of medical practice.[4]

Even when this narrow definition is used, the consultation situation remains extremely complex. It implies a prior and continuing relationship between a primary physician who requested the consultation and the patient who agreed with the primary physician that such a consultation should be sought. Any analysis must relate the rights and responsibilities of the three parties involved in a medical consultation (patient, primary physician, and consultant) to those of the two parties (patient and primary physician) in the original relationship. In turn these analyses must be related to the nature of medicine itself — its goals, practices, and organization. Since the decision to seek a medical consultation can best be understood as a specific application of the general rules guiding decision-making within a morally acceptable relationship, the consultant's responsibility will depend in large measure on the procedural adequacy and moral acceptability of the patient-physician relationship which generated the consultation in the first place. In other words, the ethical standards for medical consultation must be based upon an ethically acceptable model of both the physician-patient relationship and of decision-making in medicine, which will finally depend upon an understanding of the nature and limits of medicine itself.

I. MEDICAL CONSULTATIONS: WHAT THEY ARE AND ARE NOT

Any commentary on the rights and responsibilities of individuals involved in a medical consultation is impossible without understanding what constitutes a consultation and what does not. In efforts to discern what actions in medicine are morally acceptable, description ought to precede prescription and empirical observations ought to be a precondition to ethical analysis. Without this priority, ethical analysis lacks a firm connection with the realities of medical practice.

There are numerous types of physician-patient encounters which need to be distinguished from medical consultations. Four of the most common are: principal or primary care physician-patient relationships, care provided by health care teams, independent primary physician-patient relationships, and referrals. A brief description of each of these encounters seems in order.

First, *principal or primary care relationships* involve continuing and comprehensive care. They necessitate a long-term commitment by a physician with the consent of the patient to provide health care, including diagnosis, treatment, advice, education, and health counseling. Primary care physicians

MEDICAL CONSULTATIONS   143

may seek the opinion of one or several medical consultants and then incorporate such opinions in providing for their patients' total health care needs. In contrast, medical consultation is episodic rather than continuous and usually is limited in scope. Today, most consultants have expertise only in their own fields (for example, surgery or internal medicine), often only in a particular subspecialty (for example, thoracic surgery or endocrinology), and often only in a particular organ system (for example, the eye, the heart, or the liver).

Second, consultations differ from the *care provided by health care teams*. As Theodore Brown points out in his essay, "An Historical View of Health Care Teams," although the health care team may be composed of individuals who represent various disciplines and have different expertise, their interaction does not resemble that of a medical consultation and is not called a consultation. The hierarchic nature of such teams and the leadership role typically accorded the physician resolves the inherent ambiguity of the inter-relationships of team members. However, even on teams composed primarily or exclusively of physicians (cardiologists and cardiac surgeons who work together in the management of open heart surgery cases, or a group of physicians who jointly direct a bone marrow transplant unit), the relationship among these physicians is not considered to be a consultation. This may be because the physicians involved have an equal status and enjoy equal and comparable relationships with the patient. Alternatively, since none of the physicians on a team enjoys a primary physician-patient relationship with the patient, the situation is one in which the concept of consultation simply does not apply.

Third, many patients are followed in the outpatient setting by more than one physician simultaneously (for example, by an internist and an ophthalmologist or by an internist and a psychiatrist). Furthermore, many patients are followed by more than one primary care physician simultaneously (for example, by an internist and a family practitioner or by an internist and a gynecologist).

These situations, which may be called *multiple independent primary physician-patient relationships*, are quite different from medical consultations. In such cases the physicians often act independently and do not serve as consultants to each other. They might only learn of the existence of the other if the patient chose to communicate the fact. The patient retains almost total control over the exchange of information between the physicians and might only encourage an exchange by asking Dr. A a question such as: "Would you check with Dr. B to find out if the medicine you want to place me on can be taken safely along with the medicine he is giving me?" No one would choose to describe the relationship between Doctors A and B as that between a principal physician and consultant.

A fourth common physician-patient encounter is a *referral*. The distinction between a medical consultation and a referral and the relationship between consultations and referrals is important – and one not often appreciated even by physicians. As opposed to a medical consultation, a referral usually means that a patient is sent by a primary physician to a new physician (perhaps a "consultant" physician) for medical care.[5] In this case the "consulting physician" now becomes the patient's new primary care physician.

Referrals may be partial or complete. An example of a partial referral would be a situation in which an internist refers a patient to a surgical colleague for an operation. The referral is partial if the internist and patient plan to continue their previous relationship after the resolution of the surgical problem. It must be noted that with any referral, in contrast to a consultation, the primary physician at least temporarily relinquishes decision-making in the patient's medical care to another physician. Despite this fact, in partial referrals the primary physician remains "involved".

In a complete referral, the responsibility for the patient's care is shifted permanently to another physician or institution. One reason for this may be that the patient's medical needs have changed (for example, a patient with chronic diabetes who has been followed by an internist develops renal failure and requires a nephrologist to manage chronic hemodialysis). Another reason may be that difficulties have arisen in the primary physician-patient relationship such that either the physician or the patient now prefers to sever the relationship. The physician then makes a complete referral to a new physician.[6]

In considering the distinction between consultation and referral, it is important to realize that a consultation often may be a prelude to a long-term referral. Furthermore, in contrast with a consultation, a complete referral generates a new physician-patient relationship, a new two-person relationship. A consultation or a partial referral maintains a triangular relationship among a patient and two physicians. These are quite different situations and they generate quite different ethical conflicts.

A major point differentiating a consultation and each of the other physician-patient arrangements is that consultations are characterized by a three-way engagement in which each of the participants – patient, primary physician, and consultant – has multiple and divided obligations to each of the other two persons and to himself within the boundaries of the medical encounter. The patient's loyalty may be divided between the primary physician and the consultant. The primary physician has an ongoing commitment to the patient, but he also has obligations arising out of collegial and professional tries to the consultant. The consultant of course is divided in his loyalties and responsibilities between the physician who invited him to see the patient and the patient for whom he is now partly responsible.

By contrast, standard physician-patient relationships, multiple independent physician-patient relationships, or complete referrals retain the essential features of a two-person encounter. Team medicine often generates its own tensions, but they differ from the specific tensions created by the triangular relationship characteristic of consultations.

II. THE SPECTRUM OF MEDICAL CONSULTATIONS

After distinguishing medical consultations from other types of physician-patient encounters, it is essential to attempt to describe the many types of situations which may generate consultations and the specific details of individual consultation arrangements. The ethical questions raised regarding medical consultations and their resolution are dependent upon the details and specifications of consultation arrangements. There will be no attempt here to analyze how the details of the consultation modify the responsibilities of the various parties. Nevertheless, the description of the range and heterogeneity of medical consultations should provide a clinical framework and the necessary background to enable others to pursue the kind of systematic ethical analysis required.[7]

There are numerous factors which modify consultation arrangements and which should influence any understanding of obligations in the consultation process. The most prominent of these factors are listed below:

The Decision to Seek Consultation

Who initiated the consultation, the patient or the physician? Did the other party agree? If it was the physician's decision to seek a consultation, did the patient have the capacity to express a preference for or against the consultation?

The Selection of a Consultant

Who selected the specific consultant? Who decided what type of specialist should be chosen? If there was disagreement, how was the matter resolved? For example, consider a situation in which a patient wanted to see a cardiologist for chest pain which he feared was of cardiac origin, but his physician suggested a thoracic surgeon to evaluate the patient for the repair of a hiatus hernia, which the physician believed was causing the patient's chest pain. It would be important to note which consultant was called in and how this arrangement was negotiated between the physician and the patient. Furthermore, which of the parties — the primary physician or the patient — assumed responsibility for the consultant's skill, competence, personality, charges, and for the outcome of the consultation?

The Type of Specialist Consulting

What type of specialist has been called in? Both the special area of expertise of the consultant and the specialty training of the primary physician will have a profound effect on the nature of the consultation process. The entire dynamics of the consultative process depends on what type of specialist is seeking a consultation from what other type. Consultations to internists and surgeons differ in many respects from those to psychiatrists. To add to the complexity, consultations requested from a particular service (for example, from psychiatry) will differ according to which primary service (for example, cardiac surgery) is requesting the consultation. There are many reasons for these differences, including the nature of the medical problem, the training of the consultant, and the severity of the patient's condition.

The Severity of the Illness

How severe is the patient's illness? The answer in any particular case modifies many aspects of the consultation arrangement just as it modifies many aspects of the primary physician-patient relationship. For example, a critically ill patient may be seen by one or several consultants in an emergency situation without consenting to these arrangements and often without even being aware of them.

The Setting of the Consultation

Is the case in question an inpatient or outpatient situation? Consultations on inpatients are different from those on outpatients, and consultations in university hospital settings often differ from those in community hospitals.

MEDICAL CONSULTATIONS   147

The very fact that inpatients require hospitalization implies that they generally are sicker than outpatients. Hospitalized patients often have their care paid for by some form of third-party insurance. Consultants are more available in the hospital than in the outpatient setting, but there may be more rules and administrative requirements to obtain their services. Finally, there is more scrutiny of care in the inpatient setting than in the office. For these reasons, inpatient consultation differs from the office setting. In general, hospitalized patients are less free to choose whether to see a consultant, who the consultant will be, or whether to reject the consultant's recommendation.

The details of the consultation process will probably differ depending on whether the patient is seen in a university medical center or in a community hospital. The latter has the single mission of providing care for community residents. The university center engages in the triple mission of providing care, educating students and houseofficers, and generating new knowledge through research. Furthermore, the university hospital is often staffed with a large number of medical specialists ("consultants"), and medical practice in such university centers is often dominated by these specialists.

In addition to the factors already discussed, it is important to recognize that in a decision to seek medical consultation, the primary physician and the patient may be pursuing different goals. The most frequent goal sought in obtaining a consultation is *technical expertise*, either for diagnostic purposes (such as when a radiologist is called in to perform and interpret a CT scan) or for therapeutic purposes (such as when a plastic surgeon is called in to resect a skin lesion). When a consultation is sought to obtain technical expertise, the consultant may accept or decline the request to participate in a case, but otherwise there is not much latitude for the consultant to modify the primary physician's diagnosis or treatment plans. If the consultant declines to perform the diagnostic or therapeutic service, the primary physician must seek the assistance of another expert. In general, technical experts are interchangeable.

Another goal in consultation may involve the need for *clinical judgment*. The primary physician may call in a consultant not because the latter possesses a special technical skill, but because he wishes another opinion from someone whose clinical judgment he respects.[8]

There also may be *medical-legal reasons* for obtaining a consultation.[9] For example, a physician may be concerned about missing a condition for which he could later be sued. This is sometimes referred to as "defensive medicine". Or, he may wish to show good faith in searching for the correct diagnosis in a difficult case. In another situation the physician may wish to countermand an unwelcome recommendation from a previous consultant by getting a contrary opinion. Occasionally, consultations are sought as a means to avoid or defer taking action. Sometimes the patient is the one who calls for a consultation and the physician may feel obligated legally and morally to act on this request.

Furthermore, the physician may be required to request a consultation for *administrative reasons*. For example, some hospitals require that all patients over a certain age who are scheduled for elective surgery must be "cleared for surgery" by a cardiology consultant. In another situation, compliance with certain third-party insurance requirements may necessitate a "second opinion" before elective surgery.

Other reasons why a physician might seek a consultation are *personal*. For example, he may wish to solidify his reputation with colleagues, to reciprocate for previous referrals, to assure a patient "everything is being done," to share responsibility and potential liability for unforeseen results, or to punish a patient for non-compliance. Finally, in *preparation for a referral*, a physician may seek consultation in situations in which the disease has changed or the patient is a "problem patient".

In summary, the ethical obligations of the parties to a consultation — the patient, the primary physician, and the consultant — vary according to the specific details of the consultation itself. Therefore, the search for a single solution to the range of ethical dilemmas and conflicts which could arise in the context of medical consultations would be naive. On the basis of the preceding observations, it should be clear that the consultation process is superimposed on an existing and continuing physician-patient relationship. In contrast to many other medical engagements, it involves three persons enmeshed in a complex network of relationships. The presumptive obligations of the consultant, then, ought to coincide with the basic goals of medicine — to attempt in an ethically appropriate way to improve the health and well-being of patients, most of whom present themselves voluntarily to physicians in seeking care. As a consequence, consultants should fulfill their ethical and clinical obligations to patients by serving as exclusive agents neither to the patient nor to the primary physician, but rather *by serving the original physician-patient relationship* from which the request for consultation originated.

In practice, the consultant's presumptive obligation to serve the physician-patient relationship in order to provide the best medical care for the patient is achieved by conforming to the traditions and current modes of medical practice as regards consultation. This usually means that the consultant reports his findings to the primary physician and not directly to the patient.

In communicating to the primary physician, the consultant will be improving the stability of the underlying physician-patient relationship and the quality of health care provided the patient. To repeat: the consultant generally helps the patient achieve the goals which the patient and primary physician established by serving that original relationship rather than by serving either of the individual parties.

III. THE PHYSICIAN-PATIENT RELATIONSHIP AS THE MORAL CENTER OF MEDICINE

As suggested earlier, a proper understanding of medical consultations as distinguished from other forms of physician-patient encounters logically implies the prior existence of a primary physician-patient relationship. Medicine is an institution with ends and purposes related to caring for persons who voluntarily seek help in the care of their health. The physician-patient relationship historically has been the central means by which such care is provided. Thus, a well-constructed physician-patient relationship remains the clinical and moral center of medicine ([6], [8]).

A properly constructed physician-patient relationship should involve two persons who negotiate a voluntary, consensual, non-coercive, and mutual accommodation aimed at achieving the health care goals of the patient while remaining consistent with the conscientious beliefs of the physician both as an individual and in his role as a physician. These days there are many types of primary physician-patient relationships, many of which are neither long-standing nor stable. Some involve temporary accommodations between patient and physician limited to the details of a specific clinical situation. The strength of a physician-patient relationship depends upon the patient, the physician, the quality of their interaction, the setting in which they meet, and the nature of the patient's illness.[10]

In the gradual achievement of a long-standing, stable, primary physician-patient relationship, many issues such as patient rights and arrangements for truth-telling, decision-making, and even for the way in which consultations will be handled, may have been discussed and negotiated between the physician and the patient. These discussions and negotiated arrangements provide an ideal and morally acceptable basis for medical practice.

Medical consultations, however, resemble transient accommodations between physician and patient, and they differ profoundly from well-established, stable physician-patient relationships. The consultant cannot hope to achieve the same degree of voluntary, consensual, non-coercive, and mutual accommodation as has been developed over time between the primary physician and the patient. Duties in medicine and duties in general derive from relationships. In respect to truth-telling, the duties of the primary physician to the patient differ from the duties of a consultant.[11]

The physician-patient relationship is the moral and clinical center of medicine, and decision-making within this accommodation is the central event of the medical enterprise. The decision to seek a consultation, like any other medical decision, is made in this context. Most clinical decisions in medicine begin with the delineation of the medical goals being sought by the patient and the acquiescence by the physician to these goals. These goals might include restoration of health, relief of symptoms (physical and psychological), restoration of function or the maintenance of compromised functions, the prolongation of life, or increased knowledge about a medical problem and its prognosis. Based upon the specific goals being pursued, the primary physician's central responsibility is to use his medical expertise to respond to the patient's request for help in the care of his health by proposing a medically-indicated course of action which appears to be the best approach to the patient's problems and health care goals.

The first step in the decision-making process involves the physician's recommendations. The physician normally proposes a diagnostic or therapeutic course or suggests that nothing be done. One recommendation that a physician might make is that the patient be seen in consultation by another physician. In deciding on a specific recommendation, the primary physician will take into account the technical aspects of the case (its severity, acuity, its potential for improvement, the risks involved either in doing nothing or in taking this or another action), and also the psychological and social needs of the patient. At this point, the physician normally proposes a diagnostic or therapeutic course or suggests that nothing be done.

Chronologically, the second stage in the decision-making process is the patient's reaction to the physician's clinical suggestion. Competent patients may either accept or reject physician's recommendations. In this regard, patient preferences are the weightiest ethical consideration in decisions reached within the physician-patient relationship. If the physician proposes a consultation for medically indicated reasons, the patient is free to accept or refuse the suggestion. In the normal course of events, the patient will usually accept this recommendation. If, however, the patient rejects a recommended consultation, several events could occur. The physician might modify his recommendation and decide differently. If he chose not to do so and substantial disagreement remained, the relationship could be severed because the physician might feel that his ability to care adequately for the patient was compromised.

On the other hand, if the patient and physician were to agree to seek a consultation, the consultant would be serving them jointly and his allegiance should be to the relationship which generated the request for his services. This situation is analogous to other decisions in medicine unrelated to consultation which are made mutually, consensually, non-coercively, and voluntarily by physician and patient, but which require the services of third parties to be implemented.[12]

An Empirical Claim

The goals of medicine are achieved better and more efficiently through primary physician-patient relationships with their traditional interactions with medical consultants than by alternative arrangements which essentially by-pass the primary physician-patient relationship. This claim is empirical and thus far has not been proven by any compilation of data.[13] Nevertheless, this claim seems intuitively correct to many physicians actively practicing medicine either in ambulatory or in-patient settings. By and large, patients who have sound, well-established physician-patient relationships get better outpatient and inpatient care than do patients who are practiced upon by teams of consultants in the hospital or whose interactions in the ambulatory setting are episodic, disjointed, and involve many consultants. There are several reasons why this is so. First of all, the relationship between physician and patient in a primary healing relationship seems to be the most effective way to provide care and to achieve the goals of medicine. This primary relationship between patient and healer also appears to have historical and transcultural validation [11]. Even with all the changes in the health system which serve to undermine long-term primary physician-patient relationships, those relationships which rely as much on trust and confidence as on technical expertise are regarded both within the profession and by patients as useful and desirable.

Another reason stems from the belief that the primary care or principal physician should assume responsibility for continuous and comprehensive health care for patients. Such care should be not only technically competent and humane, but also should be directed at the entire person rather than at some isolated organ system. A principal physician should also serve as his patient's friend, advisor, and advocate within the health care system. This latter responsibility includes guiding the patient through the maze of hospitals, laboratory services, and *consultants*.

A well-established physician-patient relationship also promises better care because the primary physician cares for his patient by collating and integrating the opinions of various consultants, thereby generating a comprehensive approach. By contrast, the consultant may present a recommendation that is not appropriate in terms of the patient's total health care needs or personal wishes. The principal physician would have taken account of the whole person – his disease, personality, history, fears, wishes, beliefs, and finances. On the other hand, too many consultants have a tunnel-vision perspective in which they see the patient as a "liver" or a "heart" wrapped in human form or as a "subject" to be catheterized or biopsied or operated upon.

The primary physician should be the spokesman for all physicians involved in a particular case. This role should lessen patient confusion when several contradictory or apparently contradictory reports are presented by various consultants. (Both good news and bad news, but particularly the latter, should not be transmitted to the patient by a consultant whom the patient has met once and may never see again.)

Alternatives to the Traditional Relationship

Some individuals might prefer to negotiate arrangements with their primary physicians so that a consultant could discuss findings and suggestions directly with the patient rather than with the primary physician. If such arrangements between patients and primary physicians are reached in a voluntary, consensual manner, there should be no moral objection to this plan. As mentioned earlier, though, there remains the real concern that patient care might be compromised by such a plan.

Other individuals might prefer to bypass the entire system of primary care relationships and traditional medical consultations in favor of alternative arrangements such as multiple, independently-negotiated accommodations with numerous physicians. These individuals might refer to such arrangements as "consultations" ("I will seek a consultation from the famous surgeon, Dr. A"), but as shown earlier, those schemes more closely resemble free-standing, dyadic physician-patient relationships than the three-part arrangement characteristic of consultations.

In modern American medicine, an individual who can pay for health services may enter into multiple, voluntary, and consensual arrangements with physicians even when such arrangements bypass a preliminary primary physician-patient relationship and the model of consultation described in this essay. Although patients have such license, it seems doubtful that this

MEDICAL CONSULTATIONS   153

policy should be universalized in that society's general interest would suffer, particularly with respect to increasing health care costs. More importantly, it would limit the opportunity to achieve the goals of medicine. The policy of multiple independently-negotiated physician-patient accommodations tends to be adversarial, contentious, time-consuming, costly to patients and physicians, counter-productive in regard to medical goals, and probably would not generate additional liberty and freedom, which already exists in properly negotiated primary physician-patient relationships. The same policy would also thwart the development of trust, confidence, and hope upon which the success of the medical encounter depends [5].

Although the presumptive obligation of the consultant is to serve primarily the physician-patient relationship, a variety of circumstances could encourage the consulting physician to override this presumption and to deal directly with the patient. For example, a consultant who realizes that a true medical consultation (the three-party relationship) is not occurring, but rather that either the physician is referring the patient permanently or that the patient is seeking a second opinion independently, probably will conclude that the patient's medical interests will be served best by open and direct communication. It can also happen that the consultant may decide conscientiously that he would serve an individual patient best not by strengthening the primary physician-patient relationship but by encouraging its disruption. In this case, there would be an obligation to act accordingly. The consultant's grounds for such action might be based upon the technical inadequacies of the primary physician or upon his perception that the primary physician-patient relationship was not a morally sound arrangement. For example, if the primary physician proved incompetent or physically or emotionally impaired, and if these deficiencies could not be corrected within the framework of the institution or the profession, the consultant would be obligated to inform the patient that medical care should be sought from another, more competent physician.[14]

Another reason why a consultant might choose to deal directly with a patient would be if the basic goal of medicine were compromised. For example, if the consultant and the primary physician have irreconcilable technical differences regarding a treatment plan, and if private discussions prove unsuccessful in resolving these differences, the consultant may either confront the patient directly or announce to the patient that he is forced to withdraw from the case because of a serious difference of opinion with the primary physician. (In the latter case, the consultant should suggest to the patient that another consultation opinion be sought.)[15]

IV. ADDITIONAL VIEWPOINTS ON RESPONSIBILITIES OF CONSULTING PHYSICIANS

Besides the views discussed thus far, two additional models of the responsibilities of the consultant can be distinguished: a paternalistic model and a contractual model.

In medical practice, a paternalistic interpretation of the responsibilities of medical consultants has emphasized the primary responsibility of the consultant to the physician who asks the consultant for an opinion. If disagreements arise between the primary physician and the consultant, they usually are resolved without involving the patient in the discussions.

This paternalistic model of medical consultation is represented well in the writings of Philip Tumulty, a distinguished consulting physician at The Johns Hopkins University School of Medicine. Tumulty has written: "Obviously, the role of consultant is to help the patient by aiding his primary physician and is not to supplant him or override him or to push him aside . . . " ([9], p. 45). He is concerned that some consultants make it difficult for the primary physician to play an essential role in the care of a patient. One way consultants do so is by giving information directly to the patient or family, or by making suggestions regarding diagnosis in treatment without first getting approval from the primary physician. Tumulty believes that under no circumstances should the consultant give to the patient or his family any specific information relating to diagnosis, treatment, or prognosis unless directly requested to do so by the primary physician. Tumulty notes that when this rule is violated, " . . . doubts may be planted and confusion may begin to grow. The primary physician may start to lose control of his own patient's management . . . " ([9], p. 45). In an effort to avoid this situation, Tumulty suggests the following strategy:

If, after examining the patient, the consultant is backed into a corner by members of the family, who insist upon getting an opinion from him, it is always possible to gracefully put them off by saying something to the effect that . . . it is essential to review certain aspects of the problem with Dr. Blank before forming an opinion ([9], p. 46).

Tumulty's attitude toward medical consultation is presented explicitly with his statement that the consultant should be ever mindful of the difficult problems encountered in the everyday practice of medicine, and he should therefore make a deliberate effort to buttress the position of the primary physician ([9], p. 45).

There are several problems with Tumulty's suggestions regarding consultations. First, he emphasizes the relationship between the consultant and the

MEDICAL CONSULTATIONS   155

primary physician almost to the exclusion of the relationship of either to the patient. This focus on collegial relationships between medical professionals is more a matter of medical etiquette than medical ethics. Tumulty acknowledges that the ends being sought in a medical consultation are health care benefits for the patient, but he stresses that the consultant serves the patient's medical needs best by serving the primary physician. Tumulty argues that in situations of serious disagreement between primary physician and consultant, the consultant should strive to resolve these matters in discussions with the physician and not involve the patient in such disagreements. Even in the "worst case" scenario, when negotiations between the primary physician and consultant collapse, the protocol outlined by Tumulty again stresses primary physician-consultant actions and again minimizes discussions with the patient.

Tumulty notes that in situations in which the responsible physician persists in a manner which the consultant believes to be harmful, the consultant should explain to the patient or family that he must withdraw from the case because he can no longer be helpful to them ([9], p. 48). Tumulty further indicates that it should be made clear to the patient and family that the central matter is one of failure to agree: "They should *not* [italics in text] be told by the consultant that he is necessarily right and the other physician is wrong. It should again be stressed that medical problems are like all other problems; there is room for disagreement" ([9], p. 48). A final problem with Tumulty's analysis of medical consultations is its unabashedly paternalistic attitude, which argues that the physician knows what is best for the patient.[16] Although the ends being sought are the health of the patient, such a paternalistic stance understates the mutual, voluntary, consensual, and non-coercive arrangements between physicians and patients, which ought to be the moral basis of medical practice.

Another model of consultation emphasizes the "rights" and "freedom" of patients. On this model, the patient is squarely at the center of the encounter and all communication and decision-making is carried out with the patient. By contrast, the two physicians have only limited or minimal obligations (or perhaps no obligations to each other), and both are primarily responsible to the patient. Any disagreements which arise between primary physician and consultant are brought directly to the attention of the patient, who then makes a choice of alternative programs of management. This model might be referred to as a *contractual model* of medical consultation.

This view of medical consultations, at least with reference to liaison psychiatry, has been defended by H. Tristram Engelhardt, Jr., and Laurence

McCullough [2]. With respect to confidentiality in psychiatric liaison consultations, Engelhardt and McCullough have suggested that the consultant physician's duty is to the patient and that any "qualification of confidentiality can be made only with the permission of the patient." In their analysis, the consultant is free to divulge information to the primary physician only when given permission to do so, and the canons of explicit informed consent must be followed to insure that the patient's consent to release information about himself or herself is informed and voluntary. Engelhardt and McCullough observe that if the patient refuses to give informed consent:

... one will have paid one of the prices for respecting persons; less that optimal treatment. ... Acknowledging such freedom is central to treating patients as autonomous agents. Moreover, it allows the resolution of the morally ambiguous position of the consultant through the patient's determining the extent to which the consultant will be an agent of the patient, i.e., determined by the patient's interests.

Their contractual and libertarian model of consultation is stated explicitly:

We have here suggested that the choices [among the duties and goods the consultant seeks] should be made in favor of respect for patient autonomy both out of regard for patients as well as in order to establish a practice which supports public liberty. Such a choice, however, is made only with the loss of other goods, in particular those that would be achieved through more paternalistic practices regardless of patient wishes, i.e., divulging information to third parties insofar as communication of information is in the best interests of this patient ([2], p. 412).

Although Engelhardt and McCullough's essay concerns the specific issue of confidentiality in liaison (consultative) psychiatry rather than consultations in general, the view developed in this particular setting offers a different model of consultation. Whereas many forms of psychiatric consultation closely resemble traditional medical and surgical consultations, some psychiatric consultations, particularly those imposed upon a patient without consent – for example, as a precondition for commitment proceedings – differ in profound ways from routine medical and surgical consultations. It appears that in their analysis Engelhardt and McCullough focus on involuntary, coerced "consultation" which must be regarded as an aberration of the traditional medical model and not as its standard. As a result, Engelhardt and McCullough avoid dealing with the practical and ethical complexities of consultations by proposing a model which bears little resemblance to consultations as they currently exist or as they have been understood traditionally in medical practice.

The physician-patient encounter as described by these authors is not a consultation in that a three-person relationship does not appear to exist. In their model, there is no presumptive obligation on the part of the consultant to communicate with the primary physician or indeed to have any interaction with that physician at all. The depicted model more closely resembles a situation in which the patient has entered into several entirely independent relationships. This model ignores the primary physician and the circumstances which generated the initial physician-patient relationship and from which the decision to seek a consultation was made.

The most serious problem with this model, however, is that by depicting autonomy and rights of the patient as the highest goal of medicine and by characterizing ethics as representing "an alternative to force", the authors describe an essentially adversarial view of medical practice.[17] This adversarial vision requires contractual guarantees to protect patients entering the medical system. The goal of medicine and in particular the human needs which encourage a patient to seek help from a physician are ignored ([5], [6]).

Consultations in medicine are the result of decisions taken in pre-existing physician-patient relationships. If these original relationships were developed in accordance with the moral principles of mutuality, consensuality, voluntariness, and non-coerciveness, and if the decision to seek consultation was made in accordance with morally sound procedures, then the issues of patient "freedom" and "rights" will all have been negotiated prior to the consultation. Thus, in the absence of serious disagreement, it remains the responsibility of the consultant to try to settle differences within the context of the enduring physician-patient relationship rather than in the transient setting of the consultant-patient relationship.

V. CONCLUSION

The model of responsibility in medical consultations proposed in this essay recognizes the voluntary, mutual, consensual, and non-coercive agreements of all parties to both the consultation process and to the physician-patient relationship which generated the request for a consultation. Any party could withdraw from the consultative arrangement (or for that matter, from the physician-patient relationship) at any time and thus change what was originally a consultation to another form of physician-patient encounter.

This view rejects the position advocated by Tumulty, which supports the primary physician and attends mainly to issues of medical etiquette in the physician-consultant relationship. It also rejects the thesis advanced by Engelhardt and McCullough that consultants have a primary obligation to

158   MARK SIEGLER

patient "autonomy" (thus focusing primarily on the patient-consultant relationship). Their thesis essentially ignores the original context of care in which the consultation was sought. In practice, the view advocated here suggests that the loyalty of the consultant and of the primary physician interacts directly. Such interactions both serve and preserve the primary physician-patient relationship — the technical and moral center of medical practice. If the decision to seek a medical consultation was arrived at in the context of a morally acceptable patient-physician relationship, the consultant would act most properly by dealing mainly with the primary physician and not directly with the patient. However, when the patient's health care and health will be ill-served by the perpetuation of an ineffective or destructive (and thus morally unacceptable patient-physician relationship), it then becomes the obligation of the consultant to so inform the patient in order that the goals of medicine — the health care and health of the patient — might be better achieved through another arrangement. In general, this approach also maximizes patient benefit and permits consultants to adhere to the collegial requirements of the medical profession.

University of Chicago

NOTES

* Work on this paper was supported in part by an Interdisciplinary Incentive Award (OSS-8018097) from the Ethics and Values in Science and Technology (EVIST) Program of the National Science Foundation.
[1] I have been interested in the question of how to establish the rights of patients and the responsibilities of physicians at a time when a societal consensus no longer exists. This paper in some ways continues the work Ann Dudley Goldblatt and I did in the Ninth Trans-Disciplinary Symposium on Philosophy and Medicine [7]. We noted in the earlier paper that a morally and technically acceptable model of the physician-patient relationship would take account of the specific clinical circumstances in which doctor and patient were interacting. Thus, we described profound differences in the physician-patient relationship between situations of acute, critical illness and those of chronic, non-critical outpatient care.

As mentioned, this essay will explore the physician-patient relationship in the context of medical consultations. An earlier version of this paper was entitled "Medical Consultations: Divided Loyalties and Uncertain Responsibilities." That title reflected the commonly held view that the central ethical dilemma in the consultation process is the consultant's divided loyalties and responsibilities to both the patient and the primary physician. The issue is sometimes framed as a question: Is the consultant primarily an agent of the attending physician or is he an agent of the patient? I believe this is an oversimplified — and possibly even a wrong — rendering of the issues involved in medical consultation. Framing the question in this way ignores the historical preconditions and

MEDICAL CONSULTATIONS 159

negotiations within the physician-patient relationship that enabled a medical consultation to occur in the first place. In this paper, I will examine the issue of the responsibility of consultants not as an isolated event, but as an interaction which is best understood within the general context of physician-patient relationships which occur within our system of medicine [1].

2 This paper will not present an historical or anthropological analysis of medical consultations. Nor will it examine consultations in systems of health care different from that of the United States. For example, the relationship of general practitioners to "consultants" in the British National Health Service is a fascinating subject and was the focus of a recent book [3]. Finally, no attempt will be made to formulate new ways to practice medical consultations: rather, an attempt will be made to describe medical consultations as they are currently practiced.

3 On occasion, physicians seek assistance from health professionals such as social workers, chaplains, dieticians, occupational therapists, etc. These requests for assistance are often described as consultations. Thus, one might say: "I will obtain a social service consultation." For reasons of simplification, in this paper I will restrict my analysis to physician-physician consultations. Many of the points made in this paper should be applicable also to non-physician health professional consultations.

4 Some medical analysts, often contractarians who believe medicine can be reduced easily to the buying and selling of a product – rather like shopping for a used car – might prefer to use the term "medical consultation" to describe what they do when they seek second or third opinions or when they go "doctor shopping". Thus, such individuals might say: "Dr. A. told me I had hypertension and should be treated; I will obtain a 'medical consultation' from Doctor B." I have no quarrel either with the wish of such individuals to seek additional medical opinions or with their peculiar use of the term "medical consultation", rather than "medical opinion" or "second opinion" to describe their activities. Such activities, however, more closely resemble the establishment of multiple primary physician-patient relationships rather than medical consultations as the term is commonly understood in medicine.

Another possible use of the term "consultation" would be to describe an opinion rendered by a specialist, a so-called consultant, at a time when the specialist was interacting with the patient in a role as a primary physician and not in the role of a consultant. The differentiation between this use of the term and the way I choose to use it relates to whether the second opinion was sought by a patient independently (thus, not a true consultation) or whether the second opinion was sought within the context of a physician-patient relationship. The former situation involves two persons; the latter situation, the true consultation, involves three persons.

5 It should be noted that the term "refer" may be used to describe either the seeking of a consultation or the making of a true "referral" in the sense of sending a patient away to be cared for permanently by another physician.

6 Referrals are frequently made at the patient's request or because a patient is dissatisfied with the primary physician. In a study by Williams *et al.*, about one-third of cases of referral from a primary physician's office to a medical center were at the request of the patient [10].

7 I will suggest, however, that an analysis of responsibilities within specific consultation situations in medicine ought to take account of the three factors noted later in this essay which begin to explicate the moral basis of consultations:

160   MARK SIEGLER

(a)   the relationship of medical consultations to the original physician-patient
        relationship which generated the request for a consultation and the moral
        soundness of that original physician-patient relationship [6], [8];

(b)   the adequacy of the procedural standards which generated the decision within
        the physician-patient relationship to seek a medical consultation [4];

(c)   the likelihood that the central goal of medicine – improvement in the health
        care and health of the patient – will be achieved as a result of the consultation.

[8] It should be noted that the skills of consultants who possess keen analytic ability and discriminating clinical judgment are not interchangeable in the way in which those of technicians are. Many aspects of their medical knowledge, interpersonal and interprofessional skills, and their success as consultants, are very special and are not transferable to another individual. In many respects, this is our generic impression of what a consultant is and what he does.

[9] I am distinguishing between the *goals* and *reasons* for a consultation. I am using the term *goals* to describe decisions arrived at jointly by patient and physician based upon legitimate medical indications. By contrast, the *reasons* for seeking a consultation may be based upon medical indications, but usually also relate to non-medical factors – legal, administrative, personal – and usually are determined by the physician without patient participation. This distinction between the *goals* and *reasons* for obtaining a consultation represents a preliminary effort at the important task of describing the broad range of consultations and why they are obtained.

[10] [6]. Too many commentators tend to have an apocalyptic vision of medicine in which all patient illness is regarded as life-threatening. Such a viewpoint colors analysis of the physician-patient relationship, because the patient is invariably regarded as weak and helpless in the face of critical illness and the physician is regarded as powerful and controlling. This vision is quite different from the real world of medical practice in which most patients do not have acute, critical illness, but rather come to physicians with a complaint or for the care of non-critical, chronic diseases.

[11] For example, among the many duties which primary physicians owe to patients is the duty of veracity. If a patient develops a grave disease such as colon cancer, it is the obligation of the patient's physician to inform the patient at the proper time, in the proper manner, and in conformity with the patient's wishes. It would be outrageous and unethical if a patient were informed by a radiology consultant who performed a barium enema or by a gastroenterology consultant who performed colonoscopy that a colon cancer had been detected. Rather, the consultant's obligation was to provide a report of the consultation to the primary physician who would act on such information based upon prior agreements between himself and the patient on how matters such as these would be handled in their relationship. The special quality of the primary physician-patient relationship would mandate that a consultant work through that relationship and not outside of it in providing information to a patient. It is the difference in the quality and depth of relationships between patients and primary physicians, as contrasted with relationships between patients and consultants, that reinforces the point that the presumptive obligation of consultants is to function with the framework of the existing primary physician-patient relationship and to act in ways which maintain that primary relationship.

[12] For example, imagine a situation in which after considerable discussion and negotiation, the physician and patient decide that the patient should try a dangerous, but

potentially beneficial, drug treatment. A prescription is written by the physician and taken by the patient to a pharmacist. The presumptive obligation of the pharmacist is to dispense the medication, although he may wish to warn the patient of its potential side-effects and even perhaps telephone the physician to confirm the prescription and dosage. In general, it would not be appropriate for the pharmacist to refuse to fill the prescription or to intrude into the physician-patient relationship which resulted in the mutual decision to use this particular medication. The pharmacist would be deviating from his appropriate role as a pharmacist if he intruded into the decision which had been arrived at jointly by the physician and patient. Similarly, consultants have been invited into a case as a result of a mutual decision reached in the context of a morally acceptable physician-patient relationship. In this situation, the consultant's obligation should be to the physician-patient relationship which generated the request.

[13] My claims in this section of the paper regarding the value of primary physician-patient relationships are empirical ones and should be subjected to experimental verification. Nevertheless, I believe that the medical relationship has been organized traditionally around primary physician-patient relationships, and therefore it remains the responsibility of those who wish to argue in favor of alternative arrangements (such as multiple independently-negotiated physician-patient accommodations) to marshal data to support their proposed innovations.

[14] It should be noted that this last general obligation of the consultant to intrude into unsuccessful physician-patient relationships is a more stringent and different requirement from those previously expected of consultants. The consultant now has a duty not only to assist the patient in the care of his health by strengthening the primary physician-patient relationship when appropriate, but sometimes to assist the patient by encouraging the disruption of that relationship. The consultant may now be required to probe both into the benefits of the existing physician-patient relationship for the patient and into its potential weaknesses. There is a great risk of officiousness here.

[15] These examples of consultant-patient interaction inevitably raise the question of whether the consultant should work to reinforce the primary physician-patient relationship or to intrude upon it. Although the presumptive obligation should be to enhance the primary relationship, circumstances such as were noted here might lead a consultant to the opposite conclusion. This conclusion and many other medical decisions are reached by a process of clinical discretion [4]; others have called this process clinical judgment. Essential to this process is discretion, the ability to draw relevant distinctions, to discard extraneous facts, to penetrate to the heart of the matter, and to make choices of one course of action as the better among many possible ones. That choice can be defended as "better" not in some absolute sense but because, given the available facts and their interpretation, judicious reflection suggests it fits the actual situation more adequately than other available options. Good choices about how to provide patients with the best medical care require clinical discretion.

[16] Tumulty's paternalistic approach to medicine is evident throughout his excellent book [9]. Interested readers in particular should examine the Introduction and also Chapter I.

[17] This adversarial vision of medicine is understandable if one accepts as the standard medical encounter a situation in which a consultation is being obtained in order to restrain a patient involuntarily. Of course, this is a limited and inaccurate portrayal of most medical and psychiatric consultations.

162   MARK SIEGLER

BIBLIOGRAPHY

1. Cassell, E. J.: 1976, *The Healer's Art: A New Approach to the Doctor-Patient Relationship*, J. B. Lippincott Company, Philadelphia and New York.
2. Engelhardt, H. T., Jr. and McCullough, L. B.: 1979, 'Confidentiality in the Consultation-Liaison Process: Ethical Dimensions and Conflicts', *Psychiatric Clinics of North America* **2**, 403–413.
3. Honigsbaum, F.: 1979, *The Division of British Medicine: A History of the Separation of General Practice from Hospital Care, 1911–1968*, St. Martin's Press, New York.
4. Jonsen, A. R., Siegler, M., and Winslade, W. J.: 1982, *Clinical Ethics: A Practical Approach to Ethical Decisions in Clinical Medicine*, Macmillan Publishing Company, New York.
5. Kass, L. R.: 1980, 'Ethical Dilemmas in the Care of the Ill: What is the Physician's Service?', *JAMA* **244**, 1811–1816.
6. Siegler, M.: 1981, 'Searching for Moral Certainty in Medicine: A Proposal for a New Model of the Doctor-Patient Encounter', *Bulletin of the New York Academy of Medicine* **57**, 56–69.
7. Siegler, M. and Goldblatt, A. D.: 1981, 'Clinical Intuition: A Procedure for Balancing the Rights of Patients and the Responsibilities of Physicians', in S. F. Spicker, *et al* (eds.), *The Law-Medicine Relation: A Philosophical Exploration*, D. Reidel Publishing Company, Dordrecht and Boston, pp. 5–31.
8. Siegler, M.: 'On the Nature and Limits of Clinical Medicine: An Essay on the Doctor-Patient Accommodation', in E. J. Cassell and M. Siegler (eds.), *Changing Values in Medicine* (submitted for publication).
9. Tumulty, P. A.: 1973, *The Effective Clinician*, W. B. Saunders Co., Philadelphia.
10. Williams, T. F., White, K. L., Fleming, W. L., and Greenberg, B. G.: 1961, 'The Referral Process in Medical Care and the University Clinic's Role', *Journal of Medical Education* **36**, 899–907.
11. Young, A.: 1980, 'An Anthropological Perspective on Medical Knowledge', *Journal of Medicine and Philosophy* **5**, 102–16.

8.7 Childress JF, Siegler M (1984) Metaphors and Models of Doctor-Patient Relationships: Their Implications for Autonomy. Theoret Med 5:17–30

JAMES F. CHILDRESS AND MARK SIEGLER

METAPHORS AND MODELS OF DOCTOR-PATIENT
RELATIONSHIPS: THEIR IMPLICATIONS FOR AUTONOMY

INTRODUCTION

Many metaphors and models have been applied to relationships between patients and physicians. One example is an interpretation of physician-patient relationships as paternalistic. In this case, the physician is regarded as a parent and the patient is regarded as a child. Opponents of such a paternalistic view of medicine rarely reject the use of metaphors to interpret medical relationships; rather, they simply offer alternative metaphors, for example, the physician as partner or the patient as rational contractor. Metaphors may operate even when patients and physicians are unaware of them. Physician-patient conflicts may arise if each party brings to their encounter a different image of medicine, as, for example, when the physician regards a paternalistic model of medicine as appropriate, but the patient prefers a contractual model.

As these examples suggest, metaphors involve seeing something as something else, for example, seeing a lover as a red rose, human beings as wolves, or medical therapy as warfare. Metaphors highlight some features and hide other features of their principal subject.[1] Thus, thinking about a physician as a parent highlights the physician's care for dependent others and his or her control over them, but it conceals the patient's payment of fees to the physician. Metaphors and models may be used to describe relationships as they exist, or to indicate what those relationships ought to be. In either the descriptive or the prescriptive use of metaphors, this highlighting and hiding occurs, and it must be considered in determining the adequacy of various metaphors. When metaphors are used to describe roles, they can be criticized if they distort more features than they illuminate. And when they are used to direct roles, they can be criticized if they highlight one moral consideration, such as care, while neglecting others, such as autonomy.

Since there is no single physician-patient relationship, it is probable that no single metaphor can adequately describe or direct the whole range of relationships in health care, such as open heart surgery, clinical research, and psychoanalysis. Some of the most important metaphors that have shaped health care in recent years include: parent-child, partners, rational contractors, friends, and technician-client. We want to determine the adequacy of these metaphors to describe and to direct doctor-patient relationships in the real world. In particular, we will assess them in relation to patient and physician autonomy.

Theoretical Medicine 5 (1984) 17—30. 0167—9902/84/0051—0017 $01.40.

18   JAMES F. CHILDRESS AND MARK SIEGLER

METAPHORS AND MODELS OF RELATIONSHIPS IN HEALTH CARE

(1) The first metaphor is *paternal* or *parental*, and the model is paternalism. For this model, the locus of decision-making is the health care professional, particularly the physician, who has 'moral authority' within an asymmetrical and hierarchical relationship. (A variation on these themes appear in a model that was especially significant earlier — the priest-penitent relationship.)

Following Thomas Szasz and Marc Hollender, we can distinguish two different versions of paternalism, based on two different prototypes.[2] If we take the *parent-infant relationship* as the prototype, the physician's role is active, while the patient's role is passive. The patient, like the infant, is primarily a dependent recipient of care. This model is applied easily to such clinical situations as anesthesia and to the care of patients with acute trauma, coma, or delirium. A second version takes the *parent-adolescent child* relationship as the prototype. Within this version, the physician guides the patient by telling him or her what to expect and what to do, and the patient co-operates to the extent of obeying. This model applies to such clinical situations as the outpatient treatment of acute infectious diseases. The physician instructs the patient on a course of treatment (such as antibiotics and rest), but the patient can either obey or refuse to comply.

The paternalist model assigns moral authority and discretion to the physician because good health is assumed to be a value shared by the patient and the physician and because the physician's competence, skills, and ability place him or her in a position to help the patient regain good health. Even if it was once the dominant model in health care and even if many patients and physicians still prefer it, the paternalist model is no longer adequate to describe or to direct all relationships in health care. Too many changes have occurred. In a pluralistic society such as ours, the assumption that the physician and patient have common values about health may be mistaken. They may disagree about the *meaning* of health and disease (for example, when the physician insists that cigarette smoking is a disease, but the patient claims that it is merely a nasty habit) or about the *value* of health relative to other values (for example, when the physician wants to administer a blood transfusion to save the life of a Jehovah's Witness, but the patient rejects the blood in order to have a chance of heavenly salvation).

As a normative model, paternalism tends to concentrate on care rather than respect, patients' needs rather than their rights, and physicians' discretion rather than patients' autonomy or self-determination. Even though paternalistic actions can sometimes be justified, for example, when a patient is not competent to make a decision and is at risk of harm, not all paternalistic actions can be justified.[3]

(2) A second model is one of *partnership*, which can be seen in Eric Cassell's

DOCTOR-PATIENT RELATIONSHIPS   19

statement: "Autonomy for the sick patient cannot exist outside of a good and properly functioning doctor-patient relation. And the relation between them is inherently a *partnership*".[4] The language of collegiality, collaboration, association, co-adventureship, and covenant is also used. This model stresses that health care professionals and their patients are partners or colleagues in the pursuit of the shared value of health. It is similar to the paternalist model in that it emphasizes the shared general values of the enterprise in which the participants are involved. But what makes this model distinctive and significant is its emphasis on the equality of the participants' interpretations of shared values such as health, along with respect for the personal autonomy of all the participants.[5] The theme of equality does not, however, cancel a division of competence and responsibility along functional lines within the relationship.

Szasz and Hollender suggest that the prototype of the model of 'mutual participation' or partnership is the adult-adult relationship. Within this model the physician helps the patient to help himself, while the patient uses expert help to realize his (and the physician's) ends. Some clinical applications of this model appear in the care of chronic diseases and psychoanalysis. It presupposes that "the participants (1) have approximately equal power, (2) be mutually interdependent (i.e., need each other), and (3) engage in activity that will be in some ways satisfying to both". Furthermore, "the physician does not know what is best for the patient. The search for this becomes the essence of the therapeutic interaction. The patient's own experiences furnish indispensable information for eventual agreement, under otherwise favorable circumstances, as to what 'health' might be for him".[6]

Although this model describes a few practices, it is most often offered as a normative model, indicating the morally desirable and even obligatory direction of practice and research.[7] As a normative model, it stresses the equality of value contributions and the autonomy of both professionals and other participants, whether sick persons or volunteers for research.

(3) A third model is that of *rational contractors*. Health care professionals and their patients are related or should be related to each other by a series of specific contracts. The prototype of this model is the specific contract by which individuals agree to exchange goods and services, and the enforcement of such contracts by governmental sanctions. According to Robert Veatch, one of the strongest proponents of the contractual model in health care, this model is the best compromise between the *ideal of partnership*, with its emphasis on both equality and autonomy, and the *reality* of medical care, where mutual trust cannot be presupposed. If we could realize mutual trust, we could develop partnerships. In the light of a realistic assessment of our situation, however, we can only hope for contracts. The model of rational contracts, according to Veatch, is the only realistic way to share responsibility, to preserve both equality

20   JAMES F. CHILDRESS AND MARK SIEGLER

and autonomy under less than ideal circumstances, and to protect the integrity
of various parties in health care (e.g., physicians are free not to enter contracts
that would violate their consciences and to withdraw from them when they give
proper notice).[8]

Such a model is valuable but problematic both descriptively and normatively.
It neglects the fact that sick persons do not view health care needs as comparable
to other wants and desires, that they do not have sufficient information to
make rational contracts with the best providers of health services, and that
current structure of medicine obstructs the free operation of the marketplace
and of contracts.[9] This model may also neglect the virtues of benevolence, care,
and compassion that are stressed in other models such as paternalism and friendship.

(4) A fourth attempt to understand and direct the relationships between
health care professionals and patients stresses *friendship*. According to P. Lain
Entraglo,

Insofar as man is a part of nature, and health an aspect of this nature and therefore a natural
and objective good, the *medical relation* develops into comradeship, or association for the
purpose of securing this good by technical means. Insofar as man is an individual and his
illness a state affecting his personality, the medical relation ought to be more than mere
comradeship – in fact it should be a friendship. All dogma apart, a good doctor has always
been a friend to his patient, to all his patients.[10]

For this version of 'medical philia', the patient expresses trust and confidence in
the physician while the doctor's "friendship for the patient should consist above
all in a desire to give effective technical help – benevolence conceived and
realised in technical terms".[11] Technical help and generalized benevolence are
'made friendly' by explicit reference to the patient's personality.

Charles Fried's version of 'medical philia' holds that physicians are *limited,
special-purpose friends* in relation to their patients. In medicine as well as in
other professional activities such as law, the client may have a relationship with
the professional that is analogous to friendship. In friendship and in these
relationships, one person assumes the interests of another. Claims in both sets of
relationships are intense and demanding, but medical friendship is more limited
in scope.[12]

Of course, this friendship analogy is somewhat strained, as Fried recognizes,
because needs (real and felt) give rise to medical relationships, even if professionals are free not to meet them unless they are emergencies, because patients
pay professionals for their 'personal care', and because patients do not have
reciprocal loyalties. Nevertheless, Fried's analysis of the medical relationship
highlights the equality, the autonomy, and the rights of both parties – the 'friend'
and the 'befriended'. Because friendship, as Kant suggested, is "the union of two
persons through equal and mutual love and respect", the model of friendship has

some ingredients of both paternalism (love or care) and anti-paternalism (equality and respect).[13] It applies especially well to the same medical relationships that fit partnership; indeed, medical friendship is very close to medical partnership, except that the former stresses the intensity of the relationship, while the latter stresses the emotional reserve as well as the limited scope of the relationship.

(5) A fifth and final model views the health care professional as a *technician*. Some commentators have referred to this model as plumber, others as engineer; for example, it has been suggested that with the rise of scientific medicine the physician was viewed as "the expert engineer of the body as a machine".[14] Within this model, the physician 'provides' or 'delivers' technical service to patients who are 'consumers'. Exchange relations provide images for this interpretation of medical relations.

This model does not appear to be possible or even desirable. It is difficult to imagine that the health care professional as technician can simply present the 'facts' unadorned by values, in part because the major terms such as health and disease are not value-free and objective. Whether the 'technician' is in an organization or in direct relation to clients, he or she serves some values. Thus, this model may collapse into the contractual model or a bureaucratic model (which will not be discussed in this essay). The professional may be thought to have only technical authority, not moral authority. But he or she remains a moral agent and thus should choose to participate or not in terms of his or her own commitments, loyalties, and integrity. One shortcoming of the paternalist and priestly models, as Robert Veatch notes, is the patient's "moral abdication", while one shortcoming of the technician model is the physician's "moral abdication".[15] The technician model offers autonomy to the patient, whose values dominate (at least in some settings) at the expense of the professional's moral agency and integrity. In other models such as contract, partnership, and friendship, moral responsibility is shared by all the parties in part because they are recognized, in some sense, as equals.

RELATIONS BETWEEN INTIMATES AND BETWEEN STRANGERS

The above models of relationships between physicians and patients move between two poles: intimates and strangers.[16] In relations of intimacy, all the parties know each other very well and often share values, or at least know which values they do not share. In such relations, formal rules and procedures, backed by sanctions, may not be necessary; they may even be detrimental to the relationships. In relations of intimacy, trust rather than control is dominant. Examples include relationships between parents and children and between friends. Partnerships

22   JAMES F. CHILDRESS AND MARK SIEGLER

also share some features of such relationships, but their intimacy and shared values may be limited to a specific set of activities.

By contrast, in relations among strangers, rules and procedures become very important, and control rather than trust is dominant.[17] Of course, in most relations there are mixtures of trust and control. Each is present to some degree. Nevertheless, it is proper to speak about relations between strangers as structured by rules and procedures because the parties do not know each other well enough to have mutual trust. Trust means confidence in and reliance upon the other to act in accord with moral principles and rules or at least in accord with his or her publicly manifested principles and rules, whatever they might be. But if the other is a stranger, we do not know whether he or she accepts what we would count as moral principles and rules. We do not know whether he or she is worthy of trust. In the absence of intimate knowledge, or of shared values, strangers resort to rules and procedures in order to establish some control. Contracts between strangers, for example, to supply certain goods, represent instances of attempted control. But contractual relations do not only depend on legal sanctions; they also presuppose confidence in a shared structure of rules and procedures. As Talcott Parsons has noted, "transactions are actually entered into in accordance with a body of binding rules which are not part of the ad hoc agreement of the parties".[18]

Whether medicine is now only a series of encounters between strangers rather than intimates, medicine is increasingly regarded by patients and doctors, and by analysts of the profession — such as philosophers, lawyers, and sociologists — as a practice that is best understood and regulated *as if it were* a practice among strangers rather than among intimates. Numerous causes can be identified: First, the pluralistic nature of our society; second, the decline of close, intimate contact over time among professionals and patients and their families; third, the decline of contact with the 'whole person', who is now parcelled out to various specialists; fourth, the growth of large, impersonal, bureaucratically structured institutions of care, in which there is discontinuity of care (the patient may not see the same professionals on subsequent visits).[19]

In this situation, Alasdair MacIntyre contends, the modern patient "usually approaches the physician as stranger to stranger: and the very proper fear and suspicion that we have of strangers extends equally properly to our encounters with physicians. We do not and cannot know what to expect of them . . . ".[20] He suggests that one possible response to this situation is to develop a rule-based bureaucracy in which "we can confront *any* individual who fills a given role with exactly the same expectation of exactly the same outcomes . . . ". Our encounters with physicians and other health care professionals are encounters between strangers precisely because of our pluralistic society: several value systems are in operation, and we do not know whether the physicians we encounter share our

DOCTOR-PATIENT RELATIONSHIPS   23

value systems. In such a situation, patient autonomy is "a solution of last resort" rather than "a central moral good". Finally patients have to decide for themselves what will be done to them or simply delegate such decisions to others, such as physicians.

Just as MacIntyre recognizes the value of patient autonomy in our pluralistic society, so John Ladd recognizes the value of the concept of rights among strangers.[21] He notes that a legalistic, rights-based approach to medicine has several important advantages because rules and rights "serve to define our relationships with strangers as well as with people whom we know . . . In the medical context . . . we may find ourselves in a hospital bed in a strange place, with strange company, and confronted by a strange physician and staff. The strangeness of the situation makes the concept of rights, both legal and moral, a very useful tool for defining our relationship to those with whom we have to deal".

Rules and rights that can be enforced obviously serve as ways to control the conduct of others when we do not know them well enough to be able to trust them. But all of the models of health care relationships identified above depend on some degree of trust. It is too simplistic to suppose that contracts, which can be legally enforced, do away with trust totally. Indeed, as we have argued, a society based on contracts depends to a very great extent on trust, precisely because not everything is enforceable at manageable cost. Thus, the issue is not simply whether trust or control is dominant, but, in part, the basis and extent of trust. Trust, at least limited trust, may be possible even among strangers. There may be a presumption of trust, unless the society is in turmoil. And there may be an intermediate notion of 'friendly strangers'. People may be strangers because of differences regarding values or uncertainty regarding the other's values; they may be friendly because they accept certain rules and procedures, which may ensure that different values are respected. If consensus exists in a pluralistic society, it is primarily about rules and procedures, some of which protect the autonomy of agents, their freedom to negotiate their own relationships.

PHYSICIAN-PATIENT INTERACTIONS AS NEGOTIATIONS

It is illuminating, both descriptively and prescriptively, to view some encounters and interactions between physicians and patients as negotiations. The metaphor of negotiation has its home in discussions to settle matters by mutual agreement of the concerned parties. While it frequently appears in disputes between management and labor and between nations, it does not necessarily presuppose a conflict of interests between the parties. The metaphor of negotiation may also illuminate processes of reaching agreement regarding the terms of continuing

24   JAMES F. CHILDRESS AND MARK SIEGLER

interaction even when the issue is mainly the determination of one party's
interests and the means to realize those interests. This metaphor captures two
important characteristics of medical relationships: (1) it accents the autonomy
of both patient and physician, and (2) it suggests a process that occurs over time
rather than an event which occurs at a particular moment.

The model of negotiation can both explain what frequently occurs and
identify what ought to occur in physician-patient interactions. An example can
make this point: A twenty-eight year old ballet dancer suffered from moderately
severe asthma. When she moved from New York to Chicago, she changed
physicians and placed herself in the hands of a famed asthma specialist. He
initiated aggressive steroid therapy to control her asthma, and within several
months he had managed to control her wheezing. But she was distressed because
her dancing had deteriorated. She suspected that she was experiencing muscle
weakness and fluid accumulation because of the steroid treatment. When she
attempted to discuss her concerns with the physician, he maintained that "bringing the disease under complete control — achieving a complete remission of
wheezes — will be the best thing for you in the long run". After several months
of unhappiness and failure to convince the physician of the importance of her
personal goals as well as her medical goals, she sought another physician, insisting
that she didn't live just to breathe, but breathed so that she could dance.[22]

As in this case — and despite the claims of several commentators — people
with medical needs generally do not confront physicians as strangers and as
adversaries in contemporary health care. As we suggested earlier, even if they can
be viewed as strangers in that they often do not know each other prior to the
encounter, both parties may well proceed with a presumption of trust. Patients
may approach physicians with some trust and confidence in the medical profession, even though they do not know the physicians before them. Indeed, codes
of medical ethics have been designed in part to foster this trust by indicating
where the medical profession stands and by creating a climate of trust. Thus,
even if patients approach individual physicians as strangers, they may have some
confidence in these physicians as members of the profession as they negotiate
the particular terms of their relationship. At the other extreme, some patients
may approach physicians as adversaries or opponents. But for negotiation to
proceed, some trust must be present, even if it is combined with some degree of
control, for example, through legal requirements and the threat of legal sanctions.

The general public trust in the medical profession's values and skills
provides the presumptive basis for trust in particular physicians and can facilitate
the process of negotiation. But, as we noted earlier, in a pluralistic society, even
people who are strangers, i.e., who share very few substantive values, may be
'friendly' if they share procedural values. Certain procedural values may provide
the most important basis for the trust that is necessary for negotiation; indeed,

procedural principles and rules should structure the negotiation in order to ensure equal respect for the autonomy of all the parties.

First, the negotiation should involve adequate disclosure by both parties. In this process of communication — much broader and richer than most doctrines of informed consent recognize — both parties should indicate their values as well as other matters of relevance. Without this information, the negotiation cannot be open and fair. Second, the negotiation should be voluntary, i.e., uncoerced. Insofar as critical illness can be viewed as 'coercing' individuals through the creation of fear, etc., it may be difficult to realize this condition for patients with certain problems. However, for the majority of patients this condition is achievable. Third, the accommodation reached through the negotiation should be mutually acceptable.[23]

What can we say about the case of the ballet dancer in the light of these procedural requirements for negotiation? It appears that the relationship foundered not because of inadequate disclosure at the outset, or along the way, but because of the patient's change in or clarification of her values and the physician's inability to accommodate these other values. The accommodation reached at the outset was mutually acceptable for a time. Initially their values and their metaphors for their relationship were the same. The physician regarded himself as a masterful scientist who was capable technically of controlling a patient's symptoms of wheezing. In fact, he remarked on several occasions: "I have never met a case of asthma I couldn't help". The patient, for her part, selected the physician initially for the same reasons. She was unhappy that her wheezing persisted, and she was becoming discouraged by her chronic health problem. Because she wanted a therapeutic success, she selected an expert who would help her achieve that goal. Both the patient and the physician made several voluntary choices. The patient chose to see *this* physician and to see him for several months, and the physician chose to treat asthma aggressively with steroids.

In a short time, the patient reconsidered or clarified her values, discovering that her dancing was even more important to her than the complete remission of wheezing, and she wanted to renegotiate her relationship so that it could be more mutual and participatory. But her new metaphor for the relationship was incompatible with the physician's nonnegotiable commitment to his metaphor — which the patient had also accepted at the outset. Thus, the relationship collapsed. This case illustrates both the possibilities and the limitations of the model of negotiation. Even when the procedural requirements are met, the negotiation may not result in a satisfactory accommodation over time, and the negotiation itself may proceed in terms of the physician's and the patient's metaphors and models of the relationships, as well as the values they affirm.

Autonomy constrains and limits the negotiations and the activities of both

26   JAMES F. CHILDRESS AND MARK SIEGLER

parties: Neither party may violate the autonomy of the other or use the other merely as a means to an end. But respecting autonomy as a constraint and a limit does not imply seeking it as a *goal* or praising it as an *ideal*.[24] This point has several implications. It means, for example, that patients may exercise their autonomy to turn their medical affairs completely over to physicians. A patient may instruct the physician to do whatever he or she deems appropriate: "You're the doctor; whatever you decide is fine". This relationship has been characterized as "paternalism with permission",[25] and it is not ruled out by autonomy as a constraint or a limit. It might, however, be ruled out by a commitment to autonomy as an ideal. Indeed, commitment to autonomy as an ideal can even be paternalistic in a negative sense; it can lead the health care professional to try to force the patient to be free and to live up to the ideal of autonomy. But our conception of autonomy as a constraint and a limit prevents such actions toward competent patients who are choosing and acting voluntarily. Likewise, maintenance, restoration, or promotion of the patient's autonomy may be, and usually is, one important goal of medical relationships. But its importance can only be determined by negotiation between the physician and the patient. The patient may even subordinate the goal of autonomy to various other goals, just as the ballet dancer subordinated freedom from wheezing to the power to dance.

This view of autonomy as a limit or a constraint, rather than an ideal or a goal, permits individuals to define the terms of their relationship. Just as it permits the patient to acquiesce in the physician's recommendations, it permits the physician to enter a contract as a mere technician to provide certain medical services, as requested by the patient. In such an arrangement, the physician does *not* become a mere means or a mere instrument to the patient's ends. Rather, the physician exercises his or her autonomy to enter into the relationship to provide technical services. Such actions are an expression of autonomy, not a denial of autonomy. If, however, the physician believes that an action requested by the patient — for example, a specific mode of therapy for cancer or a sterilization procedure — is not medically indicated, or professionally acceptable, or in the patient's best interests, he or she is not obligated to sacrifice autonomy and comply. In such a case, the professional refuses to be an instrument of or to carry out the patient's wishes. When the physician cannot morally or professionally perform an action (not legally prohibited by the society) he or she may have a duty to inform the patient of other physicians who might be willing to carry out the patient's wishes. A refusal to be an instrument of another's wishes is very different from trying to prevent another from realizing his or her goals.

Negotiation is not always possible or desirable. It is impossible, or possible only to a limited extent, in certain clinical settings in which the conditions for a fair, informed, and voluntary negotiation are severely limited, often because one party lacks some of the conditions for autonomous choices. First, negotiation may be difficult if not impossible with some types of patients, such as the mentally incompetent. Sometimes paternalism may be morally legitimate or even morally obligatory when the patient is not competent to negotiate and is at risk. In such cases, parents, family members, or others may undertake negotiation with the physician, for example, regarding defective newborns or comatose adults. But health care professionals and the state may have to intervene in order to protect the interests of the patient who cannot negotiate directly. Second, the model of negotiation does not fit situations in which patients are forced by law to accept medical interventions such as compulsory vaccination, involuntary commitment, and involuntary psychiatric treatment. In such situations, the state authorizes or requires treatment against the wishes of the patient; the patient and the physician do not negotiate their relationship. Third, in some situations physicians have dual or multiple allegiances, some of which may take priority over loyalty to the patient. Examples include military medicine, industrial medicine, prison medicine, and university health service. The physician is not free in such settings to negotiate in good faith with the patient, and the patient's interests and rights may have to be protected by other substantive and procedural standards and by external control. Fourth, negotiation may not be possible in some emergencies in which people desperately need medical treatment because of the risk of death or serious bodily harm. In such cases, the physician may *presume* consent, apart from a process of negotiation, if the patient is unable to consent because of his/her condition or if the process of disclosing information and securing consent would consume too much time and thus endanger the patient. Finally, procedural standards are important for certain types of patients, such as the poor, the uneducated, or those with 'unattractive medical problems' (e.g., drug addiction, obesity, and hypochrondriasis). In such cases, there is a tendency — surely not a universal one — to limit the degree of negotiation with the patient because of social stigmatization. A patient advocate may even be appropriate.

In addition to the procedural requirements identified earlier, there are societal constraints and limits on negotiation. Some actions may not be negotiable. For example, the society may prohibit 'mercy killing', even when the patient requests it and the physician is willing to carry it out.[26] Such societal rules clearly limit the autonomy of both physicians and patients, but some of these rules may be necessary in order to protect important societal values. However, despite such notable exceptions as 'mercy killing', current societal rules provide physicians and patients with considerable latitude to negotiate their own relationship and actions within that relationship.

If negotiation is a process, its accommodations at various points can often be

28   JAMES F. CHILDRESS AND MARK SIEGLER

characterized in terms of the above models — parent-child, friends, partners, contractors, and technician-consumer. Whatever accommodation is reached through the process of negotiation is not final or irrevocable. Like other human interactions, medical relationships change over time. They are always developing or dissolving. For example, when a patient experiencing anginal chest pain negotiates a relationship with a cardiologist, he may not have given or even implied consent to undergo coronary angiography or cardiac surgery if the cardiologist subsequently believes that it is necessary. Medical conditions change, and people change, often clarifying or modifying their values over time. In medical relationships either the physician or the patient may reopen the negotiation as the relationship evolves over time and may even terminate the relationship. For example, the ballet dancer in the case discussed above elected to terminate the relationship with the specialist. That particular relationship had not been fully negotiated in the first place. But even if it had been fully negotiated, she could have changed her mind and terminated it. Such an option is essential if the autonomy of the patient is to be protected over time. Likewise, the physician should have the option to renegotiate or to withdraw from the relationship (except in emergencies), as long as he or she gives adequate notice so that the patient can find another physician.

JAMES F. CHILDRESS   MARK SIEGLER
Department of Religious Studies   *Department of Medicine,*
University of Virginia,   *University of Chicago Hospitals,*
Charlottesville, Virginia 22903,   *950 East 59th Street,*
U.S.A.   *Chicago, IL 60637, U.S.A.*

NOTES

1   On metaphor, see George Lakoff and Mark Johnson, *Metaphors We Live By* (Chicago: University of Chicago Press, 1980).

2   See Thomas S. Szasz and Marc H. Hollender, 'A contribution to the philosophy of medicine: The basic models of the doctor-patient relationship', *Archives of Internal Medicine* 97, (1956) 585—92; see also, Thomas S. Szasz, William F. Knoff, and Marc H. Hollender, 'The doctor-patient relationship and its historical context', *American Journal of Psychiatry* 115, (1958) 522—28.

3   For a fuller analysis of paternalism and its justification, see James F. Childress, *Who Should Decide? Paternalism in Health Care* (New York: Oxford University Press, 1982).

4   Eric Cassell, 'Autonomy and ethics in action', *New England Journal of Medicine* 297, (1977) 333—34. Italics added. Partnership is only one of several images and metaphors Cassell uses, and it may not be the best one to express his position, in part because he tends to view autonomy as a goal rather than as a constraint.

5   According to Robert Veatch, the main focus of this model is "an equality of dignity and respect, an equality of value contributions". Veatch, 'Models for ethical medicine in a revolutionary age', *Hastings Center Report* 2, (June 1972) 7. Contrast Eric Cassell who

DOCTOR-PATIENT RELATIONSHIPS   29

disputes the relevance of notions of "equality" and "inequality". *The Healer's Art: A New Approach to the Doctor-Patient Relationship* (Philadelphia: J. B. Lippincott Company, 1976), pp. 193–94.

6   Thomas S. Szasz and Marc H. Hollender, 'A contribution to the philosophy of medicine: The basic models of the doctor-patient relationship', pp. 586–87. (See Note 2.)

7   See, for example, Paul Ramsey, 'The ethics of a cottage industry in an age of community and research medicine', *New England Journal of Medicine* 284, (1971) 700–706; *The Patient as Person: Explorations in Medical Ethics* (New Haven: Yale University Press, 1970), esp. Chap. 1; and Hans Jonas, 'Philosophical reflections on experimenting with human subjects', Ethical Aspects of Experimentation with Human Subjects, *Daedalus* 98, (1969) 219–47.

8   Robert Veatch, 'Models for ethical medicine in a revolutionary age', p. 7. (See Note 5.)

9   See Roger Masters, 'Is contract an adequate basis for medical ethics?', *Hastings Center Report* 5, (December 1975) 24–28. See also May, 'Code and covenant or philanthropy and contract?', in *Ethics in Medicine: Historical Perspectives and Contemporary Concerns*, ed. by Stanley Joel Reiser, Arthur J. Dyck, and William J. Curran (Cambridge, Mass.: The MIT Press, 1977), pp. 65–76.

10 P. Lain Entralgo, *Doctor and Patient*, trans. from the Spanish by Frances Partridge (New York: McGraw-Hill Book Co., World University Library, 1969), p. 242.

11 *Ibid.*, p. 197.

12 See Charles Fried, *Medical Experimentation: Personal Integrity and Social Policy* (New York: American Elsevier Publishing Co., Inc., 1974), p. 76. Our discussion of Fried's position is drawn from that work, *Right and Wrong* (Cambridge, Mass.: Harvard University Press, 1978), Chap. 7, and 'The lawyer as friend: The moral foundations of the lawyer-client relation', *The Yale Law Journal* 85, (1976) 1060–89.

13 Immanuel Kant, *The Doctrine of Virtue*, Part II of *The Metaphysic of Morals*, trans. by Mary J. Gregor (New York: Harper and Row, Harper Torchbook, 1964), p. 140.

14 Thomas S. Szasz, William F. Knoff, and Marc H. Hollender, 'The doctor-patient relationship and its historical context', p. 525. See also Robert Veatch, 'Models for ethical medicine in a revolutionary age', p. 5, and Leon Kass, 'Ethical dilemmas in the care of the ill: I. What is the physician's service?', *Journal of the American Medical Association* 244, (1980) 1815 for criticisms of the technical model (from very different normative positions).

15 Veatch, 'Models for ethical medicine in a revolutionary age', p. 7.

16 See Stephen Toulmin, 'The tyranny of principles', *Hastings Center Report* 11, (December 1981) 31–39.

17 On trust and control, see James F. Childress, 'Nonviolent resistance: Trust and risk-taking', *Journal of Religious Ethics* 1, (1973) 87–112.

18 Talcott Parsons, *The Structure of Social Action* (New York: The Free Press, 1949), p. 311.

19 On the factors in the decline of trust, see Michael Jellinek, 'Erosion of patient trust in large medical centers', *Hastings Center Report* 6, (June 1976) 16–19.

20 Alasdair MacIntyre, 'Patients as agents', in *Philosophical Medical Ethics: Its Nature and Significance*, ed. by Stuart F. Spicker and H. Tristram Engelhardt, Jr. (Boston: D. Reidel Publishing Co., 1977).

21 John Ladd, Legalism and medical ethics', *The Journal of Medicine and Philosophy* 4, (March 1979) 73.

22 This case has been presented in Mark Siegler, 'Searching for moral certainty in medicine: A proposal for a new model of the doctor-patient encounter', *Bulletin of the New York Academy of Medicine* 57, (1981) 56–69.

23 See *ibid.* for a discussion of negotiation. Other proponents of a model of negotiation include Robert A. Burt, *Taking Care of Strangers: The Rule of Law in Doctor-Patient Relations* (New York: Free Press, 1979) and Robert J. Levine, *Ethics and Regulation of Clinical Research* (Baltimore: Urban and Schwarzenberg, 1981).

30   JAMES F. CHILDRESS AND MARK SIEGLER

[24] See the discussion in Childress, *Who Should Decide?*, Chap. 3.

[25] Alan W. Cross and Larry R. Churchill, 'Ethical and cultural dimensions of informed consent', *Annals of Internal Medicine* **96**, (1982) 110–113.

[26] See Oscar Thorup, Mark Siegler, James Childress, and Ruth Roettinger, 'Voluntary exit: Is there a case of rational suicide?', *The Pharos* **45**, (Fall 1982) 25–31.

8.8   Siegler M (1985) The Progression of Medicine: From Physician Paternalism to Patient Autonomy to Bureaucratic Parsimony. Arch Intern Med 145:713–15

<u>Clinical Ethics</u>

The Progression of Medicine

From Physician Paternalism to
Patient Autonomy to Bureaucratic Parsimony

Mark Siegler, MD

The language used to describe the practice of medicine and the metaphors employed to depict the relationship of patients and physicians establish conceptual boundaries for such discussions and affect the practices themselves. My colleague, James Gustafson, PhD, made a similar point recently:

How the medical staff or the ethician describes persons and their relations to each other [ie, whether as ". . . individual contractors or persons in patterns and processes of interdependence . . ."] is a matter of critical judgment. The alternative descriptions back alternative ways of construing the moral situation. How that situation is construed confines or enlarges the morally relevant features to be taken into account in patient care [unpublished work, 1984].

In recent years, medical practice has been regarded (at least by most medical ethicists and by lawyers) primarily as an impersonal encounter between two isolated and autonomous persons—the patient and the physician—whose individual interests were to be rigorously protected from each other by rules and procedural standards. This view of

See also p 716.

medicine has generated a variety of legislative and judicial initiatives intended to protect patients from physicians. It also has determined what factors were morally relevant and, in turn, what sorts of medical actions were considered moral or immoral. This narrow, limited, and somewhat sterile conception of medicine is now changing.

It is not surprising that this view never caught on with physicians and patients; it was wrong. It failed to describe the extent or complexity of the interactions that surfaced when a previously healthy individual became ill. Thus, it failed to take account of the relationship of the ill person to family and friends as well as to the physician; it also disregarded the physician's relationship to colleagues, the health care team, the institution, and society.

In this issue of the ARCHIVES, Kathryn Hunter, PhD, a sensitive observer of the medical system, describes a case that illustrates the subtlety and difficulty of reaching good

Accepted for publication June 12, 1984.

From the Center for Clinical Medical Ethics and the Department of Medicine, University of Chicago Pritzker School of Medicine.

The views expressed are those of the author and do not necessarily reflect those of the Fund for Medical Education or the Henry J. Kaiser Family Foundation.

Reprint requests to Center for Clinical Medical Ethics, University of Chicago Pritzker School of Medicine, Box 72, 950 E 59th St, Chicago, IL 60637 (Dr Siegler).

(and therefore morally appropriate) clinical decisions.[1] The metaphors of autonomy and paternalism are not sufficient to capture the complexity of the relationship of the patient to the health team; simplistic decision procedures are also found wanting. Dr Hunter recognizes that the world of medicine is a world filled with technical and human details. Decision making is a process, not an act. Moral rightness depends not only upon procedural guarantees but upon knowing all that is relevant about the patient who is receiving care and in acting rightly based upon that knowledge.

As a procedure for reaching good decisions, Dr Hunter suggests the elegant image of a Greek chorus, as represented, for example, in the plays of Sophocles. At first glance, this seems a burdensome and inefficient suggestion. Imagine a group of white-robed individuals swaying rhythmically to the clinical fortune of a seriously ill patient: expressing happiness and pleasure when the patient appears to be improving and speaking gloomily when the patient's condition deteriorates. On further reflection, however, it appears that the suggestion may not be quite so unreasonable. In fact, it may describe our hospital care system as it currently exists. Even in the hospital setting, the principal players in the drama, the physician and patient, are cushioned or buffeted from all sides by community interests that include the patient's family and friends and the house staff, the nursing staff, medical consultants, chaplains, social workers, dieticians, and hospital administrators.

Those of us who have cared for severely ill patients realize that life-and-death decisions are not reached secretly in back rooms but are arrived at through an ongoing process of discussion, reflection, and consideration, which yields a temporary conclusion that will more than likely be modified in the face of changes in the patient's condition. Most medical decisions are neither private nor irrevocable; they tend to be public and are open always to reassessment. Health professionals and the patient's family and friends together play the part of a modern-day chorus, sometimes supporting difficult decisions and other times criticizing them for technical mistakes or narrowness of vision.

PATERNALISM AND AUTONOMY

For the past 20 years, the field of bioethics has been concerned with one issue more than any other: the proper relationship between physician paternalism and patient autonomy in medical practice. This tension between autonomy and paternalism has reverberated in discussions ranging from informed consent to appropriate care for dying patients to ethically acceptable models of the physician-patient relationship. This issue was the dominating motif in the work of two recent national bioethics commissions. The modern medical era, which began triumphantly after World War II and which is now coming to an end, might be called *the Age of Autonomy*. This emphasis on autonomy was sparked by widespread political and social movements to gain entitlements and rights, to achieve equity and equality in the distribution of health services, and to dissolve the hierarchical barriers (often believed by critics of medicine to be artificial and power-oriented barriers) between the patient and the physician.

The central question that has occupied a generation of American bioethicists has been this: *Procedurally*, where should decision-making power reside, with the physician or with the patient? A quite different question, and one that has been of much greater concern to clinicians than ethicists, is this: What is the right and good decision for this particular patient in these clinical circumstances? In the bioethics literature, however, ideas of right and good decisions often have been subordinated to *procedural standards*—the allocation of power—by which such decisions are reached. In this latter view, a "good and right" decision is one that pays sufficient heed to the wishes and presumed values of the patient—that is, one that "respects the person"—even if the patient's health problems may be so severe as to limit his or her capacity to make crucial, and at times life-and-death, decisions. "Good and right" decisions, in this view, are less concerned with outcome, or with the patient's "best medical interests," than they are with the process of respecting the patient's right to control what is done to his or her body.

By contrast, traditional paternalism in medicine assigned considerable moral authority and discretion to physicians because good health was assumed to be a value shared by the patient and the physician and because physicians' competence, skills, and ability placed them in a position to help patients regain good health. This model emphasized patient care rather than patient wishes, patient needs rather than their "rights," and physician discretion rather than patient autonomy or self-determination. The central issue in a pluralistic society such as ours, and the issue that has engaged bioethicists for the past 20 years, is this: Under what circumstances can one justify paternalistic actions, which at times might ignore patients' wishes in order to save their lives? A brief review of the history of the physician-patient relationship may illuminate the question.

THREE AGES OF MEDICINE:
A PROGRESSION IF NOT "PROGRESS"

The history of the physician-patient relationship in Western medicine can be divided into three periods: *the Age of Paternalism, the Age of Autonomy,* and *the Age of Bureaucracy*.

The Age of Paternalism lasted thousands of years and represented the basic authoritarian and sacerdotal strain in medicine. The bond between patient and physician was dyadic and few outsiders could penetrate into this personal, magical realm of healing. This model of medicine—the "doctor knows best" model—was premised on trust in the physician's technical skills and moral stature, was buttressed by an attribution of magical powers to the healer, and was characterized by patient dependency and physician control.

Medical achievements during this lengthy period were rather modest. In fact, this medical system was relatively cheap and relatively ineffective. It provided symptomatic care rather than cure; it emphasized the power of information (the prognosis), which was a mystery known only to the trained physician and imparted in measured doses to the patient; it was able to deal better with psychological than with physical aspects of disease; and it taught principles of hygiene and preventive health care. In this system, the physician was the source of information, psychological support, and symptomatic relief. In light of our modern ideas of pathophysiologic medicine and of immensely effective medical and surgical therapies, we are often struck by how long this older and much less effective medical system held sway over the minds and bodies of men and women. We are thus forced to realize that for all its limitations, this traditional and relatively ineffective system of healing must have addressed and satisfied many basic human needs for the multitude of patients it served.

The Age of Autonomy, by contrast, lasted at most 40 years (1945 to the present) and, more likely, just 20 years (1965 to the present). Technically, it was an age of extraordinary advances in the understanding of physiologic and biochemical mechanisms of disease, and in the development of remarkable and often very expensive medical and surgical therapies for disease. It was a medical epoch that focused on disease. It emphasized treatment rather than prevention, cure rather than care. Cost was not seen as a relevant factor and certainly not one to be taken account of when juxtaposed against patient autonomy, patient need, or even patient desire.

During this period, the dyadic relationship between physician and patient was maintained, but the theoretical balance of power was shifting subtly from physician to patient. The informed consent legal doctrine, and the potential threat of malpractice suits for battery or negligence against physicians who failed to respect the doctrine, reflected deeper concerns. Many ethicists, legal scholars, and consumer advocates wished to assign patients control over (but not always responsibility for) decisions about their own care. This model emphasized patient education and patient rights. According to this view, practitioners should act as servants to their patients, to transmit medical information and to use clinical skills as the patient directs, without seeking to influence patients' decisions, much less actually making them.

The rhetoric of this period was libertarian and consumerist and the medical air (at least, the air in ivory towers where medical ethicists held court) was filled with cries of "autonomy . . . self-determination . . . patient sovereignty . . . freedom . . . liberty . . ." and the like. The antipaternalist movement reached a peak of sorts when it joined forces with thanatologists to defend the notion of the autonomy of the dying patient and even of those dying patients who were mentally incompetent. The idea here was that even for dying patients who lacked competence, autonomy rather than the medical interests of the patient was the principal ethical ideal to be preserved. This viewpoint led to some strange ideas that are represented, for example, in the report of the President's commission on decisions regarding life-sustaining treatment. Thus, according to the commission, cardiopulmonary resuscitation should be performed on patients who demand it—presumably to acknowledge their autonomy—even if physicians believe, and have so informed the patient, that such an exercise would be futile.[2]

The Age of Bureaucracy has arrived and it is also an Age of Parsimony. This new era will demand cost containment and cost-efficiency and will be based on bureaucratic risk-benefit analyses. Quality of care, always so hard to define, will no longer be an end in itself, but will be balanced against cost of care, which is much easier to quantify. Tradeoffs will be made. Inexpensive, even if unproved, strategies of care will be promoted by a variety of interest groups. In this new period, dyadic physician-patient relationships will become the exception. The physician will be accountable to multiple interests including employers (health maintenance organizations [HMOs], hospital corporations), hospitals, insurance companies, and government. The physician in the Age of Bureaucracy will have divided allegiances.

In the previous two eras, the patient's "good" was the dominant concern for physicians. In the Age of Paternalism, it was the patient's "best medical interest." In the Age of Autonomy, it was the patient's freedom and right of self-determination. In the new era, however, the patient's good will be balanced against other goods such as the needs of the hospital, the needs of its employees (including physicians), and the needs of society. Decision making no longer will be vested exclusively in the hands of physicians or patients. Physician paternalism and patient autonomy, particularly with respect to medical decisions, will be replaced by institutional and societal efficiency and expediency, based largely on cost concerns. These have emerged as the major elements in decision making. In contrast to the two earlier periods, the wishes of both patients and physicians are already—or will soon be—subservient to the wishes of government bureaucrats, administrators of HMOs, insurance company executives, or corporate vice-presidents of proprietary multihospital chains.

A new medical age is dawning—or has dawned already—but it is not clear that the postmodern age of bureaucratic parsimony will be better than either the old-fashioned age of professional paternalism or the more recent and short-lived age of patient autonomy. The patient and physician fought a battle, which the patient appeared to have won (eg, through the informed consent doctrine), but it was a Pyrrhic victory; in retrospect, it is clear that by becoming antagonists, they both lost. The main hope remaining is that patients and physicians resolve their conflict and that different health professional disciplines resolve theirs and join together again as natural allies—to fight not only the patient's illness but also the society's illness. Together, the physician and patients are a powerful team, who can in one circumstance combat the patient's disease and in another, combat the direction in which health care is headed, toward centralized, bureaucratic control and a resulting loss of autonomy for both physician and patient. This battle must be fought in the political arena, but patients and physicians make up a formidable lobby and one whose concerns would be given a respectful hearing by their political representatives.

INSTITUTIONAL ETHICS COMMITTEE OR GREEK CHORUS

Dr Hunter's suggestion that "management rounds" be organized on each unit rather than for the entire hospital in order to permit "community participation in difficult decisions" is one way to begin the rapprochement of patient and physician. "Management rounds" would represent a kind of Greek chorus, a community of viewpoints that would, in Gustafson's words, ". . . describe persons in patterns and processes of interdependence" (unpublished work, 1984). This metaphor of the Greek chorus is strikingly different from the individualistic language of autonomy and is a more accurate reflection of the multiple interests that enter into difficult medical and ethical decisions. This suggestion also has the advantage of both opening the decision process to involved individuals—professional and lay—and keeping the forum for decisions as close as possible to the actual patient and the immediate nursing unit.

Management rounds, like the Greek chorus, can provide counsel, guidance, and criticism to the protagonist decision maker. But decisions must not be made by a group, just as tragic choices in Greek drama were not made by the chorus. Individuals, not committees, ultimately must choose and must take responsibility for their decisions.

It has recently been suggested by the President's commission and others that hospital ethics committees might help to clarify ethical deliberations and might also improve clinicians' decision making. The precise function of such committees is not entirely clear, but in addition to serving as educational and deliberative bodies, such committees might reach decisions or at least be able to ". . . see that clearly wrong decisions are not permitted."[3] This last suggestion is disquieting. Cassel[4] recently commented on the issue of decision making by committee:

The coming together of many different perspectives and areas of expertise may provide the "crucible" in which the best (i.e., most humane and most just) decisions are made. But a committee can also provide the setting in which immoral decisions can be made for which no one has ultimate responsibility. This is most likely to occur in a setting where most persons on the committee are relatively removed from the clinical setting, where conflict of interest with administrative needs exists, and where the group dynamic is bureaucratized. Such a committee is no longer a crucible for the tempering of apparently conflicting values, but rather a bureau whose primary value is not the anguish of moral dilemma but the efficiency of decision-making, abiding by rules and adhering to regulations and legal proscriptions.

Currently, hospitals are struggling to develop administrative mechanisms to deal with clinical-ethical concerns, and good ideas deserve a try. The American Hospital Association's recent report, *Guidelines: Hospital Committees on Biomedical Ethics*,[5] encourages considerable flexibility for such committees: "Each institution should take the steps necessary to implement suitable mechanisms that will reasonably provide for sound decision-making practices and for responsible and timely assessment of medical and ethical issues." Perhaps the time is ripe to experiment both with institutional ethics committees and with Dr Hunter's suggestions for Greek choruses (ie, ward management rounds).

Dr Hunter's proposal has considerable appeal. Her suggestion that participation in management rounds be restricted to those individuals involved in a particular case still opens the discussion to many viewpoints—clinical and lay—while limiting the contributions of mere observers and uninvolved moral experts. Furthermore, her idea of many small, local deliberative bodies seems preferable to the notion of single, large, bureaucratic, institution-wide ethics committees. Finally, a Greek chorus that captures the spirit of "persons in patterns and processes of interdependence" may be a sound model to investigate for allocating limited or controversial human and capital resources at the local level.

This study was supported by grant 26/82A from the Fund for Medical Education and by a development grant from the Henry J. Kaiser Family Foundation.

References

1. Hunter KM: Limiting treatment in a social vacuum: A Greek chorus for William T. *Arch Intern Med* 1985;145:716-719.
2. *Deciding to Forego Life-Sustaining Treatment*. President's Commission for the Study of Ethical Problems in Medicine and Biomedical and Behavioral Research, 1983, p 244, Table 2.
3. Fleischman AR, Murray TH: Ethics committees for infants Doe? *Hastings Cent Rep* 1983;13:5-9.
4. Cassel CK: Deciding to forego life-sustaining treatment: Implications for policy in 1984. *Cardozo Law Review*, in press.
5. *Guidelines: Hospital Committees on Biomedical Ethics*. Chicago, American Hospital Association, 1984.

8.9 Daugherty CK, Siegler M, Ratain MJ, Zimmer G (1997) Learning from Our Patients: One participant's Impact on Clinical Trial Research and Informed Consent. Ann Intern Med 126:892–7

PERSPECTIVE

Learning from Our Patients: One Participant's Impact on Clinical Trial Research and Informed Consent

Christopher K. Daugherty, MD; Mark Siegler, MD; Mark J. Ratain, MD; and George Zimmer, PhD

This Perspective includes an essay on modifying phase I clinical trials, written by George Zimmer, who was a professor of English and a commentary on that essay. Professor Zimmer was a cancer patient who participated in the phase I clinical trial program at the University of Chicago. His ideas are eloquently expressed and have had a profound effect on our investigational research for anticancer agents. Although at times his suggestions may seem radical, Professor Zimmer urges us to reconsider the 50-year-old Nuremberg paradigm that participants in human research are ignorant and vulnerable and must be protected. Although we must protect patients who have life-threatening diseases from coercive inducements and misplaced hopes, we must also listen carefully and thoughtfully to our patients. This is particularly true when, as research participants in the face of sacrifice and the threat of a life-ending diagnosis, they have made the effort to express their concerns. With the effect of the acquired immunodeficiency syndrome movement on clinical studies and on drug research and development, a precedent has been set that allows patients to reshape their role as participants in research trials. On a personal level, the essay by Professor Zimmer has had a significant effect on our research methods and, indeed, the focus of our research efforts. Thus, it is with a sense of respect and honor that we share George Zimmer's thoughts and our comments about the influence he has had on our research practices.

Ann Intern Med. 1997;125:892-897.

From the University of Chicago, Chicago, Illinois. For current author addresses, see end of text.

T*he following essay was written by George Zimmer, a professor of English. Professor Zimmer was a cancer patient and a participant in several phase I cancer trials. He died of cancer approximately 6 months after writing the essay.*

An Idea for Modifying Phase I Clinical Trials: A Patient's View

Human participants in a protocol differ in two ways from the rats and dogs that preceded them. First, because human participants are not distinguished by breed, they do not have identical or blanket reactions to an experiment; in contrast, animals that are bred or selected for laboratory research react the same. Second, human patients have differing mental and personality characteristics. In experimental trials, doses can be adjusted in advance to accommodate the size and other physical aspects of human participants, but the trials cannot compensate for the thoughts and emotions of individual participants. These important facets of the whole person are largely ignored when trial programs are designed.

An experiment that uses brown, gray, and other rats in addition to carefully bred white rats and that adds wolfhounds and Chihuahuas to the laboratory population would approximate the varied human population that serves as protocol participants. Because different breeds would probably have different reactions, a single success would not be applicable to the general rat or dog population. Considering that, in human trials, some participants may be inclined to act at cross-purposes to the experiment, it is a wonder that any success can be validated for use.

Although physical differentiation may be impossible to overcome in most human protocols, the nonphysical differences may present a source of great utility. Because human temperament ranges quite randomly through all body types, successful results with protocol participants who share the same temperament could apply to all body sizes and shapes. The solution, it would seem, therefore rests in the recognition and use of personality traits.

Most patients do not ask to participate in protocols but rather are content to either let the disease follow its natural course or adhere to the advice of their health care providers (who in turn may be somewhat fatalistic). Patients who do seek to participate in protocols are those who question the status quo and who are most eager to alter it. These useful traits often make them the despair of those who care for them because they question the program in detail: They want to redesign the protocol to fit self-perceived needs. To a minor extent, they often do succeed in having the protocol adjusted, thereby rendering trial results still more suspect.

What would happen if a control group of more or less uncontrolled participants were permitted to change a protocol in radical ways? For example, what if participants were allowed to combine substances as long as the combination was not known to cause death? Or, what if participants were allowed to increase drug doses as long as the amount was not known to cause permanent crippling? A hundred such patients might improve the chances of finding a cure a hundredfold when the new combinations of chemicals or altered drug doses are tested. One breakthrough by a single participant could be followed by other participants who are only too eager to achieve a like cure. Gradually, the successful dose schedule could be adjusted to lessen dreaded side effects.

That some of these 100 participants would die of the effects of their medication would be unavoidable—but better that a few fall in the storming of the bastion than no storming be attempted. Without direct assault, cancer becomes a battle of attrition, with the tumors digging in ever more securely. I have come to know from experience that tumors do learn how to resist agents over time. Tumors must be kept off-balance and under constant attack by a variety of weapons. To use weapons singly or desultorily is a design for toughening tumors. They must be punished constantly, even if the price is constant pain and discomfort for the patient. Letting a patient choose the poisons (under professional guidance) adds something to the will to struggle. We who are struggling to escape cancer do not, obviously, want to die of it. We do prefer death in the struggle to life under cancer's untender rule. The enemy is not pain or even death, which will come for us in any eventuality. The enemy is cancer, and we want it defeated and destroyed.

Just before assaults on fortified positions, U.S. Civil War soldiers would pin their names and addresses to their uniforms to make it easier for the body-sorters to do their work after the battle. Patients going into these modified protocols could likewise place their names on specific protocol adjustments. Survivors could then proclaim: This is how I wanted to die—not a suicide and not passively accepting, but eagerly in the struggle.

Commentary

The Man behind the Words

Drs. Christopher K. Daugherty, Mark Siegler, and Mark J. Ratain: Professor Zimmer, a patient who had a refractory malignancy, participated in several phase I cancer clinical trials at the University of Chicago. With the consent of his widow, his essay is published in this issue of *Annals*. Professor Zimmer's perspective has helped us to better understand the motivation and vulnerability of persons who have life-threatening incurable diseases and

who choose to become involved in investigational therapies. Further, his views have encouraged us to reevaluate our attitudes toward phase I cancer trials and to initiate an ongoing research project that was designed to examine the motivations and behavior of the participants and physicians involved in clinical trials.

Although Professor Zimmer describes personal experiences encountered during his battle against cancer, his views on how some patients respond to incurable illnesses certainly apply to many other terminal diseases. Zimmer raises serious questions about basic aspects of clinical trials, including informed consent and risk-to-benefit calculations, and challenges what he considers the paternalistic attitude of clinical investigators, institutional review boards, and regulatory agencies. At one point in his essay, Professor Zimmer makes a radical suggestion: Patients who participate in phase I cancer trials should be permitted to alter a research protocol in hopes of benefiting from additional therapeutic options as well as to advance scientific knowledge in the field of cancer care. Zimmer urges us to reconsider the 50-year-old Nuremberg paradigm of clinical research. This paradigm suggests that human research participants are ignorant and vulnerable and must be protected by regulatory mechanisms from unscrupulous clinical investigators who are more concerned about advancing science and their careers than they are about providing benefits to individual patients (1).

One way to deal with Zimmer's challenges is simply to respond that because no patient can really understand the complexities of clinical trial research design and methodology, these matters are best left to experts. But this discounts the fact that some patients, such as Professor Zimmer, have a high degree of knowledge, motivation, intelligence, and comprehension. For these patients, a paternalistic response may be facile. Another response could acknowledge that although some patients may understand the foundation of clinical trials, participants should not have a role in designing or modifying research protocols. From a scientific standpoint, Zimmer's notion of allowing a "control group of more or less uncontrolled patients ... to change a protocol in radical ways" seems preposterous. His suggestions, if adopted, could generate research anarchy with little, if any, meaningful information emerging from clinical trials. In addition, if patients with cancer and other persons with incurable diseases are regarded as vulnerable individuals who are susceptible to inducements and misplaced hopes, there would be a great risk for harm to patients who volunteer to participate in loosely regulated trials that might not yield any meaningful scientific information.

Research Participants as Patient Advocates: The Lessons of AIDS

During the 1960s, 1970s, and much of the 1980s, the foremost concerns of the U.S. Food and Drug Administration (FDA) and the general public regarding clinical research and drug development were to minimize risk and protect potentially vulnerable patients from ambitious clinical investigators and from a profit-motivated pharmaceutical industry (1, 2). A social trade-off that permitted slower progress in the conquest of disease (3) was accepted to provide a safer, more closely monitored environment that protected research participants from harm. Thus, for the past three decades, the FDA and institutional review boards have been permitted to decide whether a clinical trial is scientifically worth conducting and whether the risk-to-benefit ratio is one that participants should be permitted to consider. Traditionally, patients and participants did not become involved in decisions about whether clinical research should be conducted. It is interesting to note that this paternalistic system developed and became established in clinical trials as the rest of society and other health care institutions increasingly recognized the importance of autonomy and the right of patients to decide what is in their own best interests (4).

Today, however, the medical community cannot ignore the claims of dying patients on the grounds that they are ill-informed, naive, vulnerable, or misled. With the development of the acquired immunodeficiency syndrome (AIDS) epidemic, activists have demanded modifications in the research and regulatory process, thereby challenging the Nuremberg paradigm. Such demands have resulted in major changes in clinical research, drug development, and the clinical trial process, at least with respect to drugs for the treatment of AIDS (5, 6). According to the literature, advocates emerged with fury (5) and demanded to be able to make their own risk assessments regarding investigational drugs. One mission of such organizations as ACT-UP (AIDS Coalition to Unleash Power) was to fight for the right of patients with AIDS to have access to experimental therapies. Activists claimed that persons who have life-threatening illnesses do not need protection from the potential harms of research trials. They argued that the role of the federal government and of such regulatory bodies as the FDA should be to maximize patient opportunity and choice to participate in clinical research rather than to maximize patient safety. Reforms in the research process were achieved because many patients with AIDS had a high level of motivation and knowledge; a strong political community was willing to fight policy and public relations battles; social attitudes shifted away

from paternalism, especially with regard to life-threatening or terminal illness; and pharmaceutical companies were eager to develop, market, and profit from new and effective drugs for an incurable condition for which effective therapy was not available (6, 7).

During the past decade, the FDA has responded to the pressures and criticisms of AIDS activists and patients with AIDS (5–7). Beginning in 1987, the agency developed a new set of regulations that heightened respect for patient autonomy by allowing patients and their physicians to assess the risks of experimental therapies. To be made available for further studies, drugs and therapies only had to show some evidence of substantial benefit, even if safety measures remained unknown after relatively small phase II trials that involved only a few hundred patients. The FDA has increasingly recognized the importance of surrogate markers of survival in AIDS and has created a less adversarial relationship between drug developers and representatives of regulatory agencies. The U.S. Congress subsequently enacted legislation that obliges the government to become involved in testing drugs that had previously been available only through an underground system and whose safety had not met U.S. standards (5). Other notable changes have included parallel drug research (that is, fast tracking of drugs), whereby patients could take a drug even without availability of phase II data if the agent had been proven safe and continued to be tested clinically (8). Thus, because of pressures from AIDS activists, the FDA and other branches of the U.S. government have become willing to reassess the balance between efficacy and safety. This reassessment has led to modifying the Nuremberg paradigm into the AIDS paradigm: The potential efficacy of clinical research is more important than the potential risk. The specific outcomes from changes in the policies of the FDA have included rapid approval of didanosine and, more recently, rapid approval and release of several new protease and reverse transcriptase inhibitors (9–12).

Before the emergence of AIDS and its effect on clinical trials and drug development, clinical research was perceived as a process of human experimentation that sometimes involved cruel, even inhumane, treatment (13). Today, clinical trials and access to the drug development process are viewed as valuable societal goods and rights that should be guaranteed. Previous regulatory policies that were designed to protect research participants from harm are now viewed by many as having created unnecessary paternalistic barriers to potentially lifesaving therapies. Clinical investigators and others who are involved in the process of developing drugs that are effective against AIDS have clearly learned the importance of obtaining support from the patient community, even to the extent of welcoming the involvement of patients in the design and planning of clinical trials (6, 7, 13).

Fast Tracking and Advocacy in Cancer

All patients with life-threatening diseases have certainly learned from the experience of AIDS activists and patients with AIDS. Most notably, many survivors of cancer and family members of patients who did not survive have developed strong activist and lobbying groups for their causes (7, 14, 15). Such organizations as the Breast Cancer Coalition have become involved in efforts to influence public policy and government funding that specifically targets breast cancer research and therapy (16). In addition, the regulatory changes that resulted from the AIDS movement have been extended and now apply to the approval process for anticancer drugs. The FDA has made a commitment to the same fast-track approach for anticancer drugs as has been used for the development of drugs effective against AIDS (17). The FDA has also indicated a willingness to use surrogate markers (for example, partial responses) rather than survival rates as a measure of drug effectiveness when considering the approval of anticancer agents. These policy changes have markedly reduced drug-approval processing times. Many of these drugs are now being approved in less than 6 months from the time a new drug application is submitted; in contrast, previous approval times often exceeded 1 year. An excellent example of the effect of changing regulatory policy is the recent approval by the FDA of irinotecan as second-line treatment for advanced colorectal carcinoma without data from phase III randomized clinical trials (18, 19).

Policy changes have come as a result of intense societal pressure from highly motivated groups, many of which have strong political support. In light of these recent changes, Professor Zimmer's essay is especially poignant. On one level, Zimmer eloquently raises the question of whether some individual patients who have a fatal disease could push investigators to move faster than they otherwise might prefer in conducting phase I clinical trials of potentially beneficial new drugs. On a more general level, Zimmer is asking fundamental questions about the relation between individual patients like himself—those who have incurable diseases, such as cancer or AIDS, and who are willing to become participants in clinical research—and the social and political aspects of clinical research trials.

Clinical Research: An Eloquent Request To Rethink the Traditional Approach

Clinical investigators in cancer research are aware that such differences as age, sex, race, genet-ics, previous chemotherapy regimens, disease, performance status, concomitant disease, and individual patient variations in drug metabolism create a heterogeneous population of patients. These differences can complicate attempts at identifying a maximum tolerated dose (the goal of a phase I trial) that can be applied to a broader population of patients with cancer (20, 21). Professor Zimmer realizes that the problems associated with physical heterogeneity may be insurmountable. He argues, however, that researchers could compensate for the problems by recognizing and constructively incorporating certain personal and psychological characteristics and goals of patients, including how aggressively they wish to pursue potential therapies, into phase I research trials. Zimmer's suggestion may be radical, but it highlights the importance of a patient's motivation to participate in a phase I clinical trial despite minimal chances for benefit.

Recognizing the effect of these personality traits, Zimmer points out that some patients, because of their assertiveness and awareness, "... seek to participate in protocols ... question the status quo and are most eager to alter it." Professor Zimmer argues that when such patients participate in a conventional phase I trial, investigators should consider the advantages of evaluating the suggestions of these patients on implementing modifications in the phase I study design. Zimmer describes a "control group of more or less uncontrolled patients" who are allowed "... to change a protocol in radical ways"—a suggestion that, if adopted as policy, could have alarming repercussions for clinical investigators and regulatory groups. On a more reasonable note, Zimmer encourages medical professionals to change the focus from minimizing potential risk to maximizing potential benefit if a patient has a terminal disease and is involved in a phase I trial. Zimmer's words clearly echo those of AIDS activists. Equally challenging is his suggestion that the design of such an unusual trial might be feasible and ethically acceptable if it were conducted with patients who had special characteristics, including the proper motivation, ability to understand the substantial risks involved in a radical trial, and willingness to accept such risks.

Zimmer suggests that society has persons who are adverse to risk and others who are risk takers. Perhaps the crux of his essay is to ask whether risk-taking behaviors in the scientific battle against cancer should be denied to individual patients who have incurable cancer and therefore have little to lose. Zimmer wonders why we deny the request of dying patients that they be permitted to approach death with a heroic struggle.

What if investigators could find a way to incorporate Zimmer's challenging ideas into rigorous clinical research? Such a merger might be accomplished by first studying the complex ethical and personal issues that affect the motivations of patients and their decision to participate in investigational phase I trials. A more informed and meaningful dialogue between investigators and patients who have terminal illnesses would recognize patients' vulnerability but also their autonomous decision-making ability. Innovative ways to design clinical trials, including phase I trials that consider patient motivation, understanding, and risk-taking behavior, could emerge from such a dialogue.

The process of drug development currently begins with a phase I study. Overall, the chances of response in patients in phase I cancer trials have been low (22, 23). Response rates of only 4% to 6% have been shown, and complete responses are extremely rare. Of significance, and perhaps contrary to what many persons believe, the overall chance of fatal reactions to drugs in these trials is also extremely low, approximately 0.5% to 1%. Also of importance is that most responses in these studies have occurred at 80% to 120% of the subsequently recommended dose for phase II trials, which is at or near the maximum tolerated dose. If patients were participating in phase I trials solely for altruistic reasons, that is, to advance cancer research and to help future patients, phase I trials would probably carry less ethical conflict. Professor Zimmer's essay reminds us that the ethical dilemmas presented by phase I trials and other clinical research are numerous and complex and extend beyond issues related simply to altruism and human experimentation.

Zimmer's Impact on Research Methodology

Thus, challenged and encouraged by Professor Zimmer's ideas, we have initiated a research program that has been designed to explore the motivation, understanding, and rights of patients who choose to participate in phase I cancer trials. The research began with a pilot study of patients with cancer who had given informed consent to participate in phase I trials at our institution (24). Objectives of the study were to identify and quantify factors in the ethical decision-making process of patients who had refractory malignant conditions and chose to participate in phase I trials. Oncologists who consented patients for the trials were also surveyed. Our findings led to the conclusion that patients are motivated to participate in phase I trials almost exclusively by the hope of therapeutic benefit. Although no patient in the pilot study mentioned altruism as a major motivating factor, we found evidence that some patients may have altruistic feelings toward other patients with cancer. Other conclusions from this study were that patients perceive themselves as adequately informed about the investigational nature of phase I trials. Despite this perception is the particulary concerning fact that most patients in our pilot study apparently did not know that the purpose of phase I trials is to study dose schedules, toxicity levels, or both. From information gathered on the survey that had been administered to oncologists, we concluded that many of them used phase I agents with therapeutic intent and that they believed patients derived psychological benefit by participating in clinical trials.

We have expanded our initial examination of patients and physicians involved in phase I studies by attempting to validate the findings from our pilot study (25). In addition, we have conducted a feasibility study that attempts to incorporate the personal decision-making process of patients involved in phase I trials and that allows patients to determine the amount of risk they are willing to accept in a clinical trial by giving them the option of selecting (within defined limits) their own doses of investigational agents (26). The goals of this study were to increase patient understanding and autonomy through direct participation in research decisions and to increase patient satisfaction with clinical research.

The focus of our examination of research ethics and informed consent in early clinical trials of cancer would seem extremely relevant and timely in light of the recently published report from the President's Advisory Committee on Human Radiation Experiments (27). The Committee's report, although commissioned to study previous abuses in research, includes a study of patients who were participating in clinical research. The findings echo our published results (24), as do the concluding recommendations, which call for further empirical study of the current process of informed consent by participants in human research.

Conclusion

Deficiencies in the current process of clinical trials are apparent. In cancer research, such problems include accrual, the ability of patients and physicians to make autonomous decisions, and arguments from patients and advocacy groups in favor of adequate reimbursement (27, 28). By conducting empirical research on the clinical trial process, we may begin to address some of these problems. We believe that our studies can affect not only the care of patients with cancer but also the care of patients who have other life-threatening illnesses. Our hope is that this research effort may lead to increased freedom of choice for patients with cancer who are participating in phase I trials and that this might result in greater patient satisfaction, improved patient outcome, and an increased number of patients who choose to participate in cancer clinical trials. Finally, we hope that this research initiative can shed some light on issues relating to informed consent in clinical research and human experimentation in general and on the decision-making processes of potentially vulnerable patients. Even if our research demonstrates that clinical outcomes do not change and that patients do not benefit from increased freedom of choice in research trials, we must remember that there are some patients like Professor Zimmer for whom the most important benefit may be having their personal views respected and perhaps put to use. We are also confident that clinical investigators can develop a better understanding of what motivates patients who willingly choose to participate in clinical research.

Acknowledgment: The authors thank the widow of Professor Zimmer, Mrs. Barbara Zimmer, for granting permission to publish his essay.

Grant Support: By grant PRTA-24 from the American Cancer Society; the MacLean Center for Clinical Medical Ethics; the Pew Charitable Trust; the Henry J. Kaiser Family Foundation; the Andrew W. Mellon Foundation; and public health service contract NO1-CMO7301 from the National Cancer Institute, National Institutes of Health, and U.S. Department of Health and Human Services.

Requests for Reprints: Christopher Daugherty, MD, Section of Hematology/Oncology, The MacLean Center for Clinical Medical Ethics, MC-2115, University of Chicago, 5841 South Maryland Avenue, Chicago, IL 60637-1470.

Current Author Addresses: Dr. Daugherty: Section of Hematology/Oncology, The MacLean Center for Clinical Medical Ethics, MC-2115, University of Chicago, 5841 South Maryland Avenue, Chicago, IL 60637.
Dr. Siegler: The MacLean Center for Clinical Medical Ethics, University of Chicago, 5841 South Maryland Avenue, Chicago, IL 60637.
Dr. Ratain: Section of Hematology and Oncology, the Committee on Clinical Pharmacology, Cancer Research Center, University of Chicago, 5841 South Maryland Avenue, Chicago, IL 60637.

References

1. **National Commission for the Protection of Human Subjects of Biomedical and Behavioral Research.** The Belmont Report: Ethical Principles and Guidelines for the Protection of Human Subjects of Research. 3 volumes. Washington, DC: USGPO; 1978. DHEW publication no. (OS) 78-0012/G.
2. **Levine RJ.** Ethics and Regulation of Clinical Research. 2d ed. Baltimore: Urban and Schwarzenburg; 1986.
3. **Jonas H.** Philosophical reflections on experimenting with human subjects. In: Freund PA, ed. Experimentation with Human Subjects. New York: Braziller; 1970.
4. **Faden RR, Beauchamp TL, King NM.** A History and Theory of Informed Consent. New York: Oxford Univ Pr; 1986.
5. **Arno PS, Feiden K.** Against the Odds: The Story of AIDS Drug Development, Politics, and Profits. New York: HarperCollins; 1992.
6. **Edgar H, Rothman DJ.** New rules for new drugs: the challenge of AIDS to the regulatory process. Milbank Q. 1990;68:111-42.
7. **Wachter RM.** AIDS, activism, and the politics of health. N Engl J Med. 1992;326:128-33.
8. Code of Federal Regulations. Title 21; Part 314, Subpart H; December 11, 1992.
9. **Cotton P.** FDA "pushing envelope" on AIDS drug. JAMA. 1991;266:757-8.
10. **Steele F.** AIDS drugs lurch towards market. Nat Med. 1995;1:285-6.
11. **Carter SK.** Clinical research and drug development of antivirals in HIV: an industry perspective. J Acquir Immune Defic Syndr Hum Retrovirol. 1995; 10(Suppl 2):S107-13.
12. **Carpenter CC, Fischl MA, Hammer SM, Hirsch MS, Jacobsen DM, Katzenstein DA, et al.** Antiretroviral therapy for HIV infection in 1996. Recommendations of an international panel. International AIDS Society—USA. JAMA. 1996;276:146-54.
13. **Levine RJ.** The impact of HIV infection on society's perception of clinical trials. Kennedy Institute of Ethics Journal 1994;4:93-8.
14. **McIntosh H.** AIDS lobby earns respect from cancer leaders. J Natl Cancer Inst. 1990;82:730-2.
15. **Flintor L.** Patient activism: cancer groups become vocal and politically active. J Natl Cancer Inst. 1991;83:528-9.
16. **Langer AS.** The politics of breast cancer. J Am Med Wom Assoc. 1992;47: 207-9.
17. **Stout H, McGinley L.** Cancer drugs to get speedier FDA review. The Wall Street Journal. 29 March 1996;81.
18. **Rothenberg ML, Eckardt JR, Kahn JG, et al.** Phase II trial of irinotecan in patients with progressive or rapidly recurrent colorectal cancer. J Clin Oncol. 1996;14:1128-35.
19. Transcripts from Oncology Drug Advisory Commission meeting. June 13, 1996.
20. **DeVita VT.** Principles of chemotherapy. In: DeVita VT, Hellman S, Rosenberg SA, eds. Principles and Practice of Oncology. 4th ed. 2 volumes. Philadelphia: Lippincott; 1993:276-92.
21. **Ratain MJ, Mick R, Schilsky R, Siegler M.** Statistical and ethical issues in the design and conduct of phase I and II clinical trials of new anticancer agents. J Natl Cancer Inst. 1993;85:1637-43.
22. **Decoster G, Stein G, Holdener EE.** Responses and toxic deaths in phase I clinical trials. Ann Oncol. 1990;1:175-81.
23. **Von Hoff DD, Turner J.** Response rates, duration of response, and dose response effects in phase I studies of antineoplastics. Invest New Drugs. 1991;9: 115-22.
24. **Daugherty C, Ratain MJ, Grochowski E, Stocking C, Kodish E, Mick R, et al.** Perceptions of cancer patients and their physicians involved in phase I trials. J Clin Oncol. 1995;13:1062-72.
25. **Daugherty C, Lyman K, Mick R, Siegler M, Ratain MJ.** Differences in perceptions and goals, expectations, and level of informed consent in phase I clinical trials [Abstract]. Proc Am Soc Clin Oncol. 1996;15:A1713.
26. **Daugherty C, Siegler M, Ratain MJ, et al.** A feasibility study of informed consent of medical decision making employing an interactive patient choice design in phase I trials [Abstract]. Proc Am Soc Clin Oncol. 1996;15:A352.
27. **Gotay CC.** Accrual to cancer clinical trials: directions from the research literature. Soc Sci Med. 1991;33:569-77.
28. Viability of cancer clinical research: patient accrual, coverage, and reimbursement. American Medical Association Council on Scientific Affairs. J Natl Cancer Inst. 1991;83:254-9.

8.10   Torke AM, Alexander GC, Lantos J, Siegler M (2007) The Physician-Surrogate Relationship. Arch Intern Med 167:1117–21

Reprinted with permission from the Archives of Internal Medicine, June 2007, Volume 167, Copyright 2007, American Medical Association.

The Physician-Surrogate Relationship

Alexia M. Torke, MD; G. Caleb Alexander, MD, MS; John Lantos, MD; Mark Siegler, MD

T he physician-patient relationship is a cornerstone of the medical encounter and has been analyzed extensively. But in many cases, this relationship is altered because patients are unable to make decisions for themselves. In such cases, physicians rely on surrogates, who are often asked to "speak for the patient." This view overlooks the fundamental fact that the surrogate decision maker cannot be just a passive spokesperson for the patient but is also an active agent who develops a complex relationship with the physician. Although there has been much analysis of the ethical guidelines by which surrogates should make decisions, there has been little previous analysis of the special features of the physician-surrogate relationship. Such an analysis seems crucial as the population ages and life-sustaining technologies improve, which is likely to make surrogate decision making even more common. We outline key issues affecting the physician-surrogate relationship and provide guidance for physicians who are making decisions with surrogates. *Arch Intern Med. 2007;167:1117-1121*

Good medical care depends on human relationships. Trust, mutual respect, and effective communication between patients and physicians are essential for gathering medical histories, making diagnoses, and carrying out complex treatment plans. Because of this, literally thousands of essays, theories, and educational initiatives have focused on the physician-patient relationship. Although there are many ways of thinking about what makes a good physician-patient relationship, a central element is that the physician works directly with the patient, the person most affected by the decisions.

This relationship is fundamentally altered when the patient is unable to participate in the decision-making process. In such cases, surrogates, usually close relatives, interact with physicians to make decisions for the patient. These situations have become increasingly common as life-sustaining therapies, such as mechanical ventilation, have become widely available. Furthermore, as the population ages, the prevalence of diseases that impair cognitive function, such as Alzheimer disease, will make surrogate decision making even more necessary.[1]

Current ethical standards for surrogate decision making focus first on the principle of autonomy and second on the principle of beneficence.[2,3] Using this framework, the surrogate is asked to speak for the incapacitated patient and to choose as the patient would choose. When the surrogate does not know what the patient would have wanted, the surrogate is then asked to judge what would be best for the patient. In our opinion, this is an inadequate view of surrogacy because it fails to recognize that the surrogate is an active, not a passive, agent in the interaction with a physician.

The physician and surrogate must establish a unique relationship with each other—the *physician-surrogate relationship*—that is very different from the traditional physician-patient relationship. Despite the frequent need for physicians and surrogates to make medical decisions together, little attention has been focused on

Author Affiliations: MacLean Center for Clinical Medical Ethics, University of Chicago, Chicago, Ill (Drs Torke, Alexander, Lantos, and Siegler), and Section of General Internal Medicine, Department of Medicine (Drs Torke, Alexander, and Siegler), and Department of Pediatrics (Dr Lantos), University of Chicago Hospitals, Chicago.

the physician-surrogate relationship. Reframing surrogate decision making in terms of relationships highlights the importance of each person's experience and the communication between them. It acknowledges the personhood of the individuals involved and the influence each has on the others.[4] This focus on relationships can broaden our understanding of surrogate decision making and provide a more useful clinical approach.

In this article, we highlight key similarities and differences between the physician-surrogate relationship and the physician-patient relationship that are likely to affect clinical decision making. We then recommend specific guidelines for physicians who are making difficult decisions for patients who cannot speak for themselves. We focus on surrogates who are making decisions for previously competent adults because the issues in pediatric decision making and for those with lifelong mental disabilities raise different but related issues.

PHYSICIAN-SURROGATE RELATIONSHIP: KEY ISSUES

There are 4 key issues in the physician-surrogate relationship that require analysis. First, physicians and surrogates face unique challenges in building relationships with each other. Second, the surrogate and physician must negotiate the decision-making role that each will play while also considering a third party—the patient. Third, the experience of serving as a surrogate for a loved one is fundamentally different from the experience of making decisions for oneself. Finally, there are often multiple surrogate decision makers. Relationships among various surrogates and among physicians often influence both the process and outcomes of clinical decisions.

Relationship Building

There are many aspects of the health care setting that undermine traditional physician-patient relationships, including time pressures, lack of continuity, and a focus on technology rather than on personal re-

lationships. In addition to these issues, the physician-surrogate relationship faces particular challenges. In many cases, surrogates and physicians do not meet each other until the patient has a severe illness or crisis. Such an arrangement leaves little or no basis to establish trust in advance of a major decision. With the increasing division of labor between inpatient and outpatient physicians, the physician may have never even met the patient, much less the surrogate, before the patient loses his or her decision-making capacity. This may affect the perspective of the physician; although the family may remember the patient as a vibrant individual, the physician knows the person only in his or her current state of ill health and debilitation. With a competent patient, the usual routine of daily bedside visits may enhance or be the sole basis of the physician-patient relationship in the inpatient setting. Because of these additional barriers, building a relationship with the surrogate requires extra attention.

Decision-making Roles

In spite of these challenges, the physician and surrogate must negotiate decision making together. There has been little exploration of how this occurs. Research on patients' preferences for their own care has found that most patients want to be fully informed of their diagnoses and treatment, but they vary in how much decision-making authority they desire.[5-8] In recent years, some authors[9-15] have advocated for shared decision making, in which the patient's autonomy is balanced against the caring concern and advice of the physician. Although the law requires the consent of the patient, the actual amount of authority the patient exercises may vary widely.

Negotiating these roles is more complex when the physician and surrogate are deciding for a third party, the patient. There may be even greater variation among surrogates than among patients in terms of the role they wish to play. Physicians should attend to the information needs and preferred decision-making role of each individual surrogate. Such an approach is com-

plex because, in addition to considering whether a choice is consistent with the patient's own wishes, the physician must consider the preferred decision-making role of the surrogate decision maker.

What factors should be considered in determining the balance of decision-making authority? Depending on the situation, the physician and surrogate will previously have had varying degrees of closeness to the patient. Both the surrogate's emotional ties to the patient and his or her biological or legal relationship to the patient must be considered.[16] Surrogates who have a close relationship with the patient are more likely to understand the patient's values or preferences and thus should have more leeway in decision making than those who do not know the patient well.[17] A physician who has known a patient for years is also in a different position to make decisions for that person than a physician who has cared for the patient only for a short time.

For example, a son who cares for his mother at home may bring her to the emergency department. In this case, they are probably both meeting the emergency department physician for the first time. If the patient cannot express her own wishes, the son may be able to base decisions on the patient's recent statements about her own illness or his own knowledge about her life.

In a second case, a patient may have a close relationship with her primary care physician but be estranged from the family members who are her legal next of kin. It is ethically appropriate that the physician take a more active role in decision making in this case. If the physician is familiar with the patient's wishes and values, he or she may recommend treatments that are consistent with them. In both cases, the physician is legally required to include the surrogate in decision making, but the amount of guidance the physician provides should vary based on the circumstances.

Experience of the Surrogate

The surrogate establishes a relationship with the physician in the context of each person's previous experience and previous relationship with the patient. Two crucial aspects of the surrogate's experience will likely affect decision making: the surrogate's emotions and his or her own goals and values.

Surrogates make decisions for loved ones in the context of grief, loss, and long-standing family dynamics that inevitably affect the decision-making process. Such emotional and psychological issues influence the decisions of surrogates, particularly regarding decisions about life-sustaining care. Making life-and-death decisions for oneself and a loved one, although both extremely complex and difficult, are fundamentally different experiences. Even though there is evidence that family caregivers experience emotional strain, financial hardship, and health risks,[18] there have been only a few studies[19-21] examining the experience of making major health care decisions for a loved one. One study found that surrogates struggle with tension between their own emotional experiences and convictions and the desire to make the right decision for the patient.[21]

Many of the stresses experienced by surrogates may arise from tensions between the surrogate's own values and goals and those of the patient. Such stresses cannot be adequately addressed by ethical and legal models that view the surrogate as merely a spokesperson for the patient rather than as an independent moral agent. In our clinical experience, dutifully caring for a disabled relative or not giving up on a loved one are also key considerations of surrogates but are not included in current ethical models. There is evidence that physicians also take a broader view of the proper role for the surrogate. Most physicians believe that the family's wishes should be considered, along with the patient's, in arriving at end-of-life decisions.[22,23]

Because the values and needs of family members will inevitably affect decision making, ethical and legal models of the physician-surrogate relationship should explicitly acknowledge these factors and incorporate them into the decision-making process.

Multiple Surrogates

Establishing a physician-patient relationship is more difficult when

Table. Guidelines for Physicians

Guideline	Tasks

Build a relationship early.	Initiate contact:
	  • In the hospital: talk to the surrogate on the day of admission
	  • Learn about the patient as a person
	Focus on common goals first:
	  • Discuss routine aspects of care before emotionally sensitive topics
	  • Listen to surrogate perspective on goals of care
	  • Emphasize mutual goals and values

Recognize emotions and values.	Assess and acknowledge the surrogate:
	  • Emotions
	  • Values and beliefs that affect decision making
	  • Readiness in coming to terms with the patient's illness
	Use a multidisciplinary approach:
	  • Consult social workers and chaplains to support the surrogate
	  • Consider palliative care consults, when available

Build consensus.	Identify points of agreement:
	    • Broad goals
	  • Specific therapies
	Negotiate points of conflict:
	    • Explore values
	  • Defer to future discussions
	  • Time limited trials
	    • Agree to disagree

many physicians and other health care professionals are involved in the care of the patient. Similarly, a major challenge to the physician-surrogate relationship is the usual presence of more than 1 surrogate. Although legal statutes identify a "chain of command" among family members, in practice, physicians may communicate with and relate to multiple surrogates for a given patient. In most cases, family members support each other through difficult times, and the physician can foster consensus and mutual understanding in the decision-making process. However, families may include individuals with very different belief systems and experiences that guide them to very different conclusions about medical care. Intrafamily conflict may be heightened by a family member's illness, making decision making more difficult. Many of the issues we have highlighted in surrogate decision making become magnified when there is not just 1 surrogate but 2 or more.

GUIDANCE FOR PHYSICIANS

Given the clinical and ethical importance of the physician-surrogate relationship, physicians who care for patients with diminished decision-making capacity should pay attention to 3 specific aspects of

their relationships with surrogates (**Table**).

First, when a patient lacks decision-making capacity, the physician should work to build a relationship with the surrogate or surrogates early in the patient's care before a crisis arises. For hospitalized patients, meeting with surrogates early in the hospital course to learn about the patient as a person and to discuss routine care may establish the groundwork for communication if the patient's condition worsens or end-of-life issues arise. Hospital physicians face many time pressures, and communication with family members may seem to be a low priority when the clinical decisions for the patient seem clear. We recommend communicating with the family on the first day of admission in all cases, with a focus on the patient's clinical situation and plan of care. The first conversations should be to establish a good working relationship based on mutual goals. Although it may be necessary to ask immediately about the patient's prior wishes or decisions about code status and goals of care, renegotiating these goals should be delayed, when possible, until after the first meeting with the surrogate.

Second, the physician should assess how the surrogate's own grief and other intense emotions may influence decision-making and should support the surrogate through this difficult process. Such recognition and support are both morally appropriate in their own right and may also improve the decision-making process. For the physician, this may involve acknowledging the experience of the surrogate and recognizing his or her unique role in the patient's life. It may involve allowing decisions to be delayed while loved ones come to terms with the patient's serious illness. A multidisciplinary approach, incorporating social workers, chaplains, and others, could provide support to loved ones in times of suffering and grief. The fields of palliative care and hospice have brought our attention to the need to employ a multidisciplinary approach to support families as well as patients.[24,25] The physician's obligations do not extend to providing medical care to family members but rather to considering the patient in the context of his or her family. Surrogate decision making may improve as the palliative care approach is increasingly brought into the acute care setting, including the intensive care unit. Surrogates who are supported as they cope with a loved one's illness may be better able to make decisions that are best for the patient. In addition, skilled physicians and interdisciplinary staff may be able to negotiate a consensus among family members when there is disagreement within the family.

Ethical guidelines for surrogate decision making require that both physicians and surrogates make decisions in accordance with the patient's prior wishes, if known, and with the patient's best interest. Because the surrogate's own interests or the needs of other family members may also play a role in decision making, honest discussion about the surrogate's motivations and reasoning requires trust and open communication and is crucial for good decision making. The physician should guide the surrogate to also incorporate the patient's own wishes and best interests into decision making while acknowledging other relevant considerations.

Third, physicians should approach decision making as a process of consensus building.[26] Fam-

ily members and physicians may in some cases have very different views about the goals of care and about the role of specific technologies, such as the use of ventilators or tube feeding. The physician also may need to develop consensus among multiple family members who disagree with each other. Although the law may give priority for decision making to certain relatives vs others, seeking consensus among family members, even at the cost of delaying nonurgent clinical decisions, will be better for the family and may facilitate future decisions. If conflict cannot be resolved, honoring the choice of the legal decision maker over the objection of others may be a necessary last resort.

In some cases, there may be conflict over the goals of care that are the result of differences in values or moral principles. If there is disagreement, the physician should explore the values and beliefs underlying those differences. Research on conflict in surrogate decision making suggests that although there may be disagreement early, it is usually resolved after a few days.[27] With time, the clinical scenario may become clearer, the nature of the decisions may change, and the family may come to terms with the patient's illness. If there is disagreement about whether a particular life-sustaining therapy such as ventilation is appropriate, a time-limited trial may be a compromise.

Even when communication is ideal, there may be differences in values and beliefs that cannot be resolved between physicians and surrogates. We find that such situations are particularly troubling to physicians. Although it may be hard for a physician to accept a patient's own choice when it conflicts with the physician's judgment, it is much more difficult to reconcile disagreement with a surrogate's choice. Good relationships and good communication cannot fully resolve the conflicts that occur when making decisions for others. In some cases, physicians must agree to disagree with the surrogate. It may be acceptable in some cases for the physician to provide care that he or she does not think is best if other moral principles, such as the patient's pre-

vious wishes or the surrogate's assessment of the patient's best interest, justify the decision.

In conclusion, the vast literature on the physician-patient relationship provides a useful starting point for an exploration of the relationship between physician and surrogate. Because the literature on surrogate decision making has focused so heavily on asking family members to speak for the patient, there has been too little emphasis on the physician-surrogate relationship. This relationship is part of a complex triad in which the physician and surrogate communicate with each other but focus their concerns on the incapacitated patient. We have highlighted certain unique aspects of this relationship and suggested specific guidelines for physicians. Such guidelines include improving the separate personal relationship that the physician must establish with the surrogate, supporting the surrogate emotionally as he or she navigates difficult decisions for a loved one, and employing a consensus-based approach to surrogate decision making that incorporates the values and obligations of the surrogate while maintaining the focus on the patient.

Accepted for Publication: February 11, 2007.
Correspondence: Alexia M. Torke, MD, University of Chicago, 5841 S Maryland Ave, MC 2007, Chicago, IL 60637 (atorke@medicine.bsd .uchicago.edu).
Author Contributions: *Study concept and design:* Torke, Alexander, Lantos, and Siegler. *Drafting of the manuscript:* Torke and Alexander. *Critical revision of the manuscript for important intellectual content:* Torke, Alexander, Lantos, and Siegler. *Study supervision:* Alexander, Lantos, and Siegler.
Financial Disclosure: None reported.
Funding/Support: Dr Torke is supported by a training grant from the Health Resources and Services Administration, and Dr Alexander is supported as a Robert Wood Johnson Faculty Scholar.
Role of the Sponsor: The Health Resources and Services Administration and the Robert Wood Johnson

Foundation had no role in the design and conduct of the study; in the collection, analysis, and interpretation of the data; or in the preparation, review, or approval of the manuscript.

REFERENCES

1. President's Council on Bioethics. Taking care: ethical caregiving in our aging society. http://www.bioethics.gov/reports/taking_care/index.html. Accessed March 19, 2007.
2. Buchanan B, Brock DW. *Deciding for Others: The Ethics of Surrogate Decision Making.* Cambridge, England: Cambridge University Press; 1990.
3. Emanuel EJ, Emanuel LL. Proxy decision making for incompetent patients: an ethical and empirical analysis. *JAMA.* 1992;267:2067-2071.
4. Beach MC, Inui T. Relationship-centered care: a constructive reframing. *J Gen Intern Med.* 2006; 21(suppl 1):S3-S8.
5. Arora NK, McHorney CA. Patient preferences for medical decision making: who really wants to participate. *Med Care.* 2000;38:335-341.
6. Degner LF, Sloan JA. Decision making during serious illness: what role do patients really want to play? *J Clin Epidemiol.* 1992;45:941-950.
7. Strull WM, Lo B, Charles G. Do patients want to participate in medical decision making? *JAMA.* 1984;252:2990-2994.
8. Levinson W, Kao A, Kuby A, Thisted RA. Not all patients want to participate in decision making: a national study of public preferences. *J Gen Intern Med.* 2005;20:531-535.
9. Veatch RM. Models for ethical medicine in a revolutionary age: what physician-patient roles foster the most ethical relationship? *Hastings Cent Rep.* 1972;2:5-7.
10. Siegler M. Critical illness: the limits of autonomy. *Hastings Cent Rep.* 1977;7:12-15.
11. Childress JF, Siegler M. Metaphors and models of doctor-patient relationships: their implications for autonomy. *Theor Med.* 1984;5:17-30.
12. Beauchamp TL, Childress JF. *Principles of Biomedical Ethics.* 4th ed. Oxford, England: Oxford University Press; 1994.
13. Emanuel EJ, Emanuel LL. Four models of the physician-patient relationship. *JAMA.* 1992;267: 2221-2226.
14. Balint J, Shelton W. Regaining the initiative: forging a new model of the patient-physician relationship. *JAMA.* 1996;275:887-891.
15. Quill TE, Brody H. Physician recommendations and patient autonomy: finding a balance between physician power and patient choice. *Ann Intern Med.* 1996;125:763-769.
16. Brock DW. What is the moral authority of family members to act as surrogates for incompetent patients? *Milbank Q.* 1996;74:599-618.
17. Veatch RM. Limits of guardian treatment refusal: a reasonableness standard. *Am J Law Med.* 1984; 9:427-468.
18. Rabow MW, Hauser JM, Adams J. Supporting family caregivers at the end of life: "they don't know what they don't know." *JAMA.* 2004;291:483-491.
19. Butcher HK, Holkup PA, Park M, Maas M. Thematic analysis of the experience of making a decision to place a family member with Alzheimer's disease in a special care unit. *Res Nurs Health.* 2001;24:470-480.
20. Park M, Butcher HK, Maas ML. A thematic analysis of Korean family caregivers' experiences in making the decision to place a family member with dementia in a long-term care facility. *Res Nurs Health.* 2004;27:345-356.
21. Chambers-Evans J, Carnevale FA. Dawning of awareness: the experience of surrogate decision making at the end of life. *J Clin Ethics.* 2005; 16:28-45.
22. Perkins HS, Bauer RL, Hazuda HP, Schoolfield JD. Impact of legal liability, family wishes, and other "external factors" on physicians' life-support decisions. *Am J Med.* 1990;89:185-194.
23. Hardart GE, Truog RD. Practicing physicians and the role of family surrogate decision making. *J Clin Ethics.* 2005;16:345-354.
24. National Consensus Project for Quality Palliative Care. Clinical Practice Guidelines for Quality Palliative Care: Executive Summary. http://www.nationalconsensusproject.org. Accessed March 19, 2007.
25. Doyle D, Hanks G, Cherney NI, Calman K. *Oxford Textbook of Palliative Medicine.* 3rd ed. Oxford, England: Oxford University Press; 2004.
26. Karlawish JH, Quill T, Meier DE; American College of Physicians–American Society of Internal Medicine End-of-Life Care Consensus Panel. A consensus-based approach to providing palliative care to patients who lack decision-making capacity. *Ann Intern Med.* 1999;130:835-840.
27. Prendergast TJ. Resolving conflicts surrounding end-of-life care. *New Horiz.* 1997;5:62-71.

Education and Professionalism

Laura Weiss Roberts and Mark Siegler

Abstract

This chapter contains reprinted works from Dr. Mark Siegler focusing on education, training, and professionalism within the field of clinical medical ethics. Based heavily on Dr. Siegler's extensive first-hand knowledge of training medical students in clinical medical ethics, these works present recommendations regarding how, where, and when the topic should be taught and how this type of training can improve both the physician's understanding of professionalism and patient care overall. Several of the works presented within this chapter move beyond education and training to discuss the health and care of medical students who may become patients during their training or residency. The works in this chapter are reprinted with permission.

L.W. Roberts, MD, MA (✉)
Department of Psychiatry and Behavioral Sciences,
Stanford University School of Medicine, Stanford, CA, USA
e-mail: robertsl@stanford.edu

M. Siegler, MD
Bucksbaum Institute for Clinical Excellence, MacLean Center
for Clinical Medical Ethics, University of Chicago, Pritzker School
of Medicine, Chicago, IL, USA

© Springer International Publishing AG 2017
L.W. Roberts, M. Siegler (eds.), *Clinical Medical Ethics*, DOI 10.1007/978-3-319-53875-4_9

9.1   Siegler M (1978) A Legacy of Osler: Teaching Clinical Ethics at the Bedside. JAMA 239:951–6

Special Communication

A Legacy of Osler

Teaching Clinical Ethics at the Bedside

Mark Siegler, MD

● The teaching of clinical medicine at the bedside is an enduring legacy of the Oslerian revolution in American education. The advantages of teaching clinical ethics at the bedside include dealing with actual cases to maximize personal accountability, reinforcing the relationship between technical competence and ethical decisions, involving the entire health care team, and possibly decreasing the resistance of the medical profession to formal medical ethics.

The proposal to teach clinical ethics at the bedside is intended to indicate a primary role for ethicists and clinicians at different stages in the medical curriculum. During the preclinical years of medical school, ethicist-philosophers, assisted by clinicians, should assume primary responsibility for teaching medical ethics. During the clinical years, physicians, assisted by clinically informed ethicist-philosophers, should accept the primary obligation to teach clinical ethics at the bedside.

(*JAMA* 239:951-956, 1978)

IT MAY appear simplistic to restate the obvious, but whatever else medical ethics is, it must have something to do with the practice of clinical and investigative medicine, or, at least, it should. Clinical medicine is taught at the bedside in the tradition formalized by William Osler, MD, who advocated a preceptorial exchange between student and teacher designed to identify and

---

*For editorial comment
see p 960.*

---

resolve the problems of patients. Analogously, it is suggested that clinical ethics, the component of medical ethics that has relevance for the practicing physician, health professional, and clinical investigator, should be taught at the patient's bedside. Although not strictly Oslerian, the term "bedside teaching" will be used here as a convenient shorthand to indicate all clinical teaching, which occurs during the delivery of medical services, whether in inpatient bedside settings, in outpa-

tient clinics, or in physician's offices. These observations may seem intuitive to a clinician, but they are not universally accepted. Serious questions persist among ethicists whether medical ethics must be clinically relevant and whether it is best taught at the bedside.

Further, although clinicians may agree in principle that medical ethics should be clinically relevant and should be taught at the bedside, it would be naive to assume that they would universally embrace the proposal advanced here to formalize instruction in medical ethics within the context of clinical teaching. Clinicians might argue that the practice and teaching of good clinical medicine imply the practice of moral and ethical medicine. It is, therefore, unnecessary, difficult, and possibly counterproductive to remove ethical considerations from the holistic concerns of the competent clinician.

While reviewing the development of medical ethics curricula of the past decade,[1-3] one is struck by the innovative, creative, and essentially heterogeneous approaches that have emerged from the many universities and medical schools that have entered this new field. The diversity of approaches and the critical scrutiny these new pro-

grams are receiving suggests that no single model has been found that is universally applicable. The design of medical ethics curricula remains in an experimental phase.

Many of the curricular innovations in medical ethics concentrate on creating preclinical required or elective courses for medical students. A parallel but less advanced effort has attempted to develop creative, clinically oriented programs in medical ethics. These clinical programs have included conferences, workshops, seminars, lecture series, and, most notably, ethical grand rounds.[4] Formal ethical grand rounds usually focus on actual clinical cases that raise ethical and philosophical issues; clinicians and ethicist-philosophers participate in these rounds.[4] This form of conference was tried experimentally at State University of New York at Stony Brook and at Columbia University in about 1970. It has subsequently been introduced successfully at such university medical centers as Harvard University, The University of California at Los Angeles, The University of Tennessee, The University of Virginia, Yale University, and others.

Many other experimental approaches to teaching clinical ethics have been tried, including seminars by Duncombe[5] on the chronically ill offered at Yale University, the introduction of philosophers into the teaching hospitals of the New York University Medical Center under the auspices of the Society for Philosophy and Public Affairs, and the development of elective courses in medical ethics for students during their clinical years of training.

These efforts to develop programs relating medical ethics and philosophy to clinical medicine are noteworthy, but should be distinguished from the proposal advanced here—to teach clinical ethics at the bedside in the context

---

From the Section of General Internal Medicine, University of Chicago Pritzker School of Medicine, Chicago.

Reprint requests to Section of General Internal Medicine, University of Chicago Hospitals, 950 E 59th St, Box 72, Chicago, IL 60637 (Dr Siegler).

of teaching clinical medicine. This difference is comparable to that existing between teaching clinical medicine in an amphitheater-lecture hall rather than at the bedside. Moral discourse in the context of clinical medicine will not become a legitimate enterprise for medical students and house officers until it is used by their clinical mentors at the bedside and until attention to these moral-ethical issues can be shown to improve patient care and physician satisfaction. In this regard, Otto Guttentag, MD,[6] has suggested that the teaching of medical ethics—"An inalienable hitherto neglected part of the curriculum"—should be examined from the point of view of the attending physician, "The person whom I, and everyone else, I think, considers to be the key figure of the entire profession."

The problems of developing a curriculum in clinical ethics can be surmounted by increasing the participation of clinicians while maintaining the valuable contributions of ethicist-philosophers in the education of medical students and physicians.

THE LEGACY OF OSLER

William Osler's remarkable contributions to American medical education hardly require restatement, but it is probable that his greatest and most lasting achievement emphasized the importance of practical experience in learning the physician's art by extending clinical teaching from the textbook, laboratory, and classroom to the patient's bedside. One of Osler's proudest claims was: "I taught medical students in the wards."

Osler's most complete statement of his philosophy of teaching medicine is contained in an address he delivered to the New York Academy of Medicine in 1902, in which he stated:

In what may be called the natural method of teaching, the student begins with the patient, continues with the patient, and ends his study with the patient, using books and lectures as tools, as means to an end.... For the junior student in medicine and surgery it is a safe rule to have no teaching without a patient for a text, and the best teaching is that taught by the patient himself.[7]

Osler's remarks of 1902 were visionary. Since then his educational methods have dominated American medical education. Indeed, bedside teaching remains the cornerstone of our clinical teaching for third- and fourth-year undergraduate medical students and for almost all postgraduate clinical training programs. The bedside teaching of medicine is viewed, at least in the United States, as the best way to teach clinical medicine. Even in these days of curricular revolutions and reassessments, few voices have been raised to suggest altering this system of medical education. In part, the success of this educational model has precluded its reevaluation or modification. The Oslerian system of bedside teaching has proved remarkably effective and has, therefore, endured.

ADVANTAGES
Intensity of the Bedside Situation

Actual patients and the combined medical and ethical challenges they present to physicians are found at the bedside. In contrast the ethical issues of patient care and clinical investigation are imperfectly approximated by the use of hypothetical or actual case histories in the classroom or the seminar room. In discussing how best to teach the cognitive skills of medical humanism, Pellegrino[8] has stated:

To be most effective with the goal-oriented medical student, the cognitive skills should be taught within the framework of a medical education—indeed, as an integral part of that education.... Teaching in such a context necessarily proceeds from the concrete, personal, and immediate to the abstract, general, and more ultimate concerns of mankind. It demands use of the case method and seminar rather than the lecture and reading assignment. It centers on personal involvement by the student with the specific concerns of his patient and thus gains a relevance scarcely equalled in other types of teaching.

The intensity of the clinical situation requires that moral-technical decisions be made at the bedside. Therefore, the keen pressure of personal accountability for an action with consequences for the patient is found at the bedside and not in the classroom. The clinician or clinical investigator has the ultimate responsibility for his medical and ethical decisions. Jonsen[9] recently emphasized this point when he commented on differences in responsibilities between physicians and ethicists:

The physician, engaging in medical practice at first hand, must make swift, definite, and often irrevocable decisions in which universal principles meet the rigorous challenge of actuality. Ethicists might issue their principles from their proverbial ivory tower. Physicians, immersed in the immediacy of wards, clinics, and surgical suites may find them of little value in alleviating the pain of decisions.

The physical presence of the patient demands that he be regarded as a subject rather than as an object, and this facilitates the pedagogical goal of humanizing medical care. Practically speaking the patient can participate directly in the making of decisions regarding his care. Further, the bedside teaching of medical ethics emphasizes and reinforces the Oslerian concept of the patient as teacher because the patient's values, aspirations, and wishes must be understood and acknowledged before the clinician reaches a technical decision.

For example, a 75-year-old man with severe, progressively worsening chronic obstructive pulmonary disease comes to a hospital with acute respiratory failure. After six hours of intensive medical treatment, his ventilatory status deteriorates further. A decision must be made whether to intubate the patient and begin using a respirator. Traditionally such cases provoke superb bedside clinical discussions and instruction on issues such as reversible factors in acute respiratory failure, the pathophysiology of respiratory failure, or the medical indications for artificial ventilation. To consider all the medical factors in such a case without simultaneously examining and discussing the profound ethical dilemma of using a respirator is to fail to completely teach the art of being a physician.

Consider the problem of truth-telling in medicine. Although principles of truth-telling can be taught by reference to philosophical theories of utilitarianism or deontological ethics, this subject might be taught with enhanced efficiency and relevance at the bedside when a clinician must present a grave diagnosis to a patient, or when a physician "hangs crepe," ie, deliberately offers the most pessimistic prognosis to the family of an acutely ill patient.[10] When a physician renders a prognosis or equivocates on how much information he will divulge to a patient, a potential teaching situation exists in which the clinician-teacher can begin to articulate the ethical principles that underlie his clinical behavior.

Technical Competence and Clinical Ethics

The ability to treat patients allows the physician the privilege or license to treat them, and this provides the opportunity to treat them in an ethical way. The franchise of the clinician derives from his special technical training and competence. A suffusion of compassion and empathy or an oath of allegiance to be ethical is poor recompense indeed for an inadequate treatment plan. To practice ethical medicine or humanistic medicine effectively, the physician's first and principal obligation is to become technically competent. Several years ago, the Spanish physician, P. Lain-Entralgo[11] wrote: "The doctor's friendship for the patient should consist above all in a desire to give effective technical help—benevolence conceived and realized in technical terms." More recently, Pellegrino[8] restated this observation: "Without clinical craftsmanship, the physician-humanist is without authenticity. Incompetence is inhumane because it betrays the trust the patient places in the physician's capacity to help and not to harm." Thus, the teaching of clinical ethics and human values should strive to emphasize the intimate association of the technical and ethical, and the ethical issues of caring for a patient should not be arbitrarily divorced from the act of caring for the patient.

For example, consider the case in which a group of clinical investigators wishes to compare the effect of frequent low doses of intravenously administered insulin with standard treatment programs in the management of diabetic ketoacidosis.[12] Could a student or house officer or clinical investigation committee that had not had personal experience in the care of acutely ill patients and that had not meticulously reviewed the available literature on the treatment of ketoacidosis reach an understanding of the ethical issues involved in the research proposal? The ethics of pursuing an investigation that compares experimental treatment with standard treatment is intricately intertwined with the technical-scientific advantages or disadvantages of the treatment plans. The opportunity to explore the ethics of a proposed protocol for treatment of ketoacidosis is available to teachers, medical students, and house officers any time a patient with diabetic ketoacidosis is admitted to a hospital ward. Such a teaching exercise might be less rewarding if carried out in a lecture hall, particularly if it were taught to first- and second-year students who had never taken care of patients.

Teaching Ethics to the Health Care Team

Teaching medical ethics at the bedside will provide the opportunity to teach an entire generation of medical students. In addition, house officers who may not have previously been exposed to medical ethics and medical faculty and clinical investigators who are well beyond their formal training will be provided with the most effective form of continuing medical education—that which occurs in the context of their clinical work.

When medicine is taught at the bedside, the tone of an entire medical unit changes, and there suddenly develops a pervasive atmosphere of intellectual excitement and inquiry. Further, the teaching of clinical ethics and human values in the ward and at the patient's bedside will permit the entire health care team—physicians, medical students, nurses, social workers, chaplains, dietitians, administrators, and the patient—to participate actively in the total educational experience, including the making of clinical decisions. In this regard, it is worth recalling Osler's remark concerning the teaching of medicine at the bedside: "I envy for our medical students the advantages enjoyed by the nurses, who live in daily contact with the sick."[13] In Osler's day, nurses, not medical students, learned medicine from the patient at the bedside. In our time, it is principally nurses, social workers, and chaplains, not medical students and houseofficers, who learn the ethics of medicine from the patient. The time has come to offer training in medical ethics and human values to the entire health care team.

Decreasing Professional Resistance

Much has been written lately about the so-called backlash in medical ethics, and several authors have commented on the inevitability of such a reaction.[14,15] Callahan,[14] for example, has suggested that a true tension might exist between the interests of the scientific and nonscientific community, and that this contributes to the widespread suspicion that much of the concern of ethics represents latent antiscientific feeling.

It seems clear that if an intellectual movement that impinges on the daily activities of a profession arises primarily from outside the profession and derives little of its intellectual nurture and sustenance from members of the profession, at some time, sooner rather than later, the profession will repudiate this new movement and will resist any further encroachment on its independence and freedom of action. This inevitable repudiation, resistance, or backlash will occur regardless of the validity or truth that the outside discipline brings to the old profession. The nature of a profession is to be self-regulating and to enforce its established codes, and this partly accounts for its resistance to outside agencies of control.

A potential solution to the backlash problem as it relates to medical ethics, and one that respects the concept of a profession and the unique position of the medical profession, is to incorporate valuable outside influences and make them a part of the new professional code. If clinical ethics can be incorporated into medical care and research and can be shown to improve medical care, the resistance to medical ethics will be effectively stifled because the profession will have become involved in the use of the principles of medical ethics. Medical ethics will become an integrated aspect of professional life when it is taught to medical students at the bedside and when it is no longer artificially divorced from the practice of medicine itself. Essentially by returning medical ethics to the bedside and by teaching it based on the primary contact of health provider and patient, ethics can develop as an essential component in the clinical process. Ingelfinger[15] recently wrote: "Ideally, ethics and science should in mutualistic fashion foster finer medical practice and research." This can be accomplished if the two are pursued and taught as a unity to students and not separated into the realm of science and the realm of philosophy.

DIFFICULTIES

Notwithstanding the apparent merits of teaching clinical ethics at the bedside, objections to this proposal might be raised by clinicians and ethicists. Some of the disadvantages to be considered are the following: (1) Physicians may be unqualified to teach medical ethics. (2) Medical students may be ill-prepared to learn medical ethics at the bedside. (3) Physicians may be reluctant to formally teach medical ethics at the bedside. (4) Many important issues in medical ethics may not be encountered at the bedside.

Unqualified Physicians

It has been suggested that physicians may be ill-prepared and unqualified to teach medical ethics. Robert Veatch[16] has argued that the physician's scientific-technical training is poor preparation for making moral decisions concerning patients, and it may be inappropriate for physicians to speak as experts on moral or ethical matters. Unfortunately, the moral judgment of physicians tends to be intuitive, is rarely self-reflective, and is frequently inconsistent from one patient or circumstance to another. When making decisions, many physicians fail to take into account and are often unaware of their own value system and the ways in which internalized values and beliefs contribute to their position on ethical, moral, and even medical issues. The physician's lack of formal training in ethics and his failure to clarify values may result in a distorted situational ethic, in which he struggles on each occasion to "reinvent the wheel" to reach an ethical decision.

Unprepared Students

Medical students in the wards are often overwhelmed by the amount of technical knowledge and clinical skill they must achieve. They are often too involved in their clinical work to take the time and energy necessary to reflect on medical ethics, which they perceive to be a "softer" subject, and one that is less relevant to their immediate task. In addition, in the absence of background knowledge in practical moral reasoning and value clarification, students may not be ready to appreciate the complexities of medical ethics. They may approach all problems in an ad hoc way and not develop systematic approaches to moral dilemmas. Thus if clinical ethics is to be taught at the bedside, some preliminary training is desirable. Such preliminary training would allow students an opportunity to examine the range of philosophical and ethical principles on which bedside decisions are based. Also, students would be able to consider in advance the types of moral-ethical decisions that might have to be made at the bedside. This anticipatory preconditioning might allow students to respond more effectively when actual circumstances require an immediate, irrevocable decision.

Reluctant Physicians

Physician-teachers generally share with medical students the feeling that the time allotted for clinical education is barely sufficient to impart basic clinical skills. Any attempt to incorporate the teaching of medical ethics into the clinical curriculum would require a proportional decrease in the time available to teach clinical medicine. Further, physicians might resist formalizing the teaching of medical ethics at the bedside because they believe that such a program would be redundant. If the ethical-moral concerns of medicine are integral and inseparable from its scientific-technical concerns, the teaching of clinical medicine necessarily involves the teaching of medical ethics. Therefore, as long as students are taught clinical medicine at the bedside in the Oslerian tradition, they will also be taught medical ethics there. As Eric Cassell[17] has recently written: "To conceive of a physician practicing his profession without constant ethical decision-making is to conceive of a physician operating in a cultural vacuum and caring for a collection of static facts wrapped in human form. Medicine is inherently moral."

Although it has been suggested that the teaching of medical ethics has not been structured or formalized and tends to be carried out by precept and example, in fact that is precisely how most successful clinical teaching is done at the bedside. This concept can be supported by briefly reflecting on the career of William Osler. Osler was a perfect example of the complete physician, the true scientist-humanist. His bedside teaching reflected a profound understanding of philosophical traditions and moral and ethical principles. Although his students were not offered a structured course in medical ethics, they were instructed in clinical medicine and true humanitarianism.

Undoubtedly, medicine and medical education would benefit from having more physician-teachers like Sir William Osler, but perhaps the notion of infusing a formal program of medical ethics into the curriculum is unnecessary and superfluous.

Ethical Issues May Not Be Encountered

The bedside component is one aspect of medical ethics, but many important issues are not regularly encountered at the bedside and cannot easily be taught there. Those issues that lend themselves to bedside teaching involve the criticism of principles of action such as telling patients the truth, the relationship of values to decision-making, and the relationship of technical decisions to ethical decisions. But other important ethical concerns usually transcend the bedside situation, and these include problems in justice, such as the right to health care, the allocation of scarce medical resources, problems in the limits of research such as fetal experimentation and genetic manipulation, and such apparent clinical issues as the definition of death or indications for abortion. These latter issues raise complex philosophical and political questions that have broad societal ramifications, and their resolution requires participation from medical professionals and from many nonmedical experts such as philosophers, theologians, economists, and politicians. The medical professional may have only a modest contribution to make in the total analysis of these questions, and therefore, it seems clear that not all issues in medical ethics can be effectively addressed at the bedside.

LEVELS OF MORAL DISCOURSE

Aiken's[18] important distinction of four levels of moral discourse suggests that the medical encounter could also be structured and analyzed in a parallel, if not in a strictly analogous fashion. Although the following discussion does not pretend to adhere to Aiken's categories of moral discourse with precise fidelity, this concept allows us to explore some potential inadequacies of the bedside method of teaching medical ethics. In the medical model, one might consider three levels of moral discourse: (1) at the bedside, the physician makes moral-technical decisions based on (2) a deeper set of ethical principles and values, and these are rooted in (3) more basic and general philosophical principles (Aiken's "post-ethical" level). The bedside teaching of medical ethics may necessarily focus on only the moral-technical aspects of decisions, while failing to analyze the ethical and philosophical bases of these judgments.

1. The moral-technical level of discourse is applied at the bedside and addresses the question of "How should we act? What ought we to do?" The answer to this is based on the concrete scientific-technical facts of the case, the unique attributes of the particular patient, and some basic moral rules, such as "Do not kill," "Do no harm," and "Do not lie," and perhaps also the positive injunction, "Do your duty."[19] For example, if a physician suspects a hard lump in a patient's breast to be cancer, how much is he obligated to tell about his thoughts and concerns and his surgical plans? If the biopsy specimen is positive for cancer and he is planning to do a radical mastectomy, must he inform the patient about alternative, more conservative forms of surgical and radiation therapy? Although most of us do not regularly use such clinical problems to explore the moral-value elements of medical care and medical decision-making, the potential for analyzing such cases and learning from them always exists.

2. At the ethical level of discourse, an attempt is made to understand what principles determine our response to the moral question: "What ought we to do?" Put another way, what justifies the judgment that a particular course of action is correct? Jonsen[9] has commented, "Ethical principles announce the limits of morally acceptable decisions." This ethical level of moral discourse cannot easily be taught at the bedside because it requires the preliminary examination of different systems of ethics such as natural law, utilitarianism, and deontological ethics. A preliminary examination of philosophical and ethical systems can be more expeditiously accomplished in the classroom than at the bedside.

3. The critical question at the post-ethical or philosophical level of moral discourse is to discern the basis for adhering to the principles and values on which our ethical decisions are formulated. The answer here must attempt to uncover and objectify the

basic commitments and beliefs of a society and of individuals that determine their orientation to behave and act in certain ways. For example, why should we tell patients the truth? Or why should patients be involved in decisions regarding their own bodies? The ethical decision to fully inform a patient with suspected breast cancer of all the therapeutic options to permit her to select among therapies is premised on two philosophical assumptions: First, human beings have the intellectual and moral capacity to understand such proposals. Second, they have free will to accept or reject what they understand. Again, this philosophical level of teaching is not easily performed at the bedside and requires preparation in philosophy. Pellegrino[20] has noted:

Medical decisions like all human actions, are based on the value each of us places on life, pain, health, esthetics, the purpose of human existence and all those beliefs which constitute our image of ourselves and our world. Physicians rarely, if ever, analyze the pre-logical roots of their own decisions. Critical philosophy is necessary to uncover the identity of these values, reveal their uncertainties, their ambiguities and their conflicts with other values.

Appreciation of the levels of moral discourse and how this notion applies in medical situations makes it clear that medical ethics must be learned in contexts other than at the bedside and must include preparatory training in ethical systems and philosophical principles for students to understand the grounds on which moral-technical bedside decisions are made.

Teaching Role

The teaching of clinical ethics will be best served by an ongoing collaboration between ethicist-philosophers and clinicians in the preclinical classroom years and later on the wards of teaching hospitals. Intuitively this kind of interdisciplinary effort is required, and the most successful programs to date have settled on this arrangement.[3] However, despite the virtue of joint teaching and collaboration, it is reasonable to suggest that during the preclinical years ethicist-philosophers should assume primary responsibility for teaching medical ethics, and during the clinical years, physicians should accept the primary obligation to instruct students in clinical ethics at the bedside.

Ethicist's Role

Whatever the specific program of instruction, ethicist-philosophers should be encouraged to interact formally and informally with physicians and medical students and to communicate their findings to physicians. Although such interaction might occur primarily in the preclinical years of medical school—in lectures, seminars, and formal courses—it should certainly continue during the clinical years of medical school in conferences and ethical grand rounds and at the bedside. In addition, ethicists should be encouraged to publish their findings in journals that are regularly subscribed to and read by medical students, medical practitioners, and clinician-teachers.[21]

Clinician-Teacher's Role

Clinician-teachers also should continue in their traditional and unique role of teaching ethical and humanitarian medicine in the context of practicing and teaching clinical medicine at the bedside. Such bedside teaching should concentrate on the moral-technical decisions clinicians are called on to make each day and on the ethical principles on which these decisions are based. Clinician-teachers have an obligation to become aware of the principles and issues of formal ethics that are relevant at the bedside, including the concept of levels of moral discourse, the importance of value clarification in reaching moral-technical decisions, and the ethical analysis of new problems that originate from new technology.

Where will this cadre of clinician-teachers capable of instructing in clinical ethics come from? They may already exist. As previously suggested, all physicians do some ethical teaching in the context of clinical teaching. Medical school faculties could probably identify clinicians who possess both the ability and desire to learn more about ethics and to develop special teaching skills in this area. It would be unfortunate if these teaching faculty were recruited preponderantly from such disciplines as psychiatry, public health, community medicine, and legal medicine (as some have suggested[1]) to the exclusion of the traditional clinical fields of internal medicine, surgery, pediatrics, and obstetrics and gynecology. Programs such as the National Endowment for the Humanities' Seminars for Medical Practitioners would be an ideal setting in which to provide exposure to formal ethical issues to permit the interested clinician to pursue the field as part of his own continuing medical education. Recently several universities and institutes have developed postdoctoral fellowship programs to prepare and train future teachers in the field of biomedical ethics. Perhaps the ideal solution to this problem is one that Pellegrino[22] suggested several years ago: "A number of students will need to be trained both in ethics and in medicine as some are trained now in biochemistry or physiology and medicine. . . . The Ph.D.-M.D. combined program in medical ethics deserves serious consideration as a source of future teachers in this field."

How Shall Medical Students Be Taught?

The answer is clear. They should be instructed in medical ethics and medical philosophy primarily by ethicists or philosophers, with some contributions from clinicians, either in undergraduate school or in the preclinical years of medical school, much as they are now instructed in anatomy, biochemistry, and physiology. Just as a student who understands the anatomy, bio-

chemistry, and physiology of myocardial contractility is better able to understand the clinical manifestations of congestive heart failure, so the student who has been prepared in basic ethical and philosophical doctrines will be better prepared to deal with ethical issues at the bedside. This educational experience, however, should not be regarded as an end in itself, just as for physicians the knowledge of anatomy is not an end in itself but rather is meaningful preparation in an important discipline basic to the practice of clinical medicine. Medical ethics then would become the humanistic discipline basic to the practice of clinical ethics. Clinical ethics, the applied skill, must be taught at the bedside, in the Oslerian tradition, and this instruction should be done primarily by clinicians.

References

1. Veatch RM, Sollitto S: Medical ethics teaching: Report of a national medical school survey. *JAMA* 235:1030-1033, 1976.
2. McElhinney TK (ed): *Human Values Teaching Programs for Health Professionals.* Institute on Human Values in Medicine. Philadelphia, Society for Health and Human Values, 1976.
3. Veatch RM, Gaylin W, Morgan C (eds): *The Teaching of Medical Ethics.* Hastings-on-Hudson, NY, Hastings Center, 1973.
4. Levine MD, Scott L, Curran WJ: Ethics rounds in a childrens medical center: Evaluation of a hospital-based program for continuing education in medical ethics. *Pediatrics* 60:202-208, 1977.
5. Duncombe DC: Five years at Yale: The

seminar on the chronically ill. *J Pastoral Care* 28:152-163, 1974.
6. Guttentag OE: Man's nature and finite freedom, in Veatch RM, Gaylin W, Morgan C (eds): *The Teaching of Medical Ethics.* Hastings-on-Hudson, NY, Hastings Center, 1973, pp 82-87.
7. Osler W: On the need of a radical reform in our methods of teaching medical students. *Med News* 82:49-53, 1903.
8. Pellegrino ED: Educating the humanist physician: An ancient ideal reconsidered. *JAMA* 227:1288-1294, 1974.
9. Jonsen AR: Ethicist's heyday. *Am Rev Respir Dis* 113:5-6, 1976.
10. Siegler M: Pascal's wager and the hanging of crepe. *N Engl J Med* 293:853-857, 1975.
11. Lain-Entralgo P: *Doctor and Patient,* New York, McGraw-Hill Book Co Inc, 1969, p 197.
12. Page M McB, Alberti KGMM, Greenwood R, et al: Treatment of diabetic coma with continuous low-dose infusion of insulin. *Br Med J* 2:687-690, 1974.
13. Osler W: The hospital as a college, in *Aequanimitas with Other Addresses.* Philadelphia, Blakiston Co, 1952, pp 311-325.
14. Callahan D: The ethic's backlash. *Hastings Cent Rep* 5:18, 1975.
15. Ingelfinger FJ: The unethical in medical ethics. *Ann Intern Med* 83:264-269, 1975.
16. Veatch RM: Generalization of expertise. *Hastings Cent Stud* 1:29-49, 1973.
17. Cassell EJ: Making and escaping moral decisions. *Hastings Cent Stud* 1:53-62, 1973.
18. Aiken HD: *Reason and Conduct: New Bearing in Mind Philosophy,* New York, Alfred A Knopf Inc, 1962, pp 65-87.
19. Clouser KD: What is medical ethics? *Ann Intern Med* 80:657-660, 1974.
20. Pellegrino ED: *Medicine and Philosophy.* Philadelphia, Society for Health and Human Values, 1974.
21. Ingelfinger FJ: Specialty journals in philosophy and ethics. *N Engl J Med* 295:1317-1318, 1977.
22. Pellegrino ED: Reform and innovation in medical education: The role of ethics, in Veatch RM, Gaylin W, Morgan C (eds): *The Teaching of Medical Ethics.* Hastings-on-Hudson, NY, Hastings Center, 1973, pp 150-165.

9.2   Culver C, Clouser KD, Gert B, Brody H, Fletcher J, Jonsen A, Kopelman L, Lynn J, Siegler M, Wikler D (1985) Basic Curricular Goals in Medical Ethics: The DeCamp Conference on the Teaching of Medical Ethics. N Engl J Med 312:253–56

SPECIAL REPORT

BASIC CURRICULAR GOALS IN MEDICAL ETHICS

FORMAL teaching of ethics in the medical school curriculum has increased greatly during the past 15 years. Yet, schools vary in how much attention they give the subject, and even those that do offer courses vary considerably in the form and content of their curricula. Although the result has been a notable degree of innovation and creativity in teaching methods, the diversity has also created certain impressions that require close scrutiny. A medical school dean or curriculum committee surveying the current state of education in medical ethics might conclude that nothing has evolved that might serve as a national standard for adequate instruction. They might also conclude that courses in ethics are fine so long as one or more interested faculty members want to teach them, but that no deeper institutional commitment needs to be made and that no additional resources need to be devoted to a teaching program.

To determine whether these impressions are correct or whether there is a broader area of agreement underlying the diversity of ethics teaching, we met to survey the current status of the teaching of medical ethics. We concluded that the field is now sufficiently developed and the need for the application of ethical knowledge and skills in medicine sufficiently compelling to justify a recommendation that all medical schools require basic instruction in the subject.

We believe that the basic medical-ethics curriculum should be centered on the kinds of moral problems that physicians encounter most frequently in practice rather than on sensational cases of the type that occur only rarely. The curriculum should address several different kinds of learning: the clarification of central concepts (e.g., the patient's competence to consent to or refuse treatment); the understanding of important decision-making procedures (e.g., how to determine when it is morally justified to treat an unwilling patient); the ability to apply concepts and decision-making procedures to actual cases; and the acquisition of certain interactional skills (e.g., the ability to discuss with a terminally ill patient his or her wishes about being placed on Do Not Resuscitate status).

We believe that a basic curriculum in medical ethics should go considerably beyond the goal of sensitizing students to ethical problems in medicine. It should provide practicing physicians with the conceptual, moral-reasoning, and interactional abilities to deal successfully with most of the moral issues they confront in their daily practice.

Before presenting our recommendation for a basic curriculum, we want to make explicit certain beliefs we hold about the teaching of medical ethics. First of all, we believe that the basic moral character of medical students has been formed by the time they enter medical school. A medical-ethics curriculum is designed not to improve the moral character of future physicians but to provide those of sound moral character with the intellectual tools and interactional skills to give that moral character its best behavioral expression.

Secondly, the content of the medical-ethics curriculum cannot be adequately taught in a piecemeal fashion as students rotate through clinical services and other courses. A portion of the curriculum must be set aside in which teachers with explicit training in medical ethics can present a coherent overview of the field.

Thirdly, there is no one specific system by which medical ethics should be taught. In fact, the field is currently profiting from curricular innovation and experimentation. This should not obscure the fact that there is a core of content that should be taught at some point in every program. One recommended curricular arrangement is to introduce issues, concepts, and theories in a preclinical course and then supervise students in applying the content and in learning appropriate interactional skills during their clinical years. This application is so important that medical ethics should not be limited to the preclinical years, though it may be possible for all course work to be taught during the clinical years.

Although the conceptual and theoretical content of medical ethics can be introduced through readings and lectures, it is important to provide time for small-group discussion as well. Small-group teaching is essential in at least the clinical portion of the medical-ethics curriculum. The concepts and methods of analysis of medical ethics are quite new to most medical students, as is the notion that ethical and philosophical concepts can be and must be used with precision. Students should, therefore, have multiple opportunities to practice and receive supervision in the application of their learning to actual clinical problems. Skills in this area as in all clinical areas must be developed and reinforced. Ward rounds should include discussion of ethical issues, and occasional grand rounds should address ethical topics in detail.

Fourthly, the content of the medical-ethics curriculum should be rigorous and precise. The material should be taught unapologetically and at a challenging level of difficulty. Readings should be required, and students' learning should be measured by means of reasonably difficult examinations or required papers or both.

Although the teaching should be rigorous, the teaching style should be perceived by students as being an emotionally supportive and facilitating one. It should be acknowledged to students that, just as in all other areas of medicine, there is not complete

254   THE NEW ENGLAND JOURNAL OF MEDICINE   Jan. 24, 1985

agreement on all the important topics among all the scholars in the field. The traditional medical school curriculum is coming under increasing and deserved criticism. It has been argued that the traditional style of teaching communicates many values that are antithetical to those that underlie proper instruction in medical ethics — the former emphasizing rote memorization, for instance, or the physician as an expert who always knows best. According to this line of argument, the more closely the medical-ethics curriculum adheres to the structure and tone of the overall medical curriculum, the less likely it is to have the desired impact on the student.

Furthermore, teaching should usually be interdisciplinary. Only rarely are clinicians sufficiently trained in ethics and do ethicists have sufficient clinical knowledge and experience to teach alone competently.

In addition, managing the moral aspects of medical practice requires more than learning concepts and decision-making procedures. Certain interactional skills are also necessary. It is of limited usefulness to decide that the patient must be told the truth about a certain matter and then to go into the patient's room and clumsily blurt out the truth in an insensitive and needlessly hurtful manner. If neither the ethicist nor the clinician teaching medical ethics is equipped to teach the necessary interactional skills, then a specialist in that area should be included on the teaching team at appropriate times.

Furthermore, medical-ethics teaching should be centered in the undergraduate (medical school) curriculum, but every residency program should provide further intensive training in understanding and managing the ethical issues that arise particularly often in that field.

Finally, medical ethics is a complex subject. Although it is possible to teach all physicians enough about it to enable them to manage the bulk of the ethical components of their practice, there will always be difficult cases in which they can benefit by consulting with those who have special training in the field. The majority of our group thought that every physician should have access to ethical consultations for his or her more difficult cases. This consultation should be formalized in hospitals, so that physicians would have an ethics committee or one or more ethics consultants to whom they could turn. Ethical consultation should be prominent in hospitals that train medical students or residents, so that physicians become aware of the availability, method, and importance of such consultation during their training years. One member of our group thought there were still too few data about the process and outcome of ethical consultations to recommend their widespread adoption.

CONTENT OF THE MINIMAL BASIC CURRICULUM

The curricular content described below is recommended as necessary but not sufficient. That is, we believe that by the end of their formal training, all medical students should have acquired at least the knowledge and abilities listed here. Most members of our group would have added more items, and in some cases they would hold that those additional items were equal in importance to some of the items listed here, or even more important; however, there was general agreement that all the items discussed below should be included in a basic curriculum.

Each item is described in terms of certain abilities that we believe a physician should have. Wherever possible, we have tried to divide these abilities into constituent parts. In this outline we have neither included specific teaching methods nor endorsed specific ethical theories. For example, we believe that students should have available some coherent criteria for deciding when it is morally justified to withhold information from a patient, but we do not state here what those criteria should be. Neither do we claim that having such criteria always leads to a definite answer about what one should do, though most of us believe that quite frequently it does. Although we are concerned primarily with medical ethics and not health law, we have indicated parenthetically the relevant items of law that we believe should be adjunctively taught.

The Ability to Identify the Moral Aspects of Medical Practice

The ability to identify the moral aspects of medical practice is more general than the other abilities discussed here and is in a sense imbedded in all of them. The moral aspects of medical practice are pervasive. Physicians are usually in the position of attempting to ameliorate the harm caused by illness, through the use of treatments that may themselves be harmful. Essentially all the decisions, suggestions, or actions of physicians in that position have a moral aspect. This frequently goes unnoticed because it is so often not controversial. For example, a competent patient with an obvious malady consults a physician who suggests a treatment that will almost certainly be effective. The physician informs the patient that the treatment has one minor risk; the patient asks a pertinent question about that risk and then decides to proceed. The treatment is carried out, and the patient recovers from the malady. We believe that medical students should be able to identify the salient moral components of such a case: the open communication of a risk, albeit minor; the patient's ability to understand the risk; and the validity of the consent given.

At least two benefits accrue from seeing the pervasiveness of moral considerations in medical practice. First, the simple notion is refuted that although a few cases involve ethical considerations, most do not. Second, the high degree of agreement about most of the moral aspects of any case constitutes a strong argument against the most prevalent versions of moral relativism.

The Ability to Obtain a Valid Consent or a Valid Refusal of Treatment

Physicians should know and understand the elements of valid consent, know what constitutes adequate information and be able to convey it in language a patient can understand, be able to distinguish between persuasion and coercion, and be able to assess whether a patient is, at a given time, fully competent, partially competent, or incompetent to consent to or refuse treatment. (They should also know the consent laws in their own state and the policy regarding consent, if any, in their own hospital.)

Any physician who interacts with patients must daily ask their consent for many tests, procedures, or treatments. Knowing how to obtain a valid consent or refusal seems a cornerstone of moral medical practice. In order to obtain such a consent or refusal, one must know first of all just what the concept means. There are at least two additional skills that also seem necessary: the ability to use comprehensible language in explaining a proposal to a patient, and the ability to determine whether the patient has adequately understood and appreciated the information one has attempted to convey.

Knowledge of How to Proceed if a Patient Is Only Partially Competent or Incompetent to Consent to or Refuse Treatment

Physicians should know, and be able to apply to actual cases, criteria for judging when it is morally justified to treat or not to treat patients who are less than fully competent. (They should also know the relevant statutory law, if any, in their jurisdiction pertaining to the legal authority of next of kin and the use of proxy consents or refusals, and they should know the legal definition of competence in their state.)

One of the most common ethical problems encountered in medicine is having to make treatment decisions for the patient who is not fully competent. It is common and usually morally justifiable, if not always legally sanctioned, to involve the patient's next of kin in these decisions. Next of kin are usually willing to make a proxy valid consent or valid refusal of treatment. In the event that the next of kin refuse treatment for the patient, physicians should know when it is justified to accede to a refusal, when that is not justified, and when it is best for the physician to seek legal intervention. Physicians should also know how to proceed when no close relative is available.

Knowledge of How to Proceed if a Patient Refuses Treatment

Physicians should know, and be able to apply to actual cases, criteria for determining whether a patient's refusal is rational and therefore should be respected, and criteria for the moral justification for treating an unwilling patient. (They should also know how to proceed legally if they believe that forced treatment is morally justified.)

Another common moral dilemma that physicians encounter involves the partially or fully competent patient who refuses a suggested treatment. Sometimes the refusal seems rational to everyone concerned, and no difficult issue arises. But at other times the treatment may offer substantial benefits, and the patient may refuse for what appears to be no good reason. In some of these latter kinds of cases, it seems morally justified to treat the patient against his or her wishes. The physician should be able to determine whether treatment in the face of a refusal is morally justified and should know how to proceed legally in his or her jurisdiction when this situation arises.

The Ability to Decide When It Is Morally Justified to Withhold Information from a Patient

Physicians should know criteria for the morally justified withholding of information and be able to apply those criteria to actual cases. There are many situations in which physicians are tempted not to give a patient full information — for example, in discussing the risks of a proposed treatment, revealing the patient's prognosis, or disclosing whether the local treatment staff is experienced or inexperienced in carrying out a proposed treatment. In rare cases it may be morally justified to withhold such information, though in most cases it is not. The physician should know how to decide whether withholding is morally justified.

The Ability to Decide When It Is Morally Justified to Breach Confidentiality

Physicians should know criteria for the morally justified breaching of confidentiality and be able to apply those criteria to actual cases. (They should also know the law in their jurisdiction that states the circumstances under which a physician is permitted or required to breach confidentiality.)

There are occasional situations in which physicians are tempted to breach confidentiality, either to prevent harm to the patient or for the protection of some third party. Physicians should know criteria that help to determine when such a breach is morally justified. They should also know the relevant laws governing confidentiality in their jurisdiction.

Knowledge of the Moral Aspects of the Care of Patients with a Poor Prognosis, Including Patients Who Are Terminally Ill

Physicians should know how best to inform a patient about his or her poor prognosis or terminal illness. They should know with whom and when it is morally justified to discuss limiting some forms of treatment for a patient — for example, placing the patient on Do Not Resuscitate status — and when it is morally justified to forgo or discontinue a treatment, even though this action is likely or certain to result in a patient's death. (They should also know the laws in their state, if any, and the emerging local and national court opinions having to do with the discontinuation of lifesaving treatments.)

Caring for seriously or terminally ill patients is an area of medical practice that is permeated with ethical issues and, increasingly, with emerging statutory law and judicial opinion. Physicians should know and understand ethical concepts and principles sufficiently to manage this part of their practice. They should also have learned certain interactional skills, such as how to talk with a patient about his or her terminal illness

256   THE NEW ENGLAND JOURNAL OF MEDICINE   Jan. 24, 1985

or about the possibility of the patient's being placed on Do Not Resuscitate status. How to conduct these interviews as sensitively and humanely as possible should be taught no less assiduously than the more abstract material in medical ethics. It is also important for physicians to know and to keep abreast of relevant health law in this area. It may sometimes not be clear what the law would dictate in a particular case, and one may on occasion decide that what is morally justified or required is at variance with what the law seems to require, but one should always know, as far as one can, the status of the current law.

ADDITIONAL CURRICULAR TOPICS

There were two additional topics that some but not all of the group thought were essential in a basic curriculum. One was knowledge of issues in the equitable distribution of health care. There are several subtopics that could be taught under this general heading: (1) the nature of distributive justice; the responsibilities of the government, health policy makers, patients, and physicians in achieving equity in the distribution of health care; and the effects of the pursuit of equity on the physician's role; (2) patterns of access to health care in the United States and the nature of barriers to adequate health care; (3) alternative models for achieving a more equitable distribution of health care resources; and (4) the social effects of the different incentives for care givers that arise in different models of health-care organization and funding.

The majority of the group believed that at least some of these equity issues were as important as some of the first seven topics listed or even more important. This majority believed that many features of our system of health care distribution are unjust and that the resultant preventable harm is at least as great as that associated with individual physician–patient interactions. Furthermore, these members of the group thought that as medicine in this country inevitably enters an era of cost limitation, the role of the physician may partially change; for some physicians, for example, the problem of rationing may become the central ethical issue in clinical practice. A minority of the group thought that although these issues were of great social importance, they did not impinge on the behavior of most physicians to the same degree as earlier topics and were less essential to a basic curriculum.

The second topic that some members of the group thought should be added to the basic medical-ethics curriculum was abortion. The group was about evenly divided on the inclusion of this topic in the curriculum. One argument in favor of including it was simply that it would seem odd to exclude such an important current social topic from any course in medical ethics. Some also thought that certain issues that arose in the consideration of abortion (for example, when does a fetus become a person?) were applicable in other important areas of medical ethics (for example, when does a dying patient cease to be a person?). Those in the group who did not think it necessary to include abortion in the basic curriculum thought that too small a minority of physicians were concerned with the issue in their practice.

None of the group members who were not in favor of including the last two topics in the basic curriculum were opposed to their being taught by others who believed they should be included. The disagreement concerned only the topic's relative importance to the practice of the majority of physicians. There was also universal agreement that some specialized topics should be included in pertinent kinds of residency training: for example, issues concerning abortion should be taught in obstetrics and gynecology programs, just as the morality of involuntary hospitalization should be taught to psychiatry residents.

The field of medical ethics has seen a burgeoning of ideas and effort over the past two decades. Such a burgeoning can seem disparate and unfocused; the time seemed ripe to try to consolidate the clear gains. However, we also realize that it would be premature and ultimately deleterious for any group, even if it could, to attempt to impose anything resembling rigid standards on this exciting and expanding area of scholarship and clinical acumen. Our intention in publishing this report is to offer for discussion one group's conclusions and recommendations about what should be some of the subjects and goals of any basic curriculum in medical ethics.

Dartmouth Medical
  School
Hanover, NH 03755 CHARLES M. CULVER, M.D., PH.D.

Pennsylvania State University
  College of Medicine
Hershey, PA 16802   K. DANNER CLOUSER, PH.D.

Dartmouth College
Hanover, NH 03756   BERNARD GERT, PH.D.

Michigan State University
  College of Human Medicine
East Lansing, MI 48824   HOWARD BRODY, M.D., PH.D.

National Institutes of Health
Bethesda, MD 20205   JOHN FLETCHER, PH.D.

University of California,
  San Francisco, School of
  Medicine
San Francisco, CA 94143   ALBERT JONSEN, PH.D.

East Carolina University
  School of Medicine
Greenville, NC 27834   LORETTA KOPELMAN, PH.D.

George Washington University
  School of Medicine
Washington, DC 20037   JOANNE LYNN, M.D.

Pritzker School of Medicine
Chicago, IL 60637   MARK SIEGLER, M.D.

University of Wisconsin
  Center for Health Sciences
Madison, WI 53706   DANIEL WIKLER, PH.D.

This report was based on a conference held at Dartmouth College, July 21 to 24, 1983, and supported by the generosity of the Ira W. DeCamp Foundation.

**9.3   Lane LW, Siegler M, Miles SH, Cassel
         CK, Singer PA (1988) Fellowship
         Training Programs in Clinical Ethics.
         Soc Gen Intern Med Newsletter 3:4–5**

_____Innovations and Institutions_____

Fellowship Training Programs in Clinical Ethics

The Center for Clinical Medical Ethics was established in 1984 in the University of Chicago's Department of Medicine (Division of General Internal Medicine). The goal of the Center is to improve patient care through clinical service, teaching, research, community outreach, and training programs for physician-scholars. The Center focuses on the practical problems that patients and health professionals face in their everyday encounters. This emphasis distinguishes the Center from other ethics institutions whose approach is more theoretical and less clinical. The Center hopes to train a core of academic physicians in the discipline of clinical ethics with the expectation that their work will be both credible academically and beneficial to patients and colleagues. To this end, the Center has begun two unique training programs: The Henry J. Kaiser Family Foundation Fellowship in Clinical Medical Ethics (Kaiser Fellowship Program), and The National Leadership Training Program for Physicians in Clinical Medical Ethics (National Scholars Leadership Program).

The Kaiser Fellowship Program was started in 1985 and is a traditional post-residency fellowship that prepares young physicians for academic careers in clinical ethics. Fellows receive an annual stipend and support of $26,000. By 1989, this program will have trained 11 junior faculty.

The National Scholars Leadership Program, supported by the Pew Charitable Trusts and the Henry J. Kaiser Family Foundation, trains senior physicians, nominated by their deans, to become leaders of their medical schools' ethics activities. This program provides an initial year of in-residence training at the Center and three additional years of training with financial support at the physicians' home institutions. The National Scholars Leadership Program, started in July 1988, is currently training three physician-scholars and will recruit six additional scholars during the next two years. Trainees in this program receive a stipend and support allowance of $52,000 during their year at Chicago and their home institutions receive $15,000 per year for three additional years.

Methods of Training

Trainees in both programs work together and their studies consist of four essential training experiences: (1) a core curriculum taught by an interdisciplinary faculty; (2) ethics consultations and clinical experience on "high-risk" clinical services; (3) supervised research in clinical ethics; and (4) the opportunity to teach clinical ethics to students, physicians, and staff. In addition to the core curriculum for both groups of trainees, Kaiser fellows also receive individual academic and career guidance, and the senior scholars attend weekly meetings to discuss issues relating to program administration, development, and funding.

Core Curriculum in Clinical Ethics

Trainees participate in a 15-hour per week multidisciplinary core curriculum. This weekly curriculum consists of an interdisciplinary University seminar, a similar medical school seminar, a lecture series on medical ethics and the law, a reading course on bioethics, a weekly ethics consultation review conference, and a seminar on ethics and health policy. In addition to this core, trainees have access to any course taught at the University of Chicago.

The core curriculum is taught by the Center's faculty (Drs. Mark Siegler, Steven Miles, Christine Cassel, Arthur Rubenstein, John Lantos, and Professors Stephen Toulmin and Carol Stocking) and by a distinguished group of University of Chicago Scholars including Leon Kass (Committee on Social Thought), Robin Lovin and Martin Marty (Divinity School), Edward Laumann and James Coleman (Sociology), Richard Epstein (the Law School), Neil Harris (History), and Edward Lawlor (School of Social Service Administration).

The interdisciplinary University seminars provide an opportunity for clinical and nonclinical faculty to address compelling ethical questions facing medicine. The 1985 seminar series examined questions of causation, responsibility, and liability for bad outcomes in medicine (1). In 1986, in cooperation with the Committee on Public Policy Studies, the Center organized a program called "AIDS: The Social Context of Contagion." In 1987 the series addressed medical, legal, and political dimensions of active euthanasia. This year's seminars focus on conflicts arising between medical ethics and medical economics in the health care system.

Ethics Consultation and Clinical Experience

In addition to direct patient care, trainees gain experience in applying ethical principles to clinical practice in three ways: (1) through an ethics consultation experience; (2) by rotating on services that deal with a large number of clinical-ethical dilemmas; and (3) by participating in the deliberations of the University Hospital's Pediatric Ethics Committee and the Institution Review Board.

The department of medicine has developed an ethics consultation team that is staffed by the faculty and trainees of the Center. The ethics consultation service has been invited to see more than 100 cases since it began in 1986 and to offer suggestions to patients, families, nurses, and physicians. Each week, an ethics consultation conference is held in which clinicians and University Scholars review the cases seen by the ethics consultation service and critique the recommendations made by the consultants. In answering consultations and in reviewing the recommendations, trainees are given an opportunity to apply their clinical and analytic skills in real cases.

Trainees are also given an opportunity to rotate on clinical services that present a large number of complex ethical problems. These services include the medical ICU, the neonatal ICU, transplantation surgery, medical oncology, neurosurgery, high-risk obstetrics, general medicine, and geriatrics services.

Fellows gain insight into the functions of hospital ethics committees and the potential roles of physician-ethicists by participating on the Pediatric Ethics Committee and the University Hospital's Institutional Review Board.

Clinical Ethics Research

A primary goal of the Center is to demonstrate that good clinical research can help clarify many of the ethical dilemmas that trouble physicians, patients, and health care institutions. With assistance from the Center's faculty, trainees define and pursue data-based and analytic research projects in medical ethics.

Recent data-based projects in the Center have included a survey of orthopedic surgeons' attitudes and practices concerning the treatment of patients with HIV infection; a longitudinal study of the wishes of patients with amyotrophic lateral sclerosis for information about the course of their disease and their preferences for end-of-life care; a study of how attending and housestaff physicians variously interpret the meaning of orders not to resuscitate; a study of the survival of very-low-birth-weight babies after resuscitative efforts; and a study of ethical problems
continued on next page

continued from previous page

identified by physicians and nurses caring for the same patients at a community hospital. Members of the Center and faculty from the liver transplantation service wrote a paper on ethical issues in segmental liver transplantation that won the 1987 Nellie Westerman Prize for Research in Ethics awarded by the American Federation for Clinical Research (2).

The Center's commitment to clarifying the conceptual issues and research questions in clinical ethics is reflected in the activity and productivity of its faculty and trainees. Since 1985 its staff and trainees have published or have "in press" more than 10 books and major policy documents, 20 book chapters, and 100 medical journal articles and essays.

Clinical Ethics Teaching Experience

Trainees participate extensively in clinical ethics teaching activities at the University of Chicago-Pritzker School of Medicine. On the ethics consultation service, trainees provide information to housestaff, nurses, and attending physicians. Faculty and trainees of the Center also teach clinical ethics within the medical school and serve as important role models for the students. The four-year medical student program uses a case-based approach to ethics training and is intended to help future physicians develop the skills, moral reasoning abilities, and interpersonal qualities needed to respond to the moral issues arising in patient care.

Physicians who have completed the Center's training programs have been appointed to academic positions on medical school faculties. They have assumed responsibilities as ethics consultants, teachers, leaders of hospital ethics committees, administrators of ethics programs, and clinical ethics researchers. The three trainees currently participating in the National Scholars Leadership Program — Dr. Susan Tolle (University of Oregon), Dr. Jay Jacobson (University of Utah), and Dr. Douglas Kinsella (University of Calgary) — will develop programs in clinical ethics when they return to their home institutions.

The Center for Clinical Medical Ethics at the University of Chicago has developed two innovative training programs to prepare academic physicians as scholars and leaders in the field of clinical ethics. We believe these programs will ultimately improve patient care by teaching physicians and medical students to recognize and respond effectively to ethical problems as they arise in medical settings.

Laura Weiss Lane
Mark Siegler
Steven H. Miles
Christine K. Cassel
Peter A. Singer
Chicago, Illinois

References

1. Siegler M, Toulmin SE, Zimring FE, Schaffner KF, eds. *Medical Innovation and Bad Outcomes: Legal, Social, and Ethical Responses*. Ann Arbor, Michigan: University of Michigan - Health Administration Press; 1987.
2. Singer PA, Lantos JD, Whittington P, Broelsch C, Siegler M. Equipoise and the ethics of segmental liver transplantation. *Clin Res*. 1988;36:39-45.

**9.4   Walker RM, Lane LW, Siegler M (1989)
         Development of a Teaching Program
         in Clinical Medical Ethics
         at the University of Chicago. Acad
         Med 64:723–9**

ROBERT M. WALKER, M.D., LAURA WEISS LANE, M.D., and
MARK SIEGLER, M.D.

Development of a Teaching Program in Clinical Medical Ethics at the University of Chicago

Abstract—The University of Chicago Pritzker School of Medicine has developed and evaluated an extensive teaching program in clinical ethics coordinated primarily through the Center for Clinical Medical Ethics. The program provides medical students with a foundation in medical ethics during the four years of medical school and augments the clinical ethics knowledge and teaching skills of the housestaff and clinical faculty at the University of Chicago. Together, medical student teaching and clinical faculty development have made clinical ethics an integral part of medical education at the University of Chicago. Through these efforts, the teaching program aims to incorporate clinical ethics considerations into medical decisions and in this way contribute to improving patient care. (A detailed overview of all clinical ethics instruction at the school is provided.) *Acad. Med.* 64(1989):723–729.

During the past two decades, several medical ethicists have introduced the concept of "clinical medical ethics"[1-5] and suggested that the teaching of clinical ethics could serve as a useful complement to traditional teaching programs in medical ethics. Clinical ethics is a branch of biomedical ethics that focuses on the physician-patient interaction and concerns itself primarily with the ethics and value considerations that must be taken into account in reaching individual decisions with individual patients. The goal of clinical ethics is to improve the quality of patient care by teaching medical students and physicians to identify, analyze, and resolve ethical problems that arise frequently in the practice of medicine.

In 1976, when clinical ethics teaching was introduced to medical students at the University of Chicago Pritzker School of Medicine, it was built on a foundation of theoretical ethics. That foundation is provided in a required first-year course started in 1971 by professor James Gustafson (one of the early leaders in the American bioethics movement) and Dr. Chase Kimball (a psychiatrist and medical educator).[6] Today, the teaching program in applied clinical ethics continues to rely on the theoretical framework taught in the first-year course and on the contributions of professional ethicists (including philosophers, theologians, legal scholars, humanists, and others). But it also depends quite heavily on the development of clinical faculty (primarily physicians) as teachers and role models in clinical ethics. This report describes the evolution of the ethics teaching program at the University of Chicago both for medical students and for clinical faculty.

Program Concepts

The practical approach developed for teaching clinical ethics to medical students at Chicago was informed by the work of Sir William Osler, who described the importance of a clinical emphasis in medical teaching:

> In what may be called the natural method of teaching, the student begins with the patient, continues with the patient, and ends his study with the patient, using books and lectures as tools, as a means to an end. . . . For the junior student in medicine and surgery it is a safe rule to have no teaching without a patient for a text, and the best teaching is that taught by the patient himself.[7]

This concept influenced the development of the clinical ethics teaching program at Chicago, which emphasizes "5 C's" of teaching medical students:

1. Teaching should be *C*linically based.
2. Real patient *C*ases should serve as the teaching focus.
3. Teaching should be *C*ontinuous throughout the four years of medical school.
4. Ethics teaching should be *C*oordinated with the students' other learning objectives.
5. *C*linicians should participate actively in the teaching effort both as instructors and as role models for the students.

The fifth point must be emphasized because it has shaped the development of the Chicago program. It seemed essential that role-model clinicians become more involved in ethics teaching for the following reasons:

- Physicians have clinical and teaching credibility with students, house officers, and clinical colleagues.
- Physicians could teach ethics in

Dr. Walker is assistant professor of medicine and director, Division of Medical Ethics and Humanities, the University of South Florida College of Medicine, Tampa, and formerly was a fellow in clinical medical ethics at the Center for Clinical Medical Ethics, Pritzker School of Medicine of the University of Chicago; Dr. Lane is a house officer in the Department of Psychiatry, University of New Mexico Medical Center, Albuquerque, and formerly was the director of programs at the Center for Clinical Medical Ethics, Pritzker; and Dr. Siegler is director, Center for Clinical Medical Ethics, Pritzker.

Correspondence and requests for reprints should be addressed to Dr. Siegler at the Center for Clinical Medical Ethics, Box 72, University of Chicago Hospitals, 5841 South Maryland Avenue, Chicago, IL 60637.

the clinical setting by reference to their own actual clinical cases, which is similar to the way most other effective clinical teaching is done.

- Physicians could identify subtle and troubling clinical-ethical situations that might go unrecognized by those without clinical experience and without direct responsibility for patients.

- Physicians are responsible for resolving—rather than just for analyzing—the clinical-ethical problems they identify as they struggle to reach right and good decisions with their patients.

- Physicians could describe ethical dilemmas in clinical rather than philosophical language, which would be immediately understood by students and clinical colleagues.

- Physicians could also demonstrate ethically appropriate professional attitudes and values to students so that students could learn both from the formal teaching of clinical ethics and also from their teachers' modeling of ethical behavior and professional conduct.

- Eventually, we hoped such physician-teachers could help incorporate clinical-ethical considerations into the routine practice and teaching of medicine.

While the clinical ethics program at Chicago sought to involve physicians in teaching ethics to a greater degree than in the past, it was with the understanding that physicians and professional ethicists would complement each other. During the clinical training years, the physician would demonstrate to students the conscientious exercise of moral responsibility in the clinical setting, while the professional ethicist would continue to teach fundamental ethical theory during the preclinical years and would continue to serve as a resource (for example, in interdisciplinary team teaching) during the students' clinical training.[1]

Obstacles

In implementing clinical ethics teaching 13 years ago, two major obstacles were encountered that are not unique to the University of Chicago: a lack of curricular time for clinical ethics teaching and a lack of ethics training for clinicians.

Lack of Curricular Time

Two strategies were pursued to deal with the chronic problem of inadequate curricular time for clinical ethics teaching. First, such teaching was integrated into existing course structures by direct negotiations with course directors (in the basic science years) and with clinical chairmen (during the clinical years). Thus, our teaching efforts could proceed without ever asking the curriculum committee or the dean for formal curricular time.

Second, in the clinical years, teaching goals and methods were developed to be achievable even in the face of time constraints. These goals and methods included (1) having students read a short text in clinical ethics[3]; (2) encouraging students to learn a four-step decision-making strategy for reaching clinical-ethical decisions and to apply this strategy to actual patient cases[8,9]; (3) encouraging students to both read about and gain practical patient care experience with a select set of clinical ethics skills described in the DeCamp report[10]; and finally, (4) providing students with annotated bibliographies of readily accessible journal articles and books that could quickly assist them in learning more about clinical medical ethics.[11,12]

Lack of Ethics Training for Clinicians

Many clinicians, even those who are ethically sensitive and humanistic, feel that they have not been prepared adequately to teach clinical ethics to students and colleagues. Because of this, the teaching program in clinical ethics began to develop along two almost-parallel tracks, the first for medical students and the second for

clinicians (faculty and housestaff) who wished to become instructors in clinical ethics. Our hope was that these tracks eventually would intersect (preferably before infinity), so that the clinicians would be better prepared to serve as clinical ethics teachers and role models for medical students. The following paragraphs describe these two tracks, that, after 15 years, at last seem to be converging.

Teaching Medical Students

The goal of clinical ethics teaching for medical students is to promote the conceptual, affective, and moral reasoning skills that enable students to identify and respond appropriately to the ethics issues intrinsic to patient care. In 1976, clinical ethics teaching began in the third-year medicine clerkship with the introduction of 15 required ethics conferences. The conferences were initially taught by a multidisciplinary clinical faculty (that included a physician, a nurse, the hospital chaplain, a social worker, and the hospital attorney) and are currently taught by clinical ethicists. In each conference, student participants analyze one or more of their active patient cases, particularly ones that raise troubling ethics issues. The topics covered in the conferences vary according to actual student cases, but usually address ethics problems related to end-of-life care, truth-telling, confidentiality, patients refusing treatment, the economics of health care, family-patient disagreements, and the general issue of physicians' and students' responsibilities.

These conferences have been formally evaluated by students at the end of each clerkship cycle since 1976. In addition, objective and essay questions sometimes have been included as part of the students' final examination for the medicine clerkship. These evaluation methods help identify useful teaching approaches and provide knowledge of what students learn through the conferences.[13]

The effectiveness of the case-conference model is also reflected in its longevity and its extension to other clinical clerkships. After 13 years, the clinical ethics conferences remain a component of the third-year medicine clerkship. Moreover, faculty and chairmen of other major clinical departments have worked with the University of Chicago's Center for Clinical Medical Ethics (described later in this article) to introduce similar required conferences into their clinical clerkships. For the past six years, a ten-hour required clinical ethics course has been co-taught by one of us (MS) and senior surgeons during the surgery clerkship, and for the past four years, a six-hour required course has been integrated into the obstetrics-gynecology clerkship. In the coming year, we hope to extend this teaching program into the third-year clerkship of the Department of Psychiatry and to contribute to a long-standing clinical ethics course developed independently by the Department of Pediatrics.

In recent years, teaching in clinical ethics has been extended from its original base in the third-year curriculum and is now taught as part of the required curriculum in the first two years of medical school, and as an elective subject in the fourth.[14] (See Table 1.) During the first year, in addition to their philosophical ethics course, all students participate in a six-month interviewing course that emphasizes the patient's story as the key to understanding the patient's goals and values.[15,16] Also, several instructors in the first- and second-year basic science courses have included lectures and discussions that relate ethics and basic science considerations, for example, the legal and ethical implications of different levels of the patient's consciousness (neuroanatomy course), ethics issues related to new reproductive technologies (genetics course), and ethics concerns about animal experimentation and phase-one experiments in humans (pharmacology course).

In the second year, during the six-month history and physical diagnosis course, a variety of methods are used to address issues such as truth-telling, informed consent, confidentiality, medical error, impaired health professionals, and the responsibility of health professionals to care for

patients with acquired immunodeficiency syndrome (AIDS). The methods include lectures, films, and participation in small-group seminars and role-playing exercises. Finally, during the elective fourth year, students participate in additional ethics courses or in collaborative research projects with clinical ethics faculty.

Clinical ethics is taught throughout the four years by a large number of faculty, including medical school faculty, physician-ethicists from the Center for Clinical Medical Ethics, and nonclinical university faculty from the divinity school, law school, School of Public Policy, and the divisions of the humanities and social sciences. The Center for Clinical Medical Ethics (CCME) was established in 1984 in the Department of Medicine, Section of General Internal Medicine. It is a privately funded center devoted to clinical ethics education, research, and the training of physician-ethicists. The Center coordinates much of the teaching program in clinical ethics developed at the Pritzker School of Medicine. (See Table 1.) The core faculty of the CCME include physician-ethicists such as Christine Cassel, Steven Miles, and Mark Siegler, and prominent bioethics scholars such as Leon Kass, Martin Marty, and Stephen Toulmin.

CCME members who teach ethics in clinical settings are often assisted by clinicians who have participated in the Center's faculty development activities (see the following section). These clinicians complement students' theoretical knowledge of ethics by adding a clinical perspective to ethics deliberations. More important, they demonstrate clinical ethics decision-making skills in case discussions and at the bedside, thereby reinforcing the importance of ethics considerations in caring for patients.

Teaching Faculty and House Officers

During the past ten years, several approaches have been used to develop the clinical ethics expertise and teaching abilities of clinicians who demonstrate an interest in clinical

ethics. Approximately 50 attending physicians and at least as many house officers have become seriously involved with one or more faculty development efforts in ethics. Further, many of these clinician-educators have used the knowledge they have acquired to teach clinical ethics to medical students. Each of the approaches to faculty development (described below) begins with the assumption that faculty are very busy and that they will get involved only in activities that are personally interesting, useful, or rewarding.

The same, of course, can be said for busy house officers. Even though the clinical ethics program has been aimed primarily at teaching medical students and clinical faculty, we have reached interested house officers through both of these teaching efforts; some house officers join us for student teaching sessions (particularly when their own patients are being discussed) and some participate in faculty development activities. The variety of clinical ethics activities at the University of Chicago Pritzker School of Medicine makes it likely that most house officers will become involved in the program during their training.

Four major approaches have been used to help faculty (and house officers) develop skills as clinical ethics teachers: collaborative clinical ethics teaching; joint participation in direct patient care through ethics consultations; interdisciplinary ethics seminars; and collaborative clinical ethics research and writing projects.

Collaborative Clinical Ethics Teaching

Many of the collaborative or team teaching activities take place during the third-year clinical clerkships in surgery, obstetrics-gynecology, and internal medicine. These teaching interventions, while chiefly for the benefit of students, are extremely helpful for the faculty as well. Ethicists learn of the specific problems faced by different clinical specialties; clinicians work with ethicists in analyzing and discussing their cases; and students learn that their clinical role models

Table 1

An Overview of the Four-Year Curriculum Involving Clinical Ethics, University of Chicago, Pritzker School of Medicine, 1989

Course or Intervention	Teaching Methods	Examples of Topics	Principal Faculty
First year (required hours)			
Orientation session (1–3 hours)	Presentation or videotape with lunchtime discussion	Medical student experience; doctor-patient relationship; ethical issues in medicine	Physician-ethicists
Clinical orientation program (36–72 hours)	Interview demonstrations; presentations and lectures; large and small-group discussions; readings	Doctor-patient relationship; clinical decision making; interpersonal skills; sensitivity to patient experiences	Internal medicine faculty, physician-ethicists, multidisciplinary faculty
Introduction to the Patient (15–20 hours)	Interviewing and interpersonal skills; small-group discussions; observation of student-patient interactions	Doctor-patient relationship; sensitivity to patient experiences; techniques of interviewing	Psychiatry faculty
Social and Ethical Issues in Medicine (30 hours)	Large-group presentations followed by small-group discussions; extensive readings; case discussions	Philosophical bioethics; euthanasia; abortion; research ethics; health and economics; legal issues	Psychiatry faculty, multidisciplinary faculty, physician-ethicists
Introduction to Psychiatry (20 hours)	Large-group presentations; patient interviews; demonstrations	Psychiatry; interview and interpersonal skills; physician impairment; treating cognitively impaired patients	Psychiatry faculty
Electives or research in clinical ethics	Independent and collaborative research; seminars and reading; individual guidance	See "fourth year" and in the article, "Collaborative clinical ethics research and writing projects"	Physician-ethicists, affiliated faculty
Participation in basic science curriculum (4–12 hours)	Team-taught lectures; seminars; small-group discussions	Use of the human body; genetic screening; HIV issues; health care economics; human experimentation	Basic science faculty, clinical faculty, physician-ethicists
Second year (required hours)			
Summer research program (12-week program for 2–6 students; research stipend provided)	Independent and collaborative research; seminars and reading; individual guidance	See "fourth year" and, in the article, "Collaborative clinical ethics research and writing projects"	Physician-ethicists, affiliated faculty
Introduction to Clinical Medicine (70 lecture hours; 40 small group hours; 120–200 interviewing hours)	Formal lectures; specialty small-group supervision; interview demonstrations; extensive history-taking experiences; communication and interpersonal skills; multidisciplinary sessions; DeCamp clinical-ethical skill areas	Preparation for patient care; sensitization to patient experiences; clinical ethical decision making; doctor-patient relationship; HIV issues; impaired physicians; legal issues; student experiences; professional ethics	Internal medicine faculty, surgery faculty, physician-ethicists, affiliated faculty
Electives/research in clinical ethics	Independent and collaborative research; seminars and reading; individual guidance	See "fourth year" and, in the article, "Collaborative clinical ethics research and writing projects"	Physician-ethicists, affiliated faculty
Participation in basic science curriculum (4–12 hours)	Team-taught lectures; seminars; small-group discussions	Use of the human body; Genetic screening; HIV issues; health care economics; human experimentation	Basic science faculty, clinical faculty, physician-ethicists

Table 1 — *Continued*

Course or Intervention	Teaching Methods	Examples of Topics	Principal Faculty
Third year			
Medicine rotation (14–20 hours)	Presentation of students own patient cases; formulation of clinical ethical concerns; DeCamp skill areas; extensive readings in the ethics literature	Caring for patients with terminal illness; consent; truth-telling; HIV issues; health care economics; confidentiality; legal issues; student roles/experiences	Internal medicine faculty, physician-ethicists, multidisciplinary faculty
Surgery rotation (8–16 hours)	Case presentations by surgeons and students; case discussions; readings	Consent and the surgical patient; HIV issues; ethical issues in breast surgery; trauma surgery; poor outcome	Surgery faculty, physician-ethicists, anesthesiology faculty
Obstetrics-gynecology rotation (2–6 hours)	Case presentations by students; case discussions; readings	Reproductive ethics; terminal illness; treatment of minors; socioeconomic issues in health care; HIV issues	Obstetrics-gynecology faculty, physician-ethicists
Pediatrics rotation (4–6 hours)	Presentations by faculty and students; case discussions; readings	Care of infants and children; reproductive ethics; socioeconomic factors in health care; legal issues	Pediatrics faculty, physician-ethicists, social work faculty
Fourth year (elective)			
Research in clinical medical ethics	Independent and collaborative research	Student-designed projects involving any topic in other courses	CCME faculty, clinical faculty
Readings in clinical medical ethics	Assigned material is read by a group; a discussion leader conducts weekly sessions	Extensive reading in periodical literature; essential bioethics texts; works from philosophy and humanities	CCME faculty, multidisciplinary faculty
University courses in ethics and health policy	Lectures; small-group discussions; papers	Health care delivery to the poor; HIV and health policy; health policy and ethics; medical ethics and the law	CCME faculty, multidisciplinary faculty

regard ethics discussions as an integral part of patient care rather than as an activity reserved for ethics experts. The ethics discussions begin in the classroom, and similar discussions continue on the wards, where the attending physicians, house officers, and students can apply what they have learned to the care of their patients.

Ethics Consultations

The CCME's ethics consultation service was started in 1985 with the primary purpose of helping faculty, housestaff, and students address the recurring ethics problems they encounter in caring for patients. To date, the clinical ethics consultation team has been invited to participate in more than 200 cases from many clinical departments in the University of Chicago Hospitals. Physician-ethicists from the CCME respond to consultation requests from attending physicians and try to assist them in understanding and resolving clinical-ethics dilemmas.[17,18] The clinical faculty learn through individual discussions with the consultant, through formal consultation notes in the patient's medical record, and through reading pertinent clinical ethics literature (provided by the consultant). In addition, all consultations are reviewed at a weekly interdisciplinary ethics consultation conference, which is attended by the individuals who requested the consultation and by physicians, attorneys, social workers, nurses, and philosophers.

Our group conducted a prospective evaluation of the ethics consultation service by distributing a questionnaire to 51 physicians who had requested a consultation. All the physicians completed their questionnaires; in 36 cases (71%), the requesting physician stated that the consultation was very important in patient management, in clarifying ethics issues, or in learning about medical ethics. Forty-nine of the physicians (96%) indicated that they planned to request another ethics consultation in the future.[18] Based on these evaluations, we regard the ethics consultation service as an effective approach to faculty and housestaff education in clinical ethics.

Interdisciplinary Ethics Seminars for Faculty

For the past seven years, two types of interdisciplinary ethics seminars — involving physicians, legal scholars, philosophers, theologians, and social scientists — have been a vital part of the Center's faculty development effort. The first type of seminar is university-wide and meets monthly for an entire academic year to discuss a topic of general interest to faculty participants. In recent years, some of the topics have been the physician's legal and ethical responsibilities when unanticipated bad outcomes occur after innovative therapy; the medical and political dimensions of the AIDS epidemic; euthanasia; the relationship of medical ethics to economics; and the doctor–patient relationship. These seminars have been especially well attended by both university faculty and medical school faculty.

The second faculty seminar in ethics is primarily oriented toward the clinical faculty of the medical school. In these medical school seminars, which meet weekly throughout the academic year, physicians and scientists are invited to describe their clinical and research activities and to indicate what ethics difficulties they encounter in their own work (for example, in transplantation surgery, innovative therapies for children, cancer treatment programs, research in emergency care, and other areas). The clinician's presentation then serves as the stimulus for discussion by seminar participants. Over the years, participants at these seminars have heard presentations from more than 75 different clinicians and investigators about the ethics dimen-

sions of their own work. The seminars help clinicians and clinical investigators clarify the ethical issues they encounter, improve their ability to teach ethics to students, and often lead them to collaborate with members of the CCME on ethics-related research and writing projects.

Collaborative Clinical Ethics Research and Writing Projects

The most effective approach to faculty development is realized when clinicians and clinical ethicists identify and work together on clinical ethics research or writing projects that lead to publication, and occasionally, to grant proposals. These collaborative projects require that all participants become extremely knowledgeable about the ethics literature and about the ethical aspects of their work. Often, the stimulus for these joint projects can be traced back to other interactions between clinicians and clinical ethicists, including joint teaching, faculty seminars, and ethics consultations. In recent years, members of the CCME have engaged in joint research and writing efforts with more than 25 clinicians from many specialties, including orthopedics,[19] neurology,[20] neonatology,[21] radiation oncology,[22] transplantation surgery,[23,24] pediatric hepatology,[23,24] pediatric endocrinology,[25] cardiology,[26] family practice,[27] and dentistry.[28] Clinicians participating in these projects have brought their new knowledge of clinical ethics to patient care situations and to their teaching encounters with students and housestaff.

Training Academic Physician-Ethicists

Faculty and leaders at many medical schools have been eager to develop greater expertise in clinical ethics. However, there are few physicians prepared to serve as leaders and developers of clinical ethics programs. This realization led to the development of two training programs to prepare physicians for academic careers

that combine clinical practice with research and teaching in medical ethics. With support from the Henry J. Kaiser Family Foundation and the Pew Charitable Trusts, these training programs (which have been described elsewhere)[29] were begun in 1985. By June 1990, the Center will have trained more than 20 physicians to serve as academic clinical ethicists in medical schools. By then, graduates of the training programs will direct or codirect ethics activities at many medical schools, including the Medical College of Wisconsin, the University of South Florida, the Oregon Health Sciences University, the University of Calgary; the University of Toronto; the University of Utah; the University of Cincinnati; West Virginia University; the University of California, Irvine; and Indiana University. The importance of these physician-ethicist trainees for medical students, housestaff, and clinical faculty at the University of Chicago is that the trainees participate in all of the CCME's clinical ethics teaching activities. In doing so, they extend the Center's ability to teach clinical ethics to medical students, clinical faculty, and housestaff.

The Future

As we look ahead, the major challenge facing the clinical ethics teaching program at the Pritzker School of Medicine is to demonstrate its importance for students and patients. Currently, the CCME evaluates the school's program in several ways: by attitude-survey questionnaires of students and faculty, the defining issues test,[30] and other formal evaluation efforts[13,14,17,18]; and through traditional methods of peer review (including journal publications and grant support). However, the future challenges us to show more clearly that the inclusion of clinical ethics considerations into doctor-patient decision making can improve patient care, patient satisfaction, and health outcomes, and that student and faculty education in clinical ethics can contribute to these improvements.

The authors thank the Andrew W. Mellon Foundation, the Pew Charitable Trusts, the Henry J. Kaiser Family Foundation, and the Ira W. DeCamp Foundation, who support the Center for Clinical Medical Ethics. They also thank Christine Cassel, M.D., Richard Epstein, J.D., Leon Kass, M.D., Ph.D., Thomas Krizek, M.D., John Lantos, M.D., Edward Laumann, Ph.D., Jane McAtee, J.D., Martin Marty, Ph.D., Steven Miles, M.D., Ralph Muller, Arthur Rubenstein, M.D., Carol Stocking, Ph.D., and Stephen Toulmin, Ph.D. The views expressed in this paper are those of the authors and do not necessarily represent those of the supporting foundations.

References

1. Siegler, M. A Legacy of Osler: Teaching Clinical Ethics at the Bedside. *JAMA* **239**(1978):951–956.
2. Pellegrino, E. D. Ethics and the Moment of Clinical Truth. *JAMA* **239**(1978): 960–961.
3. Jonsen, A. R., Siegler, M., and Winslade, W. J. *Clinical Ethics: A Practical Approach to Ethical Decisions in Clinical Medicine.* 2nd ed. New York: Macmillan, 1986.
4. Kass, L. R. Ethical Dilemmas in the Care of the Ill: I. What is the Physician's Service? II. What is the Patient's Good? *JAMA* **244**(1980):1811–1816; 1946–1949.
5. Toulmin, S. How Medicine Saved the Life of Ethics. *Perspect. Biol. Med.* **25**(1982): 736–750.
6. Gustafson J. M., Kimball, C. P., Tighe, P. Teaching Medical Ethics. *Medicine on the Midway* [University of Chicago alumni magazine] **30**(no. 2, 1975):16–21.
7. Osler, W. On the Need of a Radical Reform in Our Methods of Teaching Medical Students. *Med. News.* **82**(1903):49–53.
8. Siegler, M. Decision-Making Strategy for Clinical Ethical Problems in Medicine.

Arch. Intern. Med. **142**(1982):2178–2179.
9. Thomasma, D. C. Training in Medical Ethics: An Ethical Workup. *Forum on Med.* **1**(1978):33–36.
10. Clouser, K. D. et al. Basic Curricular Goals in Medical Ethics. *N. Engl. J. Med.* **312**(1985):253–256.
11. Ad Hoc Committee on Medical Ethics. American Colleges of Physicians Ethics Manual. *Ann. Intern. Med.* **101**(1984): 129–137; 263–274.
12. Siegler, M. Singer, P. A., and Schiedermayer, D. L. *Medical Ethics: An Annotated Bibliography.* Philadelphia, Pennsylvania: American College of Physicians, 1988.
13. Siegler, M. Rezler, A. G., and Connel, K. J. Using Simulated Case Studies to Evaluate a Clinical Ethics Course for Junior Students. *J. Med. Educ.* **57**(1982):380–385.
14. Lane, L. W. Clinical Ethics Training at the University of Chicago Pritzker School of Medicine. Report of the Center for Clinical Medical Ethics, University of Chicago (unpublished), 1988.
15. Coles, R. *The Call of Stories: Teaching and the Moral Imagination.* Boston, Massachusetts: Houghton Mifflin, 1989.
16. Kleinman, A. *The Illness Narratives: Suffering, Healing and the Human Condition.* New York: Basic Books, 1988.
17. La Puma, J. Consultation Clinical Ethics: Issues and Questions in 27 Cases. *West. J. Med.* **146**(1987):633–637.
18. La Puma, J., Stocking, C. B., Silverstein, M. D., DiMartini, A., and Siegler, M. Evaluation and Utilization of an Ethics Consultation Service. *JAMA* **260**(1988):808–811.
19. Arnow, P. M. Pottenger, L. A., Stocking, C. B., Siegler, M., and DeLeeuw, H. W. Orthopedic Surgeons' Attitudes and Practices Concerning Treatment of Patients with HIV Infection. *Pub. Health Rep.* **104** (1989):121–129.
20. Stocking, C. B., Silverstein, M.D., Siegler, M., and Antel, J. A Prospective Study of

ALS Patients' Knowledge, Attitudes and Decisions about Life-Sustaining Therapy. *Clin. Res.* **34**(1986):837A.
21. Lantos, J. D., Miles, S. H., Silverstein, M.D., and Stocking, C. B. Survival after Cardiopulmonary Resuscitation in Babies of Very Low Birth Weight: Is CPR Futile Therapy? *N. Engl. J. Med.* **318**(1988): 91–95.
22. Singer, P. A., et al. Sex or Survival? The Role of Patient Preference in Choosing Treatment for Prostate Cancer. *Clin. Res.* **37**(1989):326A.
23. Singer, P. A., Lantos, J. D., Whitington, P. F., Broelsch, C. E., and Siegler, M. Equipoise and the Ethics of Segmental Liver Transplantation. *Clin. Res.* **36**(1988): 539–545.
24. Singer, P. A. et al. Ethics of Liver Transplantation Using Live Donors. *N. Eng. J. Med.* **321**(1989):620–622B.
25. Lantos, J. D. Siegler, M., and Cuttler, L. Ethical Issues in Growth Hormone Therapy. *JAMA* **261**(1989):1020–1024.
26. Grim, P. S., et al. Informed Consent in Emergency Research: Prehospital Thrombolytic Therapy for Acute Myocardial Infarction. *JAMA* **262**(1989):252–255.
27. Walker, R. M., Miles, S. H., Stocking, C. B., and Siegler, M. A Prospective Study of Ethical Problems Identified by Physicians and Nurses on General Medical Services. *Clin. Res.* **36**(1988):719A.
28. Siegler, M., Bresnahan, J. F. Schiedermayer, D. L, and Roberson, P. Exploring the Future of Clinical Ethics. *J. Am. Coll. Dent.* **56**(1989):13–15.
29. Lane, L. W., Siegler, M., Miles, S. H., Cassel, C. K., and Singer, P. A. Fellowship Training Programs in Clinical Ethics. *SGIM* [Society for General Internal Medicine] *Newsletter* **3**(1989):4–5.
30. Rest, J. R. A Psychologist Looks at the Teaching of Ethics. *Hastings Center Rep.* **12**(1982):29–36.

**9.5   Jacobson JA, Tolle SW, Stocking C,
         Siegler M (1989) Internal Medicine
         Residents' Preferences
         Regarding Medical Ethics Education.
         Acad Med 64:760–4**

Internal Medicine Residents' Preferences Regarding Medical Ethics Education

JAY A. JACOBSON, M.D., SUSAN W. TOLLE, M.D., CAROL STOCKING, Ph.D., and MARK SIEGLER, M.D.

Abstract—Three hundred and twenty-three residents in six internal medicine programs in three states were surveyed concerning what they wanted to learn about medical ethics and how they would prefer to learn it; they were also asked to indicate what medical ethics education they had already received. Specifically, the residents were given a list of 35 medical ethics topics and asked to indicate whether they would like more attention to a topic, or whether it had received enough or too much attention. (They could also indicate that they thought the topic was inappropriate for attention during residency.) The residents were also given a list of 17 teaching methods for medical ethics and asked to indicate whether each method was very useful, somewhat useful, or not useful. Sixty-one percent of the residents responded. Approximately three-fourths of these had had some formal teaching about medical ethics in both medical school and residency, and nearly all indicated that they wanted more ethics training on specific topics. Certain topics were chosen as particularly suitable or unsuitable for such training; many of those judged as deserving more attention concerned legal issues and end-of-life issues. Most of the responding residents regarded standard clinical teaching formats as very useful for learning about medical ethics but regarded several other methods as not useful. The authors discuss the implications of these and related findings. *Acad. Med.* 64(1989):760–764.

Internal medicine residency is an opportune and appropriate time to teach medical ethics,[1-6] but just what to teach to residents and how to teach it remain perplexing questions. Striking variations in the residents' prior experience with ethics,[7,8] new issues arising from rapid changes in medicine, and compelling clinical demands on their time make it essential to choose topics that residents regard as important and methods that are efficient and effective.

To discover what residents want to learn about medical ethics and how they would prefer to learn it, we conducted a questionnaire survey of residents in six training programs in three states. Our principal objective was to provide program directors and ethics educators with a list of subject areas that most residents wanted to learn more about and methods of teaching that residents indicated would be most effective.

Method

We surveyed residents from six internal medicine programs: The University of Chicago and the Evanston Hospital in Illinois, the University of Utah and the LDS Hospital in Salt Lake City, Utah, and the Oregon Health Sciences University and the Good Samaritan Hospital in Portland, Oregon. We selected three university programs and three private affiliated programs. The program directors or the chief residents notified the house staff about our survey and encouraged them to participate. In February 1989, we distributed a six-page questionnaire about medical ethics education to the 332 residents in these programs. A second mailing to nonrespondents was sent in April 1989.

The 35 medical ethics topics we asked the residents about were similar to those used in a previous survey of physicians and those mentioned in the DeCamp report.[3,5] The residents we surveyed could indicate whether they would like more attention to a topic, or whether it had received enough or too much attention. They could also indicate that they thought the topic was inappropriate for attention during residency. The 17 teaching methods we offered for consideration were those discussed in the DeCamp Report or described by other educators.[9-13] The residents we surveyed were asked to indicate whether each method was very useful, somewhat useful, or not useful. Residents were also asked to indicate what medical ethics education they had received in medical school and during their residency periods.

We assured residents that their responses would be confidential and that only aggregated data would be reported. The design of the study and the questionnaire were approved by the Institutional Review Board at the University of Chicago Pritzker School of Medicine.

Results

Of the 332 residents, 202 (61%) returned their questionnaires by May 12, 1989. The sizes of their programs ranged from 33 to 77 residents, and

Dr. Jacobson and Dr. Tolle were visiting scholars, Center for Clinical Medical Ethics, Pritzker School of Medicine, University of Chicago, Chicago, Illinois, at the time of the study. Dr. Jacobson is chief, Division of Medical Ethics, LDS Hospital and University of Utah Department of Medicine in Salt Lake City, Utah; Dr. Tolle is director, Center for Ethics in Health Care, Oregon Health Sciences University, Portland, Oregon. Dr. Stocking is director of research and Dr. Siegler is director, Center for Clinical Medical Ethics, Pritzker School of Medicine.

Correspondence and requests for reprints should be addressed to Dr. Jacobson, Division of Medical Ethics, LDS Hospital, 8th Avenue and C St., Salt Lake City, UT 84143.

the response rates varied by program from 52 to 75%. Overall, 65% of the sample were men and 62% of the respondents were men. The average age of the residents was 30 years. They were approximately equally divided in terms of years of training: 37% were in their first year, 30% in their second year, and 30% in their third year. In two programs, approximately 60% of the responses came from first-year trainees. The 162 residents who identified their medical schools had graduated from 79 U.S. medical schools.

Seventy-two percent of the residents had had at least one formal course about medical ethics in medical school, usually during the preclinical years; 97% recalled some informal education about ethics as well. A majority in each program and 74% overall said they had received medical ethics teaching during their residencies (range, 57–90%). There was no significant difference in the answers to this question by the residents' years of training.

The residents' preferences about ethics topics and how to teach them are shown in Tables 1 and 2. Surprisingly, the responses regarding topics did not differ significantly between those who had had no formal ethics course in medical school and those who had had one or more. With two exceptions, the distribution of responses did not vary significantly by the residents' years of training. The first-year residents were more likely than their more senior colleagues to want more teaching about withholding life support (80% versus 64%, chi-square = 6.077, df = 2, $p = .05$), and the more senior residents more often wanted additional information about laws related to physician-patient relations (84% versus 71%, chi-square = 5.81, df = 2, $p = .055$).

Nineteen topics merit more attention, according to a majority or plurality of residents in the survey. No topic was judged to have received too much attention by more than 5% of respondents, and no topic was felt to be inappropriate by more than 13%.

Table 1 shows the 11 topics identified by 50% or more of the residents in each program as needing more at-

tention. The list suggests that residents are particularly interested in learning more about laws and decisions related to end-of-life issues and about problems of access to health care and allocation of resources.

Table 1 also contains 17 topics selected by a majority of residents in at least one program, but not by all, as needing more attention. Distributions of the responses by program differed significantly for six topics: role of an ethics consultant, functions of ethics committees, conflict resolution between resident and attending physician and conflict resolution between doctors and patients, and the family's and the patients roles in decision making (chi − square > 31.7, df = 15, $p < .01$).

Only seven topics were judged not to need more attention by a majority of residents in any program. Only four topics were considered inappropriate by at least 10% of all respondents: making admission or treatment decisions based on ability to pay, experimentation on human subjects, religious views on ethical questions, and euthanasia.

The residents' responses about the usefulnesses of various teaching methods are shown in Table 2. Although there was variation between programs, several methods were fairly strongly endorsed or rejected. Four methods were judged very useful by a majority of residents: several conferences on ethics, several lectures or grand rounds, incorporation of these issues in other presentations and discussions, and discussion with colleagues and a knowledgeable discussion leader. Only two methods were regarded as not useful by more than 50%: watching a self-instructive videotape about an ethical issue and a reading course based on novels.

Discussion

Our survey showed that most of the residents had had some medical ethics education in medical school,[7,8] that 74% also had had it during their residencies, and that nearly all wanted more ethics training in specific areas. Most regarded standard

clinical teaching formats as very useful for learning about medical ethics, but they regarded several other methods as not useful.

A majority of respondents from each program we surveyed indicated that they had had some formal teaching about ethics during their residencies. This high prevalence of ethics education may not be representative of all U.S. programs. In a 1984 survey, 40% of internal medicine residencies provided no formal exposure to medical ethics.[14] Despite some ethics education during residency, most of our respondents indicated that they would like more. These results parallel those of several earlier surveys of residents and practicing physicians.[15,16] Three conclusions, then, can be drawn from our survey.

First, residents, including those with prior exposure to teaching about medical ethics, appear receptive to more medical ethics education. However, how much time should be spent on medical ethics was not addressed in our survey.

Second, despite variations in their prior experiences and differences between their residency programs, a majority of respondents from each program chose 11 topics that they would like to learn more about. These clustered in the areas of laws and practices related to limiting life-support systems, allocation of resources, and access to medical care. Our respondents' interest in these subjects was keener than that of physicians in an earlier survey.[5] This may be because, as residents, they confront end-of-life decisions more often than many practicing physicians do and because physicians in general are more concerned today about economic issues and legal risk than they were in 1982. However, even topics not cited by most residents as meriting more attention might be of considerable interest and importance to individual residents because of their particular circumstances.

Third, some topics may be particularly well or poorly suited for individual programs. Several of the differences we encountered among programs regarding specific topics are

Table 1

Percentages of 202 Residents in Six Internal Medicine Residency Programs* Who Reported They Wanted More Attention Given to Instruction on Each of 37 Topics in Medical Ethics, 1989

Topic	% of All Respondents	Range of % by Program
Selected by 50% or more of residents in all programs		
Laws related to withdrawal of life support	84	71–95
Laws related to physician-patient relations	80	71–90
Withdrawing life-supporting treatment	75	58–88
Living wills and advance directives	73	61–95
Allocation of limited resources related to diagnosis or prognosis	73	50–86
Government policy regarding access to medical care	73	61–80
Withholding life-supporting treatment	70	52–80
Understanding rights of incompetent patients	64	53–74
Euthanasia	63	50–75
Incompetent or impaired colleagues	62	55–85
Priority for scarce organs	61	50–75
Selected by 50% or more of residents in one or more, but not all, programs		
Making admission or treatment decisions based on ability to pay	60	43–85
Selection of transplant recipients	56	34–72
Requesting organ donation	54	45–72
Do not rescitate orders	51	42–60
Withholding information from patients	49	34–63
Role of an ethics consultant†	49	16–85
Experimentation on human subjects	48	30–55
Religious views on ethical questions	45	26–80
How to care for and communicate with a dying patient	47	34–67
Functions of ethics committees†	46	26–80
How to cope with death of patient	44	36–57
Conflict resolution between resident and attending†	42	25–60
Conflict resolution between doctors and nurses	42	28–55
Conflict resolution between doctors and patients†	40	31–50
Nursing ethics	39	16–75
Confidentiality	38	22–54
Physician's conflict of interest: financial advantage versus patient welfare	34	11–50
Not selected by 50% or more of residents in any program		
Family's role in decision making†	32	10–46
Patient's role in decision making†	30	13–40
Informed consent	35	24–45
Physician's obligations to patients	34	22–45
Personal values versus patient's values	33	19–43
Guidance on expression of compassion	30	16–45
Physician's role in decision making	26	13–40

*The six programs (one in Chicago and one in Evanston, Illinois; two in Salt Lake City, Utah; and two in Portland, Oregon) had a total of 332 residents.

†Significant difference between programs, $p < .01$.

explainable and instructive. Residents at a program with a widely discussed policy regarding admission of indigent patients were less likely than others to want more attention paid to making admission or treatment decisions based on ability to pay.

Likewise, many house officers at a program with an active medical ethics consultation service desired less additional information about the role of an ethics consultant. Most residents

at a program with a newly established ethics committee, which included house staff members, indicated that they wanted more education about the function of that committee. Thus, in a particular program, awareness of issues, of the resources available, and of the frequency with which particular problems arise should help predict which topics residents would like to learn more about. A survey similar to ours could be used by an individual

program to plan its curriculum.

While our survey records residents' preferences for learning about ethical problems, it does not describe the types of ethical problems physicians encounter or their frequencies. These are important considerations for curriculum planning, and other studies have examined them.[17–20] Physicians surveyed in 1982 reported that the four most common issues they confronted were compassion, truth-tell-

Table 2

Percentages of 202 Residents in Six Internal Medicine Residency Programs* Who Rated as "Very Useful" Each of 17 Methods for Teaching Medical Ethics, 1989

Teaching Method	% of All Respondents	Range of % by Program
Several conferences on ethics†	57	33–76
Incorporation of these issues in other presentations and discussions†	57	30–78
Several lectures or grand rounds on ethics†	55	24–83
Discuss these subjects with colleagues and knowledgeable discussion leader	53	36–59
Calling on ethics consultation†	45	6–63
Special lecture course on ethics†	42	12–67
Observing attending physicians handle ethical problems with patient	40	15–56
Bringing problems to the attention of an ethics committee†	37	6–60
Independent reading	34	27–47
Discuss ethical issues with colleagues	32	23–48
Discuss ethical issues with hospital attorney	30	20–35
Workshops at professional meetings	30	15–41
An ethics manual	29	9–45
Reading aided by annotated bibliography	29	24–36
Discussing a videotape about an ethical issue with knowledgeable discussion leader	19	9–25
A reading course based on novels	9	5–16
Watching self-instructive videotape	8	0–11

*The six programs (one in Chicago and one in Evanston, Illinois; two in Salt Lake City, Utah; and two in Portland, Oregon) had a total of 332 residents. They rated the teaching methods on a Likert-type scale.

†Significant differences between programs, $p < .01$.

ing, patient's role in decision making, and obtaining informed consent.[5] On a medical inpatient service, sensitized residents most often identified as problems withholding tests or treatment, informed consent, truth-telling, relationships among physicians, and limited resources.[1] All of these problems, except informed consent, were among those categorized most often in our survey as suitable for more attention.

Our survey provides some helpful information about methods for teaching ethics. The residents clearly rejected watching instructional videotapes by themselves or reading novels, but they were not asked specifically about other uses of videotapes or about reading shorter pieces of literature. The majority of residents favored the methods by which they learn about the rest of clinical medicine. This may be because they have little experience with some of the other methods included in our survey. We do not believe that the survey results argue convincingly against using these techniques, especially in view of the wide variation in responses by program. The results, however, suggest that conventional methods, available at nearly all pro-

grams, may be quite acceptable for medical ethics teaching. Other, innovative methods not listed in our survey may also be useful.[11]

Several internal medicine departments have already described the contents and methods they are using in their ethics programs[9-13] and others do so in this issue of *Academic Medicine*. Barnard has called attention to other, perhaps neglected dimensions of medical ethics.[21]

Although the response rate of residents to our survey was better than the rate achieved in similar surveys,[5] the number of nonrespondents, the lack of information about whether they differed significantly from respondents, and the non-random selection of programs preclude broad generalizations from our results. The age and gender distributions of our participating residents, for example, are similar to those of internal medicine residents in the United States, but our survey included no acknowledged foreign medical graduates. Nevertheless, we think · the results provide some guidance, especially for programs similar to the ones we studied.

We hope our survey of residents' preferences combined with the obser-

vations, recommendations, and curricular innovations of others will help faculty provide the kind of medical ethics education that most residents seem eager to receive.

The authors thank the program directors, house staff coordinators, chief medical residents, and especially the residents themselves, for their cooperation and participation in this study; and Thelma Davis for helping in the conduct of the study. The work of the Center for Clinical Medical Ethics is supported by The Henry J. Kaiser Family Foundation, The Pew Charitable Trusts, and the Andrew W. Mellon Foundation.

References

1. Lo, B., Schroeder, M. D. Frequency of Ethical Dilemmas in a Medical Inpatient Service. *Arch. Intern. Med.* 141(1981): 1062–1064.
2. Winkenwerder, W. Jr. Ethical Dilemmas for House Staff Physicians. *JAMA* 254(1985):3454–3457.
3. Culver, C. M., et al. Basic Curricular Goals in Medical Ethics. *N. Engl. J. Med.* 312(1985):253–256.
4. Subcommittee on the Evaluation of Humanistic Qualities in the Internist, American Board of Internal Medicine. Evaluation of Humanistic Qualities of the Internist. *Ann. Intern. Med.* 99(1983): 720–724.
5. Pellegrino, E. D., Hart, R. J., Henderson, S. R., Loeb, S. E., and Edwards, G. Rele-

vance and Utility of Courses in Medical Ethics. *JAMA* **253**(1985):49–53.

6. Siegler, M. A Legacy of Osler: Teaching Clinical Ethics at the Bedside. *JAMA* **239**(1978):951–956.

7. Pellegrino, E. D., and McElhinney, T. K. Teaching Ethics, The Humanities and Human Values in Medical Schools: A Ten-Year Overview. Washington, D.C.: Institute on Human Values in Medicine and Society for Health and Human Values, 1982.

8. Bickel, J. Integrating Human Values Teaching Programs into Medical Students' Clinical Education. Washington, D.C.: Association of American Medical Colleges, 1986.

9. Radwany, S. M., and Adelson, B. H. The Use of Literary Classics in Teaching Medical Ethics to Physicians. *JAMA* **257**(1987):1629–1631.

10. Arnold, R. M., Forrow, L., Wartman, S. A., and Teno, J. Teaching Clinical Ethics: A Model Programme for Primary Care Residency. *J. Med. Ethics* **14**(1988):91–96.

11. Perkins, H. S. Teaching Medical Ethics in Internal Medicine Residency: A Rationale and a Proposal for Curricular Content and Format. *Arch. Intern. Med.* (in press).

12. Tolle, S. W., Cooney, T. G., and Hickam, D. H. A Program to Teach Residents Humanistic Skills for Notifying Survivors of a Patient's Death. *Acad. Med.* **64**(1989): 505–506.

13. Hong, H. P., Singer, P. A., Lynch, A., and Siegler, M. Teaching and Learning Clinical Medical Ethics during Residency Training. *Ann. R. Coll. Phys. Surg. Can.* **21**(1988): 2193–2198.

14. Povar, G. J., and Keith, K. J. The Teaching of Liberal Arts in Internal Medicine Residency Training. *J. Med. Ed.* **59**(1984): 714–721.

15. Kearn, D. C., Parrino, T. A., and Korst, D. R. The Lasting Value of Clinical Skills. *JAMA* **254**(1985):70–76.

16. Sheehan, T. J., et al. Teaching Humanistic Behavior. Presented at the annual meeting of the American Education Research Association, Washington, D.C., April 1987.

17. Connelly, J. D., and DalleMura, S. Ethical Problems in the Medical Office. *JAMA* **260**(1988):812–815.

18. La Puma, J. Stocking, C. B., Silverstein, M.D., DiMartini, A., and Siegler, M. An Ethics Consultation Service in a Teaching Hospital — Utilization and Evaluation. *JAMA* **260**(1988):808–811.

19. Perkins, H. S., and Saathoff, B. S. Impact of Medical Ethics Consultations on Physicians: An Exploratory Study. *Am. J. Med.* **85**(1988):761–765.

20. Brennan, T. Ethics Committees and Decisions to Limit Care, Experience at Massachusetts General Hospital. *JAMA* **260** (1988):803–807.

21. Barnard, D. Residency Ethics Teaching: A Critique of Current Trends. *Arch. Intern. Med.* **148**(1988):1836–1838.

9.6   Lane LW, Lane G, Schiedermayer DL, Spiro JH, Siegler M (1990) Caring for Medical Students as Patients. Arch Intern Med 150:2249–53

Commentaries

Caring for Medical Students as Patients

Medical students become ironically vulnerable patients. Despite their level of education, awareness of illness, and proximity to medical professionals and health institutions, unusual and largely unrecognized problems may interfere with medical student health care. The reasons for this relate both to the special characteristics of medical students and to the systems in which they receive health care. As a group, medical student–patients may ignore or deny their health problems and psychological stresses[1-4]; think themselves able to diagnose and treat their own ills[1,5-10]; believe their concerns to be unimportant or less legitimate than those of other patients[1,4]; or, like physicians, feel awkward in seeking care.[1,11-16] Further, medical students are at risk for impairing illnesses that affect physicians, including substance abuse, psychiatric disorders, and, more recently, AIDS.[2,3,6-10,17-43] These stigmatizing illnesses often discourage individuals from seeking health care.[2,42] In addition, at a system level, health care for medical students is often provided by teachers, friends, or colleagues within their own training institutions.[1,5,33,34] As a consequence, open communication between medical student–patients and their caregivers may be hampered, confidentiality may be breached, and conflicts may emerge as appropriate physician, patient, and student role distinctions become blurred.

This commentary explores how the unusual role of the medical student–patient can be both a source of vulnerability and a resource for teaching medical students how to provide excellent and humane health care.[15,16,33] We begin by exploring four problems associated with caring for medical student–patients: (1) complexities in communication between medical student–patients and physicians; (2) difficulties in protecting medical student–patient confidentiality and in resolving role conflicts between medical student–patients and their physicians; (3) special issues involved in responding to psychiatric illnesses affecting medical student–patients; and (4) problems associated with caring for medical students who are positive for human immunodeficiency virus (HIV) or who have been exposed to AIDS infection during training experiences. We conclude that providing exemplary care for medical students may not only improve the physical and psychological well-being of these future physicians, but it may also enrich and improve their caregiving skills and thus benefit future patients.

COMPLEXITIES IN COMMUNICATION

Effective communication may be less easily achieved with a medical student patient than with other patients. Initial communication problems may occur when the medical student's level of clinical experience is overestimated by the physician or misrepresented by the student. For example, the caregiver may expect the student–patient to provide spontaneously all of the medical information relevant to the health problem (ie, give a "perfect" medical history). The caregiver may also assume that certain diagnoses and therapies are well understood by the medical student–patient, who in turn may not wish to reveal the limits of his knowledge for fear of embarrassment and loss of status. As a result, medical student-patients may be inadequately informed when consenting to procedures or deciding on treatment options. While it may be unintended, in these situations the medical student is asked to apply advanced clinical judgment to his own case—in essence, to serve as his own physician.

Irrespective of one's level of medical expertise, it is difficult to be purely intellectual or objective about one's own health.[15,16] Twenty years ago, Tumulty[44] described the inherently subjective character of patienthood:

Almost all patients, regardless of intellectual capacity, are naive and simplistic when dealing with their own health problems. One should assume nothing, and start from basic facts and build upward.

Tumulty's[44] caution applies to all patients, including those with medical knowledge. Indeed, it may apply with special force to medical student–patients whose early and incomplete clinical knowledge may amplify or distort their worries. A caregiver who expects that medical students will exhibit a more detached or intellectual perspective than other patients may not understand the emotional needs of these unusual patients. Making matters more difficult, medical students themselves may believe that they should be as objective about their own symptoms as they are about other patients' health problems. Consequently, medical student patients may be reluctant to voice their concerns, believing them to be less legitimate than those of other patients because they feel that they "ought" to know their clinical facts better.[1] For all of these reasons, caregivers should interpret the clinical meanings of symptoms and signs for their student patients, remaining mindful of the intensely personal character of patienthood.

Efforts at communication are hampered when physicians "over-identify" with their medical student–patients. Believing that the medical student–patient resembles himself, for example, a physician may make incorrect assumptions about a medical student's background, responses to stress, and lifestyle. More worrisome, perhaps, is the physician who has become so accustomed to ignoring his own health concerns throughout medical training that he underestimates the medical student–patient's complaints. In these circumstances, necessary and explicit discussions of the medical student's health problems may not occur. Although the process of identification can sometimes enhance the physician-patient relationship, it may also lead to unwarranted assumptions that adversely affect care practices.

Other problems in communication arise, however, when medical student patients actually do behave in ways similar to their future colleagues. Medical students, like physicians, are known to seek health care in contexts outside of the clinic.[1,83,84] In these settings, there rarely is sufficient time for an adequate exchange of information and, consequently, curbside consultation seldom promotes an effective, supportive, and therapeutic physician-patient relationship. While the casual advice and fragmented care given in the hallway may sometimes be correct, it may also bring about misdiagnosis and mistreatment. At the very least, in such situations, the diagnostic and therapeutic efforts made on behalf of the medical student–patient are seldom documented, making future care more difficult.

Medical students, like their physician role models, may also deny or disguise their symptoms, delay seeking help, and diagnose and treat themselves.[1-10,17-21,23-26,30,87-39] Confounded, obscure, or hidden symptoms and findings (eg, appendicitis symptoms initially masked by antibiotics) may make it difficult for the clinician to determine the student-patient's actual health problem and to provide effective care. This is especially true when medical students—reputed to be but perhaps not more "hypochondriacal" than other patients[1,20,45,46]—minimize or alter their real symptoms or present with "acceptable" self-diagnoses because they are worried about more embarrassing or serious illness. Concerns about sexually transmitted diseases, chemical dependence, psychological difficulties, or even an unlikely disease process discussed in the lecture hall may actually prompt the visit to the physician. Uncovering the medical student–patient's actual reason for seeking medical attention may require continued, sensitive, and unhurried interviewing.

In the main, these obstacles to communication may be overcome when addressed through educational efforts aimed both at medical students and at the clinicians who provide health care for the medical student–population. Very early in medical school, perhaps even as part of the orientation process, medical students should be taught that it is legitimate for them to be ill at times and in need of help from health professionals. Students should be informed about the health care resources available to them several times during their training.[5,33] Each medical school should develop a cadre of health professionals who are specially prepared to care for medical student–patients with tact and thoroughness and to serve as their student-patients' advocates within the university health care context. Although these recommendations may improve some medical student-patient care practices, effective communication may be virtually impossible between medical student patients and their caregivers if the privilege of confidentiality, desired by all patients, cannot be guaranteed.

CONFIDENTIALITY AND CONFLICTING ROLES

Absolute protection of patient confidentiality is difficult in most institutional clinical settings and has been described as a decrepit concept.[47] In the care of medical student–patients who, of choice or necessity, seek health care in their own training institutions, maintaining confidentiality is particularly tenuous unless special efforts are made to ensure it.

Protecting medical student–patient confidentiality is difficult for a few reasons. Clearly, the risk of written records or laboratory data being seen by "interested" hospital employees, both unintentionally and illicitly, is increased for medical student–patients as opposed to more "anonymous" patients. Similarly, because the medical student may be seen as a colleague and friend, physicians may be less guarded about revealing confidential information to other professionals when they believe that the information is shared "among friends" who probably "already know the details." Finally, physicians within most training institutions are expected to discuss patient cases openly with colleagues, residents, and medical students while teaching and while developing diagnostic and therapeutic plans. This is not typically viewed as harming patient privacy: it is seen by patients and clinicians as an element of effective medical practice and training. In the unusual circumstance of the medical student patient, however, such discussions frequently result in significant breaches of patient confidentiality.

The whole notion of confidentiality may be moot when the medical student is placed in the position where he must reveal personal information to the person he would least wish to have it. In the past, applicants who acknowledged "emotional problems" and certain medical illnesses were rejected from medical schools presumably on the basis that these problems were incompatible with the practice of medicine.[22,34,41] Recently, it was demonstrated that a bias exists against residency applicants with a history of psychological counseling.[48] For clear reasons, the usual medical student–patient would not choose freely to see a physician-teacher about an unplanned pregnancy, an episode of depression, a drug abuse problem, a urethral discharge, or an HIV test.[21,22] Even when the medical student's health problem is less sensitive in nature, he or she may feel uncomfortable in the dual role of patient and student. In these instances, because the medical student may be com-

pelled by the student insurance plan to seek care within his own institution, these problems of confidentiality render the student particularly vulnerable.[5,20]

The caregiver sometimes finds himself in an awkward or even untenable position when responding to certain medical student health problems.[22] When the medical student–patient's work-up reveals a diagnosis that may interfere with classwork or clinical responsibilities, the caregiving physician is presented with conflicting duties to the patient, institution, and profession. Should the caregiver protect his student patient's confidentiality? Is it essential to inform medical school authorities of troubling findings such as chemical dependence, HIV positivity, or suicidal thoughts? How should the caregiver decide? These role conflicts are lessened if nonpunitive institutional guidelines have been developed previously to address the problems of medical student illnesses, particularly those that lead to impairment of thought and judgment. Such guidelines will assist the physician in determining when he is expected to report medical student health problems. They will also offer some reassurance and protection to medical students who may fear seeking care in the absence of explicit confidentiality policies.

Finally, role conflicts predictably occur when a teaching attending physician provides care for a medical student–patient. Difficult questions inevitably arise: is it ever proper for a teaching attending physician to serve also as a medical student's physician? Should an attending physician evaluate a student's academic performance when part of his knowledge is derived from a physician-patient relationship? These problems concerning role conflicts strongly indicate the need for thoughtful delineation of the responsibilities of clinicians who teach and provide care for medical students in academic institutions.[5,34,43]

To preserve confidentiality for medical students and to decrease the potential role conflicts we have described, we recommend that medical students' health insurance provide them with an option to seek care outside of the training institution. Attending physicians should be encouraged to consider whether assuming the medical care of a student will place them in an untenable role conflict. Educators at training institutions and leaders in the health care professions should address explicitly the question raised by Arnstein[20] as to whether certain illnesses are incompatible with the practice of medicine. We support the approach taken by Hays et al[17] in which strict confidentiality is observed at all times in the care of medical students (except as mandated by law) and in which a formal understanding exists such that the mental health center's evaluations of students cannot be used in assessing a medical student's academic status. We realize that these suggestions may be impossible to implement in all settings, but they may serve as the basis for developing responsive institutional policies.

RESPONDING TO PSYCHIATRIC ILLNESSES

Medical students are predisposed toward impairing psychiatric illnesses that can be difficult to identify and often have devastating consequences. Medical students have been shown to suffer from anxiety, major depression, eating disorders, adjustment disorders, and marital and interpersonal problems that may ultimately become life-threatening.[2-10,17-26,28-33,37-39,41] Several authors have described the serious risk of suicide in medical students.[10,19,31,33,35,36] Women medical students, in particular, are at a significantly increased risk for suicide.[10,21,36] As reported in 1985, the annual suicide rate for women medical students was two to three times higher (18.9 per 100 000) than the rate for women of the same age in the general population.[10,36] These issues are particularly worrisome as serious psychiatric symptoms and maladaptive behaviors sometimes emerge in response to the stresses of medical training,[1,2,9,17-21,25,26,28-30,37-39,49,50] as evidenced by the "clustering" of suicides among students occurring during the second and third years of medical school.[10]

Medical students are at risk for alcohol and polysubstance abuse and for self-treatment with psychoactive drugs.[2,3,5-8,19-21,23-32,38] Herzog et al[38] found that approximately 18% of 200 respondents to a 1987 survey were at risk for alcohol or substance abuse and nearly 7% were found to be at high risk. Conard et al[23] received surveys from 489 fourth-year students at 13 medical schools and found that 97% of medical students had used alcohol at some time; 88% had used alcohol in the preceding 30-day period; and 9% used alcohol daily. Alcohol, marijuana, and cocaine were the three most frequently used substances by medical students and alcohol and tranquilizer use was slightly higher among these students than among other cohorts in a national sample. Seventy-eight percent of 504 medical students in a study by McAuliffe et al[6] reported psychoactive drug use at some time and more medical students had used psychoactive drugs than had comparable samples of pharmacy students. Forney et al[39] found that more than 17% of medical students at four regional schools were "heavy drinkers" and that illicit drug, alcohol, and tobacco use were highly correlated.

In a longitudinal study of one medical school class, Clark et al[2] found that alcohol abuse was not uncommon and that academic performance was not influenced by students' drinking habits. Eleven percent of the students drank excessively for at least one 6-month period and 18% were identified as alcohol abusers during the first 2 years of medical school. Women medical students who drank alcohol were less likely to decrease their drinking through medical school than were their male counterparts. Interestingly, alcohol abusers had better first-year grades and overall test scores on the National Board of Medical Examiners (part one) than their classmates. These data led Clark et al[2] to comment:

... the academic success of alcohol abusers may pose a serious obstacle to their seeking help or to their receptivity to intervention measures if and when their drinking pattern becomes a reason for serious concern. Many medical students, particularly those motivated to excel, have a pronounced fear of being stigmatized or penalized in their career progress for admitting to any psychological problems or for using psychotherapy.

In light of the extensive use of psychoactive substances by medical students and the disincentives to their coming forward for help, it is disconcerting that 52 of 93 US medical schools in 1987 did not yet have a policy or program for identifying and treating substance abuse by students.[51]

Despite their proximity to health care, medical students suffering from psychiatric illnesses often do not receive adequate health care for preventable and treatable diseases, including suicidal depression and substance dependence. Do medical students deny their symptoms or are they discouraged from seeking help, fearful of academic repercussions? Are attending physicians and medical educators slow to suspect or reluctant to identify illness in medical students? To what extent is medical student abuse contributing to psychiatric illnesses in medical students?[49,50] Are the suspicions of Pepitone-Arreola-Rockwell et al[10] correct that ". . . for whatever reasons, some [medical] schools systematically underserve the mental health needs of their student bodies"? Each of these questions must be studied if we are to provide appropriate care for medical students who experience psychiatric illness.

An adequate response to psychiatric illness in medical students thus requires an awareness of the special vulnerabilities of medical student–patients and an improved ability of all physicians to identify psychiatric illness, even in highly successful medical students. It also requires a system in which appropriate interventions may be provided. We support Zoccolillo's recent proposal[37] of a practical program for the early

detection and treatment of depressed students and residents. The key elements of this proposal include: educating students and residents to the signs, symptoms, and risk factors for major depression; emphasizing that major depression is a treatable disorder and not simply a "normal" concomitant of training; stipulating that a trainee's decision to seek or receive psychiatric treatment should not, by itself, interfere with academic promotion; encouraging trainees who contemplate leaving the field of medicine to undergo a strictly confidential psychiatric evaluation; providing a confidential and convenient psychiatric service for all medical students and house officers; and developing methods to evaluate program effectiveness. Finally, Zoccolillo[37] urged that responsibility for the program should rest in a dean's office or a "similarly high position" to eliminate logistic or financial barriers involved in the care of students and residents. In an effort to prevent suicide, we also agree with Pepitone-Arreola-Rockwell et al[10] who suggest that increased attention to the mental health needs of medical students is essential; that a profile of the suicide-prone medical student should be developed; that because three quarters of suicides occur in second- and third-year medical classes, these classes should be identified as "high-risk"; and finally, that preventive and educational programs concerning suicide should be implemented early in medical school.[10,41]

AIDS AND MEDICAL STUDENT HEALTH CARE

The problems of communication, role conflict, confidentiality, and stigmatization are amplified in the medical student who develops HIV positivity from a work-related exposure, social behaviors, or other contacts. Aoun,[42] a physician who contracted AIDS from a leukemia patient during his residency training, has written a painful account of his experiences as a physician-patient. In his essay, Aoun describes his exposure to the AIDS virus (breaking a capillary tube containing HIV-infected blood); the profoundly troubling process of his diagnosis; the frightening realization that his wife and child might become infected; and the disbelief, cruelty, and rejection by members of the medical community.

Several of the issues raised by Aoun[42] relate directly to the problems of medical student health care. First, medical students, like residents and other health care workers, are at risk for developing AIDS through training experiences in the medical setting or through social behaviors during their training period. This risk may increase as the number of HIV-infected individuals grows. Medical students who become infected with the AIDS virus through social behaviors, moreover, are likely to be doubly stigmatized. Second, Aoun comments that the ambiguous status of medical students complicates the question of their compensation for training-related exposure to HIV. He has found that medical students entering residency are usually unaware of the occupational hazards they face and of the extent of their health and disability benefits.

Beyond its reputation, location, and the quality of its training, we must also examine how an institution cares for its workers and what benefits it provides. . . . [I]f we [health care workers] are to be in the front lines, then we must make sure we are better protected in all respects.[42]

Finally, Aoun describes his concern that health care workers, including residents and medical students, may hesitate to come forward for necessary medical care out of fear that they will lose their training positions, lose their income, lose their ability to find another job, and lose their self-esteem through ostracism or public humiliation.

The issue of physician impairment (discussed in the previous section) and the problem of HIV-positive medical students should encourage academic medical centers to focus renewed attention on providing adequate health care to medical students. Efforts to communicate openly, to address the issue of confidentiality directly, and to minimize role conflicts will improve the medical student–patient's ability to reveal his concerns freely and accept needed health care. While these efforts are important in the care of all medical student–patients, they become imperative in the care of medical students afflicted by potentially impairing and stigmatizing illnesses. By sensitively and competently addressing these issues, we expect that the health problems of medical students will be diagnosed and treated earlier in the course of their illnesses. We hope that some illnesses may even be prevented.[33]

LESSONS FROM PATIENTHOOD

In caring for medical student–patients, physicians are given a unique opportunity to impart clinical skills and professional values in a context of extraordinary significance. Being on the "other end" of the stethoscope from an exemplary clinician can teach more to the medical student about caregiving than perhaps any other experience in medical school.[34] Personal experience as a patient teaches the importance of communication, confidentiality, sensitivity, and thoroughness in interactions with patients: it roots empathy in the future physician.

Empathy has been defined as "the ability to accurately recognize the immediate emotional perspective of another person while maintaining one's own perspective."[52] Thus, the dual perspective necessary for empathy is paralleled in the dual perspective involved in the medical student–patient role. Inglefinger,[15] in reflecting on his experiences as a physician-patient dying of cancer, believed that physicians who have been patients themselves are likely to be more empathic in their care of others.

In medical school, students are told about the perplexity, anxiety, and misapprehension that may affect the patient as he enters the medical-care system, and in the clinical years the fortunate and sensitive student may learn much from talking to those assigned to his supervision. But the effects of lectures and conversations are ephemeral and are no substitute for actual experience. One might suggest, of course, that only those who have been hospitalized during their adolescent or adult years be admitted to medical school. Such a practice would . . . increase the number of empathic doctors . . . .

Through direct experiences as a patient, the medical student may learn the significance of voicing one's concerns and having them heard by a caring physician; the meaning of mutual decision-making between physician and patient; and the need for clinical competence in implementing diagnostic and therapeutic plans. Through such experience, the medical student–patient becomes aware of the needs of each patient and learns about the responsibilities of every physician.

CONCLUSION

We have described the unusual challenges involved in providing health care for medical students. Medical student–patients have many of the same concerns shared by all patients; some of the knowledge, susceptibilities, and attitudes of physicians; and several special vulnerabilities related to their unusual status as both students and patients. Especially when receiving health care within their own training institutions, problems may arise for medical student–patients and their physicians in communicating openly, preserving confidentiality, and resolving role conflicts. These issues, which have not received much attention in the past, become acute when medical students are afflicted by potentially impairing or stigmatizing illnesses, such as psychiatric disorders or AIDS. Furthermore, the experiences of medical students as patients may provide the most meaningful and constructive lessons of physician training.

We suggest that conscientious attention to the difficult issues surrounding the health care of medical students will

improve the quality of their care, may better their health status, and should enrich their educational experience. We believe that a capable and responsive physician working within a system designed to provide excellent care for medical student–patients is in a unique position to help and to teach future physicians.

LAURA WEISS LANE, MD
Department of Psychiatry
GEORGE LANE, PhD
Religious Studies Program
University of New Mexico, Albuquerque
DAVID L. SCHIEDERMAYER, MD
Center for the Study of Bioethics
JOANNA H. SPIRO, EdD
Student Mental Health Services
Medical College of Wisconsin, Milwaukee
MARK SIEGLER, MD
Center for Clinical Medical Ethics
University of Chicago (Ill)

This study was supported in part by grants from the Andrew W. Mellon Foundation, the Henry J. Kaiser Family Foundation, the Ira W. DeCamp Foundation, and the National Fund for Medical Education. The opinions expressed are those of the authors and do not necessarily represent those of the foundations.

This work was developed primarily at the Center for Clinical Medical Ethics, Pritzker School of Medicine, University of Chicago (Ill). We thank David Hyman, JD, Brian Roberts, MD, Jeanne Garcia, MD, and Robert Kellner, MD, for their thoughtful comments on the manuscript.

References

1. Rintels P. From hypochondriasis to denial: in doctors as patients. *Harvard Med Alumni Bull.* 1986-1987:16-44.
2. Clark DC, Eckenfels EJ, Daugherty SR, Fawcett J. Alcohol use patterns through medical school: a longitudinal study of one class. *JAMA.* 1987;257:2921-2926.
3. Marchand WR. The effect of an educational program on the desire for treatment among impaired medical students. *J Nerv Mental Dis.* 1988;176:372-373.
4. Scott CD, Hawk J. *Heal Thyself: The Health of Health Care Professionals.* New York, NY: Brunner-Mazel Publishers; 1986.
5. Westmeyer J. Mental health care for medical students and residents: current problems and evolving resources. *Minn Med.* 1987;70:565-569.
6. McAuliffe WE, Rohman M, Santangelo S, et al. Psychoactive drug use among practicing physicians and medical students. *N Engl J Med.* 1986;315:805-810.
7. McAuliffe WE, Santangelo S, Magnuson E, Sobol A, Rohman M, Weissman J. Risk factors of drug impairments in random samples of physicians and medical students. *Int J Addict.* 1987;22:825-841.
8. Kory WP, Crandall LA. Nonmedical drug use patterns among medical students. *Int J Addict.* 1984;19:871-874.
9. Drouin J. Medical students seen in psychiatry. *J Am Coll Health.* 1988;36:349-351.
10. Pepitone-Arreola-Rockwell F, Rockwell D, Core N. Fifty-two medical student suicides. *Am J Psychiatry.* 1981;138:198-201.
11. Stoudemire A, Rhoads JM. When the doctor needs a doctor: special considerations for the physician-patient. *Ann Intern Med.* 1983;98:654-659.
12. Marzuk PM. When the patient is a physician. *N Engl J Med.* 1987;317:1409-1411.
13. Mack RM. Lessons from living with cancer. *N Engl J Med.* 1984;311:1640-1644.
14. Mullan F. Seasons of survival: reflections of a physician with cancer. *N Engl J Med.* 1985;313:270-273.
15. Inglefinger F. Arrogance. *N Engl J Med.* 1980;303:1507-1511.
16. Brice JA. Empathy lost. *Harvard Med Alumni Bull.* 1986-1987:28-32.
17. Hays LR, Dickson LR, Lyles MR, Ludwig AM, Martin CA, Bird MA. Treating psychiatric problems in medical students. *Am J Psychiatry.* 1986;143:1428-1431.
18. Hamburg P, Herzog DP. Studying reports of women medical students on their eating disorders. *J Med Educ.* 1985;60:644-646.
19. Franks RD. Medical student and resident 'impairments': prediction, early recognition, and intervention: should they be rehabilitated or should they be removed? *Proc Annu Res Med Educ.* 1985;24:321-324.
20. Arnstein RL. Emotional problems of medical students. *Am J Psychiatry.* 1986;143:11.
21. Bissell L, Skoring JK. One hundred alcoholic women in medicine: an interview study. *JAMA.* 1987;257:2939-2944.
22. Callahan D, Gaylin W. Case studies in bioethics: the psychiatrist as double agent. *Hastings Cent Rep.* 1974;4:11-14.
23. Conard S, Hughes P, Baldwin DC, Ackenbach KE, Sheehan DV. Sub-

stance use by fourth year students at 13 US medical schools. *J Med Educ.* 1988;63:747-758.

24. Report of the AMA Council on Mental Health. The sick physician: impairment by psychiatric disorders, including alcoholism and drug dependence. *JAMA.* 1973;223:684-687.

25. Kelly JA, Bradlyn AS, Dubbert PM, St Lawrence JS. Stress management training in medical school. *J Med Educ.* 1982;57:91-99.

26. Blackwell B. Prevention of impairment among residents in training. *JAMA.* 1986;255;1177-1178.

27. Gorovitz S. Preparing for the perils of practice. *Hastings Cent Rep.* 1984;14:38-41.

28. Folse ML, DaRosa DA, Folse R. The relationship between stress and attitudes toward leisure among first year medical students. *J Med Educ.* 1985;60:610-617.

29. Kris K. Distress precipitated by psychiatric training among medical students. *Am J Psychiatry.* 1986;143:1432-1435.

30. Clark DC, Zeldow PB. Vicissitudes of depressed mood during four years of medical school. *JAMA.* 1988;260:2521-2528.

31. Thomas CB. What becomes of medical students: the dark side. *Johns Hopkins Med J.* 1976;138:185-195.

32. Borenstein DB, Cook K. Impairment prevention in the training years. *JAMA.* 1982;247:2700-2703.

33. Simon HJ. Mortality among medical students, 1947-1967. *J Med Educ.* 1968;43:1175-1182.

34. Earley LW, Johnson DG. Medical student health. *J Med Educ.* 1969;44:36-45.

35. Everson RB, Fraumeni JF. Mortality among medical students and young physicians. *J Med Educ.* 1975;50:809-811.

36. Ray A. Suicide in doctors. *Psychiatr Clin North Am.* 1985;8:377-387.

37. Zoccolillo M. Major depression during medical training. *JAMA.* 1988;260:2560-2561.

38. Herzog DB, Borus JF, Hamburg P, Ott IL, Concus A. Substance use,

eating behaviors, and social impairment of medical students. *J Med Educ.* 1987;62:651-657.

39. Forney PD, Forney MA, Fischer P, et al. Sociocultural correlates of substance use among medical students. *J Drug Educ.* 1988;18:97-109.

40. Steindler EM. Alcoholic women in medicine: still homeless. *JAMA.* 1987;257:2954-2955.

41. Willer B, Keill S, Isada C. Survey of US and Canadian medical schools on admissions and psychiatrically at risk students. *J Med Educ.* 1984;59:928-936.

42. Aoun H. When a house officer gets AIDS. *N Engl J Med.* 1989;321:693-696.

43. Spiro J, Roenneberg M, Maly B. Teaching doctors to treat doctors. *Med Teacher.* 1980;2:288-290.

44. Tumulty PA. What is a clinician and what does he do? *N Engl J Med.* 1970;283:20-24.

45. Kellner R, Wiggins RJ, Pathak D. Distress in medical and law students. *Compr Psychiatry.* 1986;27:220-223.

46. Kellner R, Wiggins RJ, Pathak D. Hypochondriacal fears in medical and law students. *Arch Gen Psychiatry.* 1986;43:487-489.

47. Siegler M. Confidentiality in medicine: a decrepit concept. *N Engl J Med.* 1982;301:1518-1521.

48. Oppenheimer K, Miller M, Forney P. Effect of history of psychological counseling on selection of applicants for residencies. *J Med Educ.* 1987;62:504-508.

49. Sheehan KH, Sheehan DV, White K, Leibowitz A, Baldwin DC. A pilot study of medical student 'abuse': student perceptions of mistreatment and misconduct in medical school. *JAMA.* 1990;263:533-537.

50. Silver HK, Glicken AD. Medical student abuse. *JAMA.* 1990;263:527-532.

51. Rowley BD, Baldwin DC. Datagram: substance abuse policies. *J Med Educ.* 1988;163:759-761.

52. Shea SC. *Psychiatric Interviewing: The Art of Understanding.* Philadelphia, Pa: WB Saunders Co; 1988.

9.7 Pellegrino ED, Siegler M, Singer PA (1990) Teaching Clinical Ethics. J Clin Ethics 1:175–80

VOLUME 1, NUMBER 3   THE JOURNAL OF CLINICAL ETHICS   175

FEATURES

Teaching Clinical Ethics

Edmund D. Pellegrino, Mark Siegler, and Peter A. Singer

In the first of two recent articles in this journal we offered a definition of clinical medical ethics,[1] and in the second we outlined its research content and methodology.[2] In this article we extend our observations to teaching clinical ethics, by describing its development, rationale, content, methodology and timing, personnel requirement, evaluation, and finally, the conceptual and practical obstacles such teaching may encounter.

The Development of "Clinical" Ethics

Teaching medical ethics as a systematic and critical exercise is an innovation of the last quarter century in American medical schools. Prior to that time, what formal teaching of ethics there was consisted of some combination of knowledge about the Hippocratic oath and *ethos* together with a rather heavy concentration on medical etiquette. Teaching was done by clinicians who communicated what they deemed to be the qualities of a good physician and the obligations of the patient-physician relationship. What passed as "moral philosophy" was a mixture of topics such as medical history; habits of study; cultivation of powers of observation; relationships with patients, physicians, and the public; and mastery of the art of medical writing

Edmund D. Pellegrino, MD, is Director of the Center for the Advanced Study of Ethics and John Carroll Professor of Medicine and Medical Humanities at Georgetown University, Washington, DC.
Mark Siegler, MD, is Director of the Center for Clinical Medical Ethics and Professor of Medicine at the University of Chicago.
Peter A. Singer, MD, is Assistant Professor of Medicine and Associate Director, Centre for Bioethics, University of Toronto, Toronto, Ontario, Canada.

and speaking.[3] The field of clinical ethics existed by implication only.

Professional philosophers largely ignored medical ethics as a subject of serious study. Even those physicians who had become philosophers, such as John Locke, William James, and Karl Jaspers, gave scant attention to professional ethics. The teaching of medical ethics and medical moral reasoning was, as a consequence, unreflective. Medical students learned ethics by precept from teachers who were deemed to be good physicians. Certain ways of behaving and thinking were accepted by assertion without justification or philosophical grounding.

All of this changed when serious philosophers began to examine the assumptions of the received moral wisdom of the profession. Medical ethics then took the analytical turn. Philosophers began to subject accepted and habitual behavior of physicians to systematic analysis. They began to critically assess the principles and norms underlying medical moral choices as well as relationships between physicians and patients. This occurred in the late 1960s, at the same time that a variety of professional claims of authority and expertise were subjected to scrutiny. Medical ethics was called to more stringent standards of justification than simply the authority of physicians or the profession. The need for teaching medical ethics in a new vein became apparent.

At first, medical educators taught the new perspective in medical ethics in lectures and seminars, albeit from the beginning they also used the case method. About a decade ago, some schools extended teaching to the clinical years and to the clinical setting.[4] It is on this phase of the teaching of medical ethics

that we wish to concentrate—the teaching of clinical ethics "at the bedside" to medical students, residents, faculty members, and practicing physicians. In this discussion, we shall use the term "clinical ethics," as defined in the first article in this series,[5] to refer to the identification, analysis, and resolution of ethical problems that arise in clinical practice.

The Rationale for Teaching Clinical Ethics

The teaching of ethics, like any other subject in a medical school, gets its ultimate justification from its contribution to the care of the sick. The principal goal of teaching clinical ethics is to improve the quality of patient care in terms of both the process and outcome of care. Presumably, if physicians are equipped with the skills required to reach ethical decisions, their patients will be protected against violations of their dignity as human beings. The necessity for the teaching of clinical ethics rests in the immutable fact that any serious medical decision involves two components—a technical decision requiring the application of knowledge of basic and clinical sciences to the patient's present problems, and a moral component demanding that the technically correct decision is also morally defensible. The technical component tells us what *can* be done, the moral component what *ought* to be done for this patient.

In the past, the correct medical decision—the "medical indications" for a choice of therapy—was regarded as synonymous with the medical good of the patient. The assumption no longer obtains. The objective determination of the patient's medical needs now must be reconciled with the patient's values,

176   THE JOURNAL OF CLINICAL ETHICS   FALL 1990

perception of what is good, life situation and plans, religious beliefs, and ethnic and cultural values. The successful outcome of the patient-physician relationship includes, therefore, not just traditional "hard data" end points like mortality or morbidity, but also such "soft data" as the quality of life as perceived by the patient, the patient's functional capacity, the impact of illness on the patient's family and job, the patient's satisfaction with care, and the emotional and financial "costs" of care.

This intermingling of the technical and moral dimensions in medical decisions puts a premium on shared decision making, on making decisions *with*, as well as *for* the patient. This, in turn, means that in educating the physician, emphasis must be not only on the ethics of the actual decision, but also on the ethics of the decision-making process itself. A morally good decision will be based upon sound analysis of the moral issues and their resolution as well as grounded in a morally sound decision-making process that respects the dignity, autonomy, and values of the patient, the physician, and the others who participate in a clinical decision (such as family members and other health professionals).

Ethics clearly is part of the fabric of clinical medicine. It has been since medicine's beginnings. But only in the last few decades have the skills of ethical analysis become an intrinsic part of being a good physician. Indeed, it is no exaggeration today to suggest that the skills of ethical analysis are as important to being a physician as the skills and knowledge of the basic and clinical sciences. The principal goal of teaching clinical ethics is to improve the quality of care and to optimize patient outcomes.

What Should Be Taught in Clinical Ethics?

Given the rationale for teaching clinical ethics, it seems clear that both cognitive and behavioral aspects of ethics should be taught. But these, in turn, depend upon the character of the phy-

sician who will be applying these ethical skills. The cognitive aspects of teaching should include the skills of ethical analysis and a familiarity with the literature and the research methodologies that we have described in our previous paper.[6] The behavioral aspects require that well-trained clinicians be able to apply cognitive knowledge to the care of individual patients. And finally, medical schools must be concerned about character formation in their trainees.

Cognitive Skills

The necessary and teachable cognitive skills include: recognition and definition of the ethical issue or problem; identification of the principles, duties, or obligations involved; clarification of real or potential conflicts among principles and ways of resolving such conflicts; attainment of a moral choice; identification of the possible objections and the reasons for them; and formulation of counterarguments and modification of the decision on the basis of these considerations, if necessary. There is an orderly way to work up an ethical problem, just as there is an orderly way to make a differential diagnosis, arrive at a probable diagnosis, and select a means of management. The process of analysis of a clinical ethical dilemma is as orderly and as rigorous as the process of clinical evaluation and is as readily taught.

The literature in medical ethics is growing at an extremely rapid rate. If clinical decisions are to be up-to-date, students and teachers must keep abreast of the published record of ethical discourse on the subjects of most immediate importance to clinical decisions. Here, the arguments pro and con, the weight assigned to various kinds of arguments, and the degree of congruence or disparity of opinion among ethicists are documented. Some facility in assessing the arguments of experts and their content is crucial to any physician who wishes to make his own decisions responsibly and in an informed way.

As with any major branch of medical study, students will need some

familiarity with the research methodology in the emergent field of empirical ethics. These studies detail the way patients and physicians actually make their decisions, the values they use, the preferences they express, and the manner in which conflicts among decision makers are handled. The methodology of empirical studies is usually some combination of the techniques of clinical epidemiology and the social sciences combined with the tools of ethical analysis.

The curriculum should reflect the incidence and prevalence of clinical ethical situations encountered in actual practice. Curriculum design should be based upon published studies of the epidemiology of ethical dilemmas in clinical practice. For example, Lo and Schroeder found that the incidence of ethical dilemmas among medical inpatients was 17 percent, and that these dilemmas included withholding tests or treatments, informed consent, truth telling, relationships among physicians, and limited resources.[7] In a study of an internal medicine office practice, Connelly and Dallemura found that ethical problems were present in 30 percent of patients and 21 percent of visits.[8] The most common problems were costs of care, psychological factors that influence preferences, competence and capacity to choose, refusal of treatment, and informed consent. Published studies about medical ethics consultation series also provide data on the epidemiology of ethical problems. For example, in one recent series the most frequent clinical ethical issues for which consultation was sought were withholding or withdrawing treatment, do-not-resuscitate orders (DNRs), and legal issues.[9]

The curriculum should also be targeted to meet students' needs. For example, Jacobson and colleagues surveyed residents in six internal medicine programs regarding their preferences for specific medical ethics topics.[10] A majority of residents said they wanted more emphasis on the following topics: withdrawal of life support, physician-patient relations, living wills and advance directives, allocation of limited resources related to diagnosis or prog-

VOLUME 1, NUMBER 3   THE JOURNAL OF CLINICAL ETHICS   177

nosis, government policy regarding access to medical care, understanding rights of incompetent patients, euthanasia, incompetent or impaired colleagues, and priority for scarce organs. This list of topics would be different for students at different levels of training and in different specialties.

Behavioral Skills

The assimilation and mastery of cognitive knowledge is not an end in itself for clinicians. To be effective in caring for patients, clinicians must have the behavioral skills that are necessary to put their knowledge to work in everyday clinical encounters. A physician who knows the legal and ethical requirements of writing an order not to resuscitate would also be expected to know how and when to approach patients and families in a thoughtful and sensitive way to initiate discussions about DNR status. Instruction in the behavioral skills of clinical ethics requires teaching and role modeling by experienced clinicians who can demonstrate the skills in practice. It further requires that students have the opportunity to practice these skills while supervised by experienced clinicians.

Character Development

In addition to cognitive knowledge and behavioral skills, some attention must be paid to the affective component of clinical ethics—that is to say, to the kind of person the physician should be as well as the kind of decisions he or she should make. In short, ethics requires that the physician be a person of character, one who can be expected habitually to act in the patient's interests when no one is watching. Trust is essential in the healing relationship. The norms and principles of clinical ethics must in the end be filtered through the person of the physician. The values or principles the physician chooses, the theory of ethics he espouses and the way he interprets the relationship with the patient will shape the ethical decision he makes in a given case. In order for a physician to perform in an ethically defensible way, both procedurally

and substantively, some development of his character is essential. This is the most difficult task in clinical ethics. The physician is often the last safeguard of the incompetent patient, and he is a moral accomplice if harm should befall the patient.

How and When Should Clinical Ethics Be Taught?

Since clinical ethics is so essential to medical education and practice, it should be an integral part of the physician's education at all levels in medical school, in the residency, and in continuing education. In our teaching, we emphasize the "Five C's" of teaching clinical ethics: 1) *clinically* based teaching; 2) *cases* as the teaching focus; 3) *continuous* teaching throughout the medical curriculum; 4) *coordinating* ethics teaching with the trainee's other learning objectives; and 5) *clinicians'* active participation both as coinstructors and as role models for students.

Medical School

Most medical schools today devote between ten and twenty hours of formal instruction in medical ethics sometime during the first two years. This is a minimal commitment. Reinforcement in the clinical years is necessary if students are to gain some tolerable degree of familiarity with clinical ethics. This is best accomplished by integrating teaching into the clinical clerkships. This practice disrupts the pattern of clinical education least, takes advantage of student involvement with actual ethical dilemmas, and eliminates the difficulty of designing a course to cover all the major issues encountered in all major specialties. A number of teaching opportunities will satisfy these conditions.

The first, and most important, is the arrangement of one or two sessions per week during each clerkship devoted to

ethical issues encountered on the clinical service. Here, students present cases selected for their clinical ethical implications. Students discuss cases in the usual manner—that is, they define the issue, suggest a resolution of the problem, provide reasons for this decision, and cite literature. In short, students "work up" the patient. However, they discuss the moral as well as the clinical aspects of each case. This method has the great advantage of student involvement. It is hard for students to reject

---

In short, ethics requires that the physician be a person of character.

---

ethics as too abstract if it is an integral part of the management of their own patients.

A second way to integrate clinical ethics into the medical school curriculum is through ethical grand rounds held periodically on each major clinical service. It greatly reinforces the importance and the vitality of clinical ethics if four or five times a year the topic for grand rounds in medicine, surgery, pediatrics, and other specialties is devoted to some complex ethical issue. This practice implies the sanction of the department chairman and is invaluable in impressing students with the central place ethics occupies in every specialty. Failing this, or perhaps in addition, a medical-center-wide grand rounds can be held once a month. Responsibility is rotated among the major clinical services. This has the advantage of bringing together the entire staff—students, residents, faculty, nurses, and other health professionals. Ethical issues—such as access to care, cost of care, end-of-life decisions, and research innovations—may be the only subjects of sufficient common interest still left to counter the centrifugal forces driving professions and specialties further from each other every day. These measures can be supplemented by lecture and seminar series and by reports of empirical research pertinent to clinical ethics.

There seems to be little question that clinical ethics should be integrated into every medical school course. There is some debate, however, on how this might best be done. Some educators favor teaching ethics as part of the courses medical students are already taking. When students learn about cardiopulmonary resuscitation in the cardiology course, they could also learn about do-not-resuscitate orders. When they learn about nephrology, the students could discuss how to approach decisions to withhold or withdraw dialysis. In psychiatry, students could be exposed to the concept of competency (decision-making capacity), the standards used to assess competency in clinical practice, and its central importance in clinical-ethical decision making. When students learn about solid organ transplantation, they could also discuss public policies to procure and distribute organs for transplant. In neurology, they could learn about the ethical implications of brain death and persistent vegetative state. In surgery, students could learn about issues of informed consent and ethical ways to obtain it.

Others argue that most clinical faculty members do not yet have the expertise or interest necessary to teach ethics well. They argue that it is better to teach clinical ethics as a separate course, assigned to a department or division of medical ethics staffed by clinicians and ethicists qualified to teach the subject.

Ideally, every clinical teacher should be competent to teach clinical ethics in his own manner at the bedside and in the classroom. This is unlikely to be the case for a long time to come. The optimal solution for the present is usually some combination of the integrated and block method best suited to the capabilities and interests of individual schools and their faculties.

In our experience, most physicians in practice or in academic medical centers prefer to be involved in the discussion of the ethical issues involving their specialties and patients. An excellent arrangement, therefore, is cooperative teaching, in which the clinician provides the essential clinical expertise and a trained ethicist assists in structuring the formal ethical analysis. As these teams work together they will learn one another's languages and overlap at various points in any discussion. The difference in perspective is valuable because it assures that both the clinical and the ethical aspects of teaching receive expert treatment—something we demand in the teaching of any medical school subject.

Clinicians may cooperate with ethicists in a variety of ways depending upon their interests and teaching style. Some want only to consult with ethicists, some are eager to team teach, and some may wish to turn the session over to the ethicist. Whatever the means of collaboration, prior preparation and consultation are absolutely essential.

Residency

The teaching of ethics to residents is increasingly a concern because residents are on the front line and must confront complex ethical dilemmas daily. In our experience, residents often feel frustrated by their insufficient preparation to assist them in making ethical decisions and the lack of time during residency to remedy these deficiencies. They need reinforcement of whatever teaching they may have had in medical school. This is best accomplished by practice in making ethical decisions in their own cases. This, we believe, can best be done by the same mechanisms we have described for medical students—that is, by teaching around their own cases, supplemented by rounds, seminars, and occasional discussions with ethics committees or consultants.

For medical students, residents, and fellows, clinical ethics is best taught in the same way as clinical medicine itself—by supervised experience, increased responsibility, and discussions in rounds. In this way also, the very sensitive issue of faculty education can be diplomatically circumvented. Without announcing anything so pretentious as a "faculty education program," faculty members can be drawn into the discussions, their interests stimulated, and their expertise utilized.

Continuing Medical Education

Medical practitioners who have had courses in medical ethics perceive themselves better prepared to deal with the ethical choices they must make in their daily practices.[11] Practitioners also appreciate the need to update themselves in medical ethics. As a result, postgraduate courses, conferences, and seminars in medical ethics are popular modalities of continuing education.

Concurrent with these interests, the possibilities for continuing education are increasing rapidly. We would cite as examples the following opportunities: 1) presentation of papers, both empirical and analytical, at national and local professional society meetings such as the Society for General Internal Medicine and the American College of Physicians; 2) attendance at ethics conferences, which have become regular events on the continuing medical education calendar; 3) enrollment in intensive bioethics courses from a few days to a week's duration, offered for the past sixteen years by the Kennedy Institute of Ethics and since offered by some of the more recently established centers for bioethics; 4) regular perusal of articles in all the major medical journals such as the *New England Journal of Medicine*, the *Journal of the American Medical Association*, and others; 5) participation in hospital ethics committees, informal consultation and discussion with colleagues, and journal clubs focusing on the bioethics literature.

An insufficiently appreciated source of continuing education is the care of a physician's own patients. The issues physicians face daily should prompt them to discuss cases with colleagues and to seek consultation from the literature, ethics consultants, or ethics committees. Cases involving patients in persistent vegetative states, decisions to remove life-sustaining nutrition and hydration, patient competence, living wills, and other controversial questions all provide opportunities to seek consultation and discuss ethical issues. The next article in this series (to appear in the Winter 1990 issue) will explore the educational possibilities in the use of ethics committees and ethics consultation services.

Who Should Teach Clinical Ethics?

Who should teach medical ethics in the clinical setting? Whoever can do it well. Increasingly, practicing physicians are training in clinical ethics. The Royal College of Physicians and Surgeons of Canada, for example, now formally credits ethics training as part of fellowship training. The University of Chicago's Center for Clinical Medical Ethics has trained twenty-six physician-fellows over the past six years; these physicians have returned to appointments in seventeen medical centers in the US and Canada. Thus, there is an increasing supply of practicing physicians trained in clinical ethics in North American medical centers.

Practicing physicians with adequate ethics education who teach clinical ethics at the bedside bring several advantages to their teaching: 1) they can teach using their own cases and thus can demonstrate how ethical considerations are incorporated into actual medical practice; 2) they have immediate credibility with students and house officers; 3) they can demonstrate ethically appropriate professional attitudes and values so that students learn both from the formal teaching about ethics and from their teachers' modeling of ethical and professional behavior.

But physicians are not the only ones who can teach clinical ethics at the bedside. Increasingly, medical schools and hospitals are employing philosopher-bioethicists to teach, to serve on ethics committees, and to provide ethics consultations. These individuals also begin their analyses in the cases of individual patients. They have much to contribute at the bedside. In addition, nurses and other health professionals in increasing numbers are being formally trained in bioethics and can ef-

fectively teach bedside clinical ethics. Indeed, the likelihood is high that in the future the demand for trained clinical ethicists in hospitals and medical schools will outstrip the supply.

How Should Clinical Ethics Teaching Be Evaluated?

One of the most persistent and difficult questions to answer is whether the teaching of medical ethics makes any difference in the subsequent behavior of the physician or the student. Two questions are conflated here because the aims of ethics are two: to form virtuous people and to make right and good decisions. The first is a character trait, the second a cognitive skill.

The cognitive grasp of the skills of ethical analysis can be evaluated like any other cognitive skill. Students can be asked to provide an ethical workup and analysis of actual cases. The coherence of their reasoning, their understanding of ethical terms and principles, and their perception of opposing arguments are all subject to evaluation. The students' clinical management of specific ethical situations can also be assessed. One of us (Peter Singer) is currently developing ethics stations for the objective structured clinical examination.[12]

The extremely difficult but important question -- does a course in ethics make a physician a better person in later life? -- is one that cannot be readily answered. Will physicians who have taken courses in ethics have sounder moral values and intuitions? Will they be more compassionate, more honest, more trustworthy, and less selfish?

To evaluate these end points is beyond current methods. Ideally, we would want to observe the physician in his own office when no one is watching to see how he makes moral decisions both

substantively and procedurally. Lacking such evidence, we can only conjecture that a physician's serious study of this ethics will raise sensitivities to ethical issues, lead to more explicit understanding of his own ethical values and principles as well as of those of others, and result in a greater sense of accountability.

The problem of evaluation deserves more attention than it has received. Close collaboration between teachers of medical ethics and medical educators is in order. This is an important

---

Clinical ethics is best taught in the same way as clinical medicine--by supervised experience, increased responsibility, discussions in rounds.

---

area for research in medical education. Ideally, evaluative methods should focus on how a student deals with actual cases rather than the student's response to abstract questions about ethical theory, principles, or presuppositions. The endpoint of education in ethics is whether, ultimately, the quality of moral decision making changes positively. This, in the moral arena, is the counterpart of the correct technical decision in the scientific dimensions of medicine.

Obstacles to the Teaching of Clinical Ethics

Although ethics is being taught in almost every medical school, there are practical and conceptual obstacles that remain to be overcome. One of us (Edmund Pellegrino) has responded to some of the more frequent questions in the minds of faculty colleagues about the teaching of ethics.[13] These will not be repeated here in any detail. However, it is pertinent to the thrust of this essay to comment briefly on a few selected problems.

Lack of time in the crowded curriculum is a reality. However, given the importance of the subject, the amount of time—an average of ten to twenty hours of classroom time—is pitifully small. So far as clinical ethics is concerned, the modes of teaching in the clinical setting that we have set forth here would cause very little disturbance, since they are integrated into the clerkship and residency experience.

Another serious difficulty is the lack of trained clinicians to teach ethics in the clinical setting or to act as discussion group leaders. Unfortunately, many clinicians, academic and nonacademic, believe they can teach ethics simply because they are ethical persons themselves. They may or may not be ethical persons, and it is true that they are models that medical students may emulate for good or harm. But most academic clinicians need some preparation in the skills of ethical analysis, and especially in the need for self-critical examination necessary to teach ethics adequately. Faculty retreats, orientation sessions, and intensive courses are some ways in which conscientious clinicians can, with the guidance of properly trained clinical ethicists, prepare themselves to teach ethics. Perhaps the most effective, least intrusive, and least threatening means of faculty education is regular attendance at ethical rounds, seminars, and ethics committee discussions. In sessions like these, faculty members can learn without the stigma some seem to attach to admitting they are not fully qualified, *de facto,* to teach ethics. Finally, the most persuasive way to sensitize faculty members to ethics is through their interaction with students. If ethics is taught well, the students themselves will raise the appropriate questions in other classes. This is even more effective than asking each teacher to integrate ethics into his courses.

A more difficult obstacle to overcome is the negative attitude of basic scientists and "scientific" clinicians who take the positivist stance: if one cannot weigh, smell, feel, measure, and subject knowledge to observation and experimentation, it is not knowledge but only opinion, and, therefore, not worth teaching. This is not the place to engage the serious epistemological confusion this attitude connotes. Teachers of ethics properly prepared in philoso-

phy should engage this question directly. But resolution of what is likely to be on ongoing philosophical contretemps cannot be allowed to block teaching so important a subject as clinical ethics. We must admit that some skepticism about goals and methods of this kind of teaching is justified. The presence of serious criticism by colleagues will serve to make ethical discourse and teaching more rigorous. Eventually, however, if we teach well, conduct serious research, and deal with objections rationally, skeptics will respect, even if they do not accept, our efforts.

The greatest skepticism, understandably, centers on whether virtue and character can be taught. Some say it is far too late in a person's life to teach him character in medical school. If church, family, and society have not done the job by this time, it is too late. Others say there are not methods for teaching character and that it is presumptuous for a medical school to attempt to do so. There is partial truth in these objections; however, there is evidence suggesting that it is not only worthwhile, but mandatory, to make some effort to shape the student's character as a physician.

First, there is evidence from psychological research that the strategies people use for problem solving and the values they espouse continue to change until they are well into their twenties and thirties. Indeed, such changes continue to occur as long as students remain in schools and colleges. Second, whether we like it or not, medical faculty teach character by their own behavior. Students emulate faculty models in the fields they have chosen. We all retain good and bad habits that we learned from our teachers, which we sort out later in our professional lives, as our own characters mature. This being the case, we cannot lightly dismiss the obligation to do whatever we can to shape character in positive ways.

Conclusion

The future development of teaching programs in clinical ethics should aim

to improve the quality of care and optimize patient outcomes. Quality refers to the process of identifying, analyzing, and attempting to resolve ethical dilemmas that arise in the clinical practice of medicine. It also refers to ensuring that a patient's clinical outcome reflects his or her preferences for health care. Clinical ethics is an essential component of quality health care. Teaching clinical ethics to medical students, house officers, and practicing physicians is one approach to improving the quality of patient care.

NOTES

1   M. Siegler, E.D. Pellegrino, P.A. Singer, "Clinical Medical Ethics," *The Journal of Clinical Ethics* 1 (Spring 1990): 5-9.

2   P.A. Singer, M. Siegler, and E.D. Pellegrino, "Research in Clinical Ethics," *The Journal of Clinical Ethics* 1 (Summer 1990): 95-100.

3   An American Physician, *Conferences on the Moral Philosophy of Medicine* (New York: Rebman, 1906).

4   M. Siegler, "A Legacy of Osler: Teaching Clinical Ethics at the Bedside," *Journal of the American Medical Association* 239 (1987): 951-56; and E.D. Pellegrino, "Ethics and the Moment of Clinical Truth," *Journal of the American Medical Association* 239 (1978): 960-61.

5   Siegler, Pellegrino, and Singer, "Clinical Medical Ethics."

6   Singer, Siegler, and Pellegrino, "Research in Clinical Ethics."

7   B. Lo and S.A. Schroeder, "Frequency of Ethical Dilemmas in a Medical Inpatient Service," *Archives of Internal Medicine* (1987): 1062-64.

8   J.E. Connelly and S. Dallemura, "Ethical Problems in the Medical Office," *Journal of the American Medical Association* 260 (1988): 812-15.

9   'J. La Puma, C.B. Stocking, M.D. Silverstein, et al., "An Ethics Consultation Service in a Teaching Hospital—Utilization and Evaluation," *Journal of the American Medical Association* 260 (1988): 808-11.

10   J.A. Jacobson, B.W. Tolle, C.B. Stocking, and M. Siegler, "Internal Medicine Resident's Preferences Regarding Medical Ethics Education," *Academic Medicine* 64 (1989): 760-64.

11   E.D. Pellegrino, R.J. Hart, S. Henderson, et al., "Relevance and Utility of Courses in Medical Ethics: A Survey of Physicians' Perceptions," *Journal of the American Medical Association* 253 (1985): 49-53.

12   R. Cohen, P.A. Singer, A.I. Rothman, and A. Robb, "Assessing Competency to Address Ethical Issues in Medicine," *Academic Medicine* (forthcoming, 1991).

13   E.D. Pellegrino, "Teaching Medical Ethics: Some Persistent Questions and Some Responses," *Academic Medicine* 64 (1989): 701-3.

9.8   **Roberts LW, Hardee JT, Franchini G, Stidley C, Siegler M (1996) Medical Students as Patients: A Pilot Study of their Health Care Needs, Practices, and Concerns. Acad Med 71:1225–32**

RESEARCH REPORT

Medical Students as Patients: A Pilot Study of Their Health Care Needs, Practices, and Concerns

Laura Weiss Roberts, MD, James T. Hardee, MD, Gregory Franchini, MD, Christine A. Stidley, MD, and Mark Siegler, MD

ABSTRACT

Background. The personal health experiences of medical students may contribute in important but previously unacknowledged ways to their well-being and education. This pilot study surveyed medical students about their health care needs, practices, insurance status, and concerns about seeking care.

Method. A questionnaire was developed and distributed to 151 students at the University of New Mexico School of Medicine in 1993–94. Participant privacy was protected. Responses were compiled and analyzed using logistic regression models and odds ratios.

Results. A total of 112 students responded. Most reported health care needs and half routinely received care at their training institution. One-third had informally requested prescriptions or diagnostic tests from medical school faculty and housestaff; one-fourth used such informal consultation as their "usual" method of obtaining care. Eighteen students were uninsured. The students reported that they had not sought care for several reasons, and many had experienced difficulty in obtaining care. The students indicated concern about confidentiality and

about the dual role as both student and patient at the training institution. They believed that their academic standing would be jeopardized if they developed certain health problems. When asked about hypothetical scenarios, a majority preferred to avoid the dual role of medical-student–patient. When asked about scenarios in which medical student peers exhibited suicidal depression or severe drug abuse, the students overwhelmingly preferred not to notify the medical school administration. Significant differences in responses were found with respect to gender and training level.

Conclusion. This pilot study examined the health care needs, practices (including the use of informal consultation), insurance status, and concerns of students at one medical school. The findings highlight the students' perceptions of illness and vulnerability during medical school training. Constructive implications for academic medicine are discussed regarding initiatives in the areas of policy, research, and the resources and structure of student health care services.
Acad. Med. 1996;71:1225–1232.

There are 67,072 students, including more than 27,500 women, enrolled in

Dr. Roberts is assistant professor and associate director of medical student education, Department of Psychiatry; Dr. Hardee is a resident, Department of Medicine; Dr. Franchini is assistant professor and director of medical student education, Department of Psychiatry; Dr. Stidley is director, Cancer Research and Treatment Center Biostatistics Group, and research assistant professor, Department of Family and Community Medicine; all at the University of New Mexico School of Medicine, Albuquerque; and Dr. Siegler is director, McLean Center for Clinical Medical Ethics, and professor, Department of Medicine, University of Chicago Pritzker School of Medicine, Chicago, Illinois.

Correspondence and requests for reprints should be addressed to Dr. Roberts, Department of Psychiatry, University of New Mexico, 2400 Tucker NE, Albuquerque, NM 87131-5326. e-mail: <lroberts@ salud.unm.edu>.

medical schools in the United States.[1] While becoming physicians, all of these students are at risk for developing serious illnesses, undergoing considerable stresses, and receiving inadequate health care.[2–10] Surprisingly, several aspects of medical student health care have not been explored, as past efforts have focused almost exclusively on psychiatric problems arising during medical training. The general health care of medical students merits attention, however, as it may contribute in important but previously unacknowledged ways to medical students' lives and education.

Six special issues arise in the care of medical-student–patients. First, the rig-

ors and exposures involved in medical training itself may lead to significant health problems, including stress-related physical symptoms, poor self-care, infection with the human immunodeficiency virus (HIV) and other agents, substance dependence, and depressive, anxiety, and adjustment disorders.[2–10] The stresses felt by medical students have been shown to exceed those of physicians in several areas, such as fatigue, financial strain, and interpersonal conflicts.[5] Second, women medical students appear to experience special difficulties, as reflected in their increased rate of suicide when compared with women in the general population and their higher levels of distress, more common depression, greater retention of alcohol abuse once acquired, and other problems.[2-4,6,9,10] The general health needs of women medical students have not yet been clarified.

Third, medical-student–patients may resemble physician–patients, who have difficulty obtaining appropriate care; who are known for their pattern of self-neglect, self-diagnosis, and self-treatment; and for whom communication, confidentiality, and role conflicts predictably arise.[2,8,11-13] Fourth, medical students, apprehensive about career repercussions, face serious obstacles in acknowledging personal illness and pursuing treatment at their training institutions. Their apprehension is accurate in that students who have histories of counseling are less likely to be selected by residency programs.[14] In addition, noncognitive criteria used to assess medical students favor sturdy and adaptable students, raising the question of how ill students are evaluated.[15]

Fifth, there is evidence that students engaged in preclinical and clinical training encounter different hazards that may affect their health.[2,6-8] Students' self-care behaviors and perceptions of personal health diminish, whereas their somatic complaints, depressive symptoms, and relationship problems typically increase over the preclinical years of medical school.[4,9] Second-year students appear to be at especially high risk for experiencing severe dysphoria and committing suicide.[2,4,6] Third- and fourth-year students often witness illness and suffering, develop maladaptive defenses for coping, and become exhausted by newly acquired patient care responsibilities.[2,4-7] Clinical students are also subject to possible mistreatment by teachers, with 80.6% of senior medical students at one institution reporting some form of abuse during medical school.[7]

Finally, access to care is a critical, though poorly understood, issue in medical education.[2,16] Many medical students may not have health insurance, may have insurance that limits

their care to the training institution, and may not have access to disability insurance.[2,17,18] Ambiguities also exist about insurance coverage when trainees leave educational programs for health reasons.[16,17]

These exceptional challenges involved in providing general health care to medical students have not, to our knowledge, been adequately explored. Literature in the areas of stress and impairment[3-6,9,10] does not capture the broader health issues for medical-student–patients. Compelling commentaries of physician–patients have also provided insights, but again do not fully illuminate the unique experience of being both medical trainee and patient.[11-14,17] For these reasons, we undertook a pilot survey study to examine medical students' health care needs and practices, their insurance status, and their concerns about illness and professional vulnerability.

METHOD

Design, subjects, procedure, survey instrument. A five-page self-report questionnaire was developed for this pilot project to investigate medical students' experiences and perceptions with respect to their own health care. The survey was given to a convenience sample of all 151 second- and fourth-year students at the University of New Mexico School of Medicine in 1993–94. Our study design assured participant voluntarism and confidentiality, though not anonymity. Because of its goals and subject protections, this study was deemed exempt from formal review by the human research committee at the university.

Analysis. Descriptive and frequency data were compiled and analyzed. Responses were compared across three main group variables: gender, age, and level of training (preclinical or clinical). Outcome variables of where students seek health care, insurance coverage, difficulty in obtaining health care, and students' practices of obtaining in-

formal consultation were examined with logistic regression models. All models included factors to adjust for the effects of the three main group variables. For the difficulty-obtaining-care outcome variables, the additional predictor variable of insurance status was included. Odds ratios were estimated and 95% confidence intervals were calculated. In tests of odds ratios, confidence intervals and significance levels (.05) are provided. The results are offered as descriptive and exploratory.

RESULTS

A total of 112 students, 74% of those asked, participated in this study. Forty-five (40%) of the respondents were women, closely resembling the base gender rate in the study population (44% women). Sixty-six students were in their twenties and 46 were in their thirties and forties (range 22–44 years; median = 29 years). Fifty-nine preclinical students in their second year and 53 clinical students in their fourth year of training participated, resembling the base population (74 preclinical, 77 clinical).

Health Care Needs Identified

Ninety-five of the students in our study reported needing or wanting health care during medical school. A greater proportion of the women (91%) than the men (81%) indicated health care needs (OR = 3.1). Ninety percent of the clinical students, a far greater percentage than of the preclinical students, indicated a need for health care (OR = 6.9; $p < .05$). These findings were adjusted for age. The students acknowledged a variety of health needs, including health maintenance (70%), infections (46%), depression/stress symptoms (42%); reproductive health (30%), headaches (24%), broken bones/injuries (21%), and other problems (21%), such as asthma, skin care, cancer, allergies, and eye care. Seven students reported that they had been hospitalized during medical school (six for medical or surgical problems; one for a psychiatric problem).

Not unexpectedly, the women reported the need for reproductive health care far more often (OR = 23.1; $p < .05$) and depression/stress symptoms somewhat more often (OR = 2.3; $p < .05$) than their male colleagues. The women more often acknowledged general health maintenance needs (OR = 2.4) and infections (OR = 2.1) than the men. The clinical students less often indicated depression/stress symptoms (OR = 0.3, $p < .05$) and headaches (OR = 0.6) than their preclinical colleagues, but more commonly acknowledged many "other" medical problems (OR = 5.7, $p < .05$).

Where Medical Students Obtained Care and Use of Informal Consultation

The students were asked to indicate the principal site or sites at which they "usually" sought medical care. About half of the students (58, 52%) usually sought medical care at their training institution (Table 1). Fifty-three students (47%) usually went outside of the training institution and 21 students (19%) usually obtained care through other avenues. The women reported use of more medical services, both at and outside of the training institution (ORs of 1.3 and 1.7, respectively).

Twenty-five students (22%) usually obtained care through informal consultation with attending physicians or residents at the medical school, including 27% of the women and 36% of the clinical students in the study. Use of informal consultation was clarified by asking whether students had "ever" asked a colleague informally to prescribe medications or to order diagnostic tests (Table 2). One-third of the students (38) acknowledged this event, including 45% of the clinical students and 40% of the women students. Two categories were defined statistically to look further at informal consultation: those

Table 1

Where Students Said They Usually Obtained Health Care, University of New Mexico School of Medicine, 1993–94*

	No. of Students (%)	Odds Ratio Women : Men	Odds Ratio Clinical : Preclinical
At training institution	58 (52)	1.3	2.2†
Formal relationship with a personal physician	48 (43)	1.1	1.6
Informal consultation with attending physician or resident	25 (22)	1.3	5.3†
Emergency department/urgent care	7 (6)	0.6	3.4
Outside training institution	53 (47)	1.7	0.7
Formal relationship with a personal physician	41 (37)	1.8	0.6
Emergency department/urgent care	12 (11)	1.5	0.7
Other	21 (19)	2.0	0.9

*A total of 112 second-year (preclinical) and fourth-year (clinical) students responded to a pilot survey about their health care needs, practices, and concerns. When asked to indicate where they "usually" obtained care, the students were given the option to choose more than one site (so the percentages in the table do not add up to 100%). The odds ratios in the table are derived from logistic regression models including factors for gender, age, and level of training.

†Statistically significant at the .05 level.

students who had responded positively to *both* of the questions ("ever" and "usually") concerning informal consultation and those students who had responded positively to *either* of the questions. In so doing, the common use of informal consultation by clinical students becomes more evident.

Insurance Coverage

Eighteen medical students reported that they had no health insurance, including 25% of the clinical students and 9% of the preclinical students (OR = 3.3, $p < .05$). Forty-three students stated that they had health insurance offered through the medical school, including 47% of the women and 33% of the men in the study. Thirty-two (74%) of the students with insurance offered through the medical school believed that they had no option to obtain care outside the training institution. Fifty-one students (46%) indicated that they had insurance other than the policies offered

through the medical school. A majority of these (30) were preclinical students. Seventy-two students, including 75% of the women and 63% of the men in the study, indicated that they were willing to pay "extra" for health insurance that allowed them to obtain outside medical care.

Reasons for Not Seeking Care

Sixty-two (55%) of the medical students in our study did not seek needed health care at some time because they were "too busy," and 48 (43%) did not seek care because they "thought the problem would resolve itself," a form of self-diagnosis. Thirty-five (31%) worried about cost and 13 (12%) worried about confidentiality. Fourteen students gave other reasons.

Difficulties in Obtaining Care

One-fourth of the students had experienced difficulty in obtaining necessary

Table 2

Students' Use of Informal Consultation to Obtain Health Care, University of New Mexico School of Medicine, 1993–94*			
		Odds Ratio	
	No. of Students (%)	Women:Men	Clinical:Preclinical
Students who have *ever* asked a colleague to prescribe or to order diagnostic tests	38 (34)	1.5	3.4†
Students who *usually* obtain health care through informal consultation	25 (22)	1.3	5.3†
Students who indicated *either* of the above practices	46 (41)	1.4	3.4†
Students who indicated *both* of the above practices	17 (15)	1.5	7.9†

*A total of 112 second-year (preclinical) and fourth-year (clinical) students responded to a pilot survey about their health care needs, practices, and concerns. The students were asked two questions about obtaining care through informal consultation with attending physicians or residents: (1) whether they had "ever" done so and (2) whether they "usually" did so. The odds ratios shown in the table are derived from logistic regression models including factors for gender, age, and level of training.

†Statistically significant at the .05 level.

health care during medical school. The women students (OR = 2.8, $p < .05$) and uninsured students (OR = 8.6, $p < .05$) were particularly affected.

Academic Jeopardy and Preferences for Site of Care

The students showed variability in their perceptions of academic jeopardy resulting from particular illnesses, but they often preferred to receive care from outside their training institution for problems that might be stigmatizing. (Table 3). Seventy-eight (70%) of the students acknowledged that confidentiality was a factor in their preferences for outside care. Thirty-nine (35%) of the students perceived academic jeopardy resulting from contracting HIV in one's personal life, but only 25 (22%) did so for contracting HIV in training settings. Seventy-two (65%) of the students, particularly women (OR = 3.2, $p < .05$), preferred care outside of the training institution for HIV resulting from personal-life exposure, but only 37

(33%) did so for HIV from training exposure. Seventy-five (67%) feared contracting HIV from patients during medical training.

Sixty-six students (59%) felt that their careers might be in jeopardy for problems with chemical dependence, with 87 (78%) preferring outside care. Only 20 students (18%) perceived academic jeopardy resulting from depression/stress symptoms, although 63 (57%) would request outside care, especially women students (OR = 2.4, $p < .05$). Many students also preferred outside care for reproductive health needs (51, 47%) and elective hernia surgery (46, 41%), though they commonly had no preference regarding site of care for other problems (e.g., urinary infection, chest pain).

Sensitivity to Dual Role as Both Patient and Student

The students were asked whether they would proceed with or avoid a dual relationship as both patient and student

in four hypothetical scenarios (Table 4): (1) an unmarried medical student seeks a pregnancy test from a clinic attending physician whom she discovers to be the faculty director of the obstetrics–gynecology clerkship; (2) a medical student seeks further care for ravaging gastrointestinal (GI) symptoms, previously misdiagnosed as "stress" by a faculty physician; (3) a medical student with rheumatoid arthritis discovers that her personal physician is to be her ward attending physician, responsible for supervising and grading her; and (4) a medical student needs non-emergent inguinal hernia repair and wonders whether he should seek care at the medical school. A majority of students did not wish to proceed with the dual role in the hernia scenario (86, 78%) and the pregnancy test scenario (72, 65%). Nearly half of the students did not wish to proceed with the dual role in the rheumatoid-arthritis scenario (55, 49%) and GI-symptom scenario (53, 47%).

Unwillingness to Report Seriously Ill Medical Students

The students were asked to respond to two hypothetical cases depicting medical students suffering from serious psychiatric difficulties. In the first scenario, the students were asked to imagine themselves as the university physician providing care to a third-year medical student in whom they find severe alcohol and amphetamine abuse and a pattern of erratic behavior. When asked whether they would notify the medical school administration of the problem 90 (80%) stated that they would not. Nine (8%) stated that they would, and 13 (12%) indicated that they would do nothing or take another course of action. In the second scenario, the students were asked to consider how they would respond if their anatomy lab partner exhibited severe depression and suicidality. A large majority (91, 81%) again responded that they would not notify the medical school administration, whereas 12 (11%) stated that they would. Nine (8%) would do nothing or choose another course of action. In both scenarios, the clinical students were somewhat more likely than their preclinical colleagues to notify the medical school administration.

DISCUSSION

Health Care Needs of Medical Students

The vast majority of medical students in this study needed or wanted health care during medical school. Comparison with other patient populations suggests that medical students more often report the need for care regarding infections, headaches, injuries, and other problems.[19] This is compatible with the observation of Kellner et al.[20] that medical students may be more attentive to somatic symptoms and seek more health care when compared with law students. Our study, like others, also documents relatively common experiences of depression/stress symptoms in medical students. We conclude that medical students experience significant rates of both physical and psychological symptoms and perceive a real need for health care during medical school.

Obstacles in Medical Student Health Care

Medical students appear to rely upon their training institutions for the provision of health care and medical insurance. They also encounter obstacles in pursuing their health care, as evidenced by several of our findings: students' direct reports of difficulty in obtaining care, especially in the case of uninsured students; their description of not seeking care because of being too busy, worried about cost, or concerned about confidentiality; their extensive use of informal consultation; their preferences for outside care, especially for embarrassing or

Table 3

Students' Preferences for Receiving Outside Care for Medical Problems, University of New Mexico School of Medicine, 1993–94*			
		Odds Ratio	
Medical Problem	No. of Students (%)	Women : Men	Clinical : Preclinical
Chemical dependence	87 (78)	2.4	1.8
HIV+ —contracted through personal life	72 (65)	3.2‡	1.8
Depression/anxiety	63 (57)	2.4‡	1.4
Reproductive health needs	51 (47)	1.4	1.3
Elective hernia surgery	46 (41)	1.4	1.2
HIV+ —contracted through training experience	37 (33)	2.0	0.8

*A total of 112 second-year (preclinical) and fourth-year (clinical) students responded to a pilot survey about their health care needs, practices, and concerns. The table shows the medical problems for which the students indicated they would prefer to receive care from outside their training institution. The odds ratios are derived from logistic regression models including factors for gender, age, and training level.

†HIV-human immunodeficiency virus; ‡statistically significant at the .05 level.

stigmatizing illnesses; some students' lack of health insurance, though relatively inexpensive plans are offered and some form of insurance is required by the medical school; their worries about HIV; and their concerns about dual roles, academic jeopardy, and confidentiality. These barriers may prevent early detection of illness in physicians, which is particularly unfortunate in light of the relatively favorable prognoses of certain illnesses when treated in medical students and physicians.[21]

Illness, Vulnerability, and Silence

The strong connection between illness and vulnerability is apparent in the students' worries about academic jeopardy and dual roles, preferences for outside care, and unwillingness to notify the medical school administration of serious symptoms in others. Even early in training, silence becomes the tacitly understood, culturally sanctioned response to illness. This is disquieting given the ethical imperative to intervene on the behalf of troubled colleagues and their endangered patients.

Our findings suggest that students may not seek care for themselves when they need it, nor will they intervene with compromised peers when it is imperative.

Concerns about illness and vulnerability are further suggested by the findings with respect to HIV infection, a phenomenon that has had a tremendous impact on medical practice and training. Many in our study feared contracting HIV from patients but, interestingly, perceived HIV acquired "in the line of duty" as less stigmatizing than HIV acquired in one's personal life. Sadly, the discrimination reported by physicians with HIV does not support the perception that the source of infection offers protection from stigma.[17]

Gender Differences

The responses of the women and the men in this study often differed. The women more often reported difficulty obtaining health care and more frequently identified health concerns, especially regarding reproductive health and depression/stress symptoms. The

Table 4

Students' Reluctance to Proceed with Dual Role as Patient and Student in Four Hypothetical Scenarios, University of New Mexico School of Medicine, 1993–94*			
	No. of Students	Odds Ratio	
Scenario	Responding "No" (%)	Women : Men	Clinical : Preclinical
Unmarried medical student seeks pregnancy test; attending physician in clinic that day is obstetrics–gynecology clerkship director; should student proceed?	72† (65)	5.0‡	5.0‡
Medical student misdiagnosed with "stress" by medical school faculty physician, when actually he or she has a serious gastrointestinal disease; should student proceed with this physician's care?	53 (47)	1.1	1.4
Medical student with rheumatoid arthritis learns that her personal physician is to be her ward attending physician on medicine rotation; should student proceed with this arrangement?	55 (49)	3.3‡	2.0‡
Medical student seeks non-emergent hernia repair; should student seek care at training institution?	86† (78)	3.3‡	1.1

*A total of 112 second-year (preclinical) and fourth-year (clinical) students responded to a pilot survey about their health care needs, practices, and concerns. The table shows how many of the students indicated they would not proceed with a dual relationship as both patient and student in four scenarios. The odds ratios are derived from logistic regression models including factors for gender, age, and level of training.

†111 students responded to this scenario; ‡statistically significant at the .05 level.

women also more commonly relied on the medical school for the provision of health care and insurance, used multiple sites for care, and pursued informal consultation to meet their health needs. They showed greater sensitivity to the complexities of dual relationships and to certain stigma-related issues, as reflected in their decisions not to proceed in hypothetical situations involving dual roles and their preferences for care outside the training institution for certain problems. These findings complement the extensive literature documenting the increased stresses experienced by women in medicine[2,3,6,7,10,16,22] and the emphasis women place upon certain issues, such as perceptions of safety and preservation of relationships, in personal decision making.[22,23]

Special Issues for Clinical Students

Special considerations for medical students engaged in clinical training arose in this study. They had more health needs and yet constituted a larger proportion of uninsured students. The clinical students were much more likely to use informal consultation to obtain health care. Perhaps informal consultation is more often sought by clinical students because they are more familiar with approachable physicians at the

medical school, because of an emerging pattern of self-diagnosis and self-treatment, because of inability to pay, or because of a desire to limit documentation of their health problems. Whatever the causes, the consequences of informal consultation are unknown. As an extension of "professional courtesy," informal consultation is inexpensive and may lower barriers to care. On the other hand, it is unlikely to provide opportunity for thoroughness in history gathering, diagnosis, and treatment or to allow for an adequate consent process. It is more likely to lead to "quick" solutions, including the prescription of psychotropic medications.[24] The clinical students were also more inclined to seek outside care and were more reluctant to proceed in dual relationships at the training institution. Taken together, these findings suggest that clinical experience sensitizes students to the realities of hierarchical medical relationships and of vulnerabilities associated with illness.

Limitations of the Study

Several aspects of this study limit its interpretation and generalization. First, this project was designed as a study of student perceptions and relies exclusively on self-disclosure. Second, our findings could be unique to one medical school. In particular, the supportive approach taken by the administration and faculty at the University of New Mexico may have led, for example, to increased reports of informal consultation and to lessened concerns about site of care, illness, and stigma. Third, the study's response rate of 74%, while a good level of participation for this type of project, may have created bias. Fourth, this study did not include those students who may have left medical school and for whom these issues may be particularly acute.[4,15] Finally, though there were efforts to minimize this problem, the number of statistical comparisons performed may introduce difficulties in interpretation. This study's results should be viewed as descriptive and as the basis for further inquiry.

Constructive Implications

This study has broad constructive implications for policy, research, and health care service initiatives in academic medicine.

Policy initiatives. A national discussion of appropriate policy initiatives regarding medical student illness, confidentiality, stigma and academic jeopardy, insurance and health care access, and related topics is essential at this time. Active efforts should be undertaken to define the special responsibilities of medical schools and faculty physicians in caring for students, to clarify what kinds of health problems are potentially incompatible with medical training and practice, and to create protected avenues for medical student health care. Such efforts are crucial if medical schools are to respond to the needs of medical students in an effective and authentic manner.

Research initiatives. Investigation of several aspects of medical student health care is warranted on both clinical and educational grounds, including identifying the health care needs and practices of medical students nationally; assessing the adequacy of health care access and insurance options for medical students; examining the long-term effect of confidentiality policies and protected avenues of care for medical student health; considering how work with HIV-infected patients affects medical student views; illuminating the contributions of gender, age, and race–ethnicity to medical student health care experiences; determining the consequences of informal consultation; understanding stigma in relation to physical and psychiatric illness in training; and clarifying how health care experiences influence the professional development of medical students. A consortium of collaborative investigators at 12 medical schools, led by our

University of New Mexico group, has begun work to study these and related issues in medical student health care nationally.

Health care service initiatives. This study adds to our appreciation of the importance of the resources and structure of student health care services.[2,8,16] We are reminded first that medical schools should redouble efforts to provide adequate insurance and to establish protected avenues of health care for their students. Second, the separation of educational, administrative, and care-giving roles of medical school faculty should be pursued, as this will reduce barriers to care. Third, clear and realistic discussions of professional health issues—beginning with the first day of orientation and revisited throughout the four years of training—are essential, as is the development of safe self- and peer-referral mechanisms for ill students. Finally, efforts to clarify policies and practices within the cultures of individual medical schools—such as positions on confidentiality measures, provision of informal consultation, and appropriate responses to student impairment—should be undertaken by faculty and administration at each institution.

In conclusion, attention to medical student health care issues is an important though underrecognized mission of academic medicine. If we believe, as Osler did, that the best lessons are those learned by example, our neglect of medical student health care may influence trainees to take poor care of themselves, to bring fear and mistrust to therapeutic relationships, and to provide inadequate care to future physicians and colleagues. Moreover, considering the transformative nature of patienthood, medical students' health care experiences represent extraordinarily poignant moments, personally and professionally. Capturing the power of these moments, uniquely able to engender empathy or cynicism in the young physician,[2,13,17] should be given more emphasis by medical educators. Through sustained attention to these and related issues, we believe

medical students will be better cared for, their physicians and teachers better prepared, and, ultimately, their patients better treated and protected.

The authors express their appreciation to Drs. Teresita McCarty, Scott Obenshain, Brian Roberts, Sally K. Severino, and Joel Yager.

REFERENCES

1. Bennett CT (ed). Medical School Admission Requirements, 1996–1997, United States and Canada. 46th ed. Washington, DC: Association of American Medical Colleges, 1995.
2. Lane LW, Lane G, Schiedermayer DL, Spiro JH, Siegler M. Caring for medical students as patients. Arch Int Med. 1989;150:2249–53.
3. Clark DC, Eckenfels EJ, Daugherty SR, Fawcett J. Alcohol use patterns through medical school: a longitudinal study of one class. JAMA. 1987; 257:2921–6.
4. Clark DC, Zeldow PB. Vicissitudes of depressed mood during four years of medical school. JAMA. 1988;260:2521–8.
5. McAuliffe WE, Rohman M, Santangelo S, et al. Psychoactive drug use among practicing physicians and medical students. N Engl J Med. 1986;315:805–10.
6. Pepitone-Arreola-Rockwell F, Rockwell D, Core N. Fifty-two medical students suicides. Am J Psychiatry. 1981;138:198–201.
7. Silver HK, Glicken AD. Medical student abuse: incidence, severity, and significance. JAMA. 1990;263:527–32.
8. Westmeyer J. Mental health care for medical students and residents: current problems and evolving resources. Minn Med. 1987;70:565–9.
9. Lloyd C, Gantrell NK. Psychiatric symptoms in medical students. Compr Psychiatry. 1984; 25:552–65.
10. Lloyd C, Gantrell NK. Sex differences in medical student mental health. Am J Psychiatry. 1981;138:1346–51.
11. Spiro HM, McCrea-Curren MG, Preschel E, St. James D. Empathy and the Practice of Medicine. New Haven, CT: Yale University Press, 1993.
12. Stoudemire A, Rhoads JM. When the doctor needs a doctor: special considerations for the physician patient. Ann Intern Med. 1983;98: 654–9.
13. Inglefinger F. Arrogance. N Engl J Med. 1980; 303:1507–11.
14. Oppenheimer K, Miller M, Forney P. Effect of history of psychological counseling on selection of applicants for residencies. J Med Educ. 1987; 62:504–8.
15. Miller GD, Frank D, Franks RD, Getto CJ.

Noncognitive criteria for assessing students in North American medical schools. Acad Med. 1989;64:42–5.

16. Plaut SM, Maxwell SA, Seng L, O'Brien JJ, Fairclough GF. Mental health services for medical students: perceptions of students, student affairs deans, and mental health providers. Acad Med. 1993;68:360–5.

17. Aoun H. When a house officer gets AIDS. N Engl J Med. 1989;221:694–6.

18. Siegler M. Confidentiality in medicine: a decrepit concept. N Engl J Med. 1982;301:1518–21.

19. Dorgan CA (ed.) Statistical Record of Health and Medicine. Detroit, MI: Gale Research Inc., International Thompson Publishing, 1995.

20. Kellner R, Wiggins RG, Pathak D. Hypochondriacal fears and beliefs in medical and law students. Arch Gen Psychiatry. 1986;43: 487–9.

21. Morse RM, Martin MA, Swenson WM, Niven RG. Prognosis of physicians treated for alcoholism and drug dependence. JAMA. 1984;251: 743–6.

22. Bickel J. Women in medical education. N Engl J Med. 1988;319:1579–84.

23. Gilligan C. In a Different Voice. Cambridge, MA: Harvard University Press, 1982.

24. Clark AW, Kay J, Clark DC. Patterns of psychoactive drug prescriptions by house officers for nonpatients. J Med Educ. 1988;63:44–50.

9.9   **Roberts LW, McCarty T, Lyketsos C, Hardee JT, Jacobson J, Walker R, Hough P, Gramelspacher G, Stidley C, Arambula M, Heebink DM, Zornberg GL, Siegler M (1996) What and How Psychiatry Residents at Ten Training Programs Wish to Learn About Ethics. Acad Psychiatry 20:131–43**

What and How Psychiatry Residents at Ten Training Programs Wish to Learn About Ethics

Laura Weiss Roberts, M.D., Teresita McCarty, M.D.
Constantine Lyketsos, M.D., James T. Hardee, M.D.
Jay Jacobson, M.D., Robert Walker, M.D.
Patricia Hough, M.D., Ph.D., Gregory Gramelspacher, M.D.
Christine A. Stidley, Ph.D., Michael Arambula, M.D.
Denise M. Heebink, M.D., Gwen L. Zornberg, M.D.
Mark Siegler, M.D.

The study's objective was to survey what and how psychiatry residents want to learn about ethics during residency. A 4-page questionnaire developed for this study was sent to 305 residents at 10 adult psychiatry programs in the United States. One-hundred and eighty-one (59%) of those surveyed responded. Seventy-six percent reported facing an ethical dilemma in residency for which they felt unprepared. Forty-six percent reported having received no ethics training during residency. More than 50% of the respondents requested that "more" curricular attention be paid to 19 specific ethics topics and more than 40% for 25 topics. Preferences with respect to learning methods are presented. This survey may provide guidance in structuring the content and process of ethics education for psychiatry residents. These findings should stimulate the efforts of faculty to commit time and attention to this important curricular area. (Academic Psychiatry 1996; 20:131–143)

While there is consensus that psychiatry residents should have a foundation of knowledge in medical ethics (1–6), an uncertainty exists about what and how residents should learn about the moral aspects of their clinical work. In the only study of its kind that we could find, Coverdale et al. (5) asked program directors and chief residents at adult psychiatry training programs about ethics training offered at their institutions. The researchers found that 40% of the 121 programs surveyed did not offer training in ethics through a planned course or seminar. Moreover, ethics topics identified as most worthy of formal attention were discussed in

fewer than 30% of the programs. These findings are of concern in light of the accreditation standards for postgraduate medical education that require ethics training in every psychiatry program (6) and the apparently universal view that ethics training is necessary and helpful for residents of all specialties (7–11).

Asking residents at each level of psychiatric training about their interests and per-

Dr. Roberts is assistant professor and associate director, Medical Student Education, Department of Psychiatry, University of New Mexico, Albuquerque. See acknowledgments for affiliations of other authors.

ceived needs with respect to ethics education is an approach that has received little attention. Certainly, the value of ethics training during postgraduate years hinges in part on its responsiveness to the experiences, preferences, and educational backgrounds of those being taught (9,11). The different priorities of chief residents and faculty found by Coverdale et al. (5) underscore the value of exploring rather than presuming resident perspectives.

In view of the importance of ethics training for the field of psychiatry, we undertook this study to ascertain what and how psychiatric residents wish to learn about ethics.

METHODS

Design and Subjects

We sent a survey to 305 residents in a convenience sample of 10 psychiatry programs nationwide. Characteristics of programs and residents are listed in Table 1. Half of the programs were at universities with private affiliations; half were at state universities. The 10 residencies were located in 9 states and 5 distinct geographical regions in the United States. Our study design assured participant confidentiality, though not anonymity, and was approved or exempt from review by the human research committees at our study sites.

Survey Instrument

Based on the work of Jacobson et al. (12), one of us (LWR) developed a 4-page questionnaire to determine the interests, preferred learning methods, and experiences of psychiatry residents with ethics training.

Procedure

An investigator at each site was responsible for distributing and collecting the surveys. The residents were given up to three opportunities to complete and return the surveys. The collected surveys were mailed to one of us (LWR), and four of us (LWR, CS, TM, JTH) conducted the data analysis at a central site (University of New Mexico).

Analysis

Survey data were entered into a database system and analyzed by using the Statistical Analysis Systems (SAS) (13). Descriptive and frequency information on the responses was obtained. In the areas of curricular topics and methods, resident responses were compared across four group variables: gender, age, presence of past ethics education, and level of residency training. Logistic regression (14) was used to model responses with the four group variables as predictors. Gender differences were assessed by using odds ratios and their 95% confidence intervals. Because of the descriptive nature of this study, no formal adjustment of significance levels was done for the statistical tests done. Several variables were summed, however, to reduce the number of individual comparisons and to aid in the interpretation of results.

RESULTS

Program and Respondent Characteristics

The survey response was 59.3% (181 residents). The response rates from the 10 schools ranged from 45.7% to 93.5% (Table 1). Ninety (49.7%) of the respondents were men, and 89 (49.2%) were women; 2 respondents did not answer the gender question. The percentages for gender for the surveyed population, including all residents in the study sample (i.e., respondents plus nonrespondents), were 53.8% men and 46.2% women. Most of the respondents were in their 20s ($n = 64$) and 30s ($n = 89$), and a smaller number were 40 years old or over ($n = 18$). Ten respondents (5.5%) did not give their age. The average age of responding

TABLE 1. Program characteristics and respondents' reports of ethics training during residency

Program	U.S. Region	University Affiliation	Residents in Program, n	Respondents, n (%)	Respondents Who Have Had Ethics Training in Residency, n (%)
1	SW	State	31	29 (93.5)	9 (31.0)
2	MW	Private	20	12 (60.0)	3 (25.0)
3	MW	State	37	18 (48.6)	4 (22.2)
4	E	Private	32	20 (62.5)	5 (25.0)
5	W	State	24	15 (62.5)	11 (73.3)
6	SE	State	35	18 (51.4)	13 (72.2)
7	MW	Private	21	16 (76.2)	11 (68.7)
8	SE	State	30	18 (56.7)	10 (55.6)
9	E	Private	35	16 (45.7)	7 (43.7)
10	E	Private	40	19 (47.5)	14 (73.7)
All Programs			305	181 (59.3)	87 (48.1)

women in the study was 32.0 years (range: 25–56), and the average age of the men was 32.8 years (range: 25–51). The residents were at 4 levels of postgraduate training: 23 (12.7%) at the postgraduate year (PGY)-1 level, 56 (30.9%) at the PGY-2 level, 50 (27.6%) at the PGY-3 level, and 48 (26.5%) at the PGY-4 level or beyond. Four respondents did not indicate their training level. The base rates with respect to level of training in the surveyed population, including all residents in the study sample (i.e., respondents plus nonrespondents), was 55 (18.0%) at the PGY-1 level, 70 (23.0%) at PGY-2, 80 (26.2%) at PGY-3, 80 (26.2%) at PGY-4 or beyond, and 20 (6.6%) unspecified.

Ethics Training Experiences

Eighty-three (45.9%) residents indicated they had received no ethics training in residency, whereas 87 (48.1%) reported receiving some ethics training in residency (Table 1). Eleven residents did not answer this question. The proportion of residents with ethics training occurring in residency varied widely in the 10 programs, ranging from 22.2% to 73.7%. Of the respondents who reported no ethics training in residency, 53.0%

($n = 44$) were PGY-1's and PGY-2's, and 46.8% ($n = 38$) were PGY-3's or beyond (Table 2). Of the 79 residents in our study who were at the PGY-1 and PGY-2 levels, 55.7% ($n = 44$) reported no ethics training. Of the 98 residents in our study who were at the PGY-3 level and beyond, 38.8% ($n = 38$) reported no ethics training during residency. Twelve residents had not received ethics education at any time during their medical school and residency training.

About two-thirds ($n = 122$) of the residents stated that they had received some form of ethics training during medical school, whereas one-third had not received or did not recall getting ethics training. Eighty-one residents had 1 formal course, and 41 residents had 2 or more courses in medical school. More than half of the residents who had received ethics education in medical school received this training only during the preclinical years. In particular, 34 residents did not receive ethics education during their clinical training (i.e., the latter 2 years of medical school and their residency). Nineteen percent of the residents in our study had ethics training during their third and fourth years of medical school, and 20% had such training throughout the preclinical and clinical portions of medical school. Nearly two-thirds ($n = 116$) of the respondents indicated that they had not received ethics training at another time (i.e., outside of medical school or residency curricula).

The residents reported exposure to several methods of learning about ethics during their medical school education, which included assigned readings ($n = 95$); discussions during clinical rounds ($n = 94$); conferences ($n = 92$); ethics lectures in the general curriculum ($n = 91$); and to a lesser extent, interactions with ethics consultation services ($n = 32$).

Ethics Interest

As shown in Table 3, most of the 181 residents in our study (76.2%) indicated that they had faced an ethical dilemma for which they felt unprepared during their medical training. Of the 82 residents who had not received ethics training in residency, three-quarters ($n = 62$) had faced an ethical dilemma for which they felt unprepared. On the basis of logistic regression models, the women were more likely to report having faced an ethical dilemma for which they felt unprepared, irrespective of their age, past ethics education, or level of residency training. Similarly, the residents over 30 also were

more likely to report this experience, irrespective of gender, past ethics education, or level of residency training. One-hundred and nine residents who reported this experience had one or no ethics courses in medical school or could not recall what their ethics training was during that period. Of the 35 residents who said they had not faced an ethical dilemma unprepared, 27 (77.1%) had received formal ethics training during medical school.

The residents overwhelmingly ($n=167$, or 92.3% of the respondents) indicated that ethics training helped them respond to ethical dilemmas that arise with patients. Interestingly, all of the 12 residents who had not received training at any time in their education presumed that ethics training would be helpful, as did each of the 34 residents without ethics training in either their residency or clinical years of medical school combined. Of the 181 residents in our study, only 5 indicated that ethics training is not helpful, and 9 did not answer this question.

Ethics Topics

We asked the residents to indicate whether 26 specific ethics topics should receive more, the same, or less curricular attention at their programs. The residents were

---

TABLE 2.   Lack of ethics training in psychiatric residents' medical and postgraduate education

	n	Percentage of All Respondents
No ethics training		
During residency	83	45.9
Postgraduate year (PGY)-1 and -2	44	
PGY-3 or beyond	38	
Unknown year	1	
No ethics training or could not recall ethics training during medical school	59	32.6
No ethics training during residency *and* no ethics training during clinical years of medical school	34	18.8
No ethics training ever	12	6.6
No ethics training outside of formal medical education	116	64.1

also able to indicate if they felt certain topics were "inappropriate." A large percentage of the psychiatry residents indicated interest in having more formal attention paid to each of the 26 ethics topics shown in Table 4. The women indicated interest in more topics than did the men. Odds ratios demonstrated that the odds of responding positively were between two and three times higher for the women than the men for nine topics: ethical and legal issues in withholding information, responding to colleague impairment, ethical issues in using unproven treatments, obtaining informed consent from psychotic patients for medical-surgical procedures, ethical and legal aspects of confidentiality concerning HIV-positive psychiatric patients, conflict resolution between psychiatric care providers and families, ethical issues in the trainee/therapy supervisor relationship, conflict resolution between resident and attending physician, and treatment decisions for indigent patients. Interestingly, of the 26 topics listed, the topic of physician-patient sexual contact was least likely to be chosen by the residents as needing more curricular attention. The topic of touching psychiatric patients was also relatively infrequently chosen by residents as needing more attention.

In addition, only 2 topics were identified by 10 or more residents as receiving "too much" curricular attention or were perceived as "inappropriate" curricular topics: physician-patient sexual contact ($n = 18$)

and physician-patient touching ($n = 10$). Other areas mentioned by a few residents as receiving "too much attention" include financial coverage of patient treatments related to the patient's diagnosis or prognosis ($n = 6$), confidentiality issues for HIV-positive patients ($n = 5$), accepting gifts from patients ($n = 4$), and appropriate responses to colleague impairment ($n = 4$).

Learning Methods

We asked the residents to rate as "very useful," "useful," or "not useful" 16 methods of learning about ethics. More than half of the residents identified as "very useful" 6 of the 16 specific learning methods, including 1) several conferences on ethics, 2) incorporation of ethics issues into other presentations and discussions, 3) discussions with colleagues and knowledgeable discussion leader, 4) a lecture course on ethics, 5) observation of attending physicians as they handle ethical problems, and 6) lectures or grand rounds on ethics.

When the questionnaires were compiled, the 16 learning methods were grouped into 4 logical categories, shown in Table 5, and include 1) lectures on ethics given by an expert, 2) discussions on ethics with experts, 3) integration of ethics teaching into clinical activities, and 4) independent learning. To look at resident preferences with respect to these various learning methods, we tabulated whether individual residents assessed

TABLE 3. Psychiatric residents' experience with difficult ethical dilemmas and the perceptions of helpfulness of ethics training[a]

Question	n (%)	
	Yes	No
Have you faced an ethical dilemma that you felt unprepared for during medical training?	138 (76.2)	35 (19.3)
Is ethics training helpful in responding to ethical dilemmas that arise with patients?	167 (92.3)	5 (2.8)

[a]Eight respondents (4.4%) did not answer the first question, and 9 respondents (5.0%) did not answer the second question.

TABLE 4.   Ethics topics chosen by psychiatry residents as needing more curricular attention

Area	Prefer "More" Curricular Attention			Odds Ratio[b]	95% Confidence Interval
	% of All Respondents (n = 181)[a]	% of Women Respondents (n = 89)[a]	% of Men Respondents (n = 90)[a]		
1. Ethical/legal issues involved in withholding information from patients	75.1	84.5	69.9	2.31[c]	1.05, 4.94
2. Understanding the legal rights of patients with compromised decisional capacity	72.9	77.6	72.6	1.40	0.68, 2.88
3. Financial coverage of patient treatments related to patient's diagnosis or prognosis	69.6	80.3	67.9	1.90	0.92, 3.91
4. Physician responsibilities when terminating with patients	65.7	69.1	65.5	1.21	0.62, 2.36
5. Government policies related to patient access to psychiatric care	64.6	69.5	66.7	1.05	0.54, 2.04
6. How to respond to impairment in a colleague due to substance abuse or psychiatric illness	64.6	77.4	56.0	2.77[c]	1.40, 5.46
7. Ethical issues involved in the use of psychiatric treatments that have not been clearly documented as efficacious in patients with certain diagnoses (e.g., ECT in nondepressed patients)	62.4	72.6	54.8	2.22[c]	1.15, 4.26
8. Obtaining informed consent from psychotic patients for medical-surgical procedures	61.9	73.8	53.0	2.46[c]	1.28, 4.75
9. Ethical and legal aspects of confidentiality concerning HIV-positive psychiatric patients	60.8	70.6	54.8	1.98[c]	1.04, 3.77
10. Ethical issues in assessing a patient's decisional capacity	60.8	64.7	57.1	1.35	0.72, 2.53
11. Obtaining informed consent from psychotic patients for medications, admission to locked wards, etc.	60.2	64.7	56.0	1.47	0.78, 2.77
12. When to report a patient case to adult protective services	59.1	63.5	57.1	1.23	0.65, 2.33
13. Ethical and legal aspects of confidentiality concerning violent psychiatric patients (e.g., "duty to warn")	55.2	60.0	48.8	1.66	0.89, 3.11
14. Conflict resolution between psychiatric care providers and families of patients	54.7	71.1	45.2	2.82[c]	1.48, 5.38
15. Ethical issues involved in the relationship between the trainee and psychotherapy supervisor	54.1	69.0	44.0	2.78[c]	1.47, 5.25
16. Ethical and legal aspects of confidentiality concerning "nondangerous" psychiatric patients	53.0	58.8	47.6	1.52	0.82, 2.81
17. Conflict resolution between resident and attending physician	51.9	66.3	44.0	2.37[c]	1.26, 4.47
18. Conflict resolution between physician and nonphysician psychiatric care provider	51.9	59.0	46.4	1.50	0.80, 2.83

(continued)

TABLE 4. Ethics topics chosen by psychiatry residents as needing more curricular attention *(continued)*

Area	Prefer "More" Curricular Attention				
	% of All Respondents (n = 181)[a]	% of Women Respondents (n = 89)[a]	% of Men Respondents (n = 90)[a]	Odds Ratio[b]	95% Confidence Interval
19. Ethical issues in accepting gifts from patients	50.8	59.5	46.4	1.71	0.92, 3.18
20. Psychiatric research services conducted on human subjects	49.2	55.6	45.2	1.55	0.83, 2.90
21. Ethical issues involved in touching psychiatric patients	48.6	54.1	46.4	1.26	0.68, 2.36
22. Ethical issues involved in making admission or treatment decisions for indigent patients	46.4	56.1	40.5	1.88[c]	1.00, 3.52
23. When to report a patient case to child protective services	43.1	48.8	40.5	1.40	0.74, 2.65
24. Obtaining informed consent	40.3	49.4	34.9	1.71	0.91, 3.23
25. The family's role in patient care decisions	39.2	46.4	35.7	1.52	0.80, 2.87
26. Ethical and legal issues related to sexual contact between physicians and patients	23.8	30.6	17.9	2.06	0.98, 4.34

[a]Two study participants did not specify gender.
[b]The odds ratios indicate how much more likely women are to respond positively to these topics relative to men.
[c]Statistically significant difference ($P < 0.05$) for gender, adjusted for age, level of residency training, and presence of past ethics education.

two or more methods from within the same category as "very useful." Table 5 shows this frequency data on the 4 categories and provides odds ratios and confidence intervals with respect to gender. We found that lectures by experts was identified as "very useful" twice or more often by individual residents 62.9% of the time. Integration of ethics teaching into usual clinical activities was preferred by 31.8% of the respondents, discussions on ethics with experts by 32.4% of the respondents, and independent learning by 22.4% of the residents.

The female residents were more enthusiastic about all four categories of learning methods, and all but one of the specific learning methods, independent reading. The odds ratios, shown on Table 5, controlling for age, level of residency training, and past ethics education, demonstrate the greater inter-

est of the female residents relative to the male residents.

DISCUSSION

This study documents how ethics training is perceived by 181 psychiatry residents at 10 programs in the United States. These residents clearly see ethics training as a valuable component in their psychiatric practice and education. Nearly all psychiatry residents in our study believe that ethics training is helpful in providing good patient care. They were remarkably enthusiastic about a variety of topics and learning techniques in ethics education. Despite this receptiveness to ethics training, many of the residents in our study reported receiving no formal ethics teaching during their postgraduate psychiatric education. Since trainees acquire significant aspects of their professional identities as physicians and psychiatrists, as well as establish lasting patterns of clinical conduct during residency, we consider ethics training during this phase of education to be critically important.

To understand the implications of our study in the development of educational guidelines for ethics education in psychiatry residencies, we will briefly discuss 6 aspects of our results: 1) the underdevelopment of training in ethics for psychiatry residents despite their apparent interest, 2) preferences about ethics topics and related gender differences, 3) preferences about learning methods and related gender differences, 4) a

comparison with the Jacobson et al. (12) study of internal medicine residents, 5) the study's limitations, and 6) the challenges faculty face in developing ethics training for psychiatric residency programs.

Underdevelopment of Ethics Training Despite Resident Interest

Our study has several salient and distressing findings with respect to psychiatry residents' ethics education. Essentially, half of the residents we surveyed had received no ethics training in residency despite the professional, institutional, and social imperatives that those in psychiatric practice have a

TABLE 5. Four categories of learning methods preferred by psychiatric residents

Learning Method & Item No.	Methods Identified as "Very Useful" Chosen Twice or More by			Odds Ratio[b]	95% Confidence Interval
	% of All Respondents ($n = 181$)[a]	% of Women ($n = 89$)[a]	% of Men ($n = 90$)[a]		
Lectures on ethics given by someone with expertise (e.g., ethics conferences, ethics lecture courses, individual ethics lectures or grand rounds)	62.9	70.6	55.3	1.92[c]	1.01, 3.64
Discussions on ethics with someone with expertise (e.g., group discussion with knowledgeable leader, discussing videotape with knowledgeable leader, workshops at professional meetings, and discussion with hospital attorney)	32.4	44.7	20.0	3.27[c]	1.64, 6.54
Integration of ethics teaching into usual clinical activities (e.g., ethics discussions during morning report, individual supervision, observing attending physicians handling ethical problems with patients, obtaining ethics consultation for clinical ethics problems, and ethics committee involvement)	31.8	43.5	20.0	3.13[c]	1.56, 6.27
Independent learning (e.g., an ethics manual, annotated bibliography, independent reading, discussion initiated by and with peers, and watching self-instruction videotape)	22.4	25.9	18.8	1.48	0.71, 3.10

[a]Two study participants did not specify gender.
[b]The odds ratios indicate how much more likely women are to respond positively to these kinds of learning methods relative to men.
[c]Statistically significant difference ($P < 0.05$) for gender, adjusted for age, level of residency training, and presence of past ethics education.

solid foundation in medical ethics. Because many of the trainees who reported no ethics education were already in their third year of residency or beyond, we cannot assume that they would receive such education before training completion. In addition, a surprisingly large number of the physicians in our study said they had received no ethics training at any point during their clinical training, that is, the last 2 years of medical school or residency. The majority of the respondents had not independently pursued ethics training, which suggests that formal curricula presented during medical school and residency may provide the only opportunity for systematic exposure to ethics education for many psychiatrists. That we found even a small number of residents who had not received ethics training at any time—within or outside of their medical and specialty education experiences—was remarkable, especially given the number of ethics initiatives implemented at U.S. medical schools over the past two decades (9).

Our findings also show that psychiatry residents expressed a need for ethics training: three-quarters of the residents had faced an ethical dilemma that they felt unprepared for. In addition, nearly all residents felt ethics training would help them in responding to moral problems arising in patient care. This is a dramatic finding in comparison with other studies in which physicians have expressed more uncertainty about the utility of ethics education (15). From these findings, we conclude that while psychiatry residents are interested in ethics and find it helpful and necessary, they still are probably receiving insufficient training in this area.

Ethics Topic Preferences and Gender Differences

The psychiatry residents in our study were remarkably eager to learn more about a wide variety of ethics topics. The residents were greatly interested in many ethical areas related to the fields of medicine generally and psychiatry specifically. All but 1 of the 26 ethics topics listed in the questionnaire were thought to deserve more curricular attention by 40% or more of the residents polled. Their interest often pertained to defining the boundaries of what can be done legally in responding to difficult ethical dilemmas, clarifying the ethical issues in social policy, and providing good care to psychiatric patients.

What residents were relatively less interested in is intriguing as well. Sexual contact between physicians and patients was the topic least frequently selected by residents as needing more curricular attention. Moreover, this topic, and the one of touching psychiatric patients, were both identified by 10 or more residents as already receiving more than an appropriate share of curricular time. From these results, we speculate that physician-patient intimacy may be one ethical issue already addressed intensively in psychiatric residency programs in the United States. This area has been an important one in psychiatric ethics courses and probably should be discussed repeatedly in training settings even if trainees tire of the subject. Our findings in this area serve as a valuable reminder that resident preferences may guide but should not be the sole factor governing curricular development and content.

The women in our study appeared especially concerned about ethics and seemed eager to explore issues primarily connected to the use of power in clinical and collegial relationships. This result is not unexpected, as it parallels the concern women exhibit about the ethical and judicious use of power in many professions (16–19). Several theorists have suggested that women may think differently about ethical issues than men, particularly in the workplace (19), and may have greater sensitivity or concern for the moral issues arising in human relationships (20–24). Gilligan has suggested that women more highly value choices that enhance personal connectedness and preserved relationships when considering moral judgments (22). She further argues that men are more likely to cast ethical decisions as a contest of one individual's rights over another's. These ideas may explain in part why our sample of female residents gave a higher priority than the men to ethical issues ranging from concerns about their own use of power with patients to the resolution of problems arising with supervising physicians, impaired colleagues, co-workers, and families.

Ethics Learning Methods and Gender Differences

Psychiatry residents value several learning techniques that may be used effectively in ethics curricula. Approaches that provide an opportunity to learn from experts, to explore clinically relevant ethical issues, to develop knowledge, and to share wisdom and obtain guidance with colleagues in familiar surroundings are all seen as worthwhile. That independent learning was less consistently preferred by the residents suggests the importance of access to experience and expertise and the benefit of a shared dialogue in approaching ethical issues systematically. The residents' preferences for methods that occur in the course of everyday departmental activities may be related to the vulnerability many people experience in dealing with ethical problems. The process of ethical reflection and solution may best be pursued in "ordinary" and familiar contexts with trusted friends, colleagues, and faculty members.

The women and men in our study valued some learning methods differently. In learning about ethical matters, the women appeared to be more generally positive and versatile, preferring interactive; traditional, clinically based; and independent methods. The men were less globally enthusiastic about specific methods and found only one, independent reading, more valuable than the women. Research on college students (23) and adolescents and their parents (24)

indicates that women are mainly concerned with resolving real, rather than hypothetical, ethical dilemmas. Our results complement these findings and suggest that preferences for certain learning methods are related to the resident's gender. We argue that the role of gender and related learning styles warrant consideration when designing ethics curricula for postgraduate psychiatry programs.

Comparison With Similar Internal Medicine Survey

This survey of psychiatry residents was conducted in a manner similar to a survey of internal medicine residents done in 1989 (12). A few comparisons are of interest. The percentage of internal medicine and psychiatry residents in both surveys with exposure to medical ethics education in medical school was similar: 72% and 67%, respectively. Fewer of the psychiatry residents (46%) than the internal medicine residents (74%) reported ethics training during their residency in that study. One finding was analogous in both surveys: the two topics chosen by the most residents as needing more attention involved legal issues. For the medical residents, the topics related to legal aspects of withdrawal of life-support measures and physician-patient relations; for psychiatry residents, the topics related to ethical and legal aspects of withholding information from patients and the legal rights of patients with compromised decisional capacity. These findings suggest that residents in both disciplines have a strong interest in getting guidance about what is legally permissible and ethically justifiable in clinical decision making.

Study Limitations

This study has several limitations that may influence its finding's interpretation. One problem with a survey of this type is that the results may not accurately reflect the participants' true beliefs, but instead may represent only what they are willing to report as their beliefs. This study also relies upon the perceptions of its participants, for example, what they perceive to be ethics training and what they consider to have been taught within their residency curriculum. This study does not seek to clarify how the residents defined ethics training nor does it discern between what the programs taught and what the residents actually learned.

Sampling biases may influence our findings in several areas. First, our survey sample was one of convenience, which may affect our results' generalizability. Our response rate of about 59%, while not atypical in this type of survey, is noteworthy. The percentage of men and women respondents closely resembled the base population's gender percentage, although there was a slight overrepresentation of women with, perhaps, modest effects on our findings. Our study sample was somewhat less representative with respect to level of training for study participants, with underrepresentation of PGY-1 residents and overrepresentation of PGY-2 residents. This factor reflects both the relatively fragmented schedules of PGY-1 trainees on different clinical services and the relatively centralized activities of PGY-2 trainees, often on inpatient services, at most of the 10 programs we studied. In addition, one of the residency programs in our study had a far higher response rate than the others. However, we found that this school's overall pattern of response was similar to the other programs'. Therefore, we do not believe that these response patterns affected the conclusions we drew. The 10 programs differed, however, in their trainees' responses about having received ethics training. In one program, three-quarters of the trainees received ethics training, whereas fewer than one-quarter of the trainees at another program received this training. This large discrepancy should be recalled when assessing our study.

Finally, we found greater enthusiasm for ethics training among the psychiatry residents who responded to our study than did Jacobson et al. in their survey of internal medicine residents (12), which may suggest that, in general, psychiatry residents are actually more positive about ethics training or merely that only the most enthused returned the survey. Because the Jacobson et al. study had roughly the same response rate and the residents' responses were less enthusiastic, we suspect that psychiatry residents are very interested in ethics.

Challenges Ahead for Faculty in Developing Ethics Training

This study shows that psychiatry educators have a clear invitation and a professional imperative: residents want to learn about ethics and have ideas on how they prefer to receive this education. Our inquiry and findings present new challenges for academic faculty. In the past, ethics curricula have not been as extensively implemented in psychiatry as other fields (11), in part because of the formidable institutional barriers and the relative absence of educational research in this area of psychiatry. These difficulties may be caused by a number of factors: a lack of resident interest or faculty expertise, the mistaken assumption that ethics is being taught universally in medical schools, the perception that ethics cannot be taught but only modeled by faculty mentors, the lack of consensus about appropriate curricular territory, and the paucity of administrative support and departmental advocacy for ethics in residency education. While many questions and obstacles remain, there is more information about ethics as it relates to medical education that psychiatric educators may find informative and helpful as they develop new curricular programs in this area for their residents.

Our study helps to define what and how our residents wish to learn about ethics. The challenging task that lies ahead is to use this information to shape the professional values, identities, and patterns of resident conduct during postgraduate training. Psychiatry faculty must now commit to developing an ethics curriculum in each residency program that is clinically centered, interactive, and encourages well-informed dialogue, so that our residents complete their training with the knowledge, attitudes, and skills needed to approach the ethical issues and concerns that arise in patient care.

Dr. McCarty is associate professor, Department of Psychiatry, University of New Mexico, and chief, Consultation Psychiatry, University Hospital; Dr. Lyketsos is director, Neuropsychiatry and Memory Group, Department of Psychiatry and Behavioral Sciences, The Johns Hopkins Hospital, Baltimore, Maryland; Dr. Hardee is resident, Department of Medicine, University of New Mexico; Dr. Jacobson is chief, Division of Medical Ethics, Department of Internal Medicine, Latter Day Saints' Hospital and University of Utah School of Medicine, Salt Lake City; Dr. Walker is associate professor and director, Division of Medical Ethics and Humanities, Department of Internal Medicine, University of South Florida College of Medicine, Tampa; Dr. Hough is assistant clinical professor of psychiatry, Medical College of Georgia, Atlanta; Dr. Gramelspacher is assistant professor of medicine, Indiana University School of Medicine, Indianapolis; Dr. Stidley is director, Cancer Center Biostatistics Group, University of New Mexico; Dr. Arambula is clinical assistant professor of psychiatry, The University of Texas Health Science Center at San Antonio; Dr. Heebink is attending psychiatrist, Department of Psychiatry, Cornell University Medical College, New York; Dr. Zornberg is clinical instructor of psychiatry, Harvard Medical School, Boston, Massachusetts; and Dr. Siegler is director, Center for Clinical Medical Ethics, Professor of Medicine, University of Chicago, Illinois. Address reprint requests to Dr. Roberts, Department of Psychiatry, University of New Mexico, 2400 Tucker N.E., Albuquerque, NM 87131.

The authors thank Dr. Ruth Benca for her participation in the survey study and Dr. Tina Walch for her comments in developing the survey instrument; Ms. Kay Browning Moolenijzer for her assistance with data analysis; and Ms. Elynn Cowden, Ms. Mary Davidson, Ms. Brenda Martinez, and Ms. Betty Bierner for secretarial support.

References

1. Bloch S: Teaching of psychiatric ethics. Br J Psychiatry 1980; 136:300–301
2. Michels R: Training in psychiatric ethics, in Psychiatric Ethics. Oxford, England, Oxford University Press, 1981, pp. 295–305
3. Jellinek M, Parmelee D: Is there a role for medical ethics in postgraduate psychiatry courses? Am J Psychiatry 1977; 134:1438–1439
4. Andre J: Learning to see: moral growth during medical training. J Med Ethics 1992; 18:148–152
5. Coverdale JH, Bayer T, Isbell P, et al: Are we teaching psychiatrists to be ethical? Academic Psychiatry 1992; 16:199–205
6. American Medical Association: Special Requirements for Residency Training in Psychiatry. Graduate Medical Education Directory 1993–1994. Chicago, IL, American Medical Association, 1993, pp. 121–126
7. Perkins HS: Teaching medical ethics during residency. Acad Med 1989; 64:262–266
8. Forrow L, Arnold RM, Frader J: Teaching clinical ethics in the residency years: preparing competent professionals. J Med Philos 1991; 16:93–112
9. Miles SH, Lane LW, Bickel J, et al: Medical ethics education: coming of age. Acad Med 1989; 64:705–714
10. Barnard D: Residency ethics training: a critique of current trends. Arch Intern Med 1988; 148:1836–1838
11. Lane LW: Residency ethics training in the United States: special considerations and early experience, in Symposium 1990 Proceedings of the Westminster Institute for Ethics and Human Values: Medical Ethics for Medical Students 1990, London, Ontario, Canada, pp. 21–32
12. Jacobson JA, Tolle SW, Stocking C, et al: Internal medicine residents' preferences regarding medical ethics education. Acad Med 1989; 64:760–764
13. SAS Institute, Inc: Statistical Analysis Systems, SAS/STAT Users Guide, Version 6, 4th Edition. Cary NC, SAS Institute, Inc., 1989
14. Hosmer DW, Lemeshow S: Applied Logistic Regression. New York, John Wiley & Sons, 1989
15. Pellegrino ED, Hart RJ, Henderson SR, et al: Relevance and utility of courses in medical ethics: a sur-

vey of physician's perceptions. JAMA 1985; 253:49–53

16. Kanter RM. Men and Women of the Corporation, 2nd Edition. New York, Basic Books, 1993

17. Dimen M: Surviving Sexual Contraindications. New York, Macmillan, 1986

18. Wood JT. Gendered Lives: Communication, Gender, and Culture. Belmont, WA, Wadsworth, 1994

19. Noddings N: Ethics from the standpoint of women, in Theoretical Perspectives on Sexual Difference, edited by Rhoe DL. New Haven, CT, Yale University Press, 1990

20. Bebeau M, Brabeck M: Integrating care and justice issues in professional moral education: a gender perspective. Journal of Moral Education 1987; 16:189–203

21. Noddings N: Caring: A Feminine Approach to Ethics and Moral Education. Berkeley, CA, University of California Press, 1984

22. Gilligan C: Concepts of self and morality, in In a Different Voice, edited by Gilligan C. Cambridge, MA, Harvard University Press, 1982, pp. 64–105

23. Haan N: Hypothetical and actual moral reasoning in a situation of civil disobedience. J Pers Soc Psychol 1975; 32:255–270

24. Holstein C: Development of moral judgment: a longitudinal study of males and females. Child Devel 1976; 47:51–61

9.10 Roberts LW, McCarty T, Roberts BB, Morrison N, Belitz J, Berenson C, Siegler M (1996) Clinical Ethics Teaching in Psychiatric Supervision. Acad Psychiatry 20:176–88

Clinical Ethics Teaching in Psychiatric Supervision

Laura Weiss Roberts, M.D., Teresita McCarty, M.D.
Brian B. Roberts, M.D., Nancy Morrison, M.D.
Jerald Belitz, Ph.D., Claudia Berenson, M.D.
Mark Siegler, M.D.

Supervision of psychiatric residents provides a natural context for clinical ethics teaching. In this article, the authors discuss the need for ethics education in psychiatry residencies and describe how the special attributes of supervision allow for optimal ethics training for psychiatry residents in their everyday encounters with ethical problems. Ethical decision making in clinical settings is briefly reviewed, and a 6-step strategy for clinical ethics training in psychiatric supervision is outlined. The value of the clinical ethics supervisory strategy for teaching and patient care is illustrated through four case examples. (Academic Psychiatry 1996; 20:176–188)

Ethics is not added to a clinical case by injecting into it new facts or by imposing on it some alien principles and values. The ethics of any case arises out of the facts and values imbedded in the case itself.
Jonsen, Siegler, and Winslade (1)

Ethics is not just a set of visceral sensations.
McIlhenney and Pellegrino (2)

Psychiatry, like the rest of medicine, is in part the practice of applied ethics. . . . Each day the resident must struggle with existential questions in the emergency room, in the clinic, on the wards. The questions are not simply idle exercises but must be answered; the answers intimately affect the lives of the patients.
Yager (3)

Psychiatric resident supervision provides a natural context for clinical ethics teaching. Supervision is case-based, contextual, exploratory, responsive, knowledge-driven, judgment-oriented, and evaluative. Ideally, clinical ethics teaching also possesses all of these features. Clinical ethics is an emerging academic discipline that seeks to improve patient care by incorporating the knowledge of ethics into everyday medical practice, enhancing the clinical judgment of physicians (1,4).

Describing why these attributes of supervision are so valuable to clinical ethics teaching is the first aim of this article. The second aim is to present a 6-step approach to clinical ethics teaching in psychiatric supervision, with examples of its use.

Dr. L. Roberts is associate director, Medical Student Education, and assistant professor, Department of Psychiatry, University of New Mexico School of Medicine, Albuquerque, New Mexico. See acknowledgments for affiliations of other authors. Address reprint requests to Dr. L. Roberts, The University of New Mexico, Department of Psychiatry, 2400 Tucker N.E., Albuquerque, NM 87131-5326.

THE NEED FOR ETHICS
TRAINING IN RESIDENCY

Caring for patients is an intrinsically ethical activity, and it is widely agreed that ethics training is an important component of a psychiatry resident's education (3–25). Ethics education provides knowledge, cognitive tools, and communication and behavioral skills that are useful to physicians and patients in clinical settings (2,10,15,26,27). Moreover, trainees are very interested in learning more about ethics as it applies to psychiatric practice, as was demonstrated in two studies involving psychiatry residents.

Roberts et al. found that 92% of 181 psychiatry residents at 10 training programs believed ethics training to be helpful in responding to ethical dilemmas in patient care (17). A majority of these residents wanted to learn more about 19 specific ethics topics. Coverdale et al. surveyed chief residents at psychiatry training programs across the United States who indicated interest in a number of ethics areas as well (8). Concern about ethical dilemmas created by new economic pressures in mental health care (28–29) and controversy about recent cases of ethical misconduct in psychiatric practice and research suggest that ethics curricula will continue to be important in postgraduate psychiatric education.

Curiously, physicians often do not receive much formal ethics teaching during residency (12,15,17). Seventy-six percent of 181 residents in the Roberts et al. study reported facing an ethical dilemma in residency for which they felt unprepared, and 46% reported having received no formal ethics training during residency (17). Similarly, Coverdale et al. found that 40% of 121 psychiatry residencies did not offer a formal ethics curriculum (8). These results are disturbing, as ethics training in medical schools also is not ubiquitous—one-third of residents in the Roberts et al. study could not recall receiving ethics education as medical students. Thus, it cannot be assumed that all psychiatrists will have been formally trained in ethics, even modestly, during their medical education. As a consequence, there is an imperative to develop rigorous, useful ethics curricula in psychiatry residency programs in the United States now (6,8,11,17,19,21–24,28,30).

While it has become clear that ethics should be taught to psychiatrists, the characteristics of effective ethics training have been less certain. Controversy surrounds the question of which curricular interventions have the greatest and most enduring value (9,14,15,26,27,31). This issue is particularly true during residency education, a period in which curricular development and innovation are extremely difficult (7–9,12,15,17,27–33).

In addition, with a few valuable exceptions (7,22,23), models for understanding psychiatric ethical issues have been relatively neglected in the psychiatric literature. The conceptual distinction between ethical and legal aspects of psychiatry also has been underrecognized, with negative repercussions for ethics curriculum development. Moreover, studies of the ethical issues in psychiatric practice and research have generated many new questions that have not yet been addressed empirically (34–36). Much remains to be understood about the task of teaching ethics in psychiatry.

Experience and some evidence suggest, however, that intensive, systematic approaches to clinical ethics training that build upon a foundation of knowledge and help to develop practical judgment may be especially worthwhile for physicians (1,2,4,10,12,15,17,29). Residents themselves prefer training methods and topics that integrate clinically relevant information on ethics with everyday medical activities and decision making (12,17,31). For psychiatry residents, individual supervision that extends beyond didactic teaching and includes a sustained and organized focus on ethics issues thus offers an ideal setting for ethics education.

PSYCHIATRIC SUPERVISION
AND CLINICAL ETHICS TEACHING

Several aspects of supervision make it particularly suited to clinical ethics teaching. The first is that it is case-based. Supervision focuses on the care of individual patients; clinical ethics focuses on the ethical issues arising in the care of individual patients. The intrinsic work of supervision—evaluation of patient symptoms and signs, formulation of diagnostic issues, and construction of therapeutic plans—lays the groundwork for exploring the ethical dimensions of a case (1,4,10).

Second, supervision is contextual. Supervision occurs on wards, in clinics, in therapy offices, and in emergency rooms. Supervisors at these sites are optimally attuned to the salient clinical issues, the real constraints on resident decisions, and the influences of the treatment milieu and institutional culture in each of these training settings. This contextual quality of supervision is helpful to ethics teaching for two reasons.

The first reason is that patient-care decisions, which may be complicated by context-related problems, are often identified as ethical dilemmas, a phenomenon that may be best clarified by residents in supervision. For example, a resident may grapple with what might appear to an outsider to be autonomy issues involving an "uncooperative" patient when the real problem is lack of access to psychiatric services, interfering with patient compliance. The supervisor can help the resident to see how the provision of clinical care within a particular system thus emerges as one kind of ethical conflict when it may, in fact, be another type of problem.

The second reason is that supervision itself becomes an important part of each training context. Consequently, ethics teaching in supervision is immediate, pervasive, and meaningful for the resident. This level of attention to ethical issues, taken not in isolation but in their real clinical context, has been

a highly touted but elusive goal of medical ethics education (9). For these reasons, psychiatric supervision provides an excellent opportunity for understanding and addressing the ethical dimensions of patient care.

Third, supervision is a uniquely responsive and exploratory educational experience in residency training (21,37). It is a collaborative relationship with two aims: the professional development of the resident and the optimal care of his or her patients. Ideally, through supervision, faculty explore and respond to the trainee's concerns in a manner that is genuinely helpful, promotes growth, reduces defensiveness, and encourages self-understanding. Supervision also provides information and support, appropriately addressing the troubling emotions, stresses, and challenges experienced by the resident (12,38). These qualities of supervision make for a constructive milieu in which to discuss difficult clinical ethical issues. Rather than simply reacting in challenging clinical situations, residents may carefully consider ethical problems with their supervisors, think about their choices and concerns, and then deliberately decide upon their actions. Good supervision thus promotes better individual ethical decisions and improves professional conduct by residents.

Finally, supervision is knowledge-driven, judgment-oriented, and evaluative. It offers an opportunity to gather information, reach clinical decisions, and learn from patient outcomes over time (25,37). Supervision sessions provide a structured occasion to reflect upon one's own perceptions and behavior in caring for patients (25). That is to say, supervision helps residents learn sound clinical practices and careful self-observation. In addition, as the clinical and ethical problems encountered by residents shift in emphasis (Table 1), their supervision also will evolve in content and meaning. The tasks of supervision heel closely to the clinical sophistication and professional maturation of residents, prompting both supervisors and supervisees to learn. The sum of a resident's experiences in supervision throughout their training thus constitutes a kind of apprenticeship in decision making and practical judgment. Because judgment encompasses not only clinical actions but also self-knowledge, self-evaluation, and professional conduct, the work of psychiatric supervision and of ethics training overlaps.

Supervision is an educational experience in psychiatric residencies in which ethical issues arise indigenously and clinical ethics teaching may be particularly compelling.

CLINICAL ETHICS: DECISION-MAKING STRATEGY

Valuable models for ethical reflection in clinical settings have been described by Jonsen, Siegler, and Winslade (1,4); by Beauchamp and Childress (39); by Hundert (22); by Sadler and Hulgus (23); and others. Each of these models offers a conceptual scheme for organizing the many complex, perplexing, and potentially incongruent aspects of a clinical case. The clinical ethics decision-making scheme proposed by Jonsen, Siegler, and Winslade (1,4) is presented here because, of all these models, it places the greatest emphasis on the clarification of clinical issues as the initial work of ethical reflection in patient care. It capitalizes on the clinical strengths of supervisors, and, as a model, it fits very naturally with the usual tasks of clinical supervision. Other conceptual schemes are very helpful and are not mutually exclusive, however, and can easily

TABLE 1.   Examples of ethics issues encountered by psychiatry residents during clinical activities

Clinical Activity	Examples of Ethics Issues
Inpatient ward	Autonomy and seclusion/restraint Dangerous patients and duty to warn Use of potentially harmful treatments Use of innovative, unproven treatments
Outpatient clinic	Access to care Informed consent and refusal Decisional ability Truth-telling and beneficence Mistakes
Emergency psychiatry	Coerced treatment Violence and the duty to care for difficult patients Suicide
Child psychiatry	Special protections for children Duty to report abuse and neglect Consent processes involving children and adolescents
Consultation psychiatry	Decisional capacity Refusal of treatment vs. noncompliance End-of-life care and suffering Medical care for psychiatric patients
Psychotherapy	Therapeutic boundaries Supervisor-trainee-patient relationship(s) Role appropriate empathy and advocacy
Substance treatment	Stigmatizing illness and confidentiality Resolution of conflicting values (family and societal needs vs. individual rights) Impaired colleagues
Clinical research	Protection of vulnerable research subjects Methodology Authorship and scientific integrity "Whistle-blowing"

be incorporated within the clinical ethics supervisory approach we propose.

The original strategy for clinical ethical decision making constructed by Jonsen, Siegler, and Winslade (1,4) involves four areas of consideration (Table 2). The first consideration always relates to the medical indications in the case. Medical indications include the diagnosis, prognosis, therapeutic alternatives, and, ultimately, the physician's recommendation or care plan. The second consideration chronologically, but of great significance in clinical actions, is the patient's preferences. The patient's informed and reasoned choice is of vital concern in clinical ethical decision making. The next consideration, quality-of-life factors, may take precedence when patient preferences are unknown or are unknowable, but these factors ordinarily play a lesser role in determining clinical ethical decisions. Finally, other relevant factors outside the immediate physician-patient encounter may influence clinical ethical decisions. Examples include limited medical resources for treatment of serious, chronic mental illnesses or for organ transplantation or other interventions; legal constraints of physicians with respect to coerced treatment or to patient confidentiality; and economic obstacles of patients seeking elective surgery, innovative pharmacotherapies, or other costly care. These factors typi-

cally set the conditions under which clinical ethical decisions must be made. Taken together, these four areas of consideration create a systematic but flexible framework for ethical decision making in clinical settings.

APPROACH TO CLINICAL ETHICS TEACHING IN PSYCHIATRIC SUPERVISION

We have developed a clinical ethics approach to psychiatric resident supervision that integrates direct teaching, ethical reflection, and clinical decision making. It is a 6-step strategy (Table 3), which is readily assimilated into individual resident supervision already occurring in a variety of psychiatric training contexts (Table 1). In this section, we describe how faculty may employ the supervisory method in their work with residents, and in the next we provide four illustrations of its use.

1. Define Clinical Decisions

Ethics teaching in psychiatry supervision begins with the task of helping the resident to define the issues and decisions involved in a clinical case. Guiding the resident as he or she develops a list of clinical problems, arrives at a diagnosis, and determines the goal(s) of treatment is a traditional

TABLE 2. Elements and relevant issues involved in clinical ethical decision making	
Elements	**Relevant Issues**
Medical indications	Diagnosis and prognosis Therapeutic alternatives Recommended clinical strategy
Patient preferences	Informed consent and refusal Decisional capacity Autonomy and voluntarism
Quality-of-life factors	Patient's values Other values (e.g., family, social) if patient's values areunknown
Factors external to the physician-patient encounter	Family needs Economic or legal constraints Limited medical resources Safety of society

activity in psychiatric supervision and represents the first step in clinical ethics decision making. On the ward, for instance, when considering whether to prescribe innovative neuroleptics or to perform electroconvulsive therapy, the resident should first decide whether this is a reasonable choice given the patient's diagnosed condition. It is unwarranted to debate broad philosophical principles, as too often happens in ethics discussions when basic medical concerns and clinical indications have not yet been clarified. By defining the clinical decisions involved in a case as the initial step of an ethics discussion, the supervisor and resident emphasize competent clinical care as the foundation of ethical action.

2. Identify Clinical Ethical Elements and Conflicts

The supervisor and the resident should next identify the ethical elements and conflicts present in a clinical situation. Clinical ethical elements may encompass those described in the original clinical ethics decision-making strategy, as depicted in Table 2: medical indications and imperatives; patient preferences, values, background, and decisional capacity; quality-of-life considerations; and other relevant factors, such as

---

TABLE 3.   Six-step approach to clinical ethics teaching in psychiatric supervision

1. Help the resident to define the clinical aspects of the patient's case
2. Guide the resident in the identification of ethical issues and conflicts in the clinical situation. Give the resident an opportunity to describe personal concerns and thoughts regarding the clinical case
3. Collaborate with the resident in gathering additional information and necessary expertise
4. Explore possible responses to the clinical ethical problems with the resident. Decide what acceptable choices exist and try to anticipate the outcomes of possible decisions
5. Provide guidance and support as the resident implements a decision
6. Create a context for reflection and review

---

family concerns, cultural contributions, and legal and economic parameters. Other models of medical ethics such as the principles of autonomy, beneficence, nonmaleficence, and justice described by Beauchamp and Childress (39) or the core aspects of the clinical encounter encompassing knowledge, ethics, and pragmatism in the context of a larger biopsychosocial approach described by Sadler and Hulgus (23) provide useful ways of articulating the ethical elements present in a patient case. Hundert's technique (22) for developing "lists of the conflicting values" also is an excellent exercise for supervisors and trainees in this step.

This second step draws upon the knowledge and experience of both the supervisor and the resident. While supervisors may find it helpful to familiarize themselves with one or more conceptual models of medical ethics, they need not be formal experts in ethics. Past encounters with clinical, ethical, and legal dilemmas in psychiatric practice, and their outcomes, represent an excellent in situ ethics education for supervisors. Residents also may have some knowledge of ethics derived from medical school and residency curricula, readings, and personal experience. In this step, the supervisor can help the resident to apply such knowledge in very real situations.

Beyond the supervisor's understanding of ethics is the supervisor's understanding of residents themselves. Supervisors ideally will remain mindful of the process of professional development during psychiatry training and will be attentive to the specific concerns of supervisees when considering ethical problems. Although clinical ethics discussions should not resemble psychotherapy, some understanding of the psychological and interpersonal determinants involved in the case can be helpful in establishing how ethical dilemmas are experienced. As in supervisory sessions focused on countertransference issues, a limited exploration of the resident's feelings about the situation may be necessary before it is possible to approach the patient's care in a clear-sighted manner (18). Thus, the success of this step depends upon the supervisor's sensitivity to ethical issues, cognizance of the resident's circumstance and perceptions, and willingness to explore the interplay between ethics and emotions explicitly. By illuminating the ethical aspects of a patient's case and by identifying points of conflict in this second step, supervisors may help their residents to better understand how clinical, personal, and ethical elements fit together to inform therapeutic decisions.

3. Gather Information and Consult

The supervisor and the resident next should gather information and expertise. For many ethical problems, supervisors will have developed a reasonable approach based on previous cases, and residents will already have obtained the data and knowledge needed to act in the clinical situation. In these instances, the process of gathering information may appropriately remain between supervisor and resident.

More challenging, and more instructive, is the situation in which the supervisor and the resident together must seek additional resources needed for optimal patient care. This collaboration between supervisor and trainee serves several purposes (Table 4). First, it enriches the understanding of the clinical and ethical dimensions of a patient's case. Second, it helps supervisors and resi-

dents alike to develop their current knowledge and skills and may prevent clinical and ethical mistakes. Third, observation of a respected role model as he or she learns is a salient educational event for residents (12,15). The supervisor's commitment to collecting information and expertise demonstrates to residents that clinical work entails curiosity and resourcefulness throughout one's career. Fourth, it affirms for residents that approaching clinical ethical decisions and, ultimately, making sound clinical judgments are intrinsically collaborative, process-oriented activities. They are not merely intuition, opinion, or the simple repetition of former actions. For these reasons, this third step of a supervisory approach to clinical ethical teaching is crucial.

Two kinds of resources are usually helpful at this stage: people and written documents. Patients and families often can provide additional history needed to clarify the clinical and ethical issues present. Through the process of talking with patients and their families, medical indications and patient preferences may also become more certain, simplifying clinical ethical decisions. While remaining cognizant of confidentiality boundaries, supervisors and residents may consider a variety of other "people resources," such as patient-care staff, faculty, peers, psychologists and social workers, institutional advisers (e.g., ethics consultants, attorneys, clergy, or others), and, if needed, outside experts. In all of these discussions, supervisors and residents learn incrementally and collect knowledge useful in clinical decisions.

Written documents of four kinds also may be especially informative for supervisors and residents in this step. Searching the medical, psychiatric, and ethics literatures may yield insights about important clinical indications and standards, current research efforts, resources to improve patients' quality of life despite illness, and others' experiences with similar clinical ethical dilemmas (40,41). Reviewing patient records, like gath-

---

TABLE 4.	Value of gathering information and expertise in psychiatric supervision

- Clarifying the clinical and ethical issues present in the patient's care
- Ensuring that specific clinical ethical decisions enacted are well-informed and reasonable, helping to prevent mistakes
- Developing the knowledge and expertise of faculty and residents in clinical practice, medical science, and ethics
- Demonstrating to trainees the importance of collaboration, curiosity, resourcefulness, and continuous learning in ethical decision making

ering additional history from patients directly, is a standard practice that often is helpful. Referring to formal codes of ethics may help resolve concrete ethical dilemmas for trainees by defining the standards of physician conduct and describing the ethical aspirations of a professional field (6,20,42,43). Knowledge of legal and institutional documents, such as hospital policy, may delimit or organize the options in caring for a patient (44,45). Reading is an important, if underemphasized, part of a physician's work (42,43,46). Its value becomes particularly evident when supervisors and residents must gather information about clinical ethical issues.

4. Explore Possible Ethical Responses

Next, the supervisor and the resident should explore possible responses to the clinical and ethical issues at hand. For example, while it might arguably be "medically indicated" to use physical restraints or chemical sedation or both in treating a violent patient, these decisions have different ethical meanings in the care of a given patient in a particular setting. The ramifications of such clinical decisions are best understood through a timely, exploratory dialogue with a knowledgeable, trusted supervisor. In this step, the supervisor must anticipate the range of choices faced by the resident and have a sense of what alternatives are either permissible or unacceptable in the situation, based on clinical, ethical, legal, or other factors. Helping the resident to see the problems intrinsic to a "bad" choice may, in fact, be more important for the resident's future practice than is helping the resident to see the advantages of a "good" choice in this step.

5. Provide Guidance and Support

The supervisor then provides guidance and support as the resident undertakes a course of action. As in the second step of

identifying ethical dilemmas, the resident's conflicting emotions often surface at this stage. Supervision affords an appropriate and well-defined opportunity to address the emotionally charged aspects of patient care when a tough decision must be made. While supervisors seldom should dictate resident choices, faculty expressions of direction and encouragement are important to the resident's confidence at such moments. On occasion, for institutional, political, legal, or personal reasons, it may be necessary for supervisors to intervene in patient care dilemmas so that residents are adequately supported. In this step, supervisors thus can ensure that sound clinical approaches are implemented by residents who have not had to make problematic decisions alone. This approach affirms the primary role of the resident in making treatment decisions without ignoring the reality of the supervisor's ultimate responsibility for patient care (19,44).

6. Create a Context for Reflection

Finally, the supervisor should create a context for ongoing ethical reflection and clinical case review. In this step, the supervisor and resident should consider the clinical ethical decisions made in the care of individual patients with the benefit of hindsight. Supervisors may choose to discuss how they have responded to similar ethical dilemmas in their own training and practice, commenting on their successes as well as their occasional mistakes. By demonstrating their own decisional processes, revisiting past patient cases, and offering themselves as role models, supervisors may truly mentor their residents.

CASE ILLUSTRATIONS

This approach to clinical ethics teaching is a natural extension of traditional psychiatric resident supervision. It is not difficult to implement and may already occur implicitly in meetings between supervisors and residents when they focus on ethical issues. Making the process explicit and applying it to a variety of supervisory relationships occurring in residency, however, are crucial in the effort to develop a more systematic, clinically based approach to teaching ethics in psychiatry programs. The versatility and value of this supervisory strategy for teachers of psychiatry residents becomes apparent in illustrations of its use.

Case Reports

Example One.   A resident objected on ethical grounds to filling in federal forms that routinely declaring certain psychiatric patients "decisionally incompetent." In supervision, this issue was discussed in relation to a particular psychiatric inpatient whose decisional capacity did show some significant deficits. The resident had the impression that the patient's financial benefits might be withheld if the form were not completed.

The first step in supervision was to clarify the patient's psychiatric diagnosis and related deficits in cognition and judgment. This served two aims: 1) to make certain that the patient's clinical needs were not obscured in the resident's passion to "do the right thing" by fighting institutional bureaucracy, and 2) to teach the resident about the phenomenology of the patient's illness and about ways of assessing his decisional abilities, the basic educational goals of clinical supervision in this case. The second step was to help the resident to identify the ethical issues involved, such as the resident's view of coercion by the institution, the resident's perceived duty to protect a vulnerable patient whose financial benefits were apparently in jeopardy, the limited autonomy of the patient because of psychiatric illness, confidentiality, and others. The process of clarifying the ethical binds and personal frustrations experienced by the resident made it possible to approach the patient's

care with a better separation of the therapeutic goals from the complexities of training within a certain institutional setting. The supervisor talked with the resident about the distinction between decisional capacity, a clinical assessment, and competence, a legal determination. The resident was encouraged to read about decisional capacity and neuropsychological testing and to gather more complete historical information about the patient. She also sought information from faculty and administrators at the institution about the actual use of the federal form.

Possible responses to the ethical dilemma, that is, whether and how to fill out the form, were then explored by the resident and supervisor. With support and further discussion with the attending supervisor and permission from the patient and his family, the resident made a decision to write a separate report documenting the observed strengths and deficits of the patient. The patient's benefits were not hindered. The resident worked further to change the policy requiring routine completion of the form. The resident and supervisor followed the patient case afterward and discussed the impact, both positive (special attention to clinical issues, continuation of the patient's benefits, and a modest sense of accomplishment for the resident) and negative (additional work and some disruption of routine), of the resident's choices in later supervision sessions.

Example Two.   A resident on the consultation-liaison service worried about a discharge request made by a woman who had taken an impulsive overdose of antidepressant pills during an argument with her boyfriend. She had very nearly died and was in the intensive care unit on the medicine service. The patient was the mother of two children and homeless. Of greatest concern to the resident was that the patient's boyfriend frequently and severely beat her. Although the patient asked to leave the hospital and denied suicidality, the resident felt that it was "unethical" to let the patient go.

The first step in supervision was to evaluate the clinical situation of the patient. She exhibited QRS widening on ECG and had elevated blood levels of a tricyclic antidepressant. On mental status examination, she was cooperative, sleepy, distractible, inaccurate by 4 days on the date, and unable to add or subtract even small numbers. It was clear that the patient's medical indications warranted continued hospitalization. A discussion of the ethical issues encompassed topics such as patient autonomy and preferences, decisional capacity and standards of competence, informed refusal of treatment, quality-of-life factors, the duty to report child abuse, and others. It became evident that the resident needed additional information on the children (who, as it turned out, had previously been placed with the patient's father) and on delirium, antidepressant toxicity, physical abuse, resources for battered spouses, and legal and institutional guidelines on holding patients involuntarily and on reporting domestic violence.

The resident and supervisor discussed a number of possible responses to the patient's discharge request, including, if necessary, coerced observation and treatment. An evaluation was done by the supervising attending physician who clarified that the patient was not demanding to leave the hospital immediately. The patient stated, in fact, that she wanted treatment so that she would "be ok" before returning to "the shelter." The patient agreed to remain in the hospital until she felt "a little bit better" and to accept the social work consultation. After careful assessment, the attending physician determined that the patient was capable of this level of consent in the acute situation. With the agreement of the attending supervisor, the resident decided to speak with the patient about remaining in the hospital and meeting with a social worker to help with her social situation. Over the next several hours, as the patient's cardiac toxicity and delirium cleared, she decided to return to her boyfriend. Psychiatric and social work follow-up

was arranged. When the resident and supervisor reviewed the case, the resident was still concerned about the patient's refusal of inpatient psychiatric care and her decision to return to a reportedly abusive relationship. He could, however, articulate the limits of the law, the rights of patients, standards of competence necessitated by different clinical situations, and his own thoughts about each of these issues. He believed that he had handled the case well despite its unsettling facts.

Example Three. A resident miscopied an evening insulin dose when writing the orders on an elderly patient being admitted to the psychiatric unit. She discovered the error the next day when she found that the patient's blood sugar readings were in the low 100s rather than the usual low 200s. The patient felt "fine," and the orders were corrected. She wondered how much to tell the patient and his family about the mistake in prescribing insulin.

In the first step, the patient's clinical status was investigated, and the issue was discussed with members of the treatment team who then were especially vigilant in their observation of the patient. The patient was considered to be stable and unharmed by the incident. The supervisor and resident discussed the ethical issues that surround medical mistakes, such as respect for persons, truth-telling, beneficence, justice, and the role of clinical outcomes in ethical analysis. They further talked about the resident's discomfort with the mistake. The supervisor and resident explicitly acknowledged that the resident had not made such errors before, directly addressing the resident's embarrassment. They then gathered information and read about the ethical issues surrounding medical mistakes and truth-telling and about the management of insulin-dependent diabetes mellitus. The institution's process for documenting mistakes, even for those with no clear harm inflicted, was also investigated and completed.

The choices before the resident (e.g.,

speaking with the patient and his family, or not, and talking further with the team members) were explored. The resident wished to talk about the error with the patient and treatment team immediately and with the family during their next scheduled session. The supervisor offered support to the resident as she pursued this series of discussions. Afterward, the supervisor reviewed with the resident the patient's reaction (unconcerned), the family's comments (critical), the team's response (supportive), and the resident's self-assessment (shaken but intact) and efforts to repair the situation (more than adequate). The supervisor and resident discussed this experience in the context of the resident's personal and professional development as a psychiatrist.

Example Four. A psychiatric resident was told "confidentially" by a patient that he had sexually molested and physically hurt several girls though he had never been caught. The patient said that he now had his "eye on" a girl in his apartment complex. He offered no name, though he described her, and then would neither affirm nor deny any definite intention to abuse her. The patient had been admitted to the psychiatric unit to "rule out depression" after taking an overdose shortly after his wife left him.

The first step in supervision was to clarify the patient's psychiatric diagnosis and to take measures ensuring the safety of the patient and of others on the locked ward. The supervisor and resident performed separate evaluations on this patient as a matter of ward routine. They both found that the patient had had a long history of self-destructive and difficult behaviors but had no prior psychiatric admissions. He had consistently been diagnosed with character pathology and experienced no psychotic or uniquely depressive symptomatology. He understood that sexual abuse of children was "damaging" and "wrong." He clearly stated what the consequences would be if he were caught. The patient was observed closely and be-

haved in a safe manner on the ward.

The next step in supervision involved discussing a number of ethical issues, including physician-patient boundaries and 'secrets'; physician duty-to-warn, patient privilege and confidentiality; culpability for deliberate, harmful actions by nonpsychotic psychiatric patients; dilemmas posed by 'difficult patients'; and others. The supervisor and resident next sought expertise from the hospital's attorneys, reviewed psychiatric and medical codes of ethics, and learned more about the patient's past history. With direction from the institution's legal counsel, the supervisor intervened and advised the police about the patient's vague threat to sexually abuse an unnamed, but identifiable, girl. Her family was then notified of the threat to the child. The supervisor and resident together informed the patient of this action. The supervisor and resident discussed therapeutic options for this difficult patient and considered possible responses to the many ethical dilemmas his care presented. Ultimately, the patient was discharged and referred for treatment of pedophilia. He was informed that he was regarded as accountable for his actions and the fact that he had undergone a psychiatric hospitalization did not relieve him of responsibility for his behavior toward others. In this case, the resident appreciated the collaborative approach taken by the attending supervisor and felt that he had learned in the process of the patient's care. The series of decisions in this extraordinarily challenging case were reviewed by the supervisor, resident, treatment team, and the legal counsel of the hospital, allowing for some sense of resolution if not satisfaction with the case. Additional follow-up information was not obtained, as the patient went to another state.

Each of these examples demonstrates how the everyday care of patients poses significant ethical challenges to psychiatry residents. Use of this 6-step strategy is felt to have improved the quality of resident teaching and patient care in each case. Supervisors experience the approach as straightforward and as not extending the supervisor and resident significantly beyond the usual tasks of supervision in a way that is burdensome or contrived. The strategy thus offers an excellent method for use by supervisors in their efforts to foster residents' decision-making skills and clinical judgment in ethically complex situations.

CONCLUSION

We have described why it is natural and essential to integrate ethics teaching into the individual supervision of psychiatry residents. A 6-step approach to clinical ethics teaching in psychiatric supervision, with illustrations of its use, was presented. The approach builds upon the strengths and activities of supervisors, offers opportunities for self-education for both residents and supervisors, and uses the resident's knowledge of ethics, ideally derived from a core didactic ethics curriculum during medical school and residency. The approach is presented as a method of promoting the development of sound clinical judgment in psychiatric trainees. Its ultimate aim is to improve the under-

standing and responses of psychiatry residents as they grapple with ethical issues that inevitably arise in the care of patients.

Dr. McCarty is associate professor, Department of Psychiatry, and chief, Consultation Psychiatry, University Hospital, University of New Mexico School of Medicine. Dr. B. Roberts is assistant professor, Department of Psychiatry, University of New Mexico School of Medicine, and chief, Inpatient Psychiatry Service, Veterans Affairs Medical Center, Albuquerque. Dr. Morrison is assistant professor and residency training director, Department of Psychiatry, University of New Mexico School of Medicine. Dr. Belitz is assistant professor, Division of Child and Adolescent Psychiatry, Department of Psychiatry, University of New Mexico School of Medicine. Dr. Berenson is associate professor, Division of Child and Adolescent Psychiatry, Departments of Psychiatry and Pediatrics, University of New Mexico School of Medicine. Dr. Siegler is professor, Department of Medicine, and director, Center for Clinical Medical Ethics, University of Chicago Pritzker School of Medicine, Chicago, Illinois.

The authors thank Drs. David Friar, Helene Silverblatt, Tina Walch, Sameera Teja, and Robert Suddath for their contributions in the early discussions leading to this manuscript.

References

1. Jonsen AR, Siegler M, Winslade W: Clinical Ethics: A Practical Approach to Ethical Decisions in Clinical Medicine, 2nd Edition. New York, McMillan, 1993
2. McIlhenney TK, Pellegrino ED: The Humanities and Human Values in Medical Schools: A Ten-Year Overview. Washington DC, Society for Health and Human Values, 1982
3. Yager J: A survival guide for psychiatric residents. Arch Gen Psychiatry 1974; 30:494–499
4. Siegler M: Decision-making strategy for clinical ethical problems in medicine. Arch Intern Med 1982; 142:2178–2179
5. American Medical Association: Special Requirements for Residency Training in Psychiatry. Chicago, IL, American Medical Association, Graduate Medical Education Directory 1993–1994, pp. 121–126
6. American Psychiatric Association: The Principles of Medical Ethics with Annotations Especially Applicable to Psychiatry. Washington DC, American Psychi-

atric Press, 1993
7. Bloch S: Teaching of psychiatric ethics. Br J Psychiatry 1980; 136:300–301
8. Coverdale JH, Bayer T, Isbell P, et al: Are we teaching psychiatrists to be ethical? Academic Psychiatry 1992; 16:199–205
9. Hafferty FW, Franks R: The hidden curriculum, ethics teaching, and the structure of medical education. Acad Med 1994; 69:861–871
10. Forrow L, Arnold RM, Frader J: Teaching clinical ethics in the residency years: preparing competent professionals. J Med Philos 1991; 16:93–112
11. Kantor JE: Ethical issues in psychiatric research and training, in Review of Psychiatry, Vol 13, edited by Oldham JM, Riba MB. Washington DC, American Psychiatric Press, 1994
12. Lane LW: Residency ethics training in the United States: special considerations and early experience, in Symposium 1990 Proceedings of the Westminster

Institute for Ethics and Human Values: Medical Ethics for Medical Students. London, Ontario, Canada, 1990 pp. 21–32

13. Lazarus JA (ed): Section III, Ethics, in Review of Psychiatry, Vol 13, edited by Oldham JM, Riba MB. Washington DC, American Psychiatric Press, 1994, pp. 319–459

14. Michels R: Training in psychiatric ethics, in Psychiatric Ethics, edited by Bloch S, Chodoff P. Oxford, England, Oxford University Press, 1981, pp. 295–305

15. Miles SH, Lane LW, Bickel J, et al: Medical ethics education: coming of age. Acad Med 1989; 64:705–714

16. Perkins HS: Teaching medical ethics during residency. Acad Med 1989; 64:262–266

17. Roberts LW, McCarty T, Lyketsos C, et al: What and how psychiatry residents at ten programs wish to learn about ethics. Academic Psychiatry 1996: 20:131–143

18. Sider RC, Clements C: Psychiatry's contribution to medical ethics education. Am J Psychiatry 1982; 139:498–501

19. Stone AA: Ethical and legal issues in psychotherapy supervision, in Clinical Perspectives on Psychotherapy Supervision, edited by Greben SE, Ruskin R. Washington DC, American Psychiatric Press, 1994, pp. 11–40

20. Bernal Y, Del Rio V: Psychiatric ethics and confidentiality, in Comprehensive Textbook of Psychiatry, 4th Edition, edited by Kaplan HI, Sadock BJ. Baltimore, MD, Williams & Wilkins, 1985

21. Lakin M: Coping with Ethical Dilemmas in Psychotherapy. New York, Pergamon, 1991

22. Hundert EM: A model for ethical problem solving in medicine, with practical applications. Am J Psychiatry 1987; 144:839–846

23. Sadler JZ, Hulgus YF: Clinical problem solving and the biopsychosocial model. Am J Psychiatry 1992; 149:1315–1323

24. Committee on Therapy, Group for the Advancement of Psychiatry: Psychotherapy in the Future (GAP Report No. 133). Washington DC, American Psychiatric Press, 1992

25. Ende J: Feedback in clinical medical education. JAMA 1983; 250:777–781

26. Culver CM, Clouser KD, Gert B, et al: Basic curricular goals in medical ethics. N Engl J Med 1985; 312:253–256

27. Pellegrino ED, Hart RJ, Henderson SR, et al: Relevance and utility of courses in medical ethics: a survey of physicians' perceptions. JAMA 1985; 253:49–53

28. Yager J: Psychiatric residency training and the changing economic scene. Hosp Community Psychiatry 1987; 38:1076–1081

29. Boyle PJ, Callahan D: Minds and hearts: priorities in mental health services. Report of the Hastings Center Project on Priorities in Mental Health Services. Hastings Cent Rep 1993; 23(suppl):S1–S24

30. Barnard D: Residency ethics training: a critique of current trends. Arch Intern Med 1988; 148:1836–1838

31. Jacobson JA, Tolle SW, Stocking C, et al: Internal medicine residents' preferences regarding medical ethics. Acad Med 1989; 64:777–781

32. American Medical Association: Evaluation Survey Report on the Effectiveness of Medical Ethics Training. Washington DC, American Medical Association, Ethics Resource Center, 1985

33. Arnold RM, Forrow L: Assessing competence in clinical ethics: are we measuring the right behaviors? J Gen Intern Med 1993; 8:52–54

34. Meisel A, Roth LH: What we do and do not know about informed consent. JAMA 1981; 246:2473–2477

35. Stanley BH, Sieber JE, Melton GB: Empirical studies of ethical issues in research. Am Psychol 1987; 42:735–741

36. Eichelman B, Wikler D, Hartwig A: Ethics and psychiatric research: problems and justification. Am J Psychiatry 1984; 141:400–405

37. Stein SP: Supervision of the beginning psychiatric resident, in Clinical Perspectives on Psychotherapy Supervision, edited by Greben SE, Ruskin R. Washington DC, American Psychiatric Press, 1994, pp. 73–84

38. Butterfield PS: The stress of residency: a review of the literature. Arch Intern Med 1985; 148:1428–1435

39. Beauchamp TL, Childress JF: Principles of Biomedical Ethics, 4th Edition. New York, Oxford University Press, 1994

40. Anzia DJ, LaPuma J: An annotated bibliography of psychiatric medical ethics. Academic Psychiatry 1991; 15:1–17

41. Sacks MH, Sledge WH, Warren C: Core Readings in Psychiatry: An Annotated Guide to the Literature, 2nd Edition. Washington DC, American Psychiatric Press, 1995

42. American Medical Association: Code of Medical Ethics: Current Opinions with Annotations, 1994 Edition. Chicago, IL, American Medical Association, Council on Ethical and Judicial Affairs, 1994

43. Ethical principles of psychologists and code of conduct. Am Psychol 1992; 47:1597–1611

44. Simon RI: Clinical Psychiatry and the Law, 2nd Edition. Washington DC, American Psychiatric Press, 1992

45. Reid WH: Treatment of violent patients: concerns for the psychiatrist, in Review of Psychiatry, Vol 8, edited by Tasman A, Hales RE, Frances AJ. Washington DC, American Psychiatric Press, 1989

46. Tiberius RG, Cleave-Hogg D: A database for curriculum design in medical ethics. Journal of Medical Education 1984; 59:512–513

9.11   Siegler M (2002) Training Doctors for Professionalism: Some Lessons from Teaching Clinical Medical Ethics. Mt. Sinai Med J 69:404–9

Training Doctors for Professionalism:

Some Lessons from Teaching Clinical Medical Ethics

MARK SIEGLER, M.D.

Abstract

Medical professionalism encourages physicians to place their patients' interests above self-interest. In recent years, many medical organizations, including the American Board of Internal Medicine (ABIM), Association of American Medical Colleges (AAMC), and the American Medical Association (AMA), have developed initiatives to strengthen medical professionalism. By emphasizing professionalism, supporters of these initiatives hope that medicine and physicians may recapture professional autonomy, decrease public criticism of medicine and physicians, and help physicians regain the moral high ground in the unending struggle with payers, both public and private. One crucial question facing medical educators is whether the concepts of professionalism can be taught to medical students and residents. This paper draws upon the author's thirty years of experience in teaching clinical medical ethics to provide guidance on how to teach the concepts of professionalism to students and residents.
Key Words: Professionalism, medical ethics, physician-patient relationship.

Introduction

ALTHOUGH DISAGREEMENTS PERSIST among experts as to which aspects of medical practice are captured by the term "medical professionalism," in recent years there has nevertheless been widespread agreement within academic medicine that it is essential to teach about medical professionalism to medical students and residents. Before considering whether lessons learned from teaching clinical medical ethics during the past thirty years may be applicable to teaching about medical professionalism, it would be useful to ask why medical professionalism has become the shared theme of many professional groups, such as the American Med-

ical Association (AMA), Association of American Medical Colleges (AAMC) and American Board of Internal Medicine (ABIM), which are not always in accord. There is no simple answer to explain why medical professionalism has rapidly emerged as a unifier for a desperately fragmented profession, but Wynia and colleagues recently suggested (1) that medical professionalism, which in their view consists of "devotion to service, profession of values, and negotiation within society . . . ," serves as a bulwark for medicine against two other forces competing to control medicine — market-driven and government-controlled health care.

Papers presented at the 15th Mount Sinai School of Medicine Ethics Conference, "Understanding Professionalism and Its Implications for Medical Education," suggested some of the following reasons to explain the contemporary importance of medical professionalism: (a) it may help physicians (perhaps in alliance with patients) to recapture some degree of autonomy, at least decisional autonomy; (b) it may help to break the cycle of public distrust and disrespect for physicians and medicine; (c) it may help physicians and medicine gain the high moral ground in their ongoing struggle with payers,

Lindy Bergman Distinguished Service Professor of Medicine and Director, MacLean Center for Clinical Medical Ethics, University of Chicago, Chicago, IL.

Address all correspondence to Mark Siegler, M.D., Director, MacLean Center for Clinical Medical Ethics, University of Chicago, 5841 S. Maryland Avenue, MC 6098, Chicago, IL 60637.

Presented at the Issues in Medical Ethics 2000 Conference at the Mount Sinai School of Medicine, New York, NY on November 3, 2000.

whether such payers be managed care organizations or government; and finally, (d) it may actually contribute to improving the process and outcome of patient care. My own view is that the political, economic, social and clinical struggles to recapture or at least retain important elements of doctor and patient autonomy are being fought on the battlefield of medical professionalism.

Even if there were widespread agreement on the desirability of teaching medical professionalism, some might question whether we as a profession are capable of teaching it. Such skeptics might raise the following two questions:

Is it possible to teach the elements of professionalism? For example, the American Board of Internal Medicine has identified seven negative behaviors as being violations of professionalism: abuse of power, arrogance, greed, misrepresentation, impairment, lack of conscientiousness, and conflict of interest (2). The Accreditation Council for Graduate Medical Education (ACGME) has identified positive aspects of professionalism, including respect, regard, integrity, and responsiveness to patients and society that supercede self-interest (3). Many of the elements identified by ABIM and by ACGME relate to innate character traits and the virtue of individuals; this raises the ancient issue of whether character and virtue can be taught. (See below in section entitled "What should be taught?").

Can you teach the values of medical professionalism without changing the internal culture of academic health centers and the entire health system? While many subscribe to the view that professional values are transmitted to physicians by a combination of didactic teaching and role-model mentoring, others including Dr. Ken Ludmerer (4) — and Samuel Bloom (5) — at this conference believe that the development of professional values is influenced by the values inherent in the entire health system.

Ludmerer recently wrote:

"...[S]tudies over the past four decades have documented the profound impact of the entire institutional environment of the academic health center on shaping the attitudes, values, beliefs, modes of thought, and behavior of medical students . . . . Formal coursework and mentoring represent only two of the many factors that affect the development of attitudes. An unfriendly institutional culture can easily undermine the well-intentioned efforts of those trying to impart professionalism by means of the curriculum . . . . The greatest challenge in proving the teaching of professionalism is to modify the internal culture of the academic health center so that it better reinforces the values that medical educators wish to impart. At present this represents no small task for the managed care revolution has caused medical schools and teaching hospitals to become much less friendly to patients and students than they were even a few years ago."

My own observations, based on my work as an attending physician at an academic medical center, reinforce Ludmerer's concerns. Recently, I supervised a particularly empathetic and compassionate resident who had admitted ten complex patients in the previous twelve hours, and was tired, irritable, and overwhelmed by her clinical responsibilities. I tried to serve as her teacher and mentor but found myself having less time to teach because I was forced to document patient records so that I could protect myself against possible legal cases of fraud and abuse. Also, many of the patients we care for in our health system are uninsured and, therefore, are often "neglected" medically between acute in-patient hospitalizations. Further, the teaching hospital I work at faces serious financial constraints, some of which have required the firing of nurses and other patient-care personnel, thereby adding new tasks to those of the already overworked residents. As Ludmerer suggests, it is not easy to model and teach medical professionalism in such a system, a commercial atmosphere which he says (4) " . . . does little to validate the altruism and idealism that students typically bring with them to the study of medicine."

Can the Teaching of Medical Ethics Provide Any Guidance for Developing Teaching of Medical Professionalism?

Cautionary Observations

Although medical ethics has been taught in most American medical schools since the 1970s, there is little data to document whether such ethics training has been successful in improving patient care or patient outcomes, whether the doctor-patient relationship has been strengthened, or whether improvements have occurred in the way medical decisions are reached. Very few studies, if any, have examined the impact on the quality of patient care of teaching medical ethics or of medical ethics in general. For example, one major study showed that despite medical ethics' preoccupation for thirty years with end-of-life issues, the care dying patients receive in American hospitals is inadequate both clinically, because it fails to provide sufficient pain medication and ethically, because it fails to respect the wishes of dying patients (6). Professor Leon Kass, one of the founders of the American bioethics movement, recently commented critically about the achievements of bioethics (7): "Though originally intended to improve our deeds, the practice of ethics, if truth be told, has at best improved our speech." As we move forward to develop and implement a national effort to teach medical professionalism, one lesson to be learned from teaching medical ethics relates to the failure of medical ethics to document its achievements. This suggests that in developing teaching in medical professionalism, it is essential to specify the goals of such new teaching, to demonstrate how such teaching improves the process and outcome of patient care, and to develop from the outset methods to evaluate its impact on students (8).

Positive Guidance

Based on my experience from teaching medical ethics for thirty years, I suggest that any new teaching program (for example, a program in medical professionalism) answers the five questions noted in Table 1.

I will discuss these five questions primarily in terms of clinical medical ethics and will provide tentative answers that I have arrived at with my colleagues, Edmund Pellegrino and Peter Singer (9). Whether our observa-

tions about clinical medical ethics also apply to the teaching of medical professionalism is a question I will leave for those with greater expertise than mine in the field of medical professionalism.

1. Why teach clinical medical ethics?

There are three important reasons for teaching clinical medical ethics:

- To provide students with essential and practical knowledge about issues that arise frequently when caring for patients and with which students must be familiar in order to provide good care. Such issues include, but are not limited to, informed consent, truth-telling, confidentiality, human subject protection in research trials, and end-of-life care.

- To encourage students to build upon this foundation of clinical medical ethics through life-long learning.

- To introduce students to the central importance of the physician-patient relationship and the ways in which communication occurs and decisions are reached within this relationship.

The fundamental justification for teaching clinical medical ethics (or for that matter, any medical school or residency subject) is based on its contribution to the care of patients. Therefore, the principal goal of teaching clinical ethics is to improve the quality of patient care in terms of both the process and outcome of care. If young physicians are equipped with the skills required to reach ethical decisions regarding patients, their patients will be protected from violations of their dignity. This means that in educating young physicians emphasis must be placed not only on the ethics of the actual decision but also on the ethics of the decision-making process. The skills of ethical analysis are part of the competence-set of young physicians and are a necessary complement to the physicians' knowledge base and competence in the scientific and technical aspects of clinical medicine.

Many of the reasons offered for teaching clinical medical ethics could also be applied to teaching professionalism.

2. When to teach clinical medical ethics?

If clinical medical ethics (or professionalism) is essential to medical education and prac-

TABLE 1
Teaching Clinical Medical Ethics to Medical Students and Residents

1.	Why teach?
2.	When to teach?
3.	What should be taught?
4.	How should it be taught?
5.	Who should teach?

tice, it should not only be taught as a block course (although some basic instruction is required) but it should also be continuously integrated into the young physician's education at all levels of medical school and residency training. Whenever possible, ethics teaching should be coordinated with students' other learning objectives. For example, an ideal time to teach about brain death and the vegetative state would be during a basic science course on neuroanatomy and neurophysiology. Similarly, the introductory anatomy course offers a unique opportunity to deal with issues of death, dying and respect for the dead body. The course on history taking and physical diagnosis is the optimal time to engage students on topics such as the doctor-patient relationship, truth-telling, confidentiality and informed consent.

Whatever foundational instruction is provided in clinical medical ethics during the first two years of medical school must be reinforced during the clinical years. This point was stated eloquently in 1902 by William Osler in a speech to the New York Academy of Medicine (10).

> "In what may be called the natural method of teaching, the student begins with the patient, continues with the patient, and ends his study with the patient, using books and lectures as tools, as means to an end . . . . . For the junior student in medicine and surgery it is a safe rule to have no teaching without a patient for a text, and the best teaching is that taught by the patient himself."

In the contemporary context, clinical teaching about ethics and professionalism is best accomplished by integrating the teaching into each of the students' clinical clerkships. This practice disrupts the pattern of clinical education least, takes advantage of the students' involvement with actual cases, and eliminates the problem of designing a course to cover all the major ethical and professional issues encountered in all major specialties.

3. What should be taught?

Ideally, teaching about clinical medical ethics should include three dimensions: cognitive skills (information and facts); behavioral skills; and character development and virtue.

a. Cognitive skills. Students should be introduced to the literature of clinical ethics, to the research methodologies used in ethics, and

to a practical approach for doing ethical analysis. The specific curriculum should reflect the incidence and prevalence of clinical situations that are encountered in the students' or residents' work. Curriculum design also can be based upon published studies of the epidemiology of ethical dilemmas that are seen in inpatient settings, outpatient setting, or consultation setting. Another approach to curriculum design is to target teaching to meet the perceived needs and preferences of students, which will vary depending on students' and residents' levels of training and specialties (11).

b. Behavioral skills. The assimilation and mastery of cognitive knowledge are not an end in itself for clinicians. To be effective in caring for patients, clinicians must have the behavioral skills that are necessary to put their knowledge to work in everyday clinical encounters. A physician who knows the legal and ethical requirements of writing an order not to resuscitate (DNR) should also be expected to know how and when to initiate discussions about DNR status with patients and families in a thoughtful and sensitive manner. Instruction in the behavioral skills of clinical ethics requires teaching and role modeling by experienced clinicians who can demonstrate the skills in practice. It further requires that students have the opportunity to practice these skills while being supervised by experienced clinicians.

An eloquent argument for integrating cognitive knowledge and behavioral skills is contained in an influential consensus statement (12) which concluded that students should be taught both cognitive knowledge and "interactional abilities to deal successfully with most of the moral issues they confront in their daily practice."

c. Character development. Ten years ago, in discussing the importance of character development as part of medical ethics teaching, my colleagues and I wrote the following statement, which may apply with equal force to the current goals of teaching medical professionalism (11):

> In addition to cognitive knowledge and behavioral skills, some attention must be paid to the affective component of clinical ethics — that is to say, to the kind of person the physician should be as well as the kind of decisions he or she should make. In short, ethics requires that the physician be a person of character, one who can be expected habit-

ually to act in the patient's interests when no one is watching. Trust is essential in the healing relationship. The norms and principles of clinical ethics must in the end be filtered through the person of the physician. The values or principles the physician chooses, the theory of ethics he espouses and the way he interprets the relationship with the patient will shape the ethical decision he makes in a given case. In order for a physician to perform in an ethically defensible way, both procedurally and substantively, some development of his character is essential. This is the most difficult task in clinical ethics.

A statement such as this inevitably raises the question that Plato raised in "The Meno" (13): "Can you tell me Socrates: Can virtue be taught? Or, if not, does it come by practice? Or does it come neither by practice nor by teaching, but do people get it by nature, or in some other way?"

4. How should clinical medical ethics be taught?

At the University of Chicago we emphasize the following six principles (the "Six C's") in teaching clinical medical ethics (Table 2):

I wish to elaborate here on the fifth point — that clinical medical ethics teaching should be clean (i.e., not too complex). Our model for teaching clinical medical ethics includes cognitive training in the fundamentals of ethics, with a core set of lectures on 8 – 10 important topics; a recommended text that is clinically oriented; and a basic approach to ethical decision making (11). It also provides students with a bibliography of accessible articles and reference materials for further reading. The students are also provided with opportunities to develop behavioral skills in their clinical work ("See one, do one, teach one"). For example, after reading about the core elements of informed consent, a

student observes a skilled clinician negotiating consent with a patient, and the student is then given an opportunity to elicit informed consent while the instructor observes the student-patient interaction.

5. Who should teach clinical medical ethics?

Medical ethics should be taught by those who do it well and who have the capacity to motivate students and residents to improve the quality of their patient-physician interactions and patient outcomes. These teachers could be either practicing physicians who have received training in ethics or bioethicists who have clinical experience. Role-model-teaching physicians are especially important for the following reasons:

- Physicians can teach ethics in the clinical setting by referring to actual clinical cases, as is done in most other effective clinical teaching.

- Physicians are responsible for resolving — rather than just for analyzing — clinical-ethical problems in order to reach good decisions with their patients.

- Physicians also demonstrate ethically appropriate professional attitudes and values to students so that students learn both from the formal teaching of clinical ethics and from their teachers' modeling of ethical behavior and professional conduct.

- Physician-teachers incorporate clinical-ethical considerations into the routine practice and teaching of medicine.

The five questions that have been addressed with respect to teaching clinical ethics should also be considered when developing a teaching and training program in medical professionalism. I suspect that many of the issues addressed about clinical medical ethics would apply also to teaching medical professionalism.

Two Final Thoughts on Teaching Clinical Medical Ethics and Medical Professionalism

Can Character Be Taught?

This ancient question has no easy answer. In my view, medical education and training not only provides students with a new vocabulary and a new knowledge base, but also serves as a

TABLE 2
Principles for Teaching Clinical Ethics
The 6 C's

1. Clinically based
2. Cases (real)
3. Continuous
4. Coordinated (integrated)
5. Clean (i.e., simple)
6. Clinicians as instructors

Vol. 69 No. 6 TRAINING DOCTORS FOR PROFESSIONALISM—SIEGLER 409

moral pilgrimage in which character and attitudes are molded by the experience of caring for sick patients. While most students will change during training, not every student will emerge with a set of character traits that ensures that ethical and professional standards are always maintained. This, in turn, places a heavy burden on those who help select medical students for admission to medical school. Medical school admissions committees do very well, but sadly, there is no gold standard with which to identify with precision those students whose character flaws may prevent them from developing the kind of ethical and professional attitudes that society wants and demands of its physicians. Left to myself, I would always select students based on positive character traits (if I could identify them) before GPAs or MCAT scores, but I acknowledge that such a selection process is an art, not a science (14).

The Fundamental Importance of the Doctor-Patient Relationship

After undergoing trial by fire during the last decade, the doctor-patient relationship in the US has emerged with renewed vitality and a strong endorsement from patients. This is as it should be, since the doctor-patient relationship has always, at all times, served a universal human need (i.e., helping people who turn to medicine for help) and has pursued an unchanging goal (to provide the best help it can within the scientific limits of the times). The ethics and professionalism of the modern physician is not very different from that of the ancient physician who subscribed to the following Hippocratic guidelines (15): ". . . as to diseases make a habit of two things, to help or at least to do no harm."

Almost 2500 years ago, in a remarkable passage in Book IV of "The Laws," Plato recognized that good doctor-patient relationships were required to achieve the goals of medicine. Plato described inadequate doctor-patient relationships, what he called "slave medicine," as follows (16):

"The physician never gives the slave any account of his complaints, nor asks for any; he gives some empiric treatment with an air of knowledge in the brusque fashion of a dictator, and then is off in haste to the next ailing slave . . . "

Plato contrasted this inadequate doctor-patient relationship with what he called the physician-patient relationship for free men, in which (16):

"The physician treats their disease by going into things thoroughly from the beginning in a scientific way and takes the patient and his family into confidence. Thus, he learns something from the patient. He never gives prescriptions until he has won the patient's trust, and when he has done so, he aims to produce complete restoration to health by persuading the patient to comply."

The best clinical medicine, Plato tells us, is practiced when the scientific and technical aspects of care are placed in the context of a personal and professional relationship in which the physician strives to win the patient's support and trust. In this regard, the professional and ethical values described by Plato and those that are expected of the contemporary physicians are remarkably similar. Both are based on a medical relationship with the patient in which the physician's core ethical and professional values are the foundation of good clinical care.

References

1. Wynia MK, Latham SR, Kao AC, et al. Medical professionalism in society. N Engl J Med 1999; 341:1612–1616.
2. American Board of Internal Medicine. Project professionalism. Philadelphia (PA): ABIM; 1994. p. 2.
3. ACGME. Graduate medical education directory. Chicago (IL): American Medical Association. 2001.
4. Ludmerer KM. Instilling professionalism in medical education. JAMA 1999; 282:881–882.
5. Bloom SW. Professionalism in the practice of medicine. Mt Sinai J Med 2002; 69:xxx–yyy.
6. The SUPPORT principal investigators. A controlled trial to improve care for seriously ill hospitalized patients. JAMA 1995; 274:233–237.
7. Kass LR. Practicing ethics: where's the action? Hastings Cent Rep 1990; 1:5–12.
8. Papadakis MA, Osborn EH, Cooke M, Healy K. A strategy for the detection and evaluation of unprofessional behavior in medical students. University of California, San Francisco School of Medicine Clinical Clerkships Operation Committee. Acad Med 1999; 74:980–990.
9. Siegler M, Pellegrino ED, Singer PA. Clinical medical ethics: the first decade. J Clin Ethics 1990; 1:5–9.
10. Osler W. On the need of a radical reform in our methods of teaching medical students. Medical News 1903; 82:49–53.
11. Pellegrino ED, Siegler M, Singer PA. Teaching clinical ethics. J Clin Ethics 1990; 1:175–180.
12. Culver CM, Clouser KD, Gert B, et al. Basic curricular goals in medical ethics. N Engl J Med 1985; 312:253–256.
13. Plato. The Meno. In: Warmington EH, Rouse PG. Great dialogues of Plato. New York: New American Library; 1956. pp. 28–68.
14. Siegler M. How to select medical students who will become old-fashioned docs. J Chron Dis 1983; 36:487–489.
15. Hippocrates. Hippocrates. Vol. 1. Boston (MA): Harvard University Press; 1992.
16. Plato. The laws. Tr. T. Age. London: Dent; 1943. pp. 104–105.

End-of-Life Care

10

Laura Weiss Roberts and Mark Siegler

Abstract

This chapter contains reprinted works from Dr. Mark Siegler focusing on the application of clinical medical ethics to end-of-life care and decision-making. These works acknowledge extremely challenging clinical settings, such as ones that involve life-sustaining treatments, critical illnesses, or requests for euthanasia. Each work demonstrates the application of clinical medical ethics to various end-of-life scenarios and provides insight and recommendations as to how practicing physicians can ensure that they are providing ethical care to their most vulnerable patients. The works in this chapter are reprinted with permission.

L.W. Roberts, MD, MA (✉)
Department of Psychiatry and Behavioral Sciences,
Stanford University School of Medicine, Stanford, CA, USA
e-mail: robertsl@stanford.edu

M. Siegler, MD
Bucksbaum Institute for Clinical Excellence, MacLean Center
for Clinical Medical Ethics, University of Chicago, Pritzker School
of Medicine, Chicago, IL, USA

© Springer International Publishing AG 2017
L.W. Roberts, M. Siegler (eds.), *Clinical Medical Ethics*, DOI 10.1007/978-3-319-53875-4_10

10.1   Siegler M (1975) Pascal's Wager and the Hanging of Crepe. N Engl J Med 293:853–7

SPECIAL ARTICLE

PASCAL'S WAGER AND THE HANGING OF CREPE

MARK SIEGLER, M.D.

Abstract   Hanging of crepe refers to one type of strategy employed by physicians in communicating prognoses to families of critically ill patients. This approach offers the bleakest, most pessimistic prediction of the patient's outcome, presumably in an effort to lessen the
family's suffering if the patient dies of his illness. Certain similarities exist between this technic and that
used by Pascal, the 17th-century philosopher, in formulating his wager on the belief in God, in that both attempt to develop "no-lose" strategies, in which
chances for "winning" are maximized.

A detailed analysis of these strategies indicates that
neither is truly "no-lose," and that both contain inherent disadvantages. Prognostication, an alternative approach to physician-family communication, appears to be strategically and morally superior to the
hanging-of-crepe strategy. (N Engl J Med 293:853-857,
1975)

O NE wagers when an outcome is uncertain, but always
in the hope of winning. This notion of risk and odds
underlies the excitement and thrill of gambling. When
one bets on a coin toss or a horse race, one is engaged in a
traditional risk situation in which all variables are potentially determinable, and in which odds can be calculated
precisely. However, when Blaise Pascal, the 17th-century
mathematician, physicist and religious philosopher, proposed a wager on the value of believing in God, he extended the notion of a wager from a risk situation in which odds
can be calculated to an uncertainty situation in which
variables are neither limited, given value nor defined. In
addition, Pascal added a dimension to the concept of wager when he invoked probability theory to justify a prudent course of conduct in spiritual and religious matters,
areas that previously had not been approached in these
terms.

From the Section of General Internal Medicine, Department of Medicine,
University of Chicago, Pritzker School of Medicine, Box 72, 950 E. 59th St.,
Chicago IL 60637, where reprint requests should be addressed to Dr.
Siegler.

Pascal stated: "Let us weigh the gain and loss in wager-
ing that God is. Let us estimate these two chances. If you
gain, you gain all; if you lose, you lose nothing. Wager,
then, without hesitation that He is."[1] Using the strategy of
the wager, Pascal appeared to have developed a "no-lose"
situation in which belief in God became not just a proper
moral position, but an unassailably rational stand based
upon probability theory.

This paper examines a form of physician behavior that
uses a strategy similar to Pascal's: a strategy designed to
convert an uncertainty situation into a "no-lose" situation.
The behavior in question is a form of physician-to-family
communication referred to as hanging crepe. Clear parallels exist between Pascal's wager and the physician's hanging-of-crepe strategy.

THE HANGING-OF-CREPE STRATEGY

Hanging crepe is a technic of communication used by
physicians in dealing with patients' families in specific situations in which the patient is critically ill and in which his
survival or death hangs delicately in the balance. When he

854   THE NEW ENGLAND JOURNAL OF MEDICINE   Oct. 23, 1975

employs the strategy the physician indicates that the scales are no longer in balance between life and death but are heavily weighted toward the side of inevitable death. A physician applies the strategy by informing the family that the acutely ill patient will almost certainly die of his illness, and that only an unexpected turn of events, possibly related to successful physician intervention, might, but only might, restore the scales to balance and preserve the patient's life. The strategy, like that of Pascal's wager, is designed to establish a "no-lose" situation in which the interests of the patient, his family and the physician are rigorously protected, and in which adverse consequences are minimized.

This strategy is employed in true medical or surgical emergencies rather than in cases in which a patient inevitably succumbs to a chronic, fatal disease. Certain conditions, such as metastatic cancers, or intractable heart failure at rest, or progressive respiratory insufficiency, have been sufficiently well studied to permit the physician to predict accurately that premature death will inevitably occur. For these situations, physicians may adopt a new, more humane approach to the dying patient such as that espoused by Dr. Elisabeth Kübler-Ross.[2] Dr. Ross stresses the importance of permitting each patient to confront the fact of dying in his own way, and she encourages physicians, medical personnel and families to maintain open channels of communication with the dying patient.

Without any underestimation of the importance of communicating with the dying patient, it is necessary to emphasize the difference between chronic situations in which a patient is known to be dying and the particular situation in which hanging crepe is employed. The principal difference is one of probability: in the former one is dealing with near certainty; and in the latter, the patient may either recover or die — i.e., the odds may be equal, or they may actually favor recovery. But in hanging crepe the physician artificially imposes certainty or greatly exaggerates probabilities of dying in a situation in which the outcome is uncertain.

The strategy of hanging crepe is certainly not new. For example, in the 12th century, an anonymous physician of the School of Salerno described the technic in a discourse on the doctor-patient relation:

> ...When examining the urine you should observe its color, substance, quantity, and content; after which you may promise the patient that with the help of God you will cure him. As you go away, however, you should say to his servants that he is in a very bad way, because if he recovers you will receive great credit and praise, and if he dies, they will remember that you despaired of his health from the beginning.[3]

Certain physicians, such as surgeons, cardiologists, neonatologists, and particularly house officers, frequently encounter critically ill patients and are more likely to be in situations in which this strategy is applicable. Much important communication with the families of critically ill patients is carried on by members of the house staff (or by the medical student, in teaching hospitals), since they are frequently involved in the minute-to-minute care of the patient. Thus, the attending physician who supervises house officers and students in their management of hospitalized patients, is indirectly involved in the strategy, even though he himself might never use it. Teachers of clinical medicine, whether their students are undergraduate medical students, house officers, or paramedical personnel, have an obligation to determine how their subordinates interact with patients' families in these critical situations.

THE STRATEGY OF PASCAL'S WAGER

Pascal's wager and the hanging-of-crepe strategy both use probability theory to attempt to define a course of conduct that is morally, ethically and strategically correct. Pascal's wager is a strategy of optimism and affirmation, in which the wagerer hopes for salvation. The strategy of hanging crepe is one of pessimism, in which the wagerer is preparing others for the worst possible eventuality. Both approaches appear to be heavily based upon establishing "no-lose" situations. For Pascal, belief in God, even if not a winning proposition, was not a losing one. For the physician who hangs crepe, his action seems to be moral, ethical, and entirely for the good of the patient's family; nothing appears to be lost in preparing them for the worst. It is instructive to examine both these apparent "no-lose" situations, in an effort to determine whether either or both contain unexpected detrimental features that might lead one to re-evaluate their usefulness as definitive solutions to difficult ethical problems.

Pascal's wager, which was invoked to justify a belief in God, has frequently been criticized by logicians, theologians and philosophers. The grounds for criticism have often begun by attacking the psychologic truth of Pascal's first assertion, "If God exists, and I believe in Him, I win all." Critics have questioned the psychology of the wager and have argued that one cannot induce belief merely by representing to oneself the advantages of belief. A second, more fanciful criticism has been advanced by Walter Kaufmann, who suggests that "...God might 'out-Luther' Luther. A special area in Hell might be reserved for those who go to Mass. Or God might punish those whose faith is prompted by prudence...."[4] These and similar criticisms begin to erode the notion that the wager represents absolutely prudent conduct.

Is there also a weakness in Pascal's second assertion? If God does not exist, said Pascal, and I devote a lifetime of belief in His existence, I have lost nothing. This is the essence of an apparent "no-lose" situation. The critical flaw seems to be that if God does not exist, and if one devotes all one's belief and energy to a nonexistent Deity, one has surrendered without recompense or reward the uniquely human qualities of rationality and intellectual integrity. And thus one has lived a lifetime with a lie, in intellectual darkness, and if God does not exist, one has indeed lost a great deal. Thus, on reassessment, an apparent "no-lose" situation is seen to contain the potential for weighty and important losses.

Pascal conceived the possibility of living a lifetime in disbelief, but invoked the concept of odds to dismiss as inconsequential the possibility of error:

> But there is here an infinity of an infinitely happy life to gain, a chance of gain against a finite number of chances of loss, and what you stake is finite. It is all divided; wherever the infinite is and there is not an infinity of chances of loss against that of gain, there is no time to hesitate, you must give all. And thus, when one is forced to play, he must renounce reason to preserve his life, rather than risk it for infinite gain, as likely to happen as the loss of nothingness.[1]

Pascal's arguments are powerful, particularly when he invokes the possibility of "infinite gain," and thereby transcends the limits of ordinary probability theory. But despite his willingness to renounce reason in the hope of gaining infinite happiness, the possibility remains that his was not truly a "no-lose" situation.

If the strategy of employing probability theory to determine moral and ethical conduct is not foolproof in justifying a belief in God, one suspects that a technic such as the hanging-of-crepe strategy also has inherent weaknesses. There appears to be nothing in the human situation comparable to the potential for "infinite gain" that Pascal uses in his wager strategy. It would be instructive to examine the hanging-of-crepe strategy to determine what liabilities and difficulties may result from this technic.

ADVANTAGES OF HANGING CREPE

This strategy is physician-generated, and the benefits that the physician derives from it are presumably great. With this technic, he establishes the following intellectual framework, which seems to be a "no-lose" situation:

- Nature kills (substitute for nature, God or Providence or chance, etc.).
- The physician saves, if he can.

The patient's condition and imminent death are ascribed to the inexorable progression of natural events. If, however, the physician succeeds in saving such a patient the credit belongs to him. This "no-lose" strategy provides obvious advantages to the physician. If the family perceives the physician struggling against overwhelming odds in an effort to save the patient, the physician's image cannot be tarnished. If he succeeds in his struggle to save the patient, he wins the family's gratitude; if he fails, he wins their respect for his valiant efforts. Interestingly enough, even if the patient recovers, the employment of the strategy subtly precludes attributing events to spontaneous recovery, which might be unrelated to physician action, and argues rather that the physician has saved the dying patient.

The physician's reputation and esteem may also rise among his colleagues. If a physician is frequently able to treat successfully patients who are thought to be dying, his fellow physicians, students, and other hospital personnel may consider him to be uniquely skilled in the practice of critical-care medicine. On the other hand, if such critically ill patients succumb to their disease, the health-care team will perceive that those deaths were inevitable.

The strategy can confer certain legal benefits and may protect the physician against potential malpractice suits. If a patient is said to be dying at the time of first presentation to the physician, it is obvious that the physician's action (or inaction) cannot be implicated in the death of the patient. Thus, the hanging-of-crepe technic militates against invoking alternative hypotheses — e.g., that death resulted from physician error or negligence — to account for the death of the patient.

The strategy may function as a psychologic defense for the physician, and his own self-image may benefit from the technic. If death is seen as inevitable, the physician can only benefit and not lose by struggling against the inevitable. If he comes to believe his own prognosis, he will see himself as personally blameless in the event of the patient's death. In these circumstances, the physician obviously feels human concern, but limited professional responsibility, if death actually ensues. Regardless of his action, inaction or outright error, which he performs in the faint hope of preventing death, the physician's responsibility, if death occurs, is minimal. Alternatively, if the patient chances to survive, the physician may believe that by his decisions and actions he pulled the patient through the crisis.

If the physician predicts that a fatal outcome is a virtual certainty, his own level of anxiety and tension may diminish, and his objectivity and performance may improve. When his reputation and self-esteem are no longer at stake, when he no longer feels vulnerable, and when there is no possibility of committing a major therapeutic error, he may take actions dispassionately and with enhanced preciseness.

In principle, it is the family of the dying patient who derive maximum benefit from the openness of the physician's communication to them in the hanging-of-crepe strategy. By means of this strategy the physician appears to share with them his special knowledge of the patient's condition and his perception of the inevitability of the patient's death. The family is prepared for the worst. The candor of the strategy requires that family members begin to think about the imminent possibility of death. The communication enables the family to draw closer together at a time of crisis and encourages them to provide mutual support for each other. This new perspective on the patient's condition might enable the family to interact more warmly and intimately with the dying patient. The mourning process may begin.

If the patient dies, the family is well prepared for this possibility. Alternatively, if the patient does not die, but survives to return home, the family is so relieved by its good fortune, that recriminations against the physician for his inaccurate prognosis are rare. Rather, the physician is thanked and complimented for his skill in saving a patient destined to die, and the family disperses without apparent ill-effects.

The patient is not directly involved in the hanging-of-crepe strategy except as object, and therefore the benefits that he derives are limited. The principal advantage to the patient comes from the gathering of his family and the

856   THE NEW ENGLAND JOURNAL OF MEDICINE   Oct. 23, 1975

warmth and support that they offer him. In addition, because the family perceive the seriousness of the illness, the patient may sense the critical nature of his own disease. This awareness may permit him to begin to deal directly with the fact of his dying and to prepare himself for death. If he survives he never directly encountered the crepe-hanging message and will probably suffer no long-term difficulties from its employment with his family.

DISADVANTAGES OF THE HANGING-OF-CREPE STRATEGY

The principal loss for the physician (as for the "gambler" in Pascal's wager) is the potential surrender of intellectual honesty and integrity. At its worst, the hanging-of-crepe strategy is based on a stereotyped response to certain clinical situations. When the physician hangs crepe he has abandoned reason and substituted a reflex action. If his professional forecast is given to decrease the likelihood of loss and to maximize his potential for gain, although unconsciously, he has already lost in an incalculable way. At best he has engaged in self-delusions; at worst he has abnegated his self-respect, professional judgment, and professional conduct. He has substituted premature intuition for reason.

The physician's reputation with his colleagues may suffer. If other members of the health-care team perceive a recurring pattern of physician behavior that they regard as spurious or melodramatic (like crepe-hanging), their respect for the person involved may decline.

By hanging crepe, the physician may be able to reduce his own level of anxiety and tension, but at the same time he creates a psychologic climate in which the patient's death seems inevitable. Not only physician performance but that of the entire health-care team may change in subtle ways. As a result the patient may receive less than maximal, aggressive care. A form of self-fulfilling prophecy may develop, in which the patient dies, because everyone acknowledges that he is destined to die.

If true, this latter notion has profound implications. It suggests that the hanging-of-crepe strategy may have therapeutic implications. The implicit relation of diagnosis, prognosis and therapy is an accepted convention of the clinical method. Such a relation is premised on the accuracy and rationality of each of these clinical steps. If, however, the prognosis offered is based upon the hanging-of-crepe strategy, can one be certain that the treatment that follows will relate only to the accuracy of the diagnosis, or might the choice of therapy be modified by the artificiality of the intervening prognosis? If the employment of the strategy blocks diagnostic inquiry, or subtly colors physician judgment, or alters therapy, this form of prognosis not only may be intellectually and ethically suspect but also may be detrimental to the actual management of the patient. If so, reservations about this form of physician conduct would be broadened and made more concrete.

The major disadvantage for the family relates to intense emotional stress and anguish generated by the use of this strategy. If the strategy is a stereotyped response by the physician to certain critical situations, and if a certain proportion of patients will recover rather than die, a certain number of families must endure torment unnecessarily. There is a kind of cruelty in marching a condemned prisoner to the gallows and setting the rope around his neck before commuting his sentence. In addition to the psychologic costs involved in the crepe-hanging strategy, actual costs may be incurred when family members neglect their ordinary obligations to family and jobs to be near the patient at this critical time. The family's perception that the patient is dying may alter their relation with him. As the family members begin to confront the anticipated loss of the loved one, and as they initiate the mourning process, they may unconsciously begin to withdraw their emotional support from the patient.

The strategy of hanging crepe may profoundly alter the family's perception of the role of the physician. On the one hand, if the patient dies, this strategy may serve to minimize objectivity and critical appraisal of the physician's performance. Actions, which in other circumstances might be viewed as negligent, would here be tolerated and accepted uncritically. Alternatively, if the patient recovers, the family might see the physician's role in the recovery as supernatural. Such mythologizing of the physician and his role, although flattering to the physician, prevents the public from achieving a fairer, more rational assessment of the physician's role.

The major disadvantage to the patient is that his care might be modified or compromised because the strategy was invoked. In addition, as his family and hospital personnel convey the impression that death is inevitable, the patient will surely receive the message that he is dying. This perception could induce despair or depression and the patient might give up his will to live.[5,6]

If the hanging-of-crepe strategy, like that of Pascal's wager, is not flawless, it would be appropriate to inquire whether there is an alternative approach for dealing with the family of the critically ill patient.

AN ALTERNATIVE STRATEGY OF COMMUNICATION: PROGNOSTICATION

Prognostication refers to an attempt by the physician to predict with accuracy the outcome of a patient's disease. In making the prediction, the physician uses all the available primary data, his interpretation of the data, and his ability to name the disease — i.e., to make a diagnosis. He then reviews the medical literature concerning similar diagnoses, and distinguishes the unique features of his patient (age, sex, associated medical conditions, social and economic factors, etc.) to arrive at a probable outcome in the individual case.

Feinstein has described a computer program that can help the clinician make prognoses.[7] The model that Feinstein presents is based on a library of data that have been programmed for a single disease (lung cancer) and the ability of the computer to generate data on a "resemblance group" of patients. A "resemblance group" is a set of patients with the same disease as the patient under consideration who also possess similar properties and characteristics. Thus, a resemblance group might be patients of similar age and sex who had presented with the same disease and similar symptoms and who also had similar associated diseases. In addition, Feinstein's computer program includes new classes of information that may be useful in defining a resemblance group such as "iatrotropic stimuli, clusters of symptoms, clinical stages, diagnostic attributes, prognostic co-morbidity, pre-therapeutic interval, and reasons for therapeutic decisions."[7] The availability of such a computer program can extend the clinician's own experience, which is often limited to a relatively small number of people with the ailment under consideration. It is unfortunate that Feinstein's work has not been extended by other groups who might use his model in analyzing additional diseases.

However, even the most accurate of prognoses is only an estimate of probabilities and as such may not predict the occurrence of an event in an individual case. Feinstein's method, although not denying individual variability, does not address itself to probability theory as applied to an individual case, or to the elements of physician-patient communication in matters of prognosis. The limitations of applying probability theory to an individual case were appreciated by J.M. Keynes:

> It has been pointed out already that no knowledge of probabilities, less in degree than certainty, helps us to know what conclusions are true, and that there is no direct relation between the truth of a proposition and its probability...The proposition that a course of action guided by the most probable considerations will generally lead to success, is not certainly true and has nothing to recommend it but its probability.[8]

True prognostication, although based upon the science of probability, clearly remains an exercise of the physician's art. Until extensive data (of the sort that Feinstein has gathered) are available for a wide variety of diseases, accurate prognosis will continue to be based upon thoughtful, subjective appraisals made by expert clinicians with considerable knowledge of specific diseases. This prognosis should always include, in addition to the mean survival of all similar cases, some mention of the extremes associated with any particular illness. It should acknowledge the uncertainties inherent in the collection of primary data, in the making of diagnoses, and in the implications of a diagnosis once made. Prognostication recognizes the inherent limitations of probability theory when applied to individual cases, and most importantly, admits that uncertainty and tentativeness underlie even the most detailed analysis of the individual's case.

CONCLUSIONS

The hanging-of-crepe strategy is employed only in certain specific situations, but by virtue of its extremeness, it may provide a model for analyzing the general problem of appropriate communication between physicians and families. For example, how does the physician balance his own uncertainty about outcome with the family's wish and right to know the "facts?" Do limits exist on the family's right to know all? Does a relation exist between the patient's welfare and the family's demands for information? In life-threatening situations how much information should a physician divulge? What are the relative benefits and disadvantages of total candor, circumspection, or an accounting of precise probabilities? Finally, what is to be said of the physician who for personal reasons is never able to offer a grave prognosis, and who is falsely optimistic and encouraging with the family of dying patients? Although serious reservations have been expressed concerning the use of the hanging-of-crepe strategy, it would be a misreading of this paper to assume that the alternative extreme of never conceding the possibility of death is morally or professionally superior as a strategy.

REFERENCES

1. Pascal B: Pensées: Thoughts on religion and other subjects. Edited by HS Thayer, EB Thayer. New York, Washington Square Press, 1965, pp 72-74
2. Kübler-Ross E: On Death and Dying. New York, The Macmillan Company, 1969
3. Corner GW: The rise of medicine at Salerno in the twelfth century. Ann Med Hist 3:1-16, 1931
4. Kaufmann W: Critique of Religion and Philosophy. New York, Harper Brothers Publishers, 1958, p 122
5. Engel GL: Sudden and rapid death during psychological stress. Ann Intern Med 74:771-783, 1971
6. *Idem:* Clinical observation: the neglected basic method of medicine. JAMA 192:849-852, 1965
7. Feinstein AR, Rubinstein JF, Ramshaw WA: Estimating prognosis with the aid of a conversational-mode computer program. Ann Intern Med 76:911-921, 1972
8. Keynes JM: A Treatise on Probability. New York, Harper and Row Publishers, 1962, pp 321-323

10.2 Siegler M (1977) Critical Illness: The Limits of Autonomy. Hast Cent Rep 7:12–5

Hastings Center Report, October 1977. Reprinted with permission from Wiley.

ETHICAL PROBLEMS IN CLINICAL PRACTICE

Critical Illness: The Limits of Autonomy

by MARK SIEGLER

Mr. D, a previously healthy sixty-six-year-old black man, came to a university hospital emergency room with his wife and described a three-day history of sore throat, muscle aches, fevers, chills, cough, sputum production, and blood in his urine. The patient was acutely ill with a high fever, shortness of breath, and a limited attention span. A chest X ray demonstrated a generalized pneumonia in both lungs. The clinical impression was that Mr. D was critically ill, that the cause of his lung disease was obscure, and that a low platelet count and blood in the urine were ominous signs. He was treated aggressively with three antibiotics in an effort to cure his pneumonia.

The next day his condition worsened. After reviewing the available clinical and laboratory data, the physicians caring for this man recommended that two uncomfortable but relatively routine diagnostic procedures be performed: a bronchial brushing to obtain a small sample of lung tissue to determine the cause of the pneumonia and a bone marrow examination to determine whether an infection or cancer was invading the bone marrow. The patient refused these diagnostic procedures. Separately, and together, the intern, resident, attending physician, and chaplain explained that these diagnostic tests were necessary to help the physicians formulate rational treatment plans. Mr. D became angry and agitated by this prolonged pressure, and subsequently began refusing even routine blood tests and X rays.

A psychiatrist who evaluated Mr. D concluded that although he was obviously ill and had a degree of mental impairment manifested by poor memory, he was not mentally incompetent. The psychiatrist thought that the patient understood the severity of his illness and the reasons the physicians were recommending certain tests, but that he was still making a rational choice in refusing the tests.

The patient's condition deteriorated

further and twenty-four hours later he appeared near death. I was the attending physician, and it was my opinion that the only treatment left was to place Mr. D on a respirator as a stopgap measure that might sustain him for another day or two, during which time the antibiotics and antituberculosis drugs might become effective. Mr. D refused.

The physicians expressed considerable disagreement on whether Mr. D was sufficiently rational to refuse a potentially life-saving treatment. In an effort to resolve this controversy, I spent two forty-five-minute periods at his bedside and explained as clearly as I could the reasons for our recommendations. I said that if he survived this crisis he would be able to return to a normal life and would not be an invalid or require chronic supportive care. During these two sessions, Mr. D was breathing rapidly and shallowly, and had trouble talking. But everything he said convinced me that he understood the gravity of his situation. For example, when I told him he was dying, he replied: "Everyone has to die. If I die now, I am ready." When I asked him if he came to the hospital to be helped, he stated: "I want to be helped. I want you to treat me with whatever medicine you think I need. I don't want any more tests and I don't want the breathing machine."

I gradually became convinced that despite the severity of his illness and his high fever, he was making a conscious, rational decision to selectively refuse a particular kind of treatment. In view of the frankness of our discussion, I then asked him whether he would want us to resuscitate him if he had a cardio-respiratory arrest. He turned away and said: "We've been through this before; now leave me alone." I left the bedside.

Throughout this day, despite vigorous attempts by social workers and neighbors, neither his wife nor children could be located.

Mr. D soon became semi-conscious and had a cardio-respiratory arrest. Des-

pite the objections of the houseofficers, I did not attempt to resuscitate him, and he died.

Mr. D's case raised the following questions:

1. Would this critically ill man be permitted to establish diagnostic and therapeutic limits on the care he wished to receive from a health care team in a large university hospital?

2. What were the medically and morally relevant factors that would encourage or permit physicians to respect his wishes? Or, alternatively, on what ground would physicians usurp the patient's presumed rights to liberty, autonomy, and self-determination?

One solution to moral-ethical dilemmas is to establish categorical rules of conduct which obviate the necessity for making agonizing choices in difficult situations. For example, in his writings Robert Veatch has consistently emphasized a commitment to individual freedom and self-determination, and the concomitant need to limit the power and authority of the medical profession. In discussing a patient's right to refuse treatment, Veatch makes the claim that "no competent patients have ever been forced to undergo any medical treatment for their own good no matter how misguided their refusal may have appeared." Veatch concludes that an adult may refuse any treatment as long as he is competent, and the principal determination to be made (in Veatch's view by the courts rather than by physicians) is whether the patient is competent.

In a recent paper entitled "The Function of Medicine," Eric Cassell describes an alternative attitude, and one equally familiar to clinicians. Cassell notes that in cases of acute illness [using pneumococcal meningitis as his example] ". . . it would be a rare hospital where such a patient would not be treated [even] against his will." In such a case, Cassell defends the decision to override a patient's wishes on the grounds that the refusal of treatment in acute illness is tantamount to suicide, that the physician has responsibilities to treat that cannot be relieved by the patient's refusal to accept treatment, that the patient is morally constrained not to prevent the physician from carrying out his responsibilities to treat him, and that in the face of acute illness, the physician does not have sufficient time to assess the patient's motives.

The Veatch and Cassell positions appear not to take into account the medically and morally relevant factors that physicians assess when determining whether to respect the wishes of critically ill patients. Clinical ethics is premised on the particularities of clinical circumstances, and workable clinical guidelines must necessarily take into account and reflect the extraordinary complexity of the medical model.

Factors Influencing the Physician's Decision

1. *The patient's ability to make (rational) choices about his care.* Either every critically ill patient in the hospital is incompetent to make choices concerning his care or each case must be assessed separately to determine if there are limits within which the critically ill patient retains some intellectual judgment and is capable of making choices. In the case of Mr. D, as in other critical care cases, the issue confronting conscientious physicians was not simply whether to respect a patient's wishes, but whether it was morally justifiable to accept at face value a critically ill patient's statement of his wishes.

Mr. D's case illustrates the practical difficulties in adhering to any rigid rule (either to defend "radical autonomy" for competent adults or to accept the "doctor's burden to heal" viewpoint) in critical care situations. Mr. D's wishes were forcefully stated and clear. He wished to be helped and to be relieved of his discomfort and pain, and to this end he would permit physicians to treat him with intravenous fluids, oxygen, antibiotics, and other medications. But he was also firm in establishing absolute limits on the diagnostic studies he would permit and in refusing to accept a respirator as a form of treatment. Thus, the perplexing question which continued to trouble his physicians was whether Mr. D was intel-

lectually capable of exercising such a degree of discrimination and choice. Although there was a considerable difference of opinion among the physicians caring for Mr. D—some believed that his illness impaired his thought processes and rendered him incapable of making choices—in my capacity as the attending physician responsible for his care, I decided otherwise and elected to respect Mr. D's wishes. This decision was based upon my subjective clinical judgment that despite the intensity of his illness, Mr. D retained sufficient intellect and rationality to make choices.

2. *The nature of the person making the choice.* Rather than assessing the rationality of a particular choice, one can ask an alternative question, whether Mr. D's decisions were consonant with his nature as a person. Who was Mr. D? What were his values? And did his choices in the hospital reflect those he might have made were he not ill? Was the patient acting autonomously—that is, with authenticity and independence? Alternatively, another question to be asked is: in the face of critical illness and within the narrow time-space frame characteristic of acute illness, is it ever possible to determine whether a patient's choices truly reflect his normal personality?

Obviously, if a patient and physician had previously established an ongoing relationship, the physician would be better acquainted with the personality, character, ideas, and beliefs of his patient. Another indicator to assess the validity of a patient's choice is whether it reflects a commitment expressed through time, such as the adherence to a particular religious belief (like a Jehovah's Witness refusing blood transfusions), or the signing and updating of a "living will," or the establishment of certain attitudes and behavior patterns in the course of a chronic illness. In Mr. D's case none of this information was available.

Another valuable insight into the patient as a person might be provided by the family as they describe the personality, character, and beliefs of the patient before the onset of this acute illness. The family could also be asked to offer an opinion on whether a patient is acting as he would normally act, or whether his behavior strikes them as aberrant and unusual. The family then would not be

making choices for the patient, but would be indicating to physicians the probable validity of the patient's own choices. In Mr. D's case the family was not available and thus could not provide evidence one way or the other.

Many people believe that the rights of individuals are not absolute, but must always be weighed against their responsibilities to social groups like the family or to the community at large. Unfortunately, in Mr. D's case, the absence of family input effectively limited the grounds upon which physicians would accept or reject Mr. D's wishes.

In most clinical circumstances it is possible either from previous knowledge of a patient or from the contributions of his family to assess accurately whether a particular choice made by an ill patient is consistent with his previous behavior and values. In this respect, Mr. D's case represents an extreme example, since none of this background material was available.

In the absence of supporting data, the physician must rely upon his basic skills of communication with the patient and must assess the patient's verbal and nonverbal messages. So much of clinical judgment and clinical decision-making involves the gathering of primary data through talking with patients, that this situation should be seen as an extreme variant of the basic clinical model. Further, much of clinical judgment involves "life and death" decisions, and thus this situation is not different in intensity from many others. I assessed Mr. D's personality as intelligent, proud, independent, wary of outsiders, and particularly suspicious of physicians and their motives. It seemed to me that the choices he was making were entirely consistent with his basic personality.

Of anecdotal interest, since it did not influence my decision, was some information that became available only after Mr. D's death which indicated that ten years earlier he had left the hospital "against medical advice" after first refusing to have a bone marrow examination!

3. *Age.* Mr. D's age made a difference in my decision. Had he been twenty-six years old, the factors I would use to decide whether to override his wishes would probably have remained essentially the

same—competence, the conformity of his choices to his personality, and the medical diagnosis and prognosis—but the standards I would apply to assess these might change. For example, I would have demanded a more perfect "mental status examination" and would have scrupulously checked a younger patient for evidence of a "toxic delirium" or an acute depression. My obvious wavering on this point may have something to do with the notion that wisdom and aging are associated, but more likely has to do with a concept of "natural death." The closer a patient gets to a "normal" life span, the more he has lived, and the more ready I am to let "nature take its course." Even though I appreciate the ambiguities and inconsistencies of taking age into account, I believe that I might have acted differently with a younger patient.

4. *Nature of the illness*. In this context, critical illness refers to an acute life-threatening illness. Several subdivisions of critical illness are necessary because physician behavior is premised on (a) whether the illness can be diagnosed or alternatively, whether it is obscure and refractory to diagnosis, and (b) what the prognosis is, whether or not the physician is able to make a diagnosis.

The most straightforward situation is one in which the physician can make a diagnosis that permits him to state with certainty that the prognosis of a particular disease is uniformly fatal if untreated, whereas with appropriate treatment complete recovery is possible. In addition to the infectious diseases such as pneumococcal meningitis which conform to this model, other medical emergencies such as acute respiratory failure, acute pulmonary edema, and diabetic ketoacidosis are also easily diagnosed and treated. It is precisely in such cases where diagnostic uncertainty is at a minimum and where the physician is confident about the probability of success with treatment, and the probability of death without treatment, that the physician will be most likely to usurp an ill patient's desires and treat him even against his wishes. In all other cases, however, the physician will be more inclined but not certain to respect the patient's wishes not to be treated. For example, certain diagnoses, in particular metastatic solid tumors or degenerative neurologic diseases, seem to generate a minimalist approach on the part of physicians and on occasion discourage physicians from aggressively treating patients with such diseases who may develop easily reversible acute conditions such as pneumonia.

The problem of uncertainty of diagnosis or uncertainty of prognosis is particularly disturbing. The absence of a diagnosis is a potential threat to the whole disease-oriented medical system, and generates a very aggressive, no-holds-barred approach to diagnostic testing. Mr. D's refusal to submit to certain routine but uncomfortable diagnostic procedures effectively blocked the efforts of his physicians to name his disease and surely contributed to their frustration. In cases of uncertainty, where the physician and patient are in agreement on pursuing diagnostic and therapeutic procedures, physicians will generally err on the side of diagnostic aggressiveness in an effort not to overlook a potentially reversible disease process. However, in cases of uncertainty where physicians and patients are in disagreement about diagnostic and therapeutic approaches, physician anxiety is maximized and the need for a moral-clinical decision is most urgent. In such cases, and Mr. D's case is a classic example, physicians must again rely upon their clinical judgment to assess the likelihood that a particular diagnostic study will yield a result that may permit a particular therapy which can change the outcome of the case. As the probability of a successful intervention decreases, most physicians can more easily, but not very easily conform to the patient's wishes.

In some cases, however, even if a particular intervention will guarantee success, the physician may still not usurp a patient's wishes. A frequent example of this latter situation arises in Jehovah's Witness cases where a simple blood transfusion could forestall a life-threatening emergency, but in which the physician is constrained by consistent legal precedents not to override a patient's wishes.

In the case of Mr. D, it soon became clear to me that whatever the diagnosis of his obscure illness was, it was fulminant and aggressive and would probably lead to his death. Even if we had been able to make a diagnosis from the bone marrow and bronchial brushing examinations, it was likely that no additional therapy would change his outcome. Even if he had consented to a respirator, his rapidly progressive deterioration suggested that he was not going to survive. I readily admit that my clinical judgment that the disease was rapidly progressive and almost certainly fatal further influenced me.

5. *The attitudes and values of the physician responsible for the decision*. At every point in the decision making, the responsible physician has resorted to value judgment. The judgments of whether the patient was rational, of what his baseline personality was, of what importance to ascribe to his age, and of whether his disease was potentially treatable and reversible, are all determinations that involve subjective value judgments based upon limited objective data.

Further, although physicians as a profession may share some general values and biases, they are not homogeneous in their basic value orientation. They differ in moral and religious background, in age, in experience, and in specialty training, to mention just a few factors. Specifically, what is a particular physician's attitude toward life and death? Does a physician view the death of a patient as a personal defeat, an avoidable tragedy? What is his concept of the role of the physician in the physician-patient relationship, that of a technician-scientist, or an advisor, or a friend, or a party to a contract? If the responsible physician invokes the doctrine of "do no harm," is his concept of harm that of omission or commission?

If all other factors were identical in arriving at a decision to support or override a patient's wishes not to be treated, we might discover that two physicians—one who believed in the primacy of life and another who believed in "death with dignity"—would reach entirely opposite conclusions. In Mr. D's case, my belief in the rights of individuals to determine their own destinies further encouraged me to support the patient's choices.

6. *The clinical setting*. Mr. D's case reflects some of the special problems of practicing medicine in a large, institutional, teaching setting. If a physician-patient encounter similar to the one described here had occurred in a patient's

home, or in a nursing home, or even in many community hospitals (particularly one without housestaff), there would be little question about acceding to the patient's wishes. There are at least two reasons. First, the kind of technology and expertise necessary to do many of these procedures is best represented in the large teaching hospital.

The second reason is more complex. It involves the nature of a teaching hospital in which authority and responsibility are diffused among the "health care team." Although the attending physician may ultimately be responsible for decisions, he does not care for patients in isolation. Indeed, most of the caring is performed by housestaff, students, nurses, and other health care personnel. The housestaff are very close to their patients and have very strong feelings about how best to care for them. Despite the housestaff's general lack of clinical experience, their views are often very accurate and persuasive. Further, housestaff are particularly skilled in the care of acutely ill patients. These young physicians strive diligently to not harm the patients, but when their concept of harm remains obscure, "do no harm" often means "do everything."

One interesting sidelight of this case was the houseofficers' wish to resuscitate this man after he died. They argued that at no time did the patient state he wanted to die; he did not offer a definitive "no" when asked whether he wished to be resuscitated; and clearly, after his heart and lungs stopped, he was no longer rational and decisions could then be made for him.

One final observation: this man was extremely strong and dignified in his last days. Despite his illness and fever, he resisted the onslaught of many physicians and consultants and the power of the hospital institution. He established limits for the health care team and would not permit those limits to be transgressed. The intellectual and emotional strength necessary to resist the powers of the medical system to persuade and force him to accept what they wanted to offer must have been enormous. He died a dignified death, and attempts at resuscitation would have violated the position he held while alive. It is unfortunate, and I am sadly moved, that he had to expend his last measures of intellectual and physical energy to engage in ongoing debate with his physicians. But perhaps that is the price the medical system sometimes exacts from those who would assert their independence and preserve their autonomy while suffering from critical illness.

MARK SIEGLER, M.D., *is a member of the Section of General Medicine, Department of Medicine, Division of the Biological Sciences and Pritzker School of Medicine, University of Chicago.*

10.3   Siegler M, Wikler D (1982) Brain Death and Live Birth. JAMA 248:1101–2

Reprinted with permission from the Journal of the American Medical Association, September 3, 1982, Volume 248, Copyright 1982, American Medical Association.

editorials

Brain Death and Live Birth

In this issue of *JAMA*, Dillon and colleagues (p 1089) describe two extraordinary cases. Both involved young pregnant, women who experienced profound neurological deterioration culminating in a clinical determination that they were both "catastrophically ill," with one patient meeting rigorous criteria of brain death. In both instances, the physicians responsible for these patients had to decide what their new obligations to them were. They had also to determine their obligations to the developing fetuses, whose chances for survival depended on the continuation of maternal circulation. These cases test our understanding of the nature and goals of medicine, of the responsibility of physicians, and even of the meaning of life and death. The authors should be praised for their clinical skills in successfully maintaining maternal circulation in case 2. They should also be commended for identifying the profound clinical-ethical quandaries, for resolving them according to their best clinical judgment, and, finally, for having the intellectual courage to report their actions and reasons in a scholarly medical journal.

The physicians' choices may be evaluated with respect to their effects on both the pregnant women and the fetuses. Most clinical decisions are based on the physicians' assessment of the individual medical needs of the patient and on the patient's choices for treatment. In neither of these cases, however, is there reported any wish on the part of the mother concerning treatment, and none of the medical options offered any hope of restoring the women to health or consciousness. Thus, the mothers' interests, apart from earlier desires to bear a healthy child, were not at issue. Further treatment could be considered neither beneficial nor harmful.

The choice among treatment options thus seems to have been based primarily on the interests of the fetus, with the goal of healthy life. The important factors were the viability of the fetus and the technical feasibility of maintaining the mother. In case 2, the decision to provide vigorous maternal support was based on the authors' clinical judgment that "after 24 weeks' gestation each extra week in utero increases the chance for fetal survival." The decision to withdraw support in case 1 was premised on the clinicians' belief (very recently challenged[1]) that somatic survival for more than two to four weeks after brain death was unlikely, regardless of the vigor of supportive efforts, and that the fetus might be defective because of a possible herpes virus infection and known exposure to adenine arabinoside. The authors also seem to have had cost in mind as a secondary concern. They advocate immediate cesarean section of fetuses aged 28 weeks or older because efforts to sustain the brain-dead mother would be "expensive, frustrating, and futile"; but they had earlier stressed the benefit to the fetus of continued gestation in the womb.

The chief interest of these cases, however, lies in their bearing on the concept of brain death and its relation to clinical ethics.

A close reading of the article reveals a number of apparent inconsistencies in expression. The authors endorse the brain-death definition of death but repeatedly speak of the brain-dead mother as alive. For example, they state that their goal was "to prolong maternal life in the face of brain death"; but one cannot prolong life in a dead body. The linguistic inconsistencies are, we believe, more than mere infelicities in usage. They reveal a deep—and in our view, justified—ambivalence about conventional wisdom on the definition of death, particularly the brain-death standard. These doubts are restimulated by the present case reports.

It has been known for some time that brain-dead patients, suitably maintained, can breathe, circulate blood, digest food, filter wastes, maintain body temperature, generate new tissue, and fulfill other functions as well. All of this is remarkable in a "corpse." Granted, these functions could not be maintained without artificial aid and, even so, will cease within a few weeks. However, many living patients depend on machines and will not live long; they are not thereby classified as (already) dead.

Now we are told that a brain-dead patient can nurture a child in the womb, which permits live birth several weeks "postmortem." Perhaps this is the straw that breaks the conceptual camel's back. It becomes irresistible to speak of brain-dead patients being "somatically alive" (what sort of "nonsomatic death" is the implied alternative?), of being "terminally ill," and eventually of "dying." These are different ways of saying that such patients (or, at least, their bodies[2]) are alive. The death of the brain seems not to serve as a boundary; it is a tragic, ultimately fatal loss, but not death itself. Bodily death occurs later, when integrated functioning ceases.

We should clarify and delimit our claim. Clinicians who find it congenial to speak of brain-dead patients as "terminally ill" (and the like) do not, on our interpretation, really view the bodies of these patients as dead. We endorse the view implicit

Address editorial communications to the Editor, 535 N Dearborn St, Chicago, IL 60610.

in their use of these terms: the kind of functioning reported in these cases is that of bodies that are biologically alive. It must be emphasized, however, that these judgments apply to "alive" and "dead" as categories of biomedical science. Law and morality raise separate questions. In particular, we may hold, in all consistency, the *moral* view that brain-dead bodies ought not be maintained (except in unusual circumstances, such as those in these case reports). We may also endorse a brain-death law as a solution to a *legal* problem of liability and uncertainty.[3] However, confusion and double-talk will persist unless these moral and legal issues are clearly distinguished from those of medical classification.

We should, then, look beyond the clinician-authors' inconsistent use of the labels "alive" and "dead." Their concern is not whether these patients technically belong to one category or the other; it is, quite properly, with the pressing clinical, ethical, and legal issues: How should these patients be treated? Who should decide? What matters is that a responsible decision was made, and a start was made toward developing a sound clinical policy on cases of this type. However, it is instructive that the conceptual confusion which still clouds the definition of death has so little bearing on the clinical-ethical issues facing conscientious physicians.

MARK SIEGLER, MD
Section of General Internal Medicine
Department of Medicine
University of Chicago
DANIEL WIKLER, PhD
University of Wisconsin
Program in Medical Ethics
Madison

1. Paris J, Kim RC, Collins GH, et al: Brain death with prolonged somatic survival. *N Engl J Med* 1982;1:14-16.

2. Green M, Wikler D: Brain death and personal identity. *Phil Pub Affairs* 1980;9:105-133.

3. *Defining Death*. President's Commission on the Study of Ethical Issues in Medicine and Biomedical Research and Behavioral Research, 1981.

**10.4   Siegler M, Weisbard AJ (1985)
Against the Emerging Stream: Should
Fluids and Nutritional Support
Be Discontinued? Arch Int Med
145:129–31**

Reprinted with permission from the Archives of Internal
Medicine, January 1985, Volume 145, Copyright 1985,
American Medical Association.

Against the Emerging Stream

Should Fluids and Nutritional Support Be Discontinued?

Mark Siegler, MD, Alan J. Weisbard, JD

The powerful rhetoric of "death with dignity" has gained intellectual currency and practical importance in recent years. Initially, this rhetoric was a plea for more humane and individualized treatment in the face of the sometimes cold and impersonal technologic imperatives of modern medicine. As such, it brought needed attention to the plight of dying patients and prompted legal and clinical changes that empowered such patients (and, at times, their representatives) to assert some control over the manner, if not the fact, of their dying. The death with dignity movement has advanced to a new frontier: the termination or withdrawal of fluids and nutritional support.

See also p 122 and p 125.

As recently as five years ago, or perhaps three, the idea that fluids and nutriment might be withdrawn, with moral and perhaps legal impunity, from dying patients, was a notion that would have been repudiated, if not condemned, by most health professionals. They would have regarded such an idea as morally and psychologically objectionable, legally problematic, and medically wrong. The notion would have gone "against the stream" of medical standards of care. Yet, as illustrated by the publication of the accompanying two articles[1,2] in this issue of the ARCHIVES, and by other recent contributions to the medical and bioethical literature, this practice is receiving increased support from both physicians and bioethicists. This new stream of emerging opinion is typically couched in the language of caution and compassion. But the underlying analysis, once laid bare, suggests what is truly at stake: That for an increasing number of patients, the benefits of continued life are perceived as insufficient to justify the burden and cost of care; that death is the desired outcome, and—critically—that the role of the physician is to participate in bringing this about.

This is an unexpected development and one that runs counter to the traditions of medical care. We feel compelled to speak out to prevent the all-too-rapid acceptance of this new emerging standard medical practice, that of withdraw-

ing fluids or nutritional supports from some classes of patients. This development may threaten patients, physicians, the patient-physician relationship, and other vital societal values. While we recognize that particular health care professionals, for reasons of compassion and conscience and with full knowledge of the personal legal risks involved, may on occasion elect to discontinue fluids and nutritional support, we, nevertheless, believe that such actions should generally be proscribed, pending much fuller debate and discussion than has yet taken place.

CURRENT THINKING

In this ARCHIVES, the articles by Meyers[1] and by Dresser and Boisaubin[2] review current legal and clinical thinking on the issue of withdrawing fluids and nutritional support from terminally ill or permanently unconscious patients. The conclusion by Meyers is one that finds support in a number of recent court decisions and in the majority of recent scholarly comments on this subject in the medical and medical ethics literature.[1-7]

Certainly, we are talking about relatively few cases. Nourishment should be provided in the vast majority of cases as long as physically possible. If the patient can be fed manually, he or she of course should be. However, in those rare cases where nourishment can only be provided through invasive means and cannot improve the patient's hopeless prognosis, it seems the law should not mandate continued medically provided nourishment.[1(p125)]

Dresser and Boisaubin[2] expressly limit their argument to cases of permanently unconscious patients, suggesting their approval of the New Jersey appellate court's decision in the *Conroy* case, which refused to endorse withdrawal of fluids and nutrition from a severely demented but conscious patient. Meyers goes further, arguing that fluids and nutrition may be withdrawn from the terminally ill and the nonterminally, yet seriously ill, like Mrs Conroy, as well as from the permanently unconscious. Others go further still. A group of distinguished clinicians recently published an article advocating the withholding of parenteral fluids and nutritional support from severely and irreversibly demented patients and perhaps, at times, from elderly patients with permanent mild impairment of competence (a group they refer to as the "pleasantly senile").[7]

A NEW ETHICS ISSUE

Several explanations may account for the emergence of this new clinical-ethical issue now. Several well-publicized

Accepted for publication Sept 24, 1984.

From the Section of General Internal Medicine and the Center for Clinical Medical Ethics, University of Chicago-Pritzker School of Medicine, Chicago (Dr Siegler); and the Benjamin N. Cardozo School of Law, Yeshiva University, New York (Dr Weisbard).

Reprint requests to PO Box 72, University of Chicago Hospitals, 950 E 59th St, Chicago, IL 60637 (Dr Siegler).

legal cases, including those reviewed by Meyers, helped. Additionally, however, the recent technologic revolution in methods of hydration and nutritional maintenance have changed the question. The question no longer is whether a dying patient is to be provided with a cool sip of water or even an intravenous line to maintain electrolyte balance, but whether enteral alimentation or parenteral hyperalimentation should be used at all.

Further, as nutritional support became more technical, there was a tendency to examine its use in the light of other invasive technologies, eg, respirators or dialysis machines. We had gradually learned that to provide appropriate care to dying patients and to maintain their dignity, respirators and dialysis machines were not mandated in all cases of respiratory or renal failure. Strategies for discontinuing or withholding these other high-technology life-support systems now were applied to the new high-technology methods of alimentation and hydration.

Finally, there is the matter of cost. As Callahan has noted: "Given the increasingly large pool of superannuated, chronically ill, physically marginal elderly, it ('denial of nutrition') could well become the non-treatment of choice."[8] However distasteful it might seem, the current intellectual climate dominated by notions of cost containment and death with dignity may encourage the union of these two independent themes as a way to meet several apparently desirable societal goals simultaneously.

CRITIQUE

In our remarks, we do not intend to consider either permanently unconscious patients (whose medical and legal status raise deep philosophic issues) or competent adult patients who are dying and who may direct their physicians to desist from a variety of life-prolonging interventions. Our principal focus will be on the withdrawal of fluids and nutrition from patients possessing the capacity for consciousness who have not competently rejected such support. While our concerns may seem premature in light of the qualifications and thoughtful discussions of both substantive and procedural safeguards expressed in several recent contributions to the literature, we remain troubled that the underlying analysis, once accepted by clinicians and the courts, will not long be confined within the limits initially set forth.

The emerging argument rests on the dual propositions that the provision of hydration and nutritional support is a medical intervention guided by considerations similar to those governing other treatment methods and that judgments concerning the withdrawal of such interventions should be based on a calculus of benefits and burdens associated with the intervention. This calculus is sometimes also referred to as "proportionality." These propositions, rooted in the work of the President's Commission for the Study of Ethical Problems in Medicine, were adopted by the California appellate court in the *Barber* case, and play a prominent role in the analyses of Meyers,[1] Dresser and Boisaubin,[2] and other recent contributors to the literature.

We do not dispute that the benefits-and-burdens formulation is useful in a number of contexts and marks a clear analytic improvement over earlier references to "extraordinary measures" or "artificial means," terms that have introduced much confusion into these discussions. What we find troublesome is the assertion that physicians, families, courts, or other third parties can properly conclude that the "burdens" of withdrawal of fluids and nutrition—an unconvincing catalog of potential complications or side effects—outweigh the benefits, ie, sustaining life. We recognize that in rare cases, the provision of fluids and, particularly,

nutritional support may be medically futile or even counterproductive in sustaining life. We do not recommend that such futile or counterproductive steps be mandated.

AGAINST THE STREAM

We now offer several additional arguments in an effort to stem the tide, to reverse the stream of opinion on the matter of discontinuing fluids.

Patients will be protected against diagnostic errors (the recognition that death is inevitable or that a case is "hopeless" often dawns slowly), inadequate treatment, and unscrupulous care for financial or other reasons. Although firm scientific evidence is lacking, even irreversibly dying patients may be more comfortable if they receive adequate hydration.

Physicians will not be forced to make ad hoc, value-laden, quality-of-life decisions. Nor will they be forced to act in violation of their conscience regarding standards of care. On this last point, a recent study published in the ARCHIVES[3] revealed that 73% of physicians would attempt to provide adequate hydration and electrolyte support even for a comatose patient dying of an untreatable painful malignant neoplasm. Many physicians believe discontinuation of hydration would sever the therapeutic relationship irrevocably, while maintaining hydration would reinforce the traditional goals of the physician-patient relationship: To cure sometimes, to relieve occasionally, to comfort always. Physicians also would be spared the direct causal responsibility for the death of the patient and the inevitable psychological associations of this practice with active euthanasia. Finally, physicians would not expose themselves to civil or criminal liability in an unsettled area of law.

The *medical profession* will benefit by avoiding any appearance that they are balancing quality of life or cost concerns against compassionate standards of medical care. The dedication of the profession to the welfare of patients might be severely undermined in the eyes of the public even by the apparent complicity of physicians in the deaths of the very ill, the permanently unconscious, or the pleasantly senile. The primary commitment of physicians to patients might be compromised and the image of physicians tarnished at precisely the time when physicians must reestablish the primacy of quality of care and not become overwhelmed by cost-containment efforts that run counter to good clinical medicine.

A chilling illustration of the confluence of these tendencies is the recent suggestion that all new applicants for Medicare be provided copies of "living wills" or similar documents. Our concern here is not with the encouragement of patient self-determination respecting medical care, a trend we support, but rather with the incorporation of such strategies *as a method of cost control*. As stated recently by the American Medical Association's Board of Trustees: "Living wills should be used for alleviating suffering and not linked to cost-containment objectives."

Finally, *society's* larger interest would be preserved by rejecting the movement toward discontinuation of fluid in dying patients. We have deep concerns about accepting the practice of withholding fluids from patients, because it may bear the seeds of unacceptable social consequences. We have witnessed too much history to disregard how easily a society may disvalue the lives of the "unproductive." The "angel of mercy" can become the fanatic, bringing the "comfort" of death to some who do not clearly want it, then to others who "would really be better off dead," and finally, to classes of "undesirable persons," which might include the terminally ill, the permanently unconscious, the severely senile, the pleasantly senile, the retarded, the incurably or chronically ill, and perhaps, the aged. This jeremiad may seem unnecessary, but recall the recent article by distinguished and well-motivated clinicians that began by considering the physician's responsibility to the hopelessly ill, and concluded by advising on the care of the pleasantly senile.

Our concerns are reinforced by the coming together of the emerging stream of medical and ethical opinion with the torrent of public and governmental concern with the cost of medical care. Cost-containment strategies may impose significant financial penalties on those who provide prolonged care for the impaired elderly. In the current environment, it may well prove convenient—and all too easy—to move from recognition of an individual's "right to die" (to us, an unfortunate phrasing in the first instance) to a climate enforcing a "duty to die."

Finally, we would urge that efforts in this field be rechanneled from demonstrating that some patients' quality of life is too poor, too "meaningless," to justify the burdens of continued life, toward the challenge of finding better ways to improve the comfort and quality of life for such patients. In particular, we hope the current debate will stimulate further discussion of the comparative merits of different techniques to provide fluids and nutrition. Endoscopic placement of gastrostomy tubes may prove to be more comfortable and safer for patients than nasogastric tubes, which additionally are more likely to require restraints to prevent their deliberate or accidental removal. More attention must be paid to clinical, institutional, economic, and legal implications of these alternatives.

Compassionate calls for withdrawing fluids in a few selected cases bear the seeds of great potential abuse. Little is to be lost and much may be gained by slowing down the process, by taking stock of where we have come and where we are going, by improving our methods of comforting and caring for the dying without necessarily hurrying to dispatch them on their way, and by deferring any premature legal, ethical, or professional approval and legitimation of this new course. Continuing fluids, even to dying patients, provides an important clinical, psychological, and social barrier that should be retained.

The movement for death with dignity arose in response to concerns of the public that medicine was paying inadequate attention to caring for patients, particularly dying patients. It would be sadly ironic if this latest manifestation served to undercut the image of physician as caring and nurturing servant and to undermine deep human values of caring and nurturance more broadly throughout the society. The issue is complicated, the tradition of medicine long, and therefore, a slow and conservative approach would seem advisable.

References

1. Meyers DW: Legal aspects of withdrawing nourishment from an incurably ill patient. *Arch Intern Med* 1985;145:125-128.

2. Dresser RS, Boisaubin EV Jr: Ethics, law, and nutritional support. *Arch Intern Med* 1985;145:122-124.

3. Micetich KC, Steinnecker PH, Thomasma DC: Are intravenous fluids morally required for a dying patient? *Arch Intern Med* 1983;143:975-978.

4. Lynn J, Childress JF: Must patients always be given food and water? *Hasting Cent Rep* 1983;13:17-21.

5. Annas GJ: Non-feeding: Lawful killing in California, homicide in New Jersey. *Hastings Cent Rep* 1983;13:19-20.

6. Lo B: The death of Clarence Herbert: Withdrawing care is not murder. *Ann Intern Med* 1984;101:248-251.

7. Wanzer SH, Adelstein SJ, Cranford RE, et al: The physician's responsibility toward hopelessly ill patients. *N Engl J Med* 1984;310:955-959.

8. Callahan D: On feeding the dying. *Hastings Cent Rep* 1983;13:22.

10.5 Singer PA, Siegler M (1990) Euthanasia: A Critique. N Engl J Med 322:1881–3

Vol. 322   No. 26

SOUNDING BOARD

1881

SOUNDING BOARD

EUTHANASIA — A CRITIQUE

A VIGOROUS medical and political debate has begun again on euthanasia, a practice proscribed 2500 years ago in the Hippocratic oath.[1-4] The issue has been publicized recently in three widely divergent settings: a journal article, a legislative initiative in California, and public policy in the Netherlands.

The case of "Debbie" shows that euthanasia can be discussed openly in a respected medical journal. "It's Over, Debbie" was an anonymous, first-person account of euthanasia, published on January 8, 1988, in the *Journal of the American Medical Association*,[5-8] that stimulated widespread discussion and elicited spirited replies. Later in 1988, perhaps as a result, the Council on Ethical and Judicial Affairs of the American Medical Association reaffirmed its opposition to euthanasia.[9]

In California, a legislative initiative[10,11] has shown that in the near future euthanasia may be legalized in certain U.S. jurisdictions. A bill proposing a California Humane and Dignified Death Act was an attempt to legalize euthanasia through the referendum process, which allows California voters to approve controversial issues directly. Public-opinion polls reported that up to 70 percent of the electorate favored the initiative, and many commentators flatly predicted that the initiative would succeed. Nevertheless, the signature drive failed, collecting only 130,000 of the 450,000 required signatures. Attributing the failure to organizational problems, the proponents vowed to introduce the legislation again in California and in other states in 1990.

Experience in the Netherlands has shown that a liberal democratic government can tolerate and defend the practice of euthanasia. Although euthanasia is technically illegal in the Netherlands, in fact it is part of Dutch public policy today.[1,12-16] There is agreement at all levels of the judicial system, including the

Supreme Court, that if physicians follow the procedural guidelines issued by a state commission, they will not be prosecuted for performing euthanasia.[16] The Dutch guidelines emphasize five requirements: an explicit, repeated request by the patient that leaves no doubt about the patient's desire to die; very severe mental or physical suffering, with no prospect of relief; an informed, free, and consistent decision by the patient; the lack of other treatment options, those available having been exhausted or refused by the patient; and consultation by the doctor with another medical practitioner (and perhaps also with nurses, pastors, or others).[13] The usual method of performing euthanasia is to induce sleep with a barbiturate, followed by a lethal injection of curare.[1] An estimated 5000 to 10,000 patients receive euthanasia each year in the Netherlands.[16]

In view of these developments, we urge physicians to consider some reasons for resisting the move toward euthanasia. This article criticizes the main arguments offered by proponents and presents opposing arguments. The case for euthanasia is described in detail elsewhere.[10,17]

CRITIQUE OF THE CASE FOR EUTHANASIA

In the debate about euthanasia, imprecision of language abounds. For the purposes of this article, euthanasia is defined as the deliberate action by a physician to terminate the life of a patient. The clearest example is the act of lethal injection. We distinguish euthanasia from such other acts as the decision to forgo life-sustaining treatment (including the use of ventilators, cardiopulmonary resuscitation, dialysis, or tube feeding — the issue raised in the Cruzan case[18]); the administration of analgesic agents to relieve pain; "assisted suicide," in which the doctor prescribes but does not administer a lethal dose of medication; and "mercy killing" performed by a patient's family or friends. The Dutch guidelines described above and the terms proposed in the California initiative represent two versions of euthanasia.

The case for euthanasia is based on two central claims.[10,17] First, proponents argue that patients whose illnesses cause them unbearable suffering should be permitted to end their distress by having a physician perform euthanasia. Second, proponents assert that the well-recognized right of patients to control their medical treatment includes the right to request and receive euthanasia.

Relief of Suffering

We agree that the relief of pain and suffering is a crucial goal of medicine.[19] We question, however, whether the care of dying patients cannot be improved without resorting to the drastic measure of euthanasia. Most physical pain can be relieved with the appropriate use of analgesic agents.[20] Unfortunately, despite widespread agreement that dying patients must

1882   THE NEW ENGLAND JOURNAL OF MEDICINE   June 28, 1990

be provided with necessary analgesia,[21] physicians continue to underuse analgesia in the care of dying patients because of concern about depressing respiratory drive or creating addiction. Such situations demand better management of pain, not euthanasia.

Another component of suffering is the frightening prospect of dying shackled to a modern-day Procrustean bed, surrounded by the latest forms of high technology. Proponents of euthanasia often cite horror stories of patients treated against their will. In the past, when modern forms of life-saving technology were new and physicians were just learning how to use them appropriately, such cases occurred often; we have begun to move beyond that era. The law, public policy, and medical ethics now acknowledge the right of patients to refuse life-sustaining medical treatment, and a large number of patients avail themselves of this new policy.[22-24] These days, competent patients may freely exercise their right to choose or refuse life-sustaining treatment; to carry out their preferences, they do not require the option of euthanasia.

We acknowledge that some elements of human suffering and mental anguish — not necessarily related to physical pain — cannot be eliminated completely from the dying process. These include the anticipated loss of important human relationships and membership in the human community, the loss of personal independence, the feeling of helplessness, and the raw fear of death. Euthanasia can shorten the duration of these emotional and psychological hardships. It can also eliminate fears about how and when death will occur. Finally, euthanasia returns to the patient a measure of control over the process of dying. These are the benefits of euthanasia, against which its potential harms must be balanced.

Individual Rights

The second argument in favor of euthanasia is based on the rights of the individual. Proponents contend that the right of patients to forgo life-sustaining medical treatment should include a right to euthanasia. This would extend the notion of the right to die to embrace the concept that patients have a right to be killed by physicians. But rights are not absolute. They must be balanced against the rights of other people and the values of society. The claim of a right to be killed by a physician must be balanced against the legal, political, and religious prohibitions against killing that have always existed in society generally and in medicine particularly. As the President's Commission for the Study of Ethical Problems in Medicine and Biomedical and Behavioral Research has observed, "Policies prohibiting direct killing may also conflict with the important value of patient self-determination. . . . The Commission finds this limitation on individual self-determination to be an acceptable cost of securing the general protection of human life afforded by the prohibition of direct killing."[22] We agree. In our view, the public good served by the pro-

hibition of euthanasia outweighs the private interests of the persons requesting it.

THE CASE AGAINST EUTHANASIA

The arguments against euthanasia are made from two perspectives: public policy and the ethical norms of medicine.

Euthanasia Is Perilous Public Policy

Proponents of euthanasia use the concept of individual rights to support their claim, but this same concept can be used for the opposite purpose. The argument against euthanasia on grounds of civil rights involves a consideration of the rights not just of those who would want euthanasia themselves but of all citizens. As public policy, euthanasia is unacceptable because of the likelihood, or even the inevitability, of involuntary euthanasia — persons being euthanized without their consent or against their wishes.

There are four ways in which a policy of voluntary euthanasia could lead to involuntary euthanasia. The first is "crypthanasia" (literally, "secret euthanasia").[15] In the Netherlands, for instance, it is alleged that vulnerable patients are euthanized without their consent. Dutch proponents of euthanasia disavow these reports and claim that they are unrelated to the toleration of voluntary euthanasia. We suggest, however, that a political milieu in which voluntary euthanasia is tolerated may also foster involuntary euthanasia and lead to the killing of patients without consent. The second way in which involuntary euthanasia may occur is through "encouraged" euthanasia, whereby chronically ill or dying patients may be pressured to choose euthanasia to spare their families financial or emotional strain.[25] The third way is "surrogate" euthanasia. If voluntary euthanasia were permissible in the United States, the constitutional guarantees of due process, which tend to extend the same rights to incompetent as to competent patients, might permit euthanizing incompetent patients on the basis of "substituted judgment" or nebulous tests of "burdens and benefits." Finally, there is the risk of "discriminatory" euthanasia. Patients belonging to vulnerable groups in American society might be subtly coerced into "requesting" euthanasia. In the United States today, many groups are disempowered, disenfranchised, or otherwise vulnerable: the poor, the elderly, the disabled, members of racial minorities, the physically handicapped, the mentally impaired, alcoholics, drug addicts, and patients with the acquired immunodeficiency syndrome. In a society in which discrimination is common and many citizens do not have access even to basic health care, the legalization of euthanasia would create another powerful tool with which to discriminate against groups whose "consent" is already susceptible to coercion and whose rights are already in jeopardy.

The proponents of euthanasia contend that procedural safeguards, such as the five provisions of the

Vol. 322   No. 26

SOUNDING BOARD

1883

Dutch guidelines noted above, will prevent involuntary euthanasia. They claim further that society permits many dangerous activities if adequate procedural safeguards are provided to reduce risk and protect the public. We agree that safeguards would reduce the risk of involuntary euthanasia, but they would not eliminate it entirely. In the case of euthanasia, safeguards have not been adequately tested and shown to be effective. Even in their presence, we are concerned that patients could be euthanized without their consent or even against their wishes. Even one case of involuntary euthanasia would represent a great harm. In the current era of cost containment, social injustice, and ethical relativism, this risk is one our society should not accept.

Euthanasia Violates the Norms of Medicine

In addition to being perilous as public policy, euthanasia violates three fundamental norms and standards of medicine. First, as noted above, it diverts attention from the real issues in the care of dying patients — among them, improved pain control, better communication between doctors and patients, heightened respect for the patient's right to choose whether to accept life-sustaining treatment, and improved management of the dying process, as in hospice care. The hospice movement has demonstrated that managing pain appropriately and allowing patients control over the use of life-sustaining treatments reduce the need for euthanasia.

Second, euthanasia subverts the social role of the physician as healer. Historically, physicians have scrupulously avoided participating in activities that might taint their healing role, such as capital punishment or torture. Physicians should distance themselves from euthanasia to maintain public confidence and trust in medicine as a healing profession.

Third, euthanasia strikes at the heart of what it means to be a physician.[26] Since the time of Hippocrates, the prohibition against it has been fundamental to the medical profession and has served as a moral absolute for both patients and physicians. This prohibition has freed physicians from a potential conflict of interest between healing and killing and in turn has enabled patients to entrust physicians with their lives. It has enabled physicians to devote themselves single-mindedly to helping patients achieve their own medical goals. This prohibition may even have encouraged medical research and scientific progress, because physicians, with the consent of patients, are motivated to perform risky, innovative procedures that are aggressive and sometimes painful, with a total commitment to benefit the patient.

CONCLUSIONS

Pressure to legalize euthanasia will surely increase in an era of spiraling health care costs, but it must be resisted. Euthanasia represents a development that is dangerous for many vulnerable patients and that threatens the moral integrity of the medical profession. Physicians must become more responsive to the concerns of patients that underlie the movement for euthanasia and must provide better pain management, more compassionate terminal care, and more appropriate use of life-sustaining treatments. But physicians need to draw the line at euthanasia. They and their professional associations should defend the integrity of medicine by speaking out against the practice. Finally, even if euthanasia is legalized in some jurisdictions, physicians should refuse to participate in it, and professional organizations should censure any of their members who perform euthanasia.

University of Toronto
Toronto, ON
M5S 1A8, Canada   PETER A. SINGER, M.D., F.R.C.P.C.

University of Chicago
Chicago, IL 60637   MARK SIEGLER, M.D.

REFERENCES

1. Angell M. Euthanasia. N Engl J Med 1988; 319:1348-50.
2. Singer PA. Should doctors kill patients? Can Med Assoc J 1988; 138:1000-1.
3. Kinsella TD, Singer PA, Siegler M. Legalized active euthanasia: an Aesculapian tragedy. Bull Am Coll Surg 1989; 74(12):6-9.
4. Wanzer SH, Federman DD, Adelstein SJ, et al. The physician's responsibility toward hopelessly ill patients: a second look. N Engl J Med 1989; 320:844-9.
5. It's over, Debbie. JAMA 1988; 259:272.
6. Vaux KL. Debbie's dying: mercy killing and the good death. JAMA 1988; 259:2140-1.
7. Gaylin W, Kass LR, Pellegrino ED, Siegler M. 'Doctors must not kill.' JAMA 1988; 259:2139-40.
8. Lundberg GD. 'It's over, Debbie' and the euthanasia debate. JAMA 1988; 259:2142-3.
9. The Council on Ethical and Judicial Affairs of the American Medical Association. Euthanasia. Report: C (A-88). AMA council report. Chicago: American Medical Association, 1988:1.
10. Risley RL. A humane and dignified death: a new law permitting physician aid-in-dying. Glendale, Calif.: Americans Against Human Suffering, 1987.
11. Parachini A. Mercy, murder, & morality: perspectives on euthanasia: the California Humane and Dignified Death Initiative. Hastings Cent Rep 1989; 19(1):Suppl:10-2.
12. Pence GE. Do not go slowly into that dark night: mercy killing in Holland. Am J Med 1988; 84:139-41.
13. Rigter H, Borst-Eilers E, Leenen HJJ. Euthanasia across the North Sea. BMJ 1988; 297:1593-5.
14. Rigter H. Mercy, murder, & morality: euthanasia in the Netherlands: distinguishing facts from fiction. Hastings Cent Rep 1989; 19(1):Suppl:31-2.
15. Fenigsen R. Mercy, murder, & morality: perspectives on euthanasia: a case against Dutch euthanasia. Hastings Cent Rep 1989; 19(1):Suppl:22-30.
16. de Wachter MAM. Active euthanasia in the Netherlands. JAMA 1989; 262:3316-9.
17. Humphry D, Wickett A. The right to die: understanding euthanasia. New York: Harper & Row, 1986.
18. Angell M. Prisoners of technology: the case of Nancy Cruzan. N Engl J Med 1990; 322:1226-8.
19. Cassell EJ. The nature of suffering and the goals of medicine. N Engl J Med 1982; 306:639-45.
20. Foley KM. The treatment of cancer pain. N Engl J Med 1985; 313:84-95.
21. Angell M. The quality of mercy. N Engl J Med 1982; 306:98-9.
22. President's Commission for the Study of Ethical Problems in Medicine and Biomedical and Behavioral Research. Deciding to forego life-sustaining treatment: a report on the ethical, medical, and legal issues in treatment decisions. Washington, D.C.: Government Printing Office, 1983.
23. The Hastings Center. Guidelines on the termination of life-sustaining treatment and the care of the dying: a report. Briarcliff Manor, N.Y.: Hastings Center, 1987.
24. Emanuel EJ. A review of the ethical and legal aspects of terminating medical care. Am J Med 1988; 84:291-301.
25. Kamisar Y. Some non-religious views against proposed "mercy-killing" legislation. Minn Law Rev 1958; 42:969-1042.
26. Kass LR. Neither for love nor money: why doctors must not kill. Public Interest 1989; 94(winter):25-46.

10.6   Singer PA, Siegler M (1991) Elective Use of Life-Sustaining Treatments in Internal Medicine. Adv Inter Med 36:57–79

This article was published in Advances in Internal Medicine, Singer PA, Siegler M. Elective use of life-sustaining treatments in internal medicine, Pages 57–79, Copyright Elsevier 1991. Reprinted with permission from Elsevier.

Elective Use of Life-Sustaining Treatments in Internal Medicine

Peter A. Singer, M.D., M.P.H., F.R.C.P.C.

Assistant Professor of Medicine, Associate Director, Centre for Bioethics,
University of Toronto, Toronto, Ontario, Canada

Mark Siegler, M.D.

Professor of Medicine, Director, Center for Clinical Medical Ethics, University of
Chicago Hospitals, Chicago, Illinois

Editor's Introduction

Medical ethics has now become a major subject for study and research, as life-sustaining technology affords physicians unprecedented power to prolong patients' survival from what, but a few decades ago, would have been "natural death." It is now timely to review a burgeoning medical literature, much of which has been devoted to hammering out the ethical principles surrounding patient/family/physician/ and ah, yes, government decision-making. Systematic study of the attitudes of patients and physicians toward such decision-making has begun only recently. Even more recently, the professional process and skills for such decision-making have been evolving. They must now be part of the clinical competence physicians need to promote patient autonomy. We have yet to implement these skills adequately, no less to research the outcomes of the effectiveness of the process required to activate what some call "advance directives," others call "advance preferences," and what Drs. Singer and Siegler call "elective use" of life-sustaining treatments. The elegant review of the relevant clinical literature and the current state-of-the-art recommendations for an effective clinical approach to the elective use of life-sustaining treatment presented by these authorities should be a useful guide for the complex task ahead of all of us who serve as the stewards of the life and death of our patients.

Gene H. Stollerman, M.D.

The current focus on the elective use of life-sustaining medical treatments began 15 years ago with the case of Karen Quinlan, a permanently comatose young woman. In that case, Ms. Quinlan's guardian was permitted by the New Jersey Supreme Court to authorize withdrawal of mechanical ventilation even though the court acknowledged the probability that such action would result in Ms. Quinlan's death.[1] The roots of the Quinlan case go back hundreds of years to the philosophers of the Enlightenment and the framers of the U.S. Constitution, but the case's legacy extends to current medical practice. To contemporary patients and doctors, the Quinlan case symbolizes the right of patients or their surrogates to choose to forego life-sustaining medical treatments.

The purpose of this chapter is to review current thinking about the "elective use of life-sustaining treatments." We prefer "elective use" to alternative terms, such as "euthanasia" or "decisions to forego life-sustaining treatment," because it emphasizes that not everything that *can* be done for patients *must* be done. Most treatments are not mandatory but rather elective, and the excellent practice of medicine is achieved by reaching the best possible decision in individual clinical cases. Elective use applies both to treatments that have not been started (that is, that might be withheld) and to those that have already been started but are being reconsidered in light of changed clinical circumstances (that is, that might be withdrawn). The key elements of elective use are the clinical circumstances of the individual case and the treatment preferences of the patient involved.

Clinicians are not always impressed with the pronouncements of medical ethicists. Doctors sometimes see ethicists as uninvolved parties who interfere with the private patient-doctor relationship. The perspective we take in this chapter, however, is not that of uninvolved parties. We are internists who have struggled with difficult decisions about elective use of life-sustaining treatments with patients and their families. And as clinicians, we believe that medical ethics has a central role to play in assisting physicians to care for patients at the end of life. In this chapter, our goal is to provide a clinically relevant perspective on the elective use of life-sustaining treatment.[2]

We begin by reviewing published empirical research about elective use of life-sustaining treatment. The studies are arranged according to a proposed taxonomy of life-sustaining treatments given in Table 1. Then, we describe five questions that the clinician at the bedside should ask when the issue of elective use of life-sustaining treatments arises. These questions, listed in Table 2, form the organizing framework for the remainder of the chapter.

Epidemiology of Elective Use

The proposed taxonomy in Table 1 provides a framework with which to examine the epidemiology of elective use of life-sustaining treatments. In this section, we review studies about cardiopulmonary resuscitation (CPR; do-not-resuscitate [DNR] orders), mechanical ventilation, dialysis, antibiotic therapy, and artificial nutrition. For each treatment, we examine the following questions: (1) What is the incidence of decisions to forego life-sustaining treatment? (2) What clinical and social factors are associated with these decisions? (3) What is the decision-making process involved?

TABLE 1.
Elective Life-Sustaining Treatments

Cardiopulmonary resuscitation
Mechanical ventilation
Intensive care
Surgery
Dialysis
Cancer chemotherapy
Blood transfusion
Antibiotic therapy
Artificial nutrition/hydration

(4) What are the outcomes of decisions to forego life-sustaining treatment?
(5) What are the associated costs?

DNR Orders

The best-studied decision to forego life-sustaining treatment is the DNR order. The incidence of DNR orders is 3% to 4% of all hospital admissions[3-7] and 5% to 14% of patients admitted to the intensive care unit (ICU).[8,9] Conversely, 66% to 75% of hospital deaths[5,6,10-12] and 39% of deaths in the ICU[9] are preceded by a DNR order. Factors associated with the writing of DNR orders include older age,[8,9,11,13-15] increased severity of illness,[8,9] poor preadmission functional status,[3,7-9] urinary incontinence,[3,5] abnormal mental status or a diagnosis of dementia,[3,5,10,11,14-16] residence in a nursing home,[5,10,14,15] a diagnosis of cancer* or acquired immunodeficiency syndrome (AIDS),[18] the physician's

TABLE 2.
Clinical Approach to Elective Use of Life-Sustaining Treatment

Is the patient brain dead?
What specific clinical decision is being considered?
Is the patient competent?
Are the incompetent patient's wishes known?
Are there any external factors affecting the decision?

*References 3, 5, 11, 12, 14, 15, 17, and 18.

estimates of patient quality of life,[19] and prognosis (including survival and functional status).[13] Recent surveys of elderly outpatients show that 77% to 82% would want CPR in their current health state, but only 21% to 38% would want CPR if they had severe dementia, stroke, irreversible coma, or terminal cancer.[20-22] With respect to the process of DNR decision making, studies indicate that the patient may only be involved in a minority of cases, with estimates ranging from 14% to 43%.[3-5, 7, 9, 11, 12, 23, 24] Families were consulted more frequently, in 45% to 86% of cases. Incompetency at the time of the DNR decision is a major reason for patient nonparticipation in the decision making. It appears that at the time patients are admitted to the hospital they are often capable of making decisions, but they become incompetent in the hospital before a DNR order is discussed. Interestingly, 27% to 51% of patients not in the ICU with DNR orders survive to be discharged from the hospital.[3-7, 25] Patients for whom a DNR order is written appear to consume a disproportionately large amount of resources, but resource consumption and hospital charges are reduced significantly after DNR orders are written.[6-10]

Mechanical Ventilation

There are no published data on the incidence of decisions to forego mechanical ventilation in general internal medicine practice. (A recent study of intensive care units found that "life support" was withheld from 1% and withdrawn from 5% of patients; mechanical ventilation accounted for 23% of withheld and 83% of withdrawn life-support therapies.[25a] Factors associated with the decision to withhold mechanical ventilation, for example, from a patient with chronic obstructive pulmonary disease, include the physician's estimate of the patient's quality of life, prognosis for survival, and the physician's level of training (residents were more likely to forego mechanical ventilation than private practitioners).[26, 27] One survey showed that 55% of homosexual men with AIDS would want mechanical ventilation (and transfer to ICU) if required for the treatment of *Pneumocystis* pneumonia; this number dropped to 19% if the patient had both *Pneumocystis* pneumonia and "severe memory loss."[28] Another survey of hospitalized patients with various diagnoses showed that 90% wanted "life support" (defined as transfer to ICU, and mechanical ventilation or dialysis) in their current state of health, 30% would want life support if they would be nonindependent on discharge, 16% wanted it despite a hopeless prognosis, and 6% wanted life support even if they would remain comatose.[29] There are no published data on the process, outcomes, or costs of decisions to forego mechanical ventilation.

Dialysis

Although there are no data on decisions to withhold dialysis, a large retrospective cohort study showed that dialysis was discontinued in 9% of patients being treated for end-stage renal disease.[30, 31] Stopping dialysis accounted for 22% of deaths in the cohort, and it was the second most common cause of death after cardiovascular causes. Factors associated with stopping dialysis included older age, diabetes, comorbid degenerative disorders, and residence in a nursing home. With respect to the process of decisions to stop dialysis, half the patients were competent and half were incompetent. In the competent patients, 88% made the decision to stop dialysis themselves. In the case of incompetent patients, the physician brought up the subject of stopping dialysis in 73% of cases and the family raised this issue in 27%. The availability of information about incompetent patients' prior stated wishes was not clear. Presumably, all patients who stop dialysis die. The effect of decisions to stop dialysis on cost has not been studied.

Antibiotic Therapy

There are no published studies concerning decisions to withdraw antibiotic therapy. One study published in 1979 examined the decision to withhold antibiotics.[32] This retrospective cohort study of patients in extended-care facilities showed that active treatment (antibiotics and/or hospitalization) was withheld in 43% of patients who developed fever. Factors associated with the decision to withhold antibiotics included a diagnosis of cancer, abnormal mental status, poor mobility, presence of pain or prescription of narcotics, small size of facility, familiarity of the physician with the patient, and statements in the medical record documenting deterioration in the patient's condition or plans for nontreatment of the patient. The mortality for patients from whom antibiotics were withheld was 59%, compared with a mortality of 9% among patients who received active treatment. In another study, 53% of outpatients said that, if demented, they would not want antibiotics and hospitalization for pneumonia.[33] There are no published studies examining the process of decisions to forego antibiotic therapy or the effect of such decisions on costs.

Nutrition and Hydration

There are no empirical studies that document the incidence of decisions to forego artificial nutrition/hydration. Factors associated with the decision to withhold artificial feeding, studied using clinical vignettes,[34] include patient preference, functional status, patient discomfort, life expectancy, family wishes, and age. In another study, 41% of physicians believed that informed consent should be obtained for nasogastric feeding.[35] A retrospective chart review, however, showed that patient consent was documented in only 12%, and surrogate consent in an additional 14%, of cases of tube feeding.[35] In this cohort, 69% of patients were incompetent and 53% required restraints to keep the feeding tube in place. Of patients who received tube feeding, 64% died in hospital, 25% were discharged to a nursing home, and 11% were discharged home. In another survey, 75%

of outpatients said they would not want tube feeding if they were demented.[33] There are no published data concerning the costs of decisions to forego artificial nutrition/hydration.

Clinical Approach to Elective Use

In the previous section, we showed that decisions to withhold or withdraw life-sustaining treatments are not uncommon in the clinical practice of medicine. In this section, we develop a clinical approach to the elective use of life-sustaining treatments. In approaching such cases, the clinician should ask the five questions listed in Table 2, which also serve as the organizing framework for the remainder of this chapter.

Is the Patient Brain Dead?

If the patient is brain dead, treatment may be discontinued. Further questions about the specific treatment decision, competency, patient wishes, and external factors do not generally apply. The family should be informed that the patient has died, and that mechanical ventilation and other forms of life support will be discontinued. There is no need to ask the family's permission to do so. Except for three specific circumstances, there is no longer any reason to continue life-sustaining treatment. These three circumstances, each of which requires continuing life support for only a relatively short time, include organ procurement, supporting the patient until family arrives, and maintaining a brain-dead pregnant woman in an attempt to deliver a viable baby. In none of these circumstances is continued life support mandatory. In all brain-death cases, however, the physician must remain sensitive to the emotions of the family and should counsel and support them.

The management of brain-dead patients may seem self-evident. Nevertheless, considerable confusion remains about the brain-death concept.[36] In our ethics consultation experience, we frequently encounter cases where doctors *ask* the families of brain-dead patients for consent to discontinue treatment, as though they were seeking consent for a DNR order. These experiences prompt us to include a brief discussion of brain death in this chapter on elective use of life-sustaining treatments.

A generation ago, before the development of modern medical technology, the definition of death was a simple matter. If there was no circulation or respiration, a person was declared dead. Today, however, physicians can support physiologic functions in persons who would have died in the absence of medical technology by employing, for example, intensive care, inotropic agents, and mechanical ventilation. Thus, for a variety of medical, social, and political reasons (including but not restricted to the need for transplantable organs), it was important to develop new criteria for declaring persons dead.

In 1968, the Harvard Ad Hoc Committee first recommended the brain-death standard.[37] In 1980, the Commission on Uniform State Laws proposed a model brain-death legislation, the Uniform Determination of Death Act. (This act states: "An individual who has sustained either (1) irreversible cessation of circulatory and respiratory functions, or (2) irreversible cessation of all functions of the entire brain, including the brain stem, is dead."[38]) In 1981, the President's Commission for the Study of Ethical Problems in Medicine and Biomedical and Behavioral Research recommended that all states adopt the Uniform Determination of Death Act.[38] By 1987, 39 states and the District of Columbia had adopted brain-death legislation and an additional 6 states had upheld the brain-death standard in case law.[39]

The specific clinical procedures for determining brain death are generally not prescribed by law. Often, institutional policies outline local guidelines. The key point to bear in mind is that brain death is a clinical diagnosis. The following criteria may be useful in determining brain death in adult patients: (1) absent cortical function as manifested by a patient in coma who has no spontaneous movement, no response to verbal commands, no response to deep pain and no seizures; (2) absent brain-stem function as manifested by the absence of pupillary, corneal, oculocephalic (doll's eyes) and oculovestibular (ice-water calorics) reflexes, and a negative apnea test (i.e., absent respiratory effort, hypercarbia, and acidosis in the oxygenated patient who has been taken off the ventilator for 5 to 10 minutes); (3) either the cause of coma is known (e.g., head trauma) and precludes improvement in brain function, or a sufficient period of observation has occurred to permit solid prognostication; and (4) other conditions that may be confused with brain death, such as drug intoxications, other metabolic problems, and hypothermia, have been excluded. Some institutional policies suggest a variety of confirmatory procedures: two or more separate observers, consultation with a neurologist or neurosurgeon, two separate examinations 6 to 12 hours apart, and supplementary tests including electroencephalography or cerebral blood flow studies. Most policies suggest that the declaration of death be made by physicians who are not involved in the potential transplantation of the organs of the deceased and who have no other economic or legal conflicts of interest.

What Specific Clinical Decision Is Being Considered?

The effective analysis of any medical case starts by determining the management question posed by the case. This is no less true for cases involving the elective use of life-sustaining treatment. Such cases may be categorized according to the specific treatment under consideration, as illustrated by the proposed taxonomy in Table 1. Moreover, the potential efficacy of life-sustaining treatments,[40] and the prognosis of patients in clinical states in which these treatments are usually used,[41, 42] are central issues that should be discussed with patients and their families.

Such a taxonomy of life-sustaining treatments replaces older distinctions, such as "ordinary" vs. "extraordinary," or "simple" vs. "heroic" treatment.

Several groups, including the President's Commission, have suggested that these older distinctions are vague and confusing and that they should be discarded.[43] The key problem with these distinctions is definitional: what is ordinary treatment to some observers may appear extraordinary to others.

Another frequent distinction is between withholding and withdrawing life-sustaining treatment. Withholding refers to the noninitiation of treatment. Withdrawing refers to the discontinuation of a treatment that has already been initiated. (The term *forego* refers to both withholding and withdrawing.) It is frequently asserted that there is no philosophical or legal difference between withholding and withdrawing. But, as a matter of clinical observation, physicians find it easier to withhold a treatment than to withdraw a treatment that has already begun.[25, 44] Physicians may fail to offer life-sustaining treatments at all to avoid the highly visible, emotionally challenging, and (in the view of many physicians) potentially litigable situation of treatment withdrawal.

The tendency to withhold potentially beneficial treatment to avoid withdrawing it if unsuccessful may not always work in the interest of the patient. Ideally, the patient should have the opportunity to choose a trial of a potentially beneficial treatment. If the treatment achieves its desired goals, then the patient is better off than if the treatment had been withheld. If the treatment is unsuccessful, it may be terminated after a predetermined period (usually a few weeks), and the patient is no worse off. We agree with recent guidelines that have emphasized the clinical usefulness of a time-limited trial in the elective use of life-sustaining treatments.[45]

The therapeutic trial raises another important question about elective use of life-sustaining treatments: when is treatment futile?[46] Futility is an elusive concept. Ambiguities in determining futility, arising from linguistic errors, from statistical misinterpretations, and from disagreements about the goals of therapy, undermine the use of futility claims. Futility should be separated into its two component parts: the chance that a treatment will be successful, and the goals against which success will be measured. The claim that a treatment is futile is often used to justify a shift in the physician's ethical obligation to patients. Whereas physicians have an obligation to discuss nonfutile treatments with patients, a physician may not be obliged to offer futile therapies. Because this radical shift in ethical obligations rests on an ill-defined concept, we recommend cautious application of futility claims in clinical practice.

Since patients often require more than one life-sustaining treatment over the course of an illness, it may be clinically useful to cluster these individual treatments into an overall treatment plan. In recent years, physicians have tended to focus single-mindedly on the issue of CPR (i.e., the DNR order). Research has shown that the DNR decision significantly affects decisions about elective use of other life-sustaining treatments.[25, 47] A broader focus on the full spectrum of life-sustaining treatments has recently been recommended.[48, 49] The development of a consolidated treatment care plan will require further clinical research aimed at uncovering how decisions about specific life-sustaining treatments interrelate in clinical practice.

Is the Patient Competent?

Once the treatment question posed by a case has been clarified, the next task for the physician is to determine whether the patient is competent to decide about the use of life-sustaining treatment. There is a broad ethical, legal, and medical consensus that competent adult patients have the right to determine the course of their medical care. In particular, patients have a fundamental ethical and legal right to refuse all proposed treatments including life-sustaining medical treatments.[50] In ethics, this right is based on the principle of individual autonomy. In law, it is based on the common-law right to be free from unconsented bodily invasion and the constitutional right of privacy. As a practical clinical matter, however, whether or not a patient is deemed competent will determine how the right to choose or refuse life-sustaining treatment will be effectuated. (Strictly speaking, only a court can declare a patient incompetent, but since most health care professionals speak of patient competency, even when this has been determined clinically and not judicially, we shall use this term.)

Assessment of Competency

The assessment of competency plays a pivotal role in patient management. Respect for the ethical and legal rights of patients means that doctors accede to the requests of competent patients to forego treatment, even if it results in the patient's death. On the other hand, doctors occasionally overrule requests to forego treatment, made by incompetent patients, because they do not want the patient to suffer serious harm that the patient would not intend if he or she were competent. Whether a doctor finds a patient competent or incompetent often determines whether or not the doctor honors the patient's stated wishes about life-sustaining treatment or takes steps to override the patient's decision. With so much at stake, it would be desirable to have well-developed clinical standards for the determination of competency. Unfortunately, at present, there are no clearly stipulated criteria for the determination of competency at the bedside.

The President's Commission has identified three elements of competency: possession of a set of values and goals, the ability to communicate and understand information, and the ability to reason and deliberate about one's choices.[51] The Commission also noted that competency was specific to "the person's actual functioning in situations in which a decision about health care was to be made."[51] In other words, whether the physician acts on a patient request to stop dialysis should not depend on whether the patient can name the date, but rather on whether the patient understands that he will die without dialysis treatments. More recently, Appelbaum and Grisso[52] have suggested that the competent patient should be able to communicate choices, understand relevant information, appreciate the situation and its consequences, and manipulate information rationally. An effective clinical index of patient competency to decide about life-sustaining treatment, however, would require a listing of specific questions for the physician to ask the patient, clearly stipulated criteria for the appraisal of patient responses, and a mechanism for combining the responses on individual questions into an overall assessment. Such an index is currently being developed and evaluated, but until this research has been completed, physicians must continue to rely on ad hoc assessments of competency.

Nevertheless, at the extremes, doctors can usually establish whether a patient is competent or incompetent. The patient who can adequately answer the five questions listed in Table 3 is probably competent. The patient in coma is incompetent, by definition. We recommend that physicians classify patients into three categories: (1) clearly competent, (2) competency uncertain, or (3) clearly incompetent. The management of clearly incompetent patients involves the process of "surrogate decision making" and is described in the next section. In the remainder of this section, we describe the management of patients who are clearly competent or whose competency is uncertain.

Clearly Competent

Based on the ethical and legal principles described previously, patients who are clearly competent should be permitted to forego life-sustaining medical treatments. This does not mean that the doctor must casually accept the patient's treatment refusal without further discussion. The physician should enter into a dialogue with the patient to ensure that the patient's desire to stop treatment is an authentic reflection of his or her wishes and goals. Further, the physician should try to persuade the patient to pursue a medically reasonable course of treatment. If, after such dialogue, the patient remains adamant in refusing treatment, then the doctor should respect the competent patient's wish and accede to the request to forego treatment.

Uncertain Competency

The patient with uncertain competency presents a difficult clinical challenge. In such cases, the clinician should first attempt to restore the patient's competency by addressing potentially treatable and reversible causes of cognitive dysfunction including a wide range of metabolic encephalopathies or psychoactive drug use. If such attempts prove unsuc-

---

TABLE 3.
Questions to Guide Assessment of Competency

What is your main medical problem right now?
What treatment was recommended for this problem?
If you receive this treatment, what will happen?
If you do not receive this treatment, what will happen?
Why have you decided to receive (not to receive) this treatment?

cessful, and uncertainty remains about the patient's competency, we recommend consultation with colleagues. Appropriate consultants include psychiatrists, neurologists, institutional ethics committees, ethics consultation services, or hospital attorneys. At present, it is unclear which of these groups is the preferred consultant, and this may vary in different clinical cases and institutional settings. In controversial cases, judicial review may be indicated. After competency has been determined, patient management will proceed as described either for competent patients (as described previously) or for incompetent patients (see next section).

Are the Incompetent Patient's Wishes Known?

If the patient is incompetent, the physician should search for reversible causes of cognitive dysfunction. Sometimes, the correction of electrolyte disturbances, acidemia, hypoxemia, uremia, or other metabolic, infectious, or structural causes will restore the patient's competency and allow the patient to speak for himself.

Incompetent patients whose competency cannot be restored present a troubling ethical problem. This group includes both permanently unconscious patients and patients who are conscious but who have severe and irreversible cognitive impairments (such as Alzheimer's disease or congenital mental retardation). Because incompetent patients cannot speak for themselves, courts and legislatures since the 1976 Quinlan decision have developed an approach to end-of-life decisions that allows other parties (surrogates) to decide for the incompetent person. The underlying philosophical and legal assumption that permits surrogate decision making is that incompetent patients have the same autonomy claims and right of self-determination (for example, in the refusal of treatment) that competent patients possess. This philosophical and legal fiction that views the incompetent person as a competent decision maker requires that the surrogate make choices that are in accord with the choices that the now-incompetent individual would make if he or she were competent.

In practice, surrogate decision making raises two key questions: who should decide on behalf of the incompetent patient, and on what basis should the decision be made? In addressing both these questions, it is important to remember that the goal of surrogate decision making is to project the incompetent patient's wishes onto the current clinical situation.

Who Should Decide?

The best surrogate decision maker is a person identified by the patient to represent the patient's own wishes. It is the responsibility of the physician to find out whether the patient has appointed such a surrogate. The patient may have done so formally or informally. The formal, legal mechanism involves appointing a durable power of attorney for health care. The durable power of attorney has two key advantages. First, the surrogate decision maker can be presumed to represent the patient's wishes. Second, decisions about elective use of life-sustaining treatment can be tailored to the actual clinical circumstances since a competent decision maker (i.e., the surrogate) is at hand. A formal durable power of attorney has proven particularly valuable in the context of AIDS, where many patients prefer to appoint their friends, rather than their families, as surrogate decision makers.[28] Seventeen states have laws or judicial opinions recognizing the authority of such durable powers of attorney for health care.[53]

In the absence of state legislation or a formally executed legal document, the physician should still attempt to discover whether the patient indicated his or her preferred surrogate. This may have been done through written or oral statements. Such a surrogate may not have the legal status of a durable power of attorney, but most cases of elective use of life-sustaining treatment are (and should be) resolved extrajudicially.

In many cases, the patient will have left no direct indication of his or her preference for a surrogate decision maker. Nonetheless, the physician should attempt to identify such a surrogate since this can simplify further clinical decision making. The physician may ask the family to identify a surrogate. Alternatively, the physician may try to identify the family member with the closest emotional connection to the patient. Evidence of close relationship might include frequency of contact, the types of issues the patient discussed with the potential surrogate, and the apparent concern expressed by the potential surrogate about the patient's condition in hospital. Usually, the surrogate decision maker will be the spouse, close relative, or friend of the patient. Several states have enacted laws recognizing the decisional authority of family surrogate decision makers even in the absence of a durable power of attorney.[54]

The patient with no readily identifiable surrogate decision maker presents a particularly difficult clinical management problem. Sometimes an independent physician, such as the department chairman or hospital chief of staff, serves as the surrogate for such patients. Sometimes these cases are referred for judicial review, and the court appoints a surrogate decision maker (known as a guardian ad litem). All too often, no surrogate is appointed and life-sustaining treatment is continued, well beyond the point the patient would wish to stop, simply because there is no one to authorize the withholding or withdrawing of life-sustaining treatment. There is no consensus on how to manage these difficult cases, but we offer three recommendations. First, health care facilities should address this situation prospectively in their institutional policies.[49] Second, such cases should be referred to the institutional ethics committee or consultation service.[44, 55-60] Third, clinical investigators should evaluate the functioning of ethics committees/consultants in this specific clinical situation and the researchers should report their results in the medical literature.[56, 58]

Another clinically challenging situation occurs when family members disagree about decisions to forego life-sustaining treatment. Usually, some family members will want treatment stopped but others will want it continued. In practice, treatment is usually continued in these situations pending the resolution of intrafamily conflicts. When such conflicts arise, ethics committees and consultants may provide an effective, extrajudicial mechanism for mediation. If the "ethical impasse" persists, judicial referral may be indicated.

On What Basis Should the Decision Be Made?

Once a surrogate decision maker has been identified, a second question arises: on what grounds should the surrogate reach a decision? Again, the physician should recall that the goal of surrogate decision making is to project the incompetent patient's wishes onto the current clinical situation. Thus, whenever possible, the surrogate should follow the incompetent patient's general wishes about life-sustaining treatment. The practical question becomes: with what level of certainty are the incompetent patient's wishes known?

Advance Directives.—The highest level of certainty accompanies an explicit directive, prepared by the patient while competent, that contains the patient's preference about elective use of life-sustaining treatment. The directive should cover the patient's actual clinical circumstances. A written directive is preferable, but a repeated, oral directive to family, close friends, or physician might also be acceptable. Written directives have been legally formalized as so-called living wills. Many groups endorse the living will in principle. Living wills have been endorsed by the President's Commission for the Study of Ethical Problems in Medicine and Biomedical and Behavioral Research.[43] A recent survey showed that almost 80% of physicians expressed a positive attitude toward advance directives.[61] Moreover, 67% of US hospitals have institutional policy about advance directives.[62] And, most importantly, surveys support the concept that the majority of patients welcome advance discussions about elective use of life-sustaining treatments.[21, 22, 28, 33] Since the first "living will" law was enacted in California in 1977, 40 states and the District of Columbia have passed legislation and several other states have had court decisions giving legal force to living wills.[53]

Despite this flurry of activity in state legislatures, living will laws have not fulfilled their promise of projecting competent patients' wishes into future clinical circumstances. One survey indicated that only 15% of Americans have executed a living will.[63] In our opinion, the emphasis on legislative activity has obscured the Achilles heel of current living wills: the documents are too vague, inflexible, and biased to be useful.[64] Living wills are *vague* about prognosis (for example, they often request cessation of treatment when "there is no reasonable expectation of . . . recovery from extreme physical or mental disability") and about which treatments should be stopped (referring to these as "artificial means" or "life-prolonging procedures"). They are *inflexible* because many living wills are limited to "terminally ill patients" and because some exclude artificial feeding from the spectrum of life-sustaining treatments that may be foregone. Finally, current-generation living wills are inherently *biased* because they focus on *refusal* of treatment, failing to capture the bilateral concept of the elective use of life-sustaining treatments: some patients will want certain life-sustaining treatments if there is any hope of recovery, and advance directives should allow patients to *choose or refuse* life-sustaining treatment. Advance directives should be designed to elicit the attitudes and preferences of patients toward life-sustaining treatment with the same objectivity as questionnaires in a research study.

A new living will known as the "medical directive" has recently been proposed by Emanuel and Emanuel.[64] The medical directive was designed to address the problems of vagueness, inflexibility, and bias discussed previously. We regard it as a major conceptual advance in medical ethics research. In the medical directive, the patient is offered four clinical scenarios. For each scenario, the patient is asked whether he or she would want each of 12 specific medical treatments. The patient may request or refuse each treatment, be undecided, or request a therapeutic trial. Researchers are currently studying the reliability and validity of the medical directive.

In addition to the methodologic problems of designing a reliable, valid, and clinically sensible advance directive, physicians also face an important public education challenge. We will need to discuss the elective use of life-sustaining treatments with our patients, and to elicit their wishes about end-of-life care. Public policy lessons from the field of organ procurement may be of value here. For example, institutions might develop policies of "routine inquiry" regarding elective use of life-sustaining treatment. Such policies might be mandated through legislation or "fiscal policy-making." As in organ procurement, however, the key to successful policy will lie not in the heavy hand of government regulation, but rather in persuading health care professionals to educate patients about the elective use of life-sustaining treatment and to discuss and document their patients' preferences. In current clinical practice, however, explicit statements of the patient's preferences are usually not available. In these situations, how should the surrogate decide about elective use of life-sustaining treatments?

Substituted Judgment.—In the absence of explicit written or oral prior wishes, two main standards for surrogate decision making have been developed: substituted judgment and best interests.[43, 65] The standards have been developed in legal cases and public policy guidelines, but they can also be applied in clinical practice. With substituted judgment, the surrogate applies the patient's preferences and values to the clinical situation at hand. The goal of substituted judgment is "to reach the decision that the incapacitated person would make if he or she were able to choose." A fundamental issue in cases that rely on substituted judgment is the quality of information about the patient's prior wishes.

Two evidentiary standards have evolved. The more stringent is the "clear and convincing" standard, as developed in the case of Mary O'Connor, a severely demented elderly woman sustained by artificial feeding.[66, 67] In 1988, the New York Court of Appeals stated that this more restrictive standard would require proof "that the patient held a firm and settled commitment to the termination of life supports under circumstances like those presented." The court held that this standard of evidence regarding prior wishes was required in New York State to forego life-sustaining treatments in incompetent patients. O'Connor's daughter testified that her mother had said she would never want "any sort of life support systems to maintain or prolong her life." The court held that this statement failed to meet the "clear and convincing" standard, and enjoined the O'Connor family from terminating Mrs. O'Connor's artificial feeding.

In other states, courts have held incompetent patients and their families to a more lenient standard of evidence about prior wishes. In the 1986 case of Paul Brophy, a 49-year-old man in a persistent vegetative state, the Massachusetts Supreme Court ruled, without requiring "clear and convincing" evidence, that artificial feeding may be stopped.[68, 69] (Referring to a burn victim who had died several months after a motor vehicle accident, Brophy had said, "If I'm ever like that, just shoot me, pull the plug." Before his own neurosurgery, Brophy had said, "If I can't get up to kiss one of my beautiful daughters, I may as well be six feet under.")

There is no national consensus on the quality of information required about prior wishes to forego treatment using the substituted judgment approach. Clinicians should consult with legal colleagues about the standards of evidence required in their own state. But more importantly, clinicians should ask the family and close friends of an incompetent patient for specific expressions of the patient's prior wishes. These details represent an important part of the incompetent patient's medical history, and they should be documented in the medical record. A weakness of the substituted judgment approach is recent empirical data that show low rates of agreement between patients and their likely surrogates in resuscitation and other decisions.[20, 70] Such data raise troubling questions about the adequacy of the substituted judgment approach and should provide impetus for the broader use of advance directives.

Best Interests.—Sometimes there is no available information about an incompetent patient's prior wishes. This can occur in three clinical situations. First, there may be no one for the physician to interview who has known the patient while the patient was competent. Second, the patient may never have discussed his or her preferences concerning life-sustaining treatment. Third, the patient may never have been competent, such as a patient with severe mental retardation since birth. In these situations, physicians and courts have had to rely on the "best interests" approach, wherein the surrogate chooses as a reasonable person in the patient's circumstance would choose. The best interests approach involves a balancing of benefits and burdens. It requires a set of "objective, societally shared criteria" to rank burdens and benefits. A specific formulation of the "best interests" standard was defined by the New Jersey Supreme Court in the 1985 case of Claire Conroy.[71] According to this so-called pure-objective test, treatment could be stopped if "the net burdens of the patient's life with the treatment clearly and markedly outweigh the benefits that the patient derives from life so that the recurring, unavoidable, and severe pain of the patient's life with the treatment would render life-sustaining treatment inhumane."

12 / P.A. Singer and M. Siegler

The key problem of the best interests approach is that it requires societal consensus on burdens and benefits. In a pluralistic society, such a consensus is extraordinarily difficult to achieve. The best interests approach requires one person to judge the quality of life of another.[72] This situation opens the door to discrimination against those with disabilities. There is empirical evidence that third parties undervalue the quality of life of chronically ill patients relative to the value these patients place on their own quality of life.[19, 73]

The potential for discrimination on the basis of third-party quality-of-life judgments is a serious limitation of the best interests approach. Nevertheless, as a practical matter, this may be the only approach available to effectuate the right to refuse treatment of those patients whose prior wishes are unknown. We make two recommendations. First, clinicians should consult with their local ethics committee or ethics consultation service about these difficult cases.[44, 55–60] Second, health care facilities should develop policies to address the elective use of life-sustaining treatments in those patients whose prior wishes are unknown.[49]

Are Any External Factors Affecting the Decision?

Two types of externalities affect decisions about the elective use of life-sustaining treatments. First is conscientious objection, which may be at the level of the individual health care provider, the health care facility, or the medical profession. Second is cost control, which may be at the level of the individual patient or society.

Conscientious Objection

What happens when the wishes of a patient to forego life-sustaining treatment conflict with the ethical precepts of the health care provider, health care facility, or medical profession? Such conflicts have arisen, for example, when patients (or their surrogates) have requested to forego artificial feeding. Does the patient's right to forego life-sustaining treatment oblige the provider, facility, or profession to participate in the limited treatment plan?

The right of individual health care providers to refuse to participate in treatment plans that they find morally objectionable has been well established. The President's Commission noted that a health care professional is not "obligated to accede to the patient in a way that violates . . . the provider's own deeply held moral beliefs."[51] (The health care professional may not refuse to provide emergency care.) If the provider refuses, on grounds of personal conscience, to participate in a patient's legal treatment (or nontreatment) request, then he or she should usually arrange for an alternative source of care for the patient.

The prerogative of health care facilities to refuse to provide certain treatment plans on moral grounds is more complex.[74] This prerogative has recently been challenged in the courts. For example, in the 1987 case of Nancy Jobes, a 31-year-old patient in persistent vegetative state whose family requested cessation of artificial feeding, the New Jersey Supreme

Court not only affirmed that artificial feeding might be stopped, but also ordered the objecting health care facility to care for Jobes until she died.[75] We suggest that the prerogative of health care facilities to project a particular moral vision of health care, as expressed in a statement of institutional mission, serves an important role in our morally pluralistic society.[74] We believe that a spectrum of health care facility missions is in the public interest, and that the prerogative of health care facilities to abide by their mission statements should be protected. Health care is a complex process not well captured by the impoverished language of informed consent to individual treatments. Mission statements, and the treatment philosophy they delineate, offer the promise that treatment proposals begin from shared fundamental beliefs. Health care facilities should inform patients and their families before or on admission of the facility's particular treatment philosophy. Certain providers, such as public hospitals, may not be permitted to promote sectarian views and should respond affirmatively to medically appropriate and legally permissible treatment requests.

The third level of conscientious objection is the medical profession as a whole. The fundamental premise here is that medicine is not a value-neutral business, but rather a profession with enduring, core values and virtues.[76] Certain acts, even though legal, contradict the quintessence of physicianhood. For example, it can be argued that active euthanasia—wherein the physician willfully and directly ends the life of the patient such as by administering a lethal injection—is contrary to the fundamental normative values of medicine.[77,78] Indeed, professional societies, such as the American Medical Association[79] and the American College of Physicians,[80] have deemed physician involvement in active euthanasia to be unethical. Currently, active euthanasia is illegal in the United States. There are, however, vigorous efforts to legalize it. Even if legalized, active euthanasia, like physician participation in capital punishment, would continue to be unethical from the standpoint of the norms of medicine.[77-80]

Cost Control

It is difficult to deny that the United States needs to control its health care costs. At almost 12% of gross national product, the estimated national health bill for 1990 is $661 billion. The care of patients in the year before their deaths accounts for a substantial fraction of this total expenditure. Thus, end-of-life care becomes a prime target for fiscal restraint.

The ethical question raised by the economics of terminal care is not *whether* initiatives should be pursued to control costs, but rather *what* should be the nature of these initiatives? Some have argued that the modern-day physician is responsible for the control of health care costs in the care of individual patients. Others maintain that the physician's duty is to serve the patient's good, irrespective of cost.

We favor the latter view. Throughout this chapter, we have argued that the patient's wishes about elective use of life-sustaining treatment should be determinative. We have also suggested, however, that the patient's wishes are not always elicited, and even when elicited, may not always be followed.

Each year, tens of thousands of Americans receive expensive life-sustaining treatments that they might not choose for themselves. At the same time, thousands of Americans are not offered life-sustaining treatments they might want. This situation of excess and deprivation is perpetuated by insufficient communication about patient wishes. A better match between patient wishes and the provision of life-sustaining treatments might not only promote higher-quality medical care but also control the so-called high cost of dying.

At the level of society, difficult choices must be made. The health budget must be balanced against other priorities such as education, transportation, and national defense. Within the health budget, the government must set priorities between treatment and prevention or among access, cost, and quality. These are political questions that deserve political answers. Cost control at this level has two advantages over bedside efforts. First, in accord with the principles of justice, similar cases across a state or country can be treated equally. Second, the government, which ultimately decides about the distribution of resources within a polity, can be held accountable for its decisions by the voting public.

Conclusions

The elective use of life-sustaining treatments is an integral component of clinical practice. The clinical approach to such patients can be summarized in a five-step algorithm: (1) Is the patient brain dead? (2) What specific clinical decision is being considered? (3) Is the patient competent? (4) Are the incompetent patient's wishes known? (5) Are any external factors affecting the decision?

In the brain-dead patient, treatment may be discontinued without further consideration of patient wishes. In all other cases, the patient's wishes are determinative. Competent patients can state their own wishes, and, after adequate discussions, these wishes should be followed. Incompetent patients cannot state their wishes directly; the physician must gather evidence about the patient's prior wishes. If the evidence is clear, such wishes should also be followed. Whenever possible, physicians are encouraged to discuss these matters with patients while the patient is competent.

As this chapter goes to press, the U.S. Supreme Court has handed down its opinion in the case of Nancy Cruzan.[84] As the first case involving the elective use of life-sustaining treatment in an adult to be considered by the Supreme Court, the decision will have substantial impact. Nancy Cruzan is a 32-year-old Missouri woman who has been in a persistent vegetative state since a 1983 automobile accident. With almost no chance of regaining consciousness, Cruzan is kept alive by a feeding tube. Before the accident, she had said she would not want to live if she couldn't be at least "halfway normal." Three years ago, her parents asked the hospital to remove the feeding tube, but the hospital refused, so the Cruzans took them to court. The trial judge decided in the family's favor, but the Missouri Attorney General appealed to the state Supreme Court. That court ruled 4 to 3 that feeding must continue, based on the state's strong interest in life and the lack of clear and convincing evidence of what Nancy would want done. The Cruzan family appealed to the U.S. Supreme Court. In a 5 to 4 decision, the Supreme Court upheld the Missouri court, ruling against the Cruzan family. The Court held that while a competent patient has a constitutional right to refuse life-sustaining treatment, an incompetent patient who is unable to make an informed and voluntary choice does not automatically possess this right. The Court ruled that states may establish procedural safeguards to guide such decisions for incompetent patients—and that Missouri's safeguards are acceptable. As Justice Sandra Day O'Connor wrote in her concurring opinion, "Today, we decide only that one State's practice does not violate the Constitution; the more challenging task of crafting appropriate procedures for safeguarding incompetents' liberty interests is entrusted to the laboratory of the States."

After 15 years of court decisions and legislation, culminating in the Cruzan case, we want to suggest two new directions for the area of elective use of life-sustaining treatments: research and public education. Further research is required to improve the management of patients at the end of life. A clinical index of patient competency is needed. Improved methods of eliciting and documenting patient preferences are also required. Finally, more basic research needs to be performed on the epidemiology of elective use of life-sustaining treatments.

Public education is also required. Every patient should be given the option of discussing end-of-life care with his or her physician. The United States has developed adequate public policies in the area of elective use of life-sustaining treatments. The emphasis now should shift to empirical research and public education to translate these policies into practical clinical reality.[81-83]

Acknowledgments

Dr. Singer is the recipient of a Canadian Life and Health Insurance Association Medical Scholarship; the Centre for Bioethics is supported by a Health System–Linked Research Unit Award from the Ontario Ministry of Health. The Center for Clinical Medical Ethics is supported by grants from the Henry J. Kaiser Family Foundation, the Andrew W. Mellon Foundation, and the Pew Charitable Trusts. The views expressed herein are those of the authors and may not reflect those of the supporting institutions.

References

1. *In re Quinlan*, 70 NJ 10 (1976).
2. Jonsen AR, Siegler M, Winslade WJ: *Clinical Ethics: A Practical Approach to Ethical Decisions in Clinical Medicine*, ed 3. New York, MacMillan Publishing Co Inc, 1991.

3. Uhlmann RF, McDonald WJ, Inui TS: Epidemiology of no-code orders in an academic hospital. *West J Med* 1984; 140:114–116.
4. Lo B, Saika G, Strull W, et al: "Do not resuscitate" decisions: A prospective study at three teaching hospitals. *Arch Intern Med* 1985; 145:1115–1117.
5. Schwartz DA, Reilly P: The choice not to be resuscitated. *J Am Geriatr Soc* 1986; 34:807–811.
6. Lipton HL: Do-not-resuscitate decisions in a community hospital: Incidence, implications, and outcomes. *JAMA* 1986; 256:1164–1169.
7. Stolman CJ, Gregory JJ, Dunn D, et al: Evaluation of the do not resuscitate orders at a community hospital. *Arch Intern Med* 1989; 149:1851–1856.
8. Youngner SJ, Lewandowski W, McClish DK, et al: 'Do not resuscitate orders': Incidence and implications in a medical intensive care unit. *JAMA* 1985; 253:54–57.
9. Zimmerman JE, Knaus WA, Sharpe SM, et al: The use and implications of do not resuscitate orders in intensive care units. *JAMA* 1986; 255:351–356.
10. Levy MR, Lambe ME, Shear SL: Do-not-resuscitate orders in a county hospital. *West J Med* 1984; 140:111–113.
11. Bedell SE, Pelle D, Maher PL, et al: Do not resuscitate orders for critically ill patients in the hospital: How are they used and what is their impact? *JAMA* 1986; 256:233–237.
12. Jonsson PV, McNamee M, Campion EW: The 'do not resuscitate' order: A profile of its changing use. *Arch Intern Med* 1988; 148:2373–2375.
13. Charlson ME, Sax FL, MacKenzie R, et al: Resuscitation: How do we decide? A prospective study of physicians' preferences and the clinical course of hospitalized patients. *JAMA* 1986; 255:1316–1322.
14. Farber NJ, Bowman SM, Major DA, et al: Cardiopulmonary resuscitation (CPR): Patient factors and decision making. *Arch Intern Med* 1984; 144:2229–2232.
15. Farber NJ, Weiner JL, Boyer EG, et al: Cardiopulmonary resuscitation: Values and decisions—A comparison of health care professionals. *Med Care* 1985; 23:1391–1398.
16. Witte KL: Variables present in patients who are either resuscitated or not resuscitated in a medical intensive care unit. *Heart Lung* 1984; 13:159–163.
17. Lawrence VA, Clark GM: Cancer and resuscitation: Does the diagnosis affect the decision? *Arch Intern Med* 1987; 147:1637–1640.
18. Wachter RM, Luce JM, Hearst N, et al: Decisions about resuscitation: Inequities among patients with different diagnoses but similar prognoses. *Ann Intern Med* 1989; 111:525–532.
19. Starr TJ, Pearlman RA, Uhlmann RF: Quality of life and resuscitation decisions in elderly patients. *J Gen Intern Med* 1986; 1:373–379.
20. Uhlmann RF, Pearlman RA, Cain KC: Physicians 'and spouses' predictions of elderly patients' resuscitation preferences. *J Gerontol* 1988; 43:M115–M121.
21. Shmerling RH, Bedell SE, Lilienfeld A, et al: Discussing cardiopulmonary resuscitation: A study of elderly outpatients. *J Gen Intern Med* 1988; 3:317–321.
22. Finucane TE, Shumway JM, Powers RL, et al: Planning with elderly outpatients for contingencies of severe illness: A survey and clinical trial. *J Gen Intern Med* 1988; 3:322–325.
23. Evans AS, Brody BA: The do-not-resuscitate order in teaching hospitals. *JAMA* 1985; 253:2236–2239.
24. Bedell SE, Delbanco TL: Choices about cardiopulmonary resuscitation in the

hospital: When do physicians talk with patients? *N Engl J Med* 1984; 310:1089–1093.

25. LaPuma J, Silverstein MD, Stocking LB, et al: Life-sustaining treatment: A prospective study of patients with DNR orders in a teaching hospital. *Arch Intern Med* 1988; 148:2193–2198.

25a. Smedira NG, Evans BH, Craig LS, et al: Withholding and withdrawal of life support from the critically ill. *N Engl J Med* 1990; 322:309-315.

26. Pearlman RA, Inui TS, Carter WB: Variability in physician bioethical decision making: A case study of euthanasia. *Ann Intern Med* 1982; 97:420–425.

27. Pearlman RA, Jonsen A: The use of quality-of-life considerations in medical decision making. *J Am Geriatr Soc* 1985; 33:344–352.

28. Steinbrook R, Lo B, Moulton J, et al: Preferences of homosexual men with AIDS for life-sustaining treatment. *N Engl J Med* 1986; 314:457–460.

29. Frankl D, Oye RK, Bellamy PE: Attitudes of hospitalized patients toward life-support: A survey of 200 medical inpatients. *Am J Med* 1989; 86:645–648.

30. Neu S, Kjellstrand CM: Stopping long-term dialysis: An empirical study of withdrawal of life-supporting treatment. *N Engl J Med* 1986; 314:14–20.

31. Neu S, Kjellstrand CM: Stopping long-term dialysis, letter. *N Engl J Med* 1986; 314:1451.

32. Brown NK, Thompson DJ: Nontreatment of fever in extended-care facilities. *N Engl J Med* 1979; 300:1246–1250.

33. Lo B, McCleod GA, Saika G: Patient attitudes to discussing life-sustaining treatment. *Arch Intern Med* 1986; 146:1613–1615.

34. Smith DG, Wigton RS: Modeling decisions to use tube feeding in seriously ill patients. *Arch Intern Med* 1987; 147:1242–1245.

35. Quill TE: Utilization of nasogastric feeding tubes in a group of chronically ill, elderly patients in a community hospital. *Arch Intern Med* 1989; 149:1937–1941.

36. Youngner SJ, Landefeld CS, Coulton CJ, et al: 'Brain death' and organ retrieval: A cross-sectional survey of knowledge and concepts among health professionals. *JAMA* 1989; 261:2205–2210.

37. Ad Hoc Committee of the Harvard Medical School to Examine the Definition of Brain Death: A definition of irreversible coma. *JAMA* 1968; 205:377.

38. President's Commission for the Study of Ethical Problems in Medicine and Biomedical and Behavioral Research: *Defining Death.* U.S. Government Printing Office, 1981.

39. Office of Organ Transplantation. *The Status of Organ Donation and Coordination Services: Report to the Congress for Fiscal Year 1987.* US Dept of Health and Human Services, 1987.

40. Moss AL: Informing the patient about cardiopulmonary resuscitation: When the risks outweigh the benefits. *J Gen Intern Med* 1989; 4:349–355.

41. Levy DE, Caronna JJ, Singer BH, et al: Predicting outcome from hypoxic-ischemic coma. *JAMA* 1985; 253:1420–1426.

42. Cranford RE: The persistent vegetative state: The medical reality (getting the facts straight). *Hastings Center Rep* 1988; 18(Feb/March):27–32.

43. President's Commission for the Study of Ethical Problems in Medicine and Biomedical and Behavioral Research: *Deciding to Forego Life-Sustaining Treatment: Ethical, Medical and Legal Issues in Treatment Decisions.* U.S. Government Printing Office, 1983.

44. LaPuma J, Stocking CB, Silverstein MD, et al: An ethics consultation service in a teaching hospital—Utilization and evaluation. *JAMA* 1988; 260:808–811.

78 / P.A. Singer and M. Siegler

45. The Hastings Center: *Guidelines on the Termination of Life-Sustaining Treatment and the Care of the Dying.* Briarcliff Manor, NY, The Hastings Center, 1987.

46. Lantos JD, Singer PA, Walker RM, et al: The illusion of futility in clinical practice. *Am J Med* 1989; 87:81–84.

47. Uhlmann RF, Cassel CK, McDonald WJ: Some treatment-withholding implications of no-code orders in an academic hospital. *Crit Care Med* 1984; 12:879–881.

48. Emanuel L: Does the DNR order need life-sustaining intervention? Time for comprehensive advance directives. *Am J Med* 1989; 86:87–90.

49. Miles SH, Gomez CF: *Protocols for Elective Use of Life-Sustaining Treatments.* New York, Springer-Verlag NY Inc, 1989.

50. Emanuel EJ: A review of the ethical and legal aspects of terminating medical care. *Am J Med* 1988; 84:291–301.

51. President's Commission for the Study of Ethical Problems in Medicine and Biomedical and Behavioral Research. *Making Health Care Decisions: The Ethical and Legal Implications of Informed Consent in the Patient-Practitioner Relationship,* vol 1. US Government Printing Office, 1982.

52. Appelbaum PS, Grisso T: Assessing patients' capacities to consent to treatment. *N Engl J Med* 1988; 319:1635–1638.

53. Brody JE: *New York Times,* Sept 21, 1989, Y20.

54. Areen J: The legal status of consent obtained from families of adult patients to withhold or withdraw treatment. *JAMA* 1987; 258:229–235.

55. LaPuma J, Toulmin SE: Ethics consultants and ethics committees. *Arch Intern Med* 1989; 149:1109–1112.

56. Lo B: Behind closed doors: Promises and pitfalls of ethics committees. *N Engl J Med* 1987; 317:46–50.

57. Perkins HS, Saathoff BS: Impact of medical ethics consultations on physicians: An exploratory study. *Am J Med* 1988; 85:761–765.

58. Siegler M, Singer PA: Clinical ethics consultation: Godsend or "God squad?" *Am J Med* 1988; 85:759–760.

59. Brennan TA: Ethics committees and decisions to limit care: The experience at the Massachusetts General Hospital. *JAMA* 1988; 260:803–807.

60. Brennan TA: Incompetent patients with limited care in the absence of family consent: A study of socioeconomic and clinical variables. *Ann Intern Med* 1988; 109:819–825.

61. Davidson KW, Hackler C, Caradine DR, et al: Physicians' attitudes on advance directives. *JAMA* 1989; 262:2415-2419.

62. McCrary SV, Botkin JR: Hospital policy on advance directives: Do institutions ask patients about living wills? *JAMA* 1989; 262:2411–2414.

63. Harvey LK, Shubat SC: Physician and public attitudes on health care issues. Chicago, American Medical Association, 1989.

64. Emanuel LL, Emanuel EJ: The medical directive: A new comprehensive advance care document. *JAMA* 1989; 261:3288–3293.

65. Emanuel EJ: What criteria should guide decision makers for incompetent patients? *Lancet* 1988; 1:170–171.

66. *In re O'Connor,* 531 N.E. 2d 607 (1988).

67. Annas GJ: Precatory prediction and mindless mimicry: The case of Mary O'Connor. *Hastings Center Rep* 1988; 18(Dec):31–33.

68. *Brophy v New England Sinai Hosp,* 497 NE2d 626 (Mass 1986).

69. Steinbrook R, Lo B: Artificial feeding—Solid ground, not a slippery slope. *N Engl J Med* 1988; 318:286–290.

70. Ouslander JG, Tymchuk AJ: Health Care decisions among elderly long-term care residents and their potential proxies. *Arch Intern Med* 1989; 149:1367–1372.

71. *In re Conroy,* 98 NJ 321 (1985).

72. Dresser RS, Robertson JA: Quality of life and non-treatment decisions for incompetent patients: A critique of the orthodox approach. *Law Med Health Care* 1989; 17:234–244.

73. Pearlman RA, Uhlmann RF: Quality of life in chronic diseases: Perceptions of elderly patients. *J Gerontol* 1988; 43:M25–M30.

74. Miles SH, Singer PA, Siegler M: Conflicts between patients' wishes to forego treatment and the policies of health care facilities. *N Engl J Med* 1989; 321:48–50.

75. *In re Jobes,* 108 NJ 394 (1987).

76. Kass LR: *Toward a More Natural Science: Biology and Human Affairs.* New York, Free Press, 1985.

77. Singer PA, Siegler M: Euthanasia: A critique. *N Engl J Med* 1990; 322:1881–1883.

78. Kass LR: Neither for love or money: Why doctors must not kill. *Public Interest* 1989; 94:25–46.

79. Council on Ethical and Judicial Affairs of the American Medical Association. *AMA Council Report C/A-88:1.* Chicago, American Medical Association, 1988.

80. American College of Physicians: Ethics manual, second edition: II. The physician and society; research; life-sustaining treatment; other issues. *Ann Intern Med* 1989; 111:327–335.

81. Siegler M, Singer PA, Schiedermayer DL: *Medical Ethics: An Annotated Bibliography.* Philadelphia, American College of Physicians, 1988.

82. Siegler M, Pellegrino ED, Singer PA: Clinical medical ethics. *J Clin Ethics* 1990; 1:5-9.

83. Singer PA, Siegler M, Pellegrino ED: Research in clinical ethics. *J Clin Ethics* 1990; 1:95-99.

84. Nancy Beth Cruzan, by her parents and co-guardians, Lester L. Cruzan et ux. v. Directors, Missouri Department of Health, et al. —5Ct.—, 1990 WL 84074 (U.S.)

10.7   Siegler M, Taylor RM (1993) Intimacy and Caring: The Legacy of Karen Ann Quinlan. Trends in Health Care Law Ethics 8:28–30, 38

Trends In Health Care, Law & Ethics, Volume 8, Number 1 (Winter, 1993)

I n 1563, when he was 88 years old, just a year before his death, Michelangelo wrote to Vasari, a fellow artist: "I have reached the twenty-fourth hour of my day and . . . no project arises in my brain which hath not the figure of death engraved upon it."

"The figure of death" was engraved upon Michelangelo's last work, the powerful and mysterious Rondinini Pieta. Michelangelo's correspondence documents that he was still working on this Pieta six days before his death. This last, unfinished work stands in dramatic contrast to an earlier Pieta (at St. Peter's in the Vatican) that Michelangelo had completed 60 years before.

The earlier Pieta is a marvelous yet traditional rendering of the theme. It depicts the individual figures conventionally, albeit sensuously. Mary, a monumental figure, supports the dead body of Jesus. Her closed eyes, and especially her left hand, signal acceptance and resignation. The two figures are distinct and isolated; Christ's head and eyes are tilted away from Mary.

By contrast, when Michelangelo returned to the same subject more than 60 years later, his image of the relationship of the living to the dead had changed. In the Rondinini Pieta, one sees two bodies supporting each other in mysterious ways that appear to defy the laws of physics. As the figures emerge from the marble block, it is Mary who is leaning for support on the dead body of Jesus, even while holding up and supporting her dead son. Christ's right hand and arm merge with Mary's body; the two figures are united, inseparable. In contrast to the earlier Pieta, there is a sense here of mutual support, almost a union of the living and the

Intimacy And Caring:
The Legacy Of
Karen Ann Quinlan

by Mark Siegler, M.D. and Robert M. Taylor, M.D.

dead, that brings to mind notions of the social, personal and religious contexts in which dying, and support for the dying, occur. There is a sense of intimacy and connectedness in the later Pieta that is not apparent in the earlier work.

These two sculptures provide strikingly different images of the relationship of the living to the dead and dying. These images, in turn, provide insights into two radically different conceptions of medical practice and of patient-physician relationships. One conception is of a legalistic relationship appropriate to strangers; the other conception is of a caring relationship appropriate to intimates. We wish to explore these two different conceptions of medicine by examining perhaps the best-known case in American medical ethics: the case of Karen Ann Quinlan.

The tragic events that led to Karen Ann Quinlan's coma, the legal drama that followed, and then the extraordinary supportive care that Ms. Quinlan received for ten years while in a persistent vegetative state are a moving story, now part of the collective American experience. But the legacy of Karen Ann Quinlan will depend on how we choose to tell her story, which lessons we choose to extract, and how we elect to use the story in the future. Which elements of the story will be regarded as central and which as peripheral?

The stories used to describe the practice of medicine and the metaphors used to depict the relationship between patient and physician affect the practice of medicine itself. Ethicist James Gustafson once made this

point in a lecture: "How we describe persons and their relationships to each other—whether as individual contractors or as persons in patterns and processes of interdependence— is a matter of critical judgment. The alternative descriptions back alternative ways of construing the moral situation. How that situation is construed confines or enlarges the morally relevant features taken into account in patient care." Thus, depending upon which parts of the story we choose to focus, different meanings may be extracted. We describe two alternative ways of telling the story of Karen Ann Quinlan; depending on which story one tells, the legacy derived from the case of Karen Ann Quinlan will be different.

One dramatic aspect of the Quinlan story resembles Gustafson's notion of relationships between people as "individual contractors." It is this aspect that usually comes to mind when considering the important precedent established by the intellectual force of the New Jersey Supreme Court decision handed down in 1976. Although the legal roots of the Quinlan case reach back hundreds of years to the framers of the United States Constitution, Quinlan's legal legacy has profoundly influenced current medical practice.

The court held that a patient's constitutionally-protected right to privacy includes the right to decline medical treatment under certain circumstances. Such circumstances are determined by balancing the patient's individual right to privacy against the competing state interests in the preservation of life, protection of third

Mark Siegler, M.D., is professor of Medicine and Director of the Center for Clinical Medical Ethics, Pritzker School of Medicine, University of Chicago; **Robert M. Taylor, M.D.,** is a Fellow at the Center for Clinical Medical Ethics.

parties and maintaining the ethical integrity of the medical profession. The court concluded that in the circumstances presented in the Quinlan case, the state's interest should yield to those of the patient.

The court further held that the patient's right to privacy could be exercised on behalf of an incompetent patient by an appropriate surrogate who used "substituted judgment," a judgment of what the patient herself would have wanted if she were able to speak on her own behalf. The court appointed Joseph Quinlan to make decisions for his incompetent daughter. The court concluded that health care decisions "should be controlled primarily within the patient-doctor-family relationship" and should generally be free of unwarranted judicial intervention.

Thus, one important part of the Quinlan story has to do with the legal procedures of clinical decision-making. Focusing on this aspect of the story, we can learn about patients' rights to privacy, about the use of substituted judgment for incompetent patients, about the importance of living wills and other advance directives and about procedures for deciding to withhold or withdraw medical treatments.

In this regard, the Quinlan case was a watershed in the ethical and legal debates about the treatment of permanently unconscious patients and about the rights of surrogates to make decisions for incompetent patients. The Quinlan case produced the first judicial ruling in the United States to permit the removal of life-sustaining medical treatment from a permanently incompetent patient. Prior to the Quinlan case, discussions about such decisions were carried on primarily in clinical and academic settings; since 1976, they have become part of the public discourse.

The legal side is an important part of the Quinlan story, but it is not the whole story. The other part of the story is less well known. For understandable reasons, the Quinlan family has chosen to keep private much of this other story. We refer here to the events that followed Mr. Quinlan's decision to have his daughter's ventilator discontinued. Ms. Quinlan survived almost ten more years. During that time, she must have received extraordinary nursing and supportive care, and as far as we know, she continued to be attended by her family.

If the first story of legal procedures teaches us about individual rights, then the largely untold story of the subsequent ten years of support should teach us lessons about the medical and nursing functions of caring not only for individuals who are permanently unconscious like Ms. Quinlan, but also for those who are handicapped, chronically ill, disabled or cognitively impaired. Even though neither cure nor functional improvement was ever possible for Ms. Quinlan, the supportive care and compassion she received reflect many of the traditional goals and ideals of medicine.

What are some of the lessons we learn from this side of the story, the story of ten years of care?

First, we learn something of the standard of care for profoundly neurologically-impaired individuals. The Quinlan case alerted the public and the medical profession to the difficult problem of people who are permanently unconscious. Some ethicists have responded to this problem by proposing rules and laws that might free them from legal responsibility and moral anguish by considering permanently unconscious patients as if they were dead. But there is every reason to agonize over these difficult life and death decisions. As a society, and as a profession, we must continue discussions about what our obligations are to such neurologically devastated individuals in our society. And we must recognize that limiting our obligations to permanently unconscious patients may be used as a justification for limiting our obligations to other severely disabled members of our society. The Quinlan case demonstrates that those who make difficult and wrenching proxy decisions for incompetent loved ones—including even the withdrawal of potentially life-sustaining interventions—can remain committed to the impaired person and can refrain from abandoning them.

The case also shows that families and guardians can be selective in deciding which treatments to withhold or withdraw. Even if they feel it is acceptable to withhold or withdraw a complex technology such as a ventilator or dialysis, they may choose to provide simpler forms of medical care, such as medications or artificial hydration and nutrition. Making such distinctions suggests that proxy decision-makers may withhold or withdraw medical treatments, recognizing that death my result from their decisions, while still not intending or even desiring to cause the patient's death.

Finally, the entire story, taken as a whole, affirms the importance of family and intimacy in medicine. It should be recalled that the case came to trial as a result the refusal of Ms. Quinlan's physician to withdraw her ventilator despite her father's request to do so. As a result of this refusal, Mr. Quinlan sought appointment as his daughter's legal guardian. The trial court agreed with the need for guardianship, but determined that guardianship should be bifurcated: Mr. Quinlan was appointed as "guardian of the trivial property but not the person of his daughter." Another person, a stranger to Ms. Quinlan, was instead appointed as guardian of the person, with the authority to consent to (but not refuse) medical treatments.

The opinion of the New Jersey Supreme Court provided extensive arguments for preferring that Mr. Quinlan be appointed as personal guardian for his daughter, stating: "The character and general suitability of Joseph Quinlan as guardian for his daughter, in ordinary circumstances, could not be doubted." The court also emphasized the agonizing process by which Mr. Quinlan made his fateful decision. Significantly, the court stated that medical deci-

Trends In Health Care, Law & Ethics, Volume 8, Number 1 (Winter, 1993)

sions "should be controlled primarily within the patient-doctor-family relationship" rather than the more limited doctor-patient relationship.

Thus the court affirmed the importance of intimacy and relationships in making decisions for incompetent patients, preferring the decisions of families over those of strangers. The court's opinion should be seen as encouraging physicians to recognize the special intimacy that most patients have with their families,and to give great weight to the family's judgments about the most appropriate care for incompetent patients. The care provided to Ms. Quinlan by her family after the withdrawal of the ventilator confirms the wisdom of the court's decision. Recently-enacted health care surrogacy laws also attest to the Quinlan court's prescience by restoring to families the right to make decisions for family members who are incompetent and have not completed advance directives.

Of course, it would be ideal to remember and learn from both sides of the Quinlan story and to integrate both sides into our clinical practices. We trivialize the legacy of Karen Ann Quinlan if we focus exclusively on the judicial events of 15 years ago. Unquestionably, these events are vitally important as legal milestones, but they are not the whole story, only the prologue. The body of the story consists of the nearly ten years of daily care provided, after the ventilator was discontinued, to Ms. Quinlan by her family members, nurses and aides, and physicians. Although less dramatic than the legal case, this aspect of the story has broader significance since it involves much more common features of medical practice.

The two legacies of Karen Ann Quinlan resemble the two Michelangelo visions of the Pieta: one legacy and vision relates to ordering and representing the relationships of individuals isolated from each other, while the other speaks to providing medical care within the intimacy of a family and community structure where the involved individuals know each other and are close to each other.

Some years ago, when ethicist James Childress and one of us examined various models and metaphors of the doctor-patient relationship (see Endnote), we offered some preliminary thoughts contrasting a medicine of strangers with a medicine of intimates. We noted that in relations among strangers, rules and procedures become very important and control rather than trust is dominant. Strangers, by virtue of being strangers, do not know each other well enough to have mutual trust. Thus, in the absence of intimate knowledge of each other's values, strangers resort to rules and procedures to establish control and to define their responsibilities to each other. In contrast, relations of intimacy imply that all the parties know each other very well and either share important values or at least know which values they do not share. In such relations, formal rules and procedures, backed by sanctions, are rarely necessary; indeed they are often detrimental to such relationships. In relations of intimacy, trust rather than control is dominant. Each person in such a relationship is trusted to act in a way that protects and upholds the values and interests of the others.

We are concerned that too much of what we call medical ethics has focused on the stranger model in which it is never assumed that patients, families and health care professionals share common goals. Moreover, the way that we conceive of a practice—the way we tell its stories—will influence how that practice evolves. That has surely been the case with American medicine. Because we have recently conceived of medicine as a practice of strangers, or of those who are estranged, we have chosen to control and regulate it through legal and ethical rules that attempt to provide at least minimum standards. These have replaced the trust and confidence that previously guided medical relationships. The principal legacy of cases like Karen Ann Quinlan's has been a long line of precedents aimed at defining legally-acceptable standards of medical practice. Predictably, this "legalization" of medicine has created a downward spiral in the relationship between patients and physicians. The process goes as follows: mistrust encourages rules and regulations, which, rather than inspiring more trust, tend to result in increasing suspicion and recriminations between doctor and patient.

It would be helpful to balance this process with another set of stories, particularly stories that reveal the intimate and covenantal relationships of doctors and patients and families, relationships based on promise-keeping, fidelity, virtue, and responsibility.

On his deathbed, Michelangelo said: "I regret that I have not done enough and that I am dying just as I am trying to learn the alphabet of my profession." The profound humility of this great artist should remind us that we in medicine are also just learning the alphabet of our profession, particularly with respect to the implications of the new and awesome technology we have at our disposal. The story of Karen Ann Quinlan provides us with many lessons, not least among them the extraordinary sense of how medicine frequently involves communal concerns of caring and nurturing and supporting, how often it involves "persons in patterns and processes of interdependence," the image revealed in Michelangelo's late Rondinini Pieta.

The perspective implicit in Michelangelo's later Pieta serves as an apt metaphor for the other legacy, the untold story, of Karen Ann Quinlan. This legacy embodies the lessons that we the living can learn from the dying, because so often it is the dying who teach us about caring, comfort, dignity, and respect.

The movement for "death with dignity" arose in response to concerns of the public that medicine was

(Continued on page 38)

Trends In Health Care, Law & Ethics, Volume 8, Number 1 (Winter, 1993)

the values that are important to what we decide with those that we believe are essential to how we decide.

What values should an expanded vision of consent include? In addition to protecting liberty and preserving life, they should include: (1) respect for the patient's human dignity; (2) promoting rational decision-making; (3) encouraging professional self-scrutiny; (4) avoiding deceit and coercion; (5) involving intimate others; and (6) educating the public.[3] These values are integral for a number of reasons. First, meaningful decision- making absent any one of them is unimaginable. Second, their inclusion insures that clinical decision-making occurs democratically. Third, if "pro-choice" and "pro-life" groups agree that we mustn't make medical decisions as the Nazis did, then they should welcome a model of decision-making that includes the principles espoused in the Nuremberg Code.

We should also incorporate into our legal fiction a presumption in favor of family decision-making. Why? Because the truth is that we have more reason to place our faith in believing that the family knows best than in what we know to be a falsehood, namely, that the state knows best. There are enough statutory and other safeguards (including the scrutiny families receive from health-care professionals) to allow us to believe and to ensure that family decision-making works properly.

Finally, we need to go back to the drawing board and explain how and

why surrogate decision-making is tied to what it means to demonstrate respect for persons by analyzing its components in terms of how consent is related to what it means to represent someone. Much of what passes for ethical theorizing is so removed from the political foundations of modern thought that it is little wonder that surrogate decision-making is in its current sorry state.

Conclusion

The only way to insure that decisions about who lives and who dies are suitably made is to see to it that what we mean by consent remains connected to what we mean by democracy. Otherwise, we will never be able to reach a consensus about limiting treatment or agreement about forgoing it. We have unwittingly allowed ourselves to believe that we can decide what ought to be done without paying close attention to how such decisions are made. Unless we wish to forgo our democratic principles, then we must rethink consent.

ENDNOTES:

[1] G Calabresi, P Bobbitt, <u>Tragic Choices</u>. New York:Norton & Co,. 1978.

[2] LR Churchill, RLB Pinkus. The use of anencephalic organs: historical and ethical dimensions. Milbank Quarterly 1990;68:147-169.

[3] J Katz, AM Capron. <u>Catastrophic Diseases: Who Decides What?</u>. New Brunswick, NJ: Transaction Books, 1982.

10.8   Helft P, Siegler M, Lantos J (2000) The Rise and Fall of the Futility Movement. N Engl J Med 343:293–6

Sounding Board

THE RISE AND FALL OF THE FUTILITY MOVEMENT

BETWEEN 1987 and 1996, the concept of "medical futility" was debated in the medical community with a vehemence that few philosophical concepts elicit. Before 1987, the concept was virtually unrecognized. Interest in the concept peaked in 1995, when 134 articles on the topic were published, and has subsequently waned; a Medline search of the key word "futility" for the year 1999 yielded only 31 articles.

The movement to establish a policy on futile treatment was an attempt to convince society that physicians could use their clinical judgment or epidemiologic skills to determine whether a particular treatment would be futile in a particular clinical situation. The idea was that once such a determination had been made, the physician should be allowed to withhold or withdraw the treatment, even over the objections of a competent patient.

In this article, we analyze the rise and fall of the "futility movement." Broadly speaking, discussions of futility can be grouped into four categories: attempts to define medical futility, attempts to resolve the debate with the use of empirical data, discussions that cast the debate as a struggle between the autonomy of patients and the autonomy of physicians, and attempts to develop a process for resolving disputes over futility.

Futile care in hospitals is still very much an issue, yet doctors today are no more empowered to declare a treatment futile unilaterally than they were 15 years ago.

ATTEMPTS TO DEFINE FUTILITY

In articles that attempted to define medical futility,[1-8] the underlying assumption was that a precise definition, if found, could be applied in cases in which the issue arose.

Schneiderman et al. defined futility on the basis of what they claimed were common-sense notions and widely accepted statistical assumptions about acceptable levels of probability, hoping that such a definition would gain broad acceptance.[1] Their definition distinguished between qualitative futility and quantitative futility. According to Schneiderman et al., "when physicians conclude (either through personal experience, experiences shared with colleagues, or consideration of reported empiric data) that in the last 100 cases, a medical treatment has been useless, they should regard that treatment as futile."[1] Qualitatively futile treatment is any treatment that "merely preserves permanent unconsciousness or that fails to end a patient's total dependence on intensive medical care."[1]

Using these definitions, Schneiderman et al. argued that once a treatment has been deemed futile, medical professionals have no ethical obligation to provide it. Their underlying assumption was that just because a treatment has an effect on the patient, it does not necessarily benefit the patient. This distinction between an effect and a benefit became an influential notion. Veatch and Spicer noted, for example, that "in order to establish that care is futile, the clinician must claim that even though the care predictably will have some effect that changes the way that the patient dies, the effect is not beneficial on balance."[9] Critics raised objections and pointed out exceptions to each of the thoughtful definitions offered by Schneiderman et al. and others, and as a result, no consensus was achieved.

Several authors shifted the debate away from definitions of futility to rationing. They believed it would be easier to achieve a consensus about rationing and that it expressed the essential problem — limited medical resources — in a more explicit way.[10-12] Many objected, however, that solutions based on rationing, though potentially viable, addressed a different set of issues. Decisions about futility involved moral judgments about right or good care. Decisions about rationing, in contrast, addressed the question of how limited resources should best be used. Such decisions therefore derived from the principle of distributive justice.

EMPIRICAL ASSESSMENTS OF FUTILITY

Several authors sought consensus by attempting to determine empirically the threshold for a physician's judgment that further treatment would be futile. In various studies, the threshold, expressed in terms of the physician's prediction of the chance of survival, ranged from 0 to 60 percent, although responses tended to cluster around 5 percent.[13-16] Critics argued that the great variability in responses would make consensus on a specific threshold for decisions about futility unlikely.

Other authors tried to develop rigorous quantitative physiologic measures for predicting which patients would die. The most influential attempt was the Acute Physiology and Chronic Health Evaluation (APACHE) system. Three versions of the system were developed with the use of successively larger sample sizes. The third version was reported in 1991. Based on data from 17,440 unselected admissions to intensive care units at 40 hospitals, it proved to be a highly predictive prognostic system.[17] As the authors recognized, however, such systems provided accurate prognostication for groups rather than for individuals, so the information was thought to represent an adjunct to discussions of futility, not a solution to the problem of defining the level at which a treatment might be called futile.

The New England Journal of Medicine

Empirical research has been conducted about the effects on survival of a number of medical treatments, such as cardiopulmonary resuscitation,[18-21] pediatric and neonatal intensive care,[22,23] and intensive care for patients with hematologic cancers,[24] including patients undergoing bone marrow transplantation.[25] Such efforts improved physicians' ability to make accurate predictions about several homogeneous groups of patients. Despite the rigor of these data, however, they could not be used to determine the level of probability that would justify calling a treatment futile. These systems of prognostication also did not take into account the other goals that various treatments might be capable of achieving, such as remaining alive to see loved ones again.

PATIENTS' AUTONOMY VERSUS PHYSICIANS' AUTONOMY

Frustrated that a consensus on futility might never be achieved, another group of authors began to focus on the issue of who has the right — that is, the power — to decide whether medical care is futile. They sought consensus through an examination of the competing interests of patients' autonomy and physicians' autonomy, often taking up the cause of one side or the other. In a 1989 article, "The Illusion of Futility in Clinical Practice,"[26] we argued that no one is better able to make judgments about what is beneficial to patients than patients themselves. The illusion of futility is the mistaken assumption that it is an objective entity. Instead, we suggested, futility must be determined in the light of the subjective views and goals of patients.

Several other authors supported this view.[9,27-29] Veatch, for example, pointed out that, though physicians may be more qualified than patients to make technical judgments about medical treatments, they have no particular expertise in making decisions about such subjective matters as futility.[27] Brett and McCullough wrote, "When a patient requests an intervention that has a finite potential for both benefit and harm, the patient's weighing of various possible strategies and outcomes should take precedence."[28] Youngner argued that all judgments, "except for physiologic futility and an absolute inability to postpone death, also involve value judgments. Physicians may be best suited to frame the choices by describing prognosis and quality of life. Beyond that, they run the risk of 'giving opinions disguised as data.'"[29]

Others have argued in favor of physicians' autonomy — that is, that there are limits to physicians' obligations to provide care that they believe has no benefit.[30-38] Paris and Reardon stated this view most clearly in arguing that complete respect for patients' autonomy reduces the physician from a moral agent to an extension of the patient's wishes.[36] Furthermore, they claimed that offering futile treatment may actually undermine patients' autonomy by making them believe there are choices when there are none. Brody argued that some territory on what he called the "moral island" of futility decisions must be reserved for professional integrity and that society cannot dictate to medical professionals the practice of their integrity.[31]

These arguments for the supremacy of one group's rights over the rights of another group also failed to achieve a consensus on futility. In the end, both sides may have been right: autonomy is not a zero-sum game but a complex network of relational obligations, which can be negotiated in one way under certain circumstances and in another way when the situation changes.

DEVELOPING A PROCESS TO RESOLVE DISPUTES OVER FUTILITY

As it became clear that efforts to achieve a consensus on futility through definition, through empirical data, or through arguments about autonomy had failed, some authors focused on developing a framework for the process of discussing futility with patients and their families.

One proposal, the so-called preventive-ethics approach, was to resolve potential conflicts over futile treatment in advance. According to this approach, primary care physicians must take responsibility for discussing decisions about futile treatment with patients before clinical circumstances call for such decisions.[39,40] The argument is that these discussions will be much more fruitful and less prone to conflict if they take place in the context of a doctor–patient relationship based on trust and at a time when the exigencies of illness do not weigh so heavily on the minds of both patients and their caregivers. This approach is clearly underused.[41] Moreover, patients' views about care before they are sick may be quite different from their views when they are acutely ill.

Other authors have argued that discussions with patients and their families should be initiated as circumstances require. Careful, step-by-step approaches to such discussions have been outlined.[42-46] Most of these approaches recommend assessing the goals of the physician, patient, and family; clarifying information and beginning to negotiate; acknowledging differences in values; and arriving at a compromise, sometimes with the help of ethics committees or the courts.

The arguments in favor of a process-based approach to discussions of futility culminated in the attempt to develop hospital and regional policies for resolving conflicts over futility. Two important examples are the Guidelines for the Use of Intensive Care in Denver[47] and the Houston Citywide Policy on Medical Futility.[48,49] These policies acknowledge the difficulty of trying to reach a consensus on futility and instead outline steps for conflict resolution. Each policy prohibits unilateral decision making by physicians, provides for the use of multidisciplinary

SOUNDING BOARD

committees before resorting to the courts, and leaves open the possibility of transferring the patient's care to another physician or institution, if no resolution can be reached. Such policies conform to the practices of many physicians and institutions, which may explain, in part, the declining interest in an issue that for a time generated heated debate.

CONCLUSIONS

Although the debate over medical futility has waned, the problem of making decisions about treatments that are of minimal benefit has not disappeared. This issue galvanized discussion for several reasons. First, the establishment of other national medical policies, such as the effort to define brain death, gave many hope that a similar effort to define medical futility would lead to changes in policy and practice.[50] Second, advances in medical technology have made it possible to prolong life in the intensive care unit and in the operating room. Youngner argued convincingly that these advances give patients the "illusion of control" over life and death.[51] Third, changes in the financing of health care services probably played a part in the debate over futility, by creating an environment in which the restriction of services was placed at a premium in an attempt to control costs.

The reasons for the declining interest in the issue of medical futility are more elusive. One explanation is that the courts did not recognize the right of physicians to act unilaterally in cases in which they thought care would be futile. As one review concluded, "To date, in nearly every known case in which the patient has sought treatment and the doctor has objected on the grounds that the treatment offers no medical benefit, courts have found in favor of the patient."[30] The notable exception is *Gilgunn* v. *Massachusetts General Hospital.*[52] This case, which involved the death of a comatose 71-year-old woman, ended in a decision by a jury, not by the court. The jury found that the hospital and doctors had not been negligent in issuing a do-not-resuscitate order for the woman over the objection of her daughter. Two aspects of this exceptional decision are relevant. First, it was a retrospective evaluation of a medical decision that had already been made. Second, because it was a jury decision, there is no official record of the reasons for the decision.

We believe the reason the courts have not upheld the right of physicians to make unilateral judgments about the futility of medical care is that the medical community could not agree on underlying principles. As we have discussed, there was no consensus on a specific definition of futility or on an empirical basis for deciding that further care would be futile. Those who argued that the critical issue was autonomy could not agree on whether patients or physicians should have the final say.

The problem of making decisions about futility, as practicing physicians know, persists. Doctors all recognize clinical situations in which intervention will be futile and should tell patients and families when they believe further treatment is futile. In many situations, the term "futile" is an extremely useful descriptor of how the physician feels about the patient's care. However, the fall of the futility movement reminds us that using a descriptive concept as the foundation for a policy is highly problematic and does not relieve us of our obligation to talk to patients and their families and to explain why we think further treatment will have no benefit. The judgment that further treatment would be futile is not a conclusion — a signal that care should cease; instead, it should initiate the difficult task of discussing the situation with the patient. Thus, the most recent attempts to establish a policy in this area have emphasized processes for discussing futility rather than the means of implementing decisions about futility. Talking to patients and their families should remain the focus of our efforts.

PAUL R. HELFT, M.D.
MARK SIEGLER, M.D.
JOHN LANTOS, M.D.
University of Chicago
Chicago, IL 60637

REFERENCES

1. Schneiderman LJ, Jecker NS, Jonsen AR. Medical futility: its meaning and ethical implications. Ann Intern Med 1990;112:949-54.
2. Jecker NS, Schneiderman LJ. Futility and rationing. Am J Med 1992; 92:189-96.
3. Schneiderman LJ, Jecker NS. Futility in practice. Arch Intern Med 1993; 153:437-41.
4. Schneiderman LJ. The futility debate: effective versus beneficial intervention. J Am Geriatr Soc 1994;42:883-6.
5. Callahan D. Necessity, futility, and the good society. J Am Geriatr Soc 1994;42:866-7.
6. Brody BA, Halevy A. Is futility a futile concept? J Med Philos 1995;20: 123-44.
7. Smith GP II. Restructuring the principle of medical futility. J Palliat Care 1995;11:9-16.
8. Jecker NS, Schneiderman LJ. Judging medical futility: an ethical analysis of medical power and responsibility. Camb Q Healthc Ethics 1995;4:23-35.
9. Veatch RM, Spicer CM. Medically futile care: the role of the physician in setting limits. Am J Law Med 1992;18:15-36.
10. Cotler MP, Gregory DR. Futility: is definition the problem? Camb Q Healthc Ethics 1993;2:219-24.
11. Gatter RA Jr, Moskop JC. From futility to triage. J Med Philos 1995; 20:191-205.
12. Truog RD, Brett AS, Frader J. The problem with futility. N Engl J Med 1992;326:1560-4.
13. Solomon MZ. Life and death decisions: physician perspectives and their implications for professional education. Ann Arbor, Mich.: University Microfilms International, 1991.
14. Poses RM, Bekes C, Copare FJ, Scott WE. The answer to "What are my chances, doctor?" depends on whom is asked: prognostic disagreement and inaccuracy for critically ill patients. Crit Care Med 1989;17:827-33.
15. Curtis JR, Park DR, Krone MR, Pearlman RA. Use of the medical futility rationale in do-not-attempt-resuscitation orders. JAMA 1995;273: 124-8.
16. McCrary SV, Swanson JW, Youngner SJ, Perkins HS, Winslade WJ. Physicians' quantitative assessments of medical futility. J Clin Ethics 1994; 5:100-5.
17. Knaus WA, Wagner DP, Draper EA, et al. The APACHE III prognostic system: risk prediction of hospital mortality for critically ill hospitalized adults. Chest 1991;100:1619-36.

The New England Journal of Medicine

18. Bedell SE, Delbanco TL, Cook EF, Epstein FH. Survival after cardio-pulmonary resuscitation in the hospital. N Engl J Med 1983;309:569-76.

19. Kellermann AL, Staves DR, Hackman BB. In-hospital resuscitation following unsuccessful prehospital advanced cardiac life support: "heroic efforts" or an exercise in futility? Ann Emerg Med 1988;17:589-94.

20. Faber-Langendoen K. Resuscitation of patients with metastatic cancer: is transient benefit still futile? Arch Intern Med 1991;151:235-9.

21. Vitelli CE, Cooper K, Rogatko A, Brennan MF. Cardiopulmonary resuscitation and the patient with cancer. J Clin Oncol 1991;9:111-5.

22. Tilford JM, Fiser DH. Futile care in the pediatric intensive care unit: ethical and economic considerations. J Pediatr 1996;128:725-7.

23. Meadow W, Katznelson J, Rosen T, Lantos J. Putting futility to use in the NICU: ethical implications of non-survival after CPR in very low-birth-weight infants. Acta Paediatr 1995;84:589-92.

24. Schuster DP, Marion JM. Precedents for meaningful recovery during treatment in a medical intensive care unit: outcomes in patients with hematologic malignancy. Am J Med 1983;75:402-8.

25. Rubenfeld GD, Crawford SW. Withdrawing life support from mechanically ventilated recipients of bone marrow transplants: a case for evidence-based guidelines. Ann Intern Med 1996;125:625-33.

26. Lantos JD, Singer PA, Walker RM, et al. The illusion of futility in clinical practice. Am J Med 1989;87:81-4.

27. Veatch RM. Why physicians cannot determine if care is futile. J Am Geriatr Soc 1994;42:871-4.

28. Brett AS, McCullough LB. When patients request specific interventions: defining the limits of the physician's obligation. N Engl J Med 1986; 315:1347-51.

29. Youngner SJ. Who defines futility? JAMA 1988;260:2094-5.

30. Daar JF. Medical futility and implications for physician autonomy. Am J Law Med 1995;21:221-40.

31. Brody H. The physician's role in determining futility. J Am Geriatr Soc 1994;42:875-8.

32. Tomlinson T, Brody H. Futility and the ethics of resuscitation. JAMA 1990;264:1276-80.

33. Johnson DH. Helga Wanglie revisited: medical futility and the limits of autonomy. Camb Q Healthc Ethics 1993;2:161-70.

34. Emson HE. Rights, duties, and the limits of autonomy. Camb Q Healthc Ethics 1995;4:7-11.

35. Paris JJ, Schreiber MD, Statter M, Arensman R, Siegler M. Beyond autonomy — physicians' refusal to use life-prolonging extracorporeal membrane oxygenation. N Engl J Med 1993;329:354-7.

36. Paris JJ, Reardon FE. Physician refusal of requests for futile or ineffective interventions. Camb Q Healthc Ethics 1992;1:127-34.

37. Layson RT, McConnell T. Must consent always be obtained for a do-not-resuscitate order? Arch Intern Med 1996;156:2617-20.

38. Jecker NS. Is refusal of futile treatment unjustified paternalism? J Clin Ethics 1995;6:133-7.

39. Wear S, Logue G. The problem of medically futile treatment: falling back on a preventive ethics approach. J Clin Ethics 1995;6:138-48.

40. Doukas DJ, McCullough LB. A preventive ethics approach to counseling patients about clinical futility in the primary care setting. Arch Fam Med 1996;5:589-92.

41. The SUPPORT Principal Investigators. A controlled trial to improve care for seriously ill hospitalized patients: the study to understand prognoses and preferences for outcomes and risks of treatments (SUPPORT). JAMA 1995;274:1591-8. [Erratum, JAMA 1996;275:1232.]

42. Zawacki BE. The "futility debate" and the management of Gordian knots. J Clin Ethics 1995;6:112-27.

43. Truog RD. Progress in the futility debate. J Clin Ethics 1995;6:128-32.

44. Tong R. Towards a just, courageous, and honest resolution of the futility debate. J Med Philos 1995;20:165-89.

45. Youngner SJ. Medical futility. Crit Care Clin 1996;12:165-78.

46. Prendergast TJ. Resolving conflicts surrounding end-of-life care. New Horiz 1997;5:62-71.

47. Murphy DJ, Barbour E. GUIDe (Guidelines for the Use of Intensive Care in Denver): a community effort to define futile and inappropriate care. New Horiz 1994;2:326-31.

48. Halevy A, Brody BA. A multi-institution collaborative policy on medical futility. JAMA 1996;276:571-4.

49. The Council on Ethical and Judicial Affairs, American Medical Association. Medical futility in end-of-life care: report of the Council on Ethical and Judicial Affairs. JAMA 1999;281:937-41.

50. Cranford RE. Medical futility: transforming a clinical concept into legal and social policies. J Am Geriatr Soc 1994;42:894-8.

51. Youngner SJ. Applying futility: saying no is not enough. J Am Geriatr Soc 1994;42:887-9.

52. Gilgunn v. Massachusetts General Hospital. Mass. Sup. Ct., April 21, 1995. (No. 92-4820.)

©2000, Massachusetts Medical Society.

Clinical Innovation

Laura Weiss Roberts and Mark Siegler

Abstract

This chapter contains reprinted works from Dr. Mark Siegler focusing on the application of clinical medical ethics to various clinical innovations and advancements throughout the previous three decades. The included works identify the ethical issues facing physicians in clinical cases that involve growth hormone therapy, living organ donations, and patients with HIV. The application of clinical medical ethics to these topics provides physicians with insight into the benefits and risks associated with these and other related procedures. The works in this chapter are reprinted with permission.

L.W. Roberts, MD, MA (✉)
Department of Psychiatry and Behavioral Sciences, Stanford
University School of Medicine, Stanford, CA, USA
e-mail: robertsl@stanford.edu

M. Siegler, MD
Bucksbaum Institute for Clinical Excellence, MacLean Center for
Clinical Medical Ethics, University of Chicago, Pritzker School of
Medicine, Chicago, IL, USA

© Springer International Publishing AG 2017
L.W. Roberts, M. Siegler (eds.), *Clinical Medical Ethics*, DOI 10.1007/978-3-319-53875-4_11

11.1 Lantos JD, Siegler M, Cuttler L (1989) Ethical Issues in Growth Hormone Therapy. JAMA 261:1020–4

Special Communication ▰

Ethical Issues in Growth Hormone Therapy

John Lantos, MD; Mark Siegler, MD; Leona Cuttler, MD

Pediatricians face clinical and ethical dilemmas about therapy to augment growth in short children who do not meet classic criteria for growth hormone (GH) deficiency. Biologic norms of health are unhelpful because of the uncertain relationship between stature, GH secretion, health, and disease. Instead, we suggest that GH therapy be evaluated from the perspective of cultural norms. We compare GH therapy for short normal children with currently accepted therapies for non–life-threatening pediatric conditions such as well-child care, cosmetic therapy, treatment of psychological problems, and invasive outpatient therapy for chronic conditions. Based on this analysis, we argue that the burdens of therapy, the uncertainty about long-term risks and benefits, the unclear therapeutic end point, and the implications for child health policy place routine GH therapy for children without documented deficiency of GH secretion outside current pediatric ethical norms. Such therapy is properly administered within a comprehensive clinical research protocol.

(*JAMA* 1989;461:1020-1024)

THE ABILITY to produce synthetic growth hormone (GH) by recombinant DNA technology has enabled the manufacture of GH in potentially unlimited quantities.[1] This has greatly facilitated the treatment of GH-deficient children.[2,3] Synthetic GH is currently approved only for the treatment of growth failure due to a lack of adequate endogenous GH, but it has also been used to treat short children who are not classically GH deficient. Recent reports[4-6] indicate that GH therapy may augment linear growth in these children, although the efficacy of GH in changing the final adult height of children without GH deficiency is not known.[7,8] Nevertheless, the use of such therapy is of great interest to companies that manufacture GH,[9] to parents of short children (*New York Times*, Feb 10, 1987, p 19),[10] and to physicians.

Physicians who consider using GH

therapy for non–GH-deficient children, however, confront intertwined clinical and ethical dilemmas.[11,12] The clinical dilemmas involve questions of efficacy and safety, ie, who will grow in response to GH and what are the risks of such therapy. The ethical issues concern whether medical intervention for short non–GH-deficient children is justified, even if it is safe and effective. Should GH therapy for short non–GH-deficient children be accepted as an attempt to maximize a child's physical potential and to prevent psychosocial sequelae that may be associated with short stature?[13,14] Alternatively, should short stature be considered a normal human variation for which treatment represents unwarranted tampering with nature?[15]

Because of the potential magnitude of the problem, physicians' decisions about the treatment of short stature will have far-reaching implications for society. Of the 3 million children born in the United States annually, 90 000 will, by definition, be below the third percentile for height. These children may be labeled as having short stature and may be candidates for GH treatment. Growth hormone currently costs about $20 000 per year for a 30-kg child and a

treatment course may last five years. If all children who are less than the third percentile for height receive a five-year course of GH therapy, GH for height augmentation therapy will cost at least $8 billion to $10 billion per year. If not all children are to be treated, physicians will need criteria for determining whom to treat in such a way as to equitably distribute both the benefits and the risks of GH therapy.

Both clinical and ethical issues concerning GH treatment will be important in the ultimate formation of physicians' prescribing habits. These intertwined issues require general discussion at this time. In this article, we will consider GH therapy for non–GH-deficient but otherwise healthy short children. We will focus on recent controversies about the diagnosis of GH deficiency, the known risks and benefits of GH therapy, and the ethical implications of decisions regarding GH treatment. We will examine these issues within the framework of two established philosophic perspectives that have been used to evaluate controversial ethical issues in medicine.

In the first perspective, the major goal for medicine is the preservation of health. Health is perceived as a biologic norm, "of bodily excellence or fitness, relative to each species and to some extent to individuals, recognizable if not definable, and to some extent attainable."[16] Disease, in this perspective, is simply a deviation from the biologic norm of health. Medical interventions are ethically acceptable only if they preserve health or restore it by preventing or treating a disease or illness. By this approach, if a child with short stature is shown to deviate from a biologic norm and thus to have a disease, and if treatment would restore health, then treatment would be acceptable. We will discuss the practical controversies and theoretical difficulties in classifying ei-

From the Center for Clinical Medical Ethics (Drs Lantos and Siegler), the Sections of Pediatric Chronic Disease (Dr Lantos) and Pediatric Endocrinology (Dr Cuttler), Department of Pediatrics, and the Section of General Medicine (Dr Siegler), University of Chicago Pritzker School of Medicine.
Reprint requests to Department of Pediatrics, University of Chicago Pritzker School of Medicine, 5841 S Maryland Ave, Chicago, IL 60637 (Dr Cuttler).

ther subtle abnormalities of GH secretion or relative short stature as diseases; in our opinion, these limit the applicability of this philosophic model.

The second approach accepts that medicine has many goals, defined not only by biologic norms but also by personal and cultural values. In this approach, the ethical acceptability of a treatment is determined by a negotiation process between a physician and a competent patient.[17] This negotiation considers the goals, efficacy, risks, and burdens of treatment.[18] The negotiation proceeds within boundaries derived from societal expectations and the moral norms of the medical profession. Because children are not competent, application of this approach to the question of GH therapy for non–GH-deficient short children, or to any pediatric therapy, must proceed by analogy. We must ask whether analogous treatments are considered ethically acceptable by parents and pediatricians.

GROWTH HORMONE AND BIOLOGIC NORMS OF HEALTH
When Is GH Deficiency a Disease?

In 1985, GH produced by recombinant DNA technology was approved by the Food and Drug Administration for the long-term treatment of children who have growth failure due to a lack of adequate endogenous GH secretion.[19] If classic criteria for diagnosing GH deficiency were applied, this would appear to limit GH distribution to those children with a subnormal growth rate (typically <4 to 5 cm/y) and peak GH levels of less than 7 or less than 10 μg/L after provocative testing.[12,20,21] The situation has, however, become much more complex. The Food and Drug Administration's criteria blend two indications—the morphological abnormality of growth failure and the biochemical abnormality of inadequate growth hormone—that are both relative rather than absolute. As a result, delineating the point at which variations become diseases requires both sophisticated biochemical assays and delicate clinical judgments.

Although there is widespread agreement about the criteria for diagnosing classic GH deficiency, endocrinologists question whether these criteria delineate the entire spectrum of GH-deficient states. For example, there is disagreement about what constitutes a normal peak GH response to provocative pharmacologic stimuli in the gray zone between 7 and 10 μg/L[21,22] and about the implications of substantial systematic variation between laboratory methods for determining GH levels.[21,23] More difficult questions are be-

ing asked about whether the GH response to any provocative stimulus can adequately assess spontaneous GH secretion.[24,25]

In response to the latter concern, many researchers and pediatric endocrinologists have begun to use serial measurements of circulating GH (every 20 to 30 minutes for 12 to 24 hours) to assess spontaneous GH secretory reserve. These studies provide a powerful means of assessing GH secretion and have led to an expanded conception of the disease GH deficiency to include disorders of GH secretion as well as those of GH production.

The usefulness and clinical applicability of spontaneous GH secretion studies are, however, uncertain. Some data suggest that tests of spontaneous GH secretion are neither more sensitive nor more specific than provocative testing.[26] Furthermore, interpretation of the results of these tests for the individual child is difficult, in part because there are no universally accepted norms and also because methods of measurement and data analysis (ie, continuous vs intermittent blood sampling and average GH secretion vs GH pulse analysis) remain controversial.[27-30] It has recently been suggested that the variability in GH levels reflects the fact that the distribution of spontaneous GH secretion is a continuum.[31] If this is so, then the division between normal children and those with GH neurosecretory disorders may be quite arbitrary and therapy would not be ethically justifiable according to the model of medicine based on biologic norms.

Because of the uncertainty about the criteria for a diagnosis of GHD, some endocrinologists have suggested that neither provocative tests nor tests of spontaneous GH secretion are adequate and that the ultimate test of GH deficiency is an increased growth velocity in response to a therapeutic trial of GH.[12,32] There are, however, potential problems with this approach. Criteria defining a significant improvement in growth velocity have not been systematically established, and the precise relationship between short-term growth velocity and long-term improvement in growth potential is uncertain. A therapeutic trial of GH may trade the uncertainties of borderline GH responses to provocative stimuli for the uncertainties of borderline alterations of growth velocity. Furthermore, an increase in growth rate in response to GH may be dose dependent[33] and may not necessarily constitute evidence of GH deficiency, since children with GH excess due to GH-secreting pituitary adenomas show accelerated linear growth.

Research into the range of GH disorders will likely result in improved methods for the diagnosis of subtle disorders of GH secretion. New groups of children with previously unrecognized forms of GH dysfunction are likely to emerge from such research. We may develop a new "gold standard" for diagnosing GH deficiency. Nevertheless, disagreement may persist about whether children with borderline test results really have a disease. In addition, there will likely be short children with no evidence of disordered GH secretion. We must therefore consider the propriety of GH supplementation for short children who do not appear to have GH deficiency.

Is Short Stature a Disease?

It may be argued that children with short stature, regardless of etiology, have a biologic abnormality and should be treated, especially when predicted adult height will be below the third percentile and parental wishes for treatment are strong. The argument for treating such children rests on the association between short stature and psychosocial morbidity[13,14,34] and on the implicit assumption that GH-induced growth will relieve the psychosocial morbidity. There are two problems with this approach. First, the data showing the relationship between short stature and psychosocial problems are inadequate to define the population of short non–GH-deficient children at risk for problems or to determine the efficacy of GH therapy in alleviating those problems. Second, the degree of short stature required to label a child as having a disease and the end point of GH therapy, either for an individual or for children in general, are both undefined.

The evidence for an association between short stature and psychosocial morbidity is based either on studies of GH-deficient children[35,36] or on population studies.[37,38] Growth hormone–deficient children with extreme short stature may suffer social isolation and are at risk for depression and low self-esteem.[39] The population of non–GH-deficient children with low-normal height does not appear to have psychosocial problems, although few studies of this population have been reported.[36,40]

It is not clear to what extent GH relieves psychosocial problems in GH-deficient children. Some studies suggest that it does not.[41] There is currently no evidence that GH treatment alleviates psychosocial morbidity in non–GH-deficient short children, even if it increases height. The use of GH for an otherwise normal short child might itself result in psychosocial morbidity, in the form of stigmatization, reinforcing self-perception as abnormal, and subsequent loss of self-esteem. If GH fails to increase height, both the child and parents may suffer from feelings of failure.[42]

Questions about the efficacy of GH in relieving short stature–associated psychosocial morbidity could be addressed by large randomized, placebo-controlled trials, with extensive follow-up. Such studies, which are under way in some populations, raise a different set of ethical issues. Since GH is widely available, few parents who wanted treatment for their short children would consent to participation in a study in which their child might receive a placebo. Endocrinologists might have difficulty maintaining a state of equipoise, or genuine uncertainty about the therapeutic merits of GH vs a placebo, which is an ethical prerequirement for physician participation in research.[43] In addition, it will be difficult to perform a study of the size and duration necessary to detect subtle improvements or rare side effects. Thus, for the foreseeable future, there will be uncertainty about the efficacy of GH as a treatment for the psychosocial sequelae of short stature.

Even if we knew that GH could increase adult height and mitigate the psychosocial morbidity associated with short stature, questions would arise about its proper use. What should be the end point of therapy be? Short stature is relative and can only be defined in relation to the rest of the population. Treatment of all children below the fifth percentile for height, even if it were effective, would not eliminate short stature. It would only create a new population of relatively short children. Should these children also be treated? If untreated, would they not be at risk for the same psychosocial problems as "naturally" short children?

If we recommend treatment for all short children, we face problems of distributive justice. If GH is made available to all short children without regard to ability to pay, it may divert funding from other child health needs. If it is allocated based on ability to pay, then any morbidity associated with short stature will disproportionately affect poor children. Pediatricians cannot remedy all the inequalities in society, but we should not advocate a treatment that selectively allocates morbidity to poor children.

Furthermore, short stature is, to some extent, a natural variation, and the associated psychosocial morbidity results from cultural prejudice.[44] We do not usually call prejudice-induced conditions, which confer cultural disadvantages but have no intrinsic negative health effects, diseases.

These considerations highlight the potential problems of a model that defines short stature as a disease. They also force our inquiry into a new area. With the exception of growth failure that is clearly related to severe GH deficiency, we cannot unambiguously define a population that has a "disease" based either on biochemical tests for GH or on height. An alternative approach to this problem is to examine the ethical norms of pediatric practice and consider whether GH therapy for non–GH-deficient short children fits those norms.

GROWTH HORMONE, CULTURAL VALUES, AND THE NORMS OF PEDIATRICS

Physicians can evaluate the ethical acceptability of new therapies by comparing them with analogous established therapies and, by inference, with currently accepted ethical standards of practice. Growth hormone therapy for non–GH-deficient but otherwise healthy short children should not be compared with the treatment of life-threatening disease, but with pediatric treatments given to children with problems that are not life threatening. Three areas of pediatrics deal with such problems. First, the area of preventive well-child care: if GH therapy were begun at the first evidence of slow growth to prevent later problems, it could be considered a form of preventive well-child care. Second, GH therapy might be compared with treatments designed to alleviate psychosocial problems or improve school performance. A third approach may consider GH treatment as a cosmetic therapy, which should be evaluated in reference to other cosmetic therapies. We will compare GH with treatments now used in each of these areas.

GH Therapy as a Form of Preventive Well-Child Care

Pediatricians implicitly evaluate three aspects of preventive treatments to determine whether they are ethically acceptable. First, the benefits must be high and the risks low. When the risk of serious morbidity approaches 1/300 000, as in the case of pertussis vaccine, the treatment has been considered justified only because it prevents a life-threatening disease.[45] Second, the burdens of treatment, or the subjective assessment by the patient of the suffering involved in complying with treatment, must be low. In well-child care, routine immunization, requiring seven injections over five years, is probably the most burdensome routine procedure. Finally, while well-child care is elective, it is considered so clearly beneficial that

it is recommended for all children.

The risks and benefits of GH therapy are currently not known precisely. The short-term risks include slipped capital femoral epiphysis and hypothyroidism in children with classic GH deficiency and autoantibodies to GH, which may or may not affect the activity of GH.[32,46] The long-term risks are currently not known. Excessive GH may contribute to diabetes, hypertension, and an increased incidence of atherosclerotic heart disease.[11,46] A recent report[47] suggests an increased incidence of leukemia in patients treated with GH, but the existence of such an association remains unproved.[48,49] With any new therapy, there is always the risk of late unforeseen complications, such as the vaginal carcinomas that occurred in some children of mothers treated with diethylstilbestrol[50] or the thyroid cancer that occurred in children who received tonsillar irradiation for thymic enlargement or tonsillitis.[51,52] The benefits of GH in altering adult height or improving psychosocial adaptation will not be known for some time. In addition, the burden of a therapy that involves parenteral injections three to seven times per week is relatively high. These considerations, in our judgment, place GH therapy outside current norms for preventive well-child care.

GH Therapy as a Treatment for Psychosocial Problems

Although somewhat controversial among both physicians[53,54] and parents,[55,56] there is precedent for using drug therapy to treat children with abnormal behavior or poor school performance.[57] Such interventions may be likened to GH therapy, since both therapies could use psychosocial criteria, such as school performance, as one measure of benefit.[58,59] Therapies for psychosocial problems involve only oral medication and would probably be unacceptable to parents and pediatricians if they required parenteral therapy. Even so, the ratio of benefits to burdens in these therapies tips in favor of treatment only for children who have psychosocial symptoms, not children who are merely at risk for problems but have not shown any symptoms.

These medical therapies also differ from GH in that they are clearly given to produce a change in behavior. With GH, the outcome usually measured is height. If GH therapy is to be justified by its beneficial effect on school performance or psychosocial adjustment, then these should be the outcomes measured in deciding whether treatment is effective. Until studies show that GH improves psychosocial adjustment in short non–GH-deficient children, GH use cannot be justified by claiming that it provides psychosocial benefits.

GH Therapy as a Form of Cosmetic Therapy

There are precedents for using cosmetic therapies for children for social reasons, to augment natural beauty in a child without major deformities, or to repair major deformities.

Onetime surgical procedures, like ear piercing or circumcision, may be performed for social reasons. Because of the duration of treatment and the potential long-term risks, GH therapy is less acceptable than a onetime surgical intervention.

Sustained or more burdensome interventions are sometimes given to augment beauty. Such therapies, including orthodontic procedures for dental alignment or comedonal extractions for acne, are usually undertaken in adolescent patients who can participate in the treatment decisions. If the subjective burden of daily GH injections is considered comparable to the burden of orthodontia, then GH therapy might be considered acceptable for children old enough to consent to treatment.

Some congenital anomalies are considered so deforming that risky and burdensome treatment is ethically acceptable, even for children too young to consent. Surgery for cleft lip, for example, is generally viewed as appropriate and is initiated soon after birth. For most pediatricians, the treatment of classic GH deficiency is acceptable precisely because the short stature is so severe that it is considered a major deformity and because the efficacy is proved.

Other anomalies are more controversial. Surgery to alter the minor stigmata of congenital disease, such as the facies or tongue size of children with Down syndrome, is sometimes performed.[60] Many physicians feel that the burdens of such surgery outweigh the benefits,[61] but others either recommend such therapy or accede to parental demands. Most pediatricians would view cosmetic surgery to alter the shape of a preadolescent child's nose unacceptable, since the anomaly would not be considered a major deformity and the child would be unable to understand the risks and benefits of treatment well enough to give valid informed consent. Similarly, GH therapy for a child of normal height to make him or her a better basketball player would be unacceptable, because the child has no deformity.

Judgments about the acceptability of such cosmetic therapies are largely dependent on judgments about the severity of the deformity to be treated. Criteria for deciding when short stature is sufficiently deforming to warrant burdensome and potentially risky therapy are needed to formulate rational and ethically acceptable criteria for GH therapy. Such criteria might be easier to develop if data were available on the psychosocial benefits of cosmetic alterations, such as data that have recently been reported regarding rhinoplasty.[62]

GH Therapy Compared With Equally Burdensome Treatments

Another way to analyze whether GH therapy fits into the ethical norms of pediatric practice is to describe the sorts of problems for which comparably burdensome therapies are considered acceptable. Diabetic children and some infants with congenital adrenal hyperplasia require regular injections. Children with sickle-cell disease who have suffered strokes may be given monthly blood transfusions. Children with short-gut syndrome may be treated with home hyperalimentation and children with cancer or osteomyelitis may be given parenteral outpatient therapy. In all of these cases, the only alternatives to therapy are prolonged hospitalization or serious morbidity or mortality. The seriousness of the consequences of untreated disease in these cases justifies the burdens of therapy. There is little precedent in pediatrics for the use of long-term parenteral injections for non–life-threatening conditions.

SUGGESTIONS FOR THERAPEUTIC USE OF GH

Physicians who must decide whether to recommend GH therapy for non–GH-deficient patients must deal with three separate issues. First, the risks and benefits are unknown. Second, currently available diagnostic techniques do not always unambiguously delimit a population with a disease. Third, the treatment goal requires a method of treatment that is relatively burdensome. The availability of GH and the strength of parental demands for height augmentation therapy ensure that decisions about whom to treat will be required before definitive risk-benefit calculations or prognostic categories can be established. Although absolute criteria for GH use are not possible, the following principles emerge from analysis of the ethical issues in GH therapy.

At this time, we would consider GH therapy ethically acceptable treatment for children who have classically defined GH deficiency. These children have a biochemical abnormality that causes short stature so severe that it predictably causes psychosocial morbidity. For such children, the benefits of therapy clearly outweigh the burdens of therapy. In addition, the efficacy of GH in increasing adult height for these children is established.

For children who are relatively short but have no documented GH abnormality, normal growth velocity, and predicted adult height above the fifth percentile, we suggest that GH therapy is not routinely indicated. This condition does not fit any current concept of a disease state, there is no good evidence that such children are at risk for psychosocial morbidity, and their appearance would not be so abnormal that burdensome and potentially risky cosmetic therapy would be justified.

Perhaps the thorniest issues concern children without classic evidence of GH deficiency but with marginal growth velocity and subnormal predicted adult height. This group includes children with idiopathic short stature. These children do not have a clear biochemical abnormality and it is not clear whether their stature will predictably cause psychosocial morbidity. For such children, the risks and benefits of GH treatment are unknown and the end point of therapy is unclear. We believe that GH treatment for these children should not be accepted as routine at this time.

Research should focus on this third group of children. Such research should try to determine which subgroups of these children show increased final adult height in response to GH therapy. Research should also focus on the psychosocial aspects of treatment, including the morbidity associated with short stature, the degree to which GH can alleviate this morbidity, and the morbidity associated with GH therapy. If no psychosocial benefit accrues from GH therapy, then it should be acknowledged as a form of cosmetic therapy, rather than a treatment for a disease, and pediatricans should discourage its use.

These recommendations reflect an attempt to balance the facts as they are now known about GH deficiency and short stature, the benefits and burdens of GH therapy, and the ethical norms of pediatrics. Future developments might tip the balance of considerations a different way. If the benefits of GH therapy were more reliably documented, or the physical and economic burdens of therapy were lower, or the data showing minimal risks from GH therapy were firmer, then the arguments against therapy would weaken. There would then be more room for parental discretion in deciding whether GH therapy was truly in a child's best interest. Parental wishes might reflect cultural and ethnic attitudes or sexual stereotypes, as they do now for decisions about other cosmetic interventions.

The GH dilemma may be paradigmatic for a type of challenge that pediatricians will face frequently in the near future. New therapies may be directed not at health maintenance or disease prevention but at the augmentation of health, beauty, or well-being. Pediatricians must decide when and whether these therapies are ethically acceptable. Such decisions should reflect both biologic norms of health and disease and cultural values and the ethical norms of the profession. If pediatricians do not respond to these dilemmas thoughtfully, carefully, and forcefully, other decision makers, whose decisions may reflect political, social, or market forces, may then respond in ways that do not reflect the best interests of children.

This investigation was supported in part by Public Health Service Clinical Research Center Clinical Associate Physician Award RR00055, Public Health Service grant DK-40221, and a Basil O'Connor Award of the March of Dimes Defect Foundation to Dr Cuttler and by a grant from the Max Goldenberg Foundation to Dr Lantos. The Center for Clinical Medical Ethics is supported by grants from the Henry J. Kaiser Family Foundation, the Pew Memorial Trusts, and the Andrew W. Mellon Foundation.

References

1. Glasbrenner K: Technology spurt resolves growth hormone problem, ends shortage. *JAMA* 1986;255:581-584, 587.
2. Milner RDG: Growth hormone 1985. *Br Med J* 1985;291:1593-1594.
3. Fryklund LM, Bierich JR, Ranke MB: Recombinant human growth hormone. *Clin Endocrinol Metab* 1986;15:511-535.
4. Gertner JM, Genel M, Gianfredi SP, et al: Prospective clinical trial of human growth hormone in short children without growth hormone deficiency. *J Pediatr* 1984;104:172-176.
5. Van Vliet G, Styne DM, Kaplan SL, et al: Growth hormone treatment for short stature. *N Engl J Med* 1983;309:1016-1022.
6. Albertsson-Wikland K: Growth hormone treatment in short children. *Acta Paediatr Scand Suppl* 1986;325:64-70.
7. Underwood LE: Growth hormone treatment for short children. *Pediatrics* 1984;104:237-239.
8. Dean HJ, Friesen HG: Growth hormone therapy in Canada: End of one era and beginning of another. *Can Med Assoc J* 1986;135:297-301.
9. Kolata G: New growth industry in human growth hormone. *Science* 1986;236:22-24.
10. Benjamin M, Muyskens J, Saenger P: Short children, anxious parents: Is growth hormone the answer? *Hastings Cent Rep* 1984;14(April):5-9.
11. Ad Hoc Committee on Growth Hormone Usage, The Lawson Wilkens Pediatric Endocrine Society, and Committee on Drugs: Growth hormone in the treatment of children with short stature. *Pediatrics* 1983;72:891-894.
12. Bercu BB: Growth hormone treatment and the short child: To treat or not to treat? *J Pediatr* 1987;110:991-995.
13. Pollitt E, Money J: Studies in the psychology of dwarfism: I. Intelligence quotient and school achievement. *J Pediatr* 1964;63:415-421.
14. Gordon M, Crouthamel C, Post E, et al: Psychosocial aspects of constitutional short stature: Social competence, behavior problems, self-esteem and family functioning. *J Pediatr* 1982;101:477-480.
15. King LS: What is disease? in Caplan AL, Engelhardt HT, McCartney JJ (eds): *Concepts of Health and Disease: Interdisciplinary Perspectives*. Reading, Mass, Addison-Wesley Publishing Co, 1981, pp 107-118.
16. Kass L: The end of medicine and the pursuit of health, in Kass L: *Toward a More Natural Science*. New York, Free Press, 1985, pp 157-186.
17. Siegler M: The doctor-patient encounter and its relationship to theories of health and disease, in Caplan AL, Engelhardt HT, McCartney JJ (eds): *Concepts of Health and Disease: Interdisciplinary Perspectives*. Reading, Mass, Addison-Wesley Publishing Co, 1981, pp 627-644.
18. Siegler M: The doctor-patient accommodation: A central event in clinical medicine. *Ann Intern Med* 1982;142:1899.
19. *Physician's Desk Reference*. Oradell, NJ, Medical Economics Co Inc, 1988, pp 999, 1193.
20. Frasier SD: A review of growth hormone stimulation tests in children. *Pediatrics* 1974;53:929-939.
21. Bercu BB, Shulman D, Root AW, et al: Growth hormone (GH) provocative testing frequently does not reflect endogenous GH secretion. *J Clin Endocrinol Metab* 1986;63:709-716.
22. Schaff-Blass E, Burstein S, Rosenfield RL: Advances in the diagnosis and treatment of short stature, with special reference to the role of growth hormone. *J Pediatr* 1984;104:801-813.
23. Reiter EO, Morris AH, MacGillivray MH, et al: Variable estimates of serum growth hormone concentration by different radioassay systems. *J Clin Endocrinol Metab* 1988;66:68-71.
24. Spiliotis BE, August GP, Hung W, et al: Growth hormone neurosecretory dysfunction: A treatable cause of short stature. *JAMA* 1984;251:2223-2230.
25. Zadik Z, Chalew SA, Raiti S, et al: Do short children secrete insufficient growth hormone? *Pediatrics* 1985;76:355-360.
26. Rose SR, Ross JL, Uriate M, et al: The advantage of measuring stimulated as compared with spontaneous growth hormone levels in the diagnosis of growth hormone deficiency. *N Engl J Med* 1988;319:201-207.
27. Evans WS, Faria ACS, Christiansen E, et al: Impact of intensive venous sampling on characterization of pulsatile GH release. *Am J Physiol* 1987;252:E549-E556.
28. Bercu BB, Diamond FB: Growth hormone neurosecretory dysfunction. *Clin Endocrinol Metab* 1986;15:537-590.
29. Merriam GR: Methods of characterizing episodic hormone secretion, in Crowley WF, Hofler JG (eds): *The Episodic Secretion of Hormones*. New York, Churchill Livingstone Inc, 1987, pp 47-65.
30. Van Cauter E: Estimating false-positive and false-negative errors in analyses of hormone pulsatility. *Am J Physiol* 1988;254:E786-E794.
31. Brook CGD, Hindmarsh PC, Smith PJ: Is growth hormone deficiency a useful diagnosis? *Acta Paediatr Scand Suppl* 1987;331:70-75.
32. Milner RDG: Which children should have growth hormone therapy? *Lancet* 1986;1:483-485.
33. Hindmarsh PC, Brook CGD: Effect of growth hormone on short normal children. *Br Med J* 1987;295:573-577.
34. Meyer-Bahlburg HFL: Psychosocial management of short stature, in Shaffer D, Ehrhardt AA, Greenhill LL (eds): *The Clinical Guide to Child Psychiatry*. New York, Free Press, 1985, pp 110-144.
35. Steinhausen HC, Stahnke N: Psychoendocrinological studies in dwarfed children and adolescents. *Arch Dis Child* 1976;51:778-783.
36. Krims MB: Observations on children who suffer from dwarfism. *Psychiatr Q* 1968;42:430-443.
37. Lee PDK, Rosenfeld RG: Psychosocial correlates of short stature and delayed puberty. *Pediatr Clin North Am* 1987;34:851-863.
38. Wilson DM, Hammer LD, Duncan PM, et al: Growth and intellectual development. *Pediatrics* 1986;78:646-650.
39. Rotnem D, Genel M, Hintz RL, et al: Personality development in children with growth hormone deficiency. *J Am Acad Child Adolesc Psychiatry* 1977;16:412-426.
40. Law CM: The disability of short stature. *Arch Dis Child* 1987;62:855-859.
41. Dean HJ, McTaggart TL, Fish DG, et al: The educational, vocational, and marital status of growth hormone deficient adults treated with growth hormone during childhood. *AJDC* 1985;135:1105-1110.
42. Rotnem D, Cohen D, Hintz R, et al: Psychological sequelae of relative 'treatment failure' for children receiving human growth hormone replacement. *J Am Acad Child Adolesc Psychiatry* 1979;18:505-520.
43. Freedman B: Equipoise and the ethics of clinical research. *N Engl J Med* 1987;317:141-145.
44. Grumbach MM: Growth hormone therapy and the short end of the stick. *N Engl J Med* 1988;319:238-240.
45. Hinman AR, Koplan JP: Pertussis and pertussis vaccine. *JAMA* 1984;251:3109-3113.
46. Underwood LE: Report of the conference on uses and possible abuses of biosynthetic human growth hormone. *N Engl J Med* 1984;311:606-608.
47. Watanabe S, Tsunematsu Y, Fujimoto J, et al: Leukemia in patients treated with growth hormone. *Lancet* 1988;1:1159.
48. Fisher DA, Job JC, Preece M, et al: Response to Watanabe et al, leukemia in patients treated with growth hormone. *Lancet* 1988;1:1159-1160.
49. Gellis SS: On growth hormone and leukemia. *Pediatr Notes* 1988;12:82.
50. Herbst AL, Ulfelder H, Poskanzer DC: Adenocarcinoma of the vagina: Association of maternal stilbestrol therapy with tumor appearance in young women. *N Engl J Med* 1971;284:878-881.
51. Simpson CL, Hemplemann H, Fuller LM: Neoplasia in children treated with x-rays in infancy for thymic enlargement. *Radiology* 1955;64:840-845.
52. Siegler M, Sheldon M: Paying the price of medical progress: Causation, responsibility, and liability for bad outcomes after innovative medical care, in Siegler M, Toulmin S, Zimrig FE, et al (eds): *Medical Innovation and Bad Outcomes: Legal, Social and Ethical Responses*. Ann Arbor, Mich, Health Administration Press, 1987, pp 1-17.
53. Copeland L, Wolraich M, Lindgren S, et al: Pediatricians' reported practices in the assessment and treatment of attention deficit disorders. *J Dev Behav Pediatr* 1987;8:191-197.
54. Cowart VS: The Ritalin controversy: What's made this drug's opponents hyperactive? *JAMA* 1988;259:2521-2523.
55. Summers JA, Caplan PJ: Lay people's attitudes toward drug treatment for behavioral control depend on which disorder and which drug. *Clin Pediatr* 1987;26:258-263.
56. Silver LB: Controversial approaches to treating learning disabilities and attention deficit disorder. *AJDC* 1986;140:1045-1052.
57. Rapport MD, Stoner G, DuPaul GJ, et al: Methylphenidate in hyperactive children: Differential effects of dose on academic, learning, and social behavior. *J Abnorm Child Psychol* 1985;13:227-234.
58. Famular R, Fenton T: The effect of methylphenidate on school grades in children with attention deficit disorder without hyperactivity: A preliminary report. *J Clin Psychiatry* 1987;48:112-114.
59. Wilson DM, Duncan PM, Dornbusch SM, et al: The effects of growth on intellectual function in children and adolescents, in Stabler B, Underwood LE (eds): *Slow Grows the Child: Psychosocial Aspects of Growth Delay*. Hillsdale, Calif, Lawrence Erlbaum Associates, 1986, pp 27-45.
60. Rozner L: Facial plastic surgery for Down's syndrome. *Lancet* 1983;1:245.
61. Gellis SS: Comment on facial plastic surgery for Down's syndrome. *Pediatr Notes* 1983;7:121.
62. Robin AA: Reshaping the psyche: The concurrent improvement in appearance and mental state after rhinoplasty. *Br J Psychiatry* 1988;152:539-543.

11.2   Arnow P, Pottenger L, Stocking C, Siegler M, DeLeeuw H (1989) Orthopedic Surgeons' Attitudes and Practices Concerning Treatment of Patients with HIV Infection. Public Health Reports 104:121–9

Orthopedic Surgeons' Attitudes and Practices Concerning Treatment of Patients with HIV Infection

PAUL M. ARNOW, MD
LAWRENCE A. POTTENGER, MD, PhD,
CAROL B. STOCKING, PhD
MARK SIEGLER, MD
HENRY W. DeLEEUW, MD

Dr. Arnow is Associate Professor of Medicine and Hospital Epidemiologist; Dr. Pottenger is Associate Professor of Surgery; Dr. Stocking is Research Associate and Director of Research at the Center for Clinical Medical Ethics, Department of Medicine; and Dr. Siegler is Professor of Medicine and Director of the Center for Clinical Medical Ethics, Department of Medicine; all of the University of Chicago. Dr. DeLeeuw is Resident, Department of Orthopedic Surgery, University of Pittsburgh.

The paper was presented in part at the Third International Conference on AIDS, Washington, DC, June 1987.

Tearsheet requests to Paul M. Arnow, MD, University of Chicago Medical Center, Department of Medicine, 5841 S. Maryland Ave., Box 11, Chicago, IL 60637.

Synopsis..................................

Concern regarding an occupational risk of acquiring human immunodeficiency virus (HIV) infection may influence surgeons' willingness to operate. A questionnaire survey of all orthopedists in the five cities with the most cases of acquired immunodeficiency syndrome (AIDS) was conducted to assess attitudes and practices. Questionnaires were completed anonymously by 325 of 510 orthopedists. In the previous year, 43 percent had examined or operated on an HIV-infected patient, and at least 90 percent who had had an opportunity to operate on an HIV-infected patient had chosen to do so.

Decisions to operate did not appear to be based on hospital requirements, perceived ethical obligations, or knowledge of HIV transmissibility. Most orthopedists (85 percent) claimed the right to order preoperative HIV testing of high-risk patients, but such testing was ordered infrequently. Although most orthopedists believed they could not be compelled to operate and that ethically they could refuse when their health was threatened, they almost always were willing to treat HIV-infected patients.

THE GROWING PUBLIC HEALTH problem of providing care to those infected with the human immunodeficiency virus (HIV) is increasing the numbers of health care providers concerned about possible occupational risks of becoming infected themselves.

Basic statistics reported by the Centers for Disease Control show that by November 23, 1987, 47,022 cases of acquired immunodeficiency syndrome (AIDS) had been reported (1), and 13,097 of the cases were reported during 1986 (2). It has been estimated that at least 1 million other persons in the country are infected with HIV (3). Cases of AIDS have been reported in all 50 States. By November 1987, 30 States each had reported more than 100 cases (1). As the number of persons infected by HIV increases, more health care workers are being called upon to treat them.

Concern regarding a possible occupational risk of acquiring HIV infection has caused anxiety among health care workers and has engendered a general reluctance to provide direct care to infected patients (4–6). Decisions about rendering treatment to HIV-infected patients may be especially difficult for surgeons. HIV can be transmitted by percutaneous inoculation of blood (7–10), and punctures in gloves that can result in inoculation occur frequently during surgery (11,12). Moreover, the occupational risk of acquiring hepatitis B infection, which is transmitted in hospitals by the same route as HIV, is higher for surgeons than for most other health care workers (13,14). Attitudes of surgeons toward the occupational risk of HIV infection appear particularly important because of the highly specialized services that surgeons provide and their leadership role in many hospitals.

'When respondents were asked how transmissible they believed HIV to be by accidental needlestick, 9 percent reported·that they thought it to be highly transmissible, 26 percent thought it to be moderately transmissible, 30 percent correctly reported that HIV has very low transmissibility, and 34 percent were not sure.'

As part of a hospital effort to develop policies concerning management of patients with HIV infection, we surveyed surgeons in other cities to learn their attitudes and practices. We chose orthopedic surgeons because a high proportion of their patients are young and middle-aged men, and because orthopedic surgeons are at substantial risk of skin puncture injuries during operative procedures.

Methods

Questionnaires were mailed to all orthopedists in the 1985 American Academy of Orthopedic Surgery (AAOS) Directory with office addresses in the five cities that had reported the largest number of AIDS cases as of December 31, 1985. The cities were New York (5,277 cases), San Francisco (1,826 cases), Los Angeles (1,439), Miami (505 cases), and Washington, DC (496 cases). Demographic information about all orthopedists in these cities was requested from AAOS, but the information could not be provided.

Questionnaires initially were mailed in March 1986 to 571 orthopedists. During the next 4 months, repeat mailings of the questionnaire were sent to nonrespondents as many as 3 times, as necessary. Other followup techniques, such as telephoning nonrespondents, were considered too aggressive and were not attempted. Sixty-one orthopedists were removed from the survey population because they had retired or died, or their questionnaires were returned as undeliverable.

Specific topics addressed by the questionnaire included

• their level of experience with HIV-infected patients
• their previous decisions to operate on HIV-infected patients

• their willingness to operate on HIV-infected patients in various risk groups
• their opinion of appropriate restrictions to place upon the professional activities of an HIV-infected surgeon
• their knowledge about the transmissibility of HIV by accidental needlestick, and
• precautions that they would take when operating on an HIV-infected patient.

Respondents also were asked to indicate their strength of agreement or disagreement with a series of Likert-type statements concerning

• a surgeon's obligation to operate on an HIV-infected patient in various situations
• the right of hospitals to require surgeons to operate on HIV-infected patients
• preoperative testing of patients for HIV antibodies
• the obligation of surgeons to have themselves tested for HIV infection, and
• the patient's right to know if his or her surgeon is infected.

Other items included in the questionnaire were not evaluated for this report. A copy of the questionnaire is available from the authors.

The virus currently designated HIV was known as HTLV-III/LAV at the time the questionnaire was prepared and distributed. The name HTLV-III was used in the questionnaire, but in this report the newer designation, HIV, is used. The questionnaires were completed anonymously and were not coded or numbered for record keeping. The only personal identifiers were age (by decade), marital status, and type of practice. Respondents were provided with an identifying postcard to be mailed separately to the study director when they sent back their completed questionnaires; 324 postcards and 325 questionnaires were received.

Orthopedic surgeons' attitudes and practices (dependent variables) were examined using city, age, type of practice, and two constructed variables as independent variables. The first constructed variable, experience with HIV-infected patients in the previous year, combined four questions and was scored as zero when respondents had neither examined nor operated on an HIV-infected patient, as one when they had examined but did not operate on an HIV-infected patient, and as two when they had operated on one or more such patients during the preceding year.

The second constructed variable concerned

knowledge about transmissibility of HIV. Answers to two questions were summed; responses were scored as two when both answers were correct, as one when one answer was correct, and as zero when neither answer was correct. "Strongly agree" and "agree" responses to Likert-type statements were combined as "agreed" in the data presented subsequently. Most null findings were not reported. The chi-square test or McNemar's test were used to assess whether differences in proportions were statistically significant. The two-sample t-test was used to compare continuous variables.

Results

Survey response. Questionnaires were completed by 325 (64 percent) of the 510 orthopedists surveyed. Response rates by city were Miami, 72 percent (36 of 50); San Francisco, 71 percent (75 of 106); Washington, DC, 67 percent (35 of 52); New York, 60 percent (107 of 178); and Los Angeles, 58 percent (72 of 124).

Respondent characteristics. All respondents were currently practicing surgeons; 38 percent were in solo private practice, 33 percent were in private orthopedic group practice, 24 percent were in academic full-time practice, and 5 percent were in multi-specialty groups. Fifty-seven percent performed 3 to 5 operations per week, 17 percent performed 6 to 8 operations per week, and 11 percent reported performing more than 8 operations per week. Sixty-eight percent of the respondents were between 40 and 59 years old, and 19 percent were 60 or older. Eighty-seven percent were currently married.

Experience with HIV-infected patients. Seventy respondents (22 percent) reported having operated on at least 1 patient with AIDS, AIDS-related complex (ARC), or asymptomatic HIV infection within the past year. An additional 68 (21 percent) had examined but had not operated on such a patient. There were 26 respondents who had examined or operated on 6 or more HIV-infected patients during the past year. The number of operations on HIV-infected patients by each orthopedist was reported as a range (zero, 1–5, > 5). Based on the lower boundary of the range, the minimum number of operations on HIV-infected patients during the previous year was 175.

Experience with HIV-infected patients differed by city. Fifty-nine percent of respondents in San Francisco had examined or operated on an HIV-infected patient, compared to 49 percent in Washington, 39 percent in Los Angeles, 36 percent in New York, and 31 percent in Miami (chi-square = 16.52, $P < 0.05$).

Knowledge of HIV transmissibility. When respondents were asked how transmissible they believed HIV to be by accidental needlestick, 9 percent reported that they thought it to be highly transmissible, 26 percent thought it to be moderately transmissible, 30 percent correctly reported that HIV has very low transmissibility, and 34 percent were not sure.

Respondents were asked to compare the transmissibility of HIV by needlestick to that of hepatitis B virus. Three percent thought HIV was more transmissible, 26 percent thought it was equally transmissible, 33 percent correctly responded that it was less transmissible, and 38 percent were not sure.

Overall, 60 percent of respondents did not answer either question about HIV transmissibility correctly, 18 percent answered one question correctly, and 22 percent answered both correctly. Knowledge about transmissibility did not differ significantly between those who responded early in the survey and those who responded later (chi-square = 1.235, $P > 0.5$).

Respondents were given a list of possible precautions that might be taken during surgery and were asked to indicate which they would use when operating on an HIV-infected patient. Ninety-three percent reported they would wear extra gloves, 73 percent would wear goggles, 63 percent would require experienced assistants, and 55 percent would proceed more slowly during the operation. Thirty-eight percent would wear an extra mask or gown, measures which the authors believe are not useful in preventing HIV transmission.

Sixty-one percent of respondents would use 3 or more of the above precautions, and 32 percent would use at least 4 of the precautions when operating on a patient with HIV infection. The number of precautions that each respondent would use did not vary significantly with experience with HIV-infected patients or knowledge about transmissibility of HIV ($P > 0.1$ for each comparison, chi-square test).

Restrictions on an infected surgeon. Orthopedists were asked what restrictions should be placed on a surgeon who becomes HIV-infected. Forty-nine percent responded that there should be no restrictions, 7 percent thought an infected surgeon should

Table 1. Survey of orthopedists' opinions regarding a surgeon's ethical obligation to operate on HIV- infected patients in different situations (percentage distribution)

Situation	Number of respondents	Strongly agree	Agree	Don't know	Disagree	Strongly disagree
Emergency	322	40	41	8	7	4
When surgery will greatly affect quality of life	318	26	35	15	17	7
In all situations when surgery is indicated	318	12	23	15	32	19

avoid only major surgery, 39 percent thought all surgery should be avoided, and 5 percent responded that an infected surgeon should discontinue practice. Those who answered that an infected surgeon should avoid major surgery, avoid all surgery, or discontinue practice are included in the analysis as favoring restrictions.

Opinions about the need for restrictions on the professional activities of infected surgeons varied with knowledge about transmissibility of HIV. Thirty-eight percent of orthopedists who correctly answered both knowledge questions favored restrictions, compared to 64 percent of those who answered 1 question correctly and 53 percent of those who answered neither correctly (chi-square = 8.88, $P < 0.025$).

We examined whether respondents who favored restrictions would take more precautions when operating than would other respondents. The mean number (+ SD) of precautions that would be taken by the former group was 3.1 ($\pm$ 1.4), compared to 2.6 ($\pm$ 1.3) by respondents who did not think that the professional activities of infected surgeons should be restricted ($P > 0.5$, two sample t-test). However, respondents who favored restrictions were significantly more likely than others to use all 5 precautions (21 percent versus 7 percent, chi-square = 9.45, $P < 0.005$).

Obligation to operate. As shown in table 1, 81 percent of respondents agreed that an orthopedist is ethically obligated to operate on HIV-infected patients in emergency situations, 61 percent agreed that an orthopedist is ethically obligated to operate in situations in which surgery will greatly affect the patient's quality of life, and 35 percent agreed that an orthopedist is ethically obligated to operate in all situations in which surgery is indicated.

The percent of respondents who agreed that surgeons are obligated to operate in all situations when surgery is indicated differed among cities. The proportion of respondents who agreed with the statement was 44 percent in San Francisco, 38

percent in New York, 35 percent in Los Angeles, 26 percent in Washington, DC, and 11 percent in Miami (chi-square = 13.60, $P < 0.01$).

Responses to questions concerning the surgeon's obligation to operate were examined in relation to knowledge of HIV transmissibility. For each of the situations presented in table 1, responses did not differ significantly among respondents with different levels of knowledge (coded as zero, 1, or 2) of HIV transmissibility ($P > 0.1$, chi-square test).

Perceived ethical obligation to operate was examined in relation to beliefs concerning the need for restrictions on the professional activities of HIV-infected surgeons. Twenty-seven percent of respondents who favored restrictions agreed that an orthopedist is ethically obligated to operate in all situations in which surgery is indicated, 57 percent when surgery would greatly affect quality of life, and 79 percent in emergency situations.

Among respondents who did not favor restrictions, the rates of agreement with ethical obligation in these three situations were 45 percent, 69 percent, and 84 percent. Differences in responses among orthopedists who favored restrictions and those who did not were significant for each of the first two situations (when surgery was indicated, chi-square = 9.20, $P < 0.005$; when quality of life would be affected, chi-square = 4.04, $P < 0.05$).

Refusal to operate. Sixty-nine percent of respondents agreed that an orthopedic surgeon may ethically refuse to operate on HIV-infected patients if operating may endanger the health of the surgeon or the surgeon's family. Agreement with this statement was not associated with independent variables such as marital status or practice type, but was inversely related to responses to questions concerning ethical obligations to operate. For example, 79 percent of respondents who did not believe surgeons are obligated to operate in all situations in which surgery is indicated agreed that a surgeon may ethically refuse in order to protect himself or his family. Only 47 percent of respondents who believed that the surgeon is ethically obligated in all situations also believed a surgeon ethically can refuse (chi-square = 32.15, $P < 0.005$).

Fourteen respondents (4 percent) at some time had declined to operate on an HIV-infected patient. Six of the 14 had, however, operated on other HIV-infected patients. We examined the 14 surgeons' responses to questions concerning ethical obligation to operate. Fifty-seven percent believed themselves obligated to operate in emergencies, 14 percent in situations in which quality of life would be greatly affected, and 7 percent of all situations in which surgery is indicated. Each of the latter two rates differed significantly from the corresponding rate for respondents who always had operated on patients with HIV infection (each P value < 0.05, chi-square test).

The rate of agreement about whether a surgeon may ethically refuse to operate did not differ significantly among surgeons who had operated and those who had declined to operate on HIV-infected patients. The belief that a surgeon may ethically refuse to operate to avoid endangering his health or the health of his family was affirmed by 59 percent of orthopedists who had always operated on HIV-infected patients, 63 percent of those who had always declined to operate, and 100 percent of those who had both operated and declined to operate.

Knowledge of HIV transmissibility did not differ significantly among orthopedists who had ever declined to operate compared to other orthopedists. Twenty-one percent of those who declined answered both questions correctly, and 57 percent answered at least one question correctly. None of the 14 who declined had characterized HIV as "highly transmissible by accidental needlestick" or "more transmissible by needlestick than hepatitis B virus."

Twelve of the respondents who had ever declined to operate answered the question concerning restrictions that they believed should be placed on the professional activities of a surgeon who becomes infected with HIV. All 12 believed that a surgeon who becomes infected should either discontinue practice or avoid all surgery (table 2). However, only 49 percent of other respondents believed restrictions are necessary (chi-square = 9.98, $P < 0.005$).

Respondents were asked whether they would be "less likely to operate" on an HIV-infected patient, based on the risk group to which the patient belonged (table 3). The purpose of the question was to assess whether risk group membership

Table 2. Survey of orthopedists' opinions concerning restrictions on the professional activities of HIV-infected surgeons

Previous experience with HIV-infected patients	Number of respondents	Percent of respondents favoring restrictions
Neither operated nor declined	214	51
Operated and never declined	59	41
Both operated and declined	4	100
Declined and never operated	8	100

Table 3. Survey of orthopedists' attitudes toward operating on HIV-infected patients from various risk groups

Previous experience with HIV-infected patients	Number of respondents	Percent of respondents "less likely to operate" on HIV-infected patients from each specific risk group		
		Hemophiliac	Homosexual	IV drug abuser
Neither operated nor refused	247	24	26	35
Operated and never refused	64	18	16	27
Refused [1]	14	42	67	78
Total	325	23	25	35

[1] 6 respondents had operated on at least 1 HIV-infected patient.

would bias an orthopedist's willingness to operate. Regardless of previous experience with HIV-infected patients, respondents were biased more often against operating on IV drug abusers than either hemophiliacs (chi-square = 28.17, $P < 0.005$, McNemar's test) or homosexuals (chi-square = 22.75, $P < 0.005$, McNemar's test). Those respondents who previously had declined to operate on an HIV-infected patient were biased more often than were other orthopedists against operating on HIV-infected patients, regardless of the risk group to which the patient belonged.

Only 12 percent of all respondents thought that a hospital may require surgeons to operate on infected patients.

Preoperative testing. Seventy-one percent of respondents agreed that surgeons have the right to demand that all patients be tested preoperatively for HIV infection. Eighty-five percent agreed that surgeons have the right to test members of high-risk groups. Respondents who believed that surgeons have the right to test all patients agreed less often than other respondents with the statement that a surgeon is obligated to operate on HIV-infected patients (table 4).

Only 2 percent of respondents reported that in

Table 4. Survey of attitudes concerning obligation to operate on HIV-infected patients among orthopedists with differing attitudes toward preoperative HIV testing of patients

Surgeon's right to test all patients	Percent of respondents who agree that a surgeon is ethically obligated to operate in specified situation		
	Emergency	When surgery will greatly affect quality of life	In all situations when surgery is indicated
Agree	77	55	30
Do not agree	89	70	46

NOTE: In all 3 situations, the proportion of respondents who agreed that a surgeon is ethically obligated to operate was significantly lower among those who agreed, compared with those who did not agree that surgeons have the right to test all patients preoperatively (all *P* values < 0.025, chi-square test).

practice they routinely request preoperative testing of all patients for HIV antibodies. Twenty-three percent reported that they routinely request preoperative testing of patients at high risk of HIV infection.

Testing of patients in high-risk groups was requested most often by orthopedists who operated on HIV-infected patients. Thirty-six percent of respondents who had operated on an HIV-infected patient tested high risk patients routinely, compared to 22 percent of respondents who had examined an HIV-infected patient and 18 percent of respondents who had not examined or operated on an HIV-infected patient (chi-square = 9.15, $P < 0.025$).

Sixty-five percent of respondents who routinely tested high risk patients, compared to 47 percent of those who did not, thought that an orthopedic surgeon should restrict his clinical activities if he became infected (chi-square = 5.81, $P < 0.025$). Use of routine preoperative testing did not differ significantly among respondents with different levels of knowledge (coded as zero, 1, or 2) of HIV transmissibility.

Self-testing by surgeons. Seventy-nine percent of respondents thought that orthopedic surgeons should have themselves tested for HIV infection after a possible HIV inoculation. Fifty-one percent thought that they should have themselves tested if their practice included patients in high risk groups. Only 7 percent felt that they should have themselves tested annually no matter where they lived or practiced.

Patients' right to know if their surgeon is HIV-positive. Forty-three percent of respondents agreed that patients have the right to know if their surgeon is HIV-positive, 31 percent disagreed, and 26 percent did not know. Those who agreed that

patients have the right to know were more likely than others to agree that the clinical activities of an infected surgeon should be restricted (64 percent *versus* 42 percent (chi-square = 12.91, $P < 0.005$), and that a surgeon should have himself tested annually if he treats high risk patients (72 percent *versus* 35 percent (chi-square = 41.97, $P < 0.005$). Opinion as to whether a patient has a right to know if his surgeon is infected did not differ significantly by experience with HIV-infected patients or knowledge of HIV transmissibility.

Discussion

The risk to hospital workers of occupationally acquiring HIV infection has been of concern since the AIDS epidemic was recognized. As of March 1986, when questionnaires for the present study were mailed, one instance of documented needlestick HIV seroconversion in a nurse had been reported (9) and three studies of HIV infection in exposed hospital personnel had been published (15–17). Two studies examined seroprevalence and instances of HIV infection in 75 workers with no other apparent risk factors who had percutaneous or mucus membrane exposure to HIV-infected blood. The third study, by the Centers for Disease Control, was prospective, and researchers found no instances of HIV seroconversion in 40 health care workers followed after percutaneous or mucus membrane exposure to body fluids of AIDS patients. Subsequently, a substantial number of cases of occupationally acquired HIV infection in health care workers has been recognized, and these cases recently were summarized by the Centers for Disease Control (18).

Worldwide, including the nurse mentioned above, 15 health care workers have developed HIV infection indicated by the timing of seroconversion to have been caused by occupational exposure to the blood of HIV-infected patients. Most of the cases involved percutaneous exposure to blood, such as by needlestick, but four cases apparently resulted from infective blood splashing onto mucous membranes or transiently contacting nonintact skin (19,20).

In response to concerns about possible nosocomial transmission of HIV, the Centers for Disease Control (20,21) and other groups (4,5,22,23) formulated infection control guidelines for health care workers. The guidelines describe precautions for patients with proven or suspected HIV infection, and most of the guidelines explicitly state that there is no basis for healthy hospital personnel to be excused from providing care to these patients (4,5,22,24). Nonetheless, some personnel remain concerned about an occupational risk of HIV transmission, and this concern may affect care given to patients. A survey of 1,194 workers in a Washington, DC, hospital showed that 35 percent actively avoided involvement with AIDS patients and one-third believed they should be permitted to refuse to care for AIDS patients (25). In another hospital, where 267 nursing personnel responded to a questionnaire, about 10 percent of those who had been called upon to care for AIDS patients indicated that they had refused (26). In a survey of Los Angeles physicians in various specialties, 22 percent believed that their staff would quit if asked to treat AIDS patients (27).

Our analysis shows that in the five cities with the greatest number of AIDS patients, orthopedic surgeons frequently treated patients with HIV infections. In the previous year, 43 percent of respondents had examined or operated on an HIV-infected patient, and at least 175 operations on such patients were performed. We considered orthopedic surgeons who had operated on an HIV-infected patient to be willing to operate, even if they had declined to operate on another patient. By this method, 90 percent (70 of 78) of the surgeons with HIV-infected patients for whom surgery was considered were willing to operate. This rate may actually underestimate willingness to operate, because the question about experience operating on HIV-infected patients addressed only the previous year, while the question about declining to operate covered all previous years.

The reasons for declining to operate were not determined and may have been based on prognosis or other medical issues, rather than on the surgeon's fear of becoming infected. To our knowledge, rates of refusal to operate on HIV-infected patients have not been reported for other surgeons. However, a survey of health professionals in an area of Britain with many HIV-infected patients found that 18 percent of surgeons, and an even higher percentage of other physicians, favored transfer of HIV-positive patients to special units when invasive procedures were required (6). In a Los Angeles survey, 81 percent of physicians agreed that special clinics staffed by physicians with particular expertise should be established to treat AIDS patients and 77 percent indicated that they would refer patients they diagnosed (27).

Testing to detect HIV infection was utilized infrequently by orthopedists we surveyed. Fewer than one-fourth routinely tested high-risk patients

'Our data indicate that orthopedists do not believe they can be compelled to operate, but at most only a small percentage would decline to operate, on HIV-infected patients in situations in which surgery would be beneficial.'

preoperatively, even though 85 percent of respondents believed surgeons have the right to order such testing. Thus, operations on HIV-infected patients may have been performed much more often than was recognized.

The high rate of willingness to operate is striking, in view of the perception by most respondents that HIV infection is highly or moderately transmissible by accidental needlestick. Only 26 percent of the 70 surgeons who operated answered both knowledge questions correctly, while 37 percent considered HIV to be more transmissible than it is. A lower rate of willingness to operate might have been expected, based on the belief by 69 percent of all respondents and 63 percent of the orthopedists who had operated on an HIV-positive patient, that a surgeon may ethically refuse to operate if he feels it may endanger his health or that of his family.

Respondents were not asked directly why they had operated or declined to operate on HIV-infected patients. Instead, attitudes were examined to assess whether factors other than a patient's medical condition might be important. Perceived ethical obligation apparently played a role, in that orthopedists who had operated on HIV-infected patients were more likely to feel an obligation to operate in specified situations than were orthopedists who had declined. However, ethical obligation clearly was not the primary motivation for at least some of 70 orthopedists who had operated, because 12 (17 percent) of them did not feel ethically obligated to operate in any of the situations described in the questionnaire. For these orthopedists, and probably for many others, factors such as peer pressure, or a desire to maintain referral networks, may have been the dominant considerations. Most orthopedists, including more than 60 percent of those who had operated on HIV-infected patients, considered it ethical for a surgeon to refuse to operate, based on concern for his health and that of his family. The conflict in ethical obligations to patients and to self is illustrated by the observation that 47 percent of orthopedists who believed that a surgeon is ethically obligated to operate on an HIV-infected patient in all situations in which surgery is indicated also believed that a surgeon may ethically refuse to operate to protect his health or that of his family.

Although one survey of physicians showed that they tend to stigmatize AIDS patients (28), few orthopedists in the present survey declined to operate on HIV-infected patients, and reasons for these decisions are not known. However, a decreased a priori willingness to operate is suggested by responses to two questions. First, orthopedists who had ever declined to operate were more likely not to operate on members of HIV risk groups than other orthopedists. This attitude was acknowledged most often about IV drug abusers (83 percent) and homosexuals (67 percent), but it also was reported about hemophiliacs (42 percent). Second, orthopedists who had declined to operate considered restrictions on the professional activities of a surgeon to be a necessary consequence of that surgeon having acquired HIV infection. This concern about a serious effect of HIV infection on the livelihood of surgeons apparently reflected personal views, because recommendations of the Centers for Disease Control released prior to the survey did not address the topic of infected health care workers who perform invasive procedures (19), and subsequent recommendations announced during the survey did not advocate restrictions (29). Nonetheless, attitudes about operating on members of risk groups and a high level of concern about the potential consequences of acquiring HIV infection may explain why knowledge of HIV transmissibility did not differ between orthopedists who operated and those who declined. Given that the risk of intraoperative transmission to surgeons is low, a surgeon still might choose not to accept even a low risk if he views the patient with disfavor or if he views the consequences of infection to be devastating personally or professionally.

A responsibility of each physician to treat patients with AIDS has been asserted widely (4,30). The basis for these assertions appears to have been a moral viewpoint rather than a legal duty or a specific covenant set forth by a medical association. A physician's legal duty to treat arises from a mutual accommodation and a consensual transaction between patient and physician (31). In American medicine, except in emergencies or instances where a doctor-patient relationship has been established previously, physicians may choose whom they will serve (32). In November 1987, the Council on Ethical and Judicial Affairs of the American

Medical Association said that this principle "does not permit categorical discrimination against a patient based solely on his or her seropositivity" and reasserted the tradition that physicians must risk their own health in epidemics (24).

The results of this study may not be applicable to all orthopedists or to other groups of surgeons. The survey queried only orthopedists in major cities with large numbers of AIDS cases and the response rate was 64 percent. While this rate compares favorably with those of other mail surveys of physicians (33–35), information is still lacking concerning a sizable minority of orthopedists. Because the questionnaires were completed anonymously, we consider it unlikely that orthopedists who had attitudes that they feared were unpopular comprised a disproportionately large share of the nonrespondents.

Our data indicate that orthopedists do not believe they can be compelled to operate, but at most only a small percentage would decline to operate on HIV-infected patients in situations in which surgery would be beneficial. The risk of infection of the surgeon appears quite small, and pressures other than moral arguments are considerable. These pressures include availability of other orthopedists to do the surgery, the natural reluctance of surgeons to use personal feelings as a basis for refusing to operate, and desire to avoid adverse peer judgment.

References ....

1. Centers for Disease Control: Acquired immunodeficiency syndrome (AIDS). Weekly Surveillance Report, United States, Nov. 23, 1987.
2. Centers for Disease Control: Acquired immunodeficiency syndrome (AIDS). Weekly Surveillance Report, United States, Dec. 29, 1987.
3. Public Health Service: Coolfont report: a PHS plan for prevention and control of AIDS and AIDS virus. Public Health Rep 101:341–347, July-August 1986.
4. Eickhoff, T. C. et al.: A hospitalwide approach to AIDS: recommendations of the Advisory Committee on Infections within Hospitals, American Hospital Association. Infection Control 5:242–248, May 1984.
5. Conte, J. E., Jr., Nadley, W. K., and Sande, M.: Infection-control guidelines for patients with the acquired immunodeficiency syndrome (AIDS). N Eng J Med 309:740–744, Sept. 22, 1983.
6. Searle, E. S.: Knowledge, attitudes, and behavior of health professionals in relation to AIDS. Lancet 1:26–28, Jan. 3, 1987.
7. McCray, E.: Occupational risk of the acquired immunodeficiency syndrome among health care workers. N Eng J Med 314: 1127–1132, Apr. 24, 1986.
8. Stricof, R. L., and Morse, D. L.: HTLV-III/LAV sero-

conversion following deep intramuscular needlestick injury. N Eng J Med 314:1115, Apr. 24, 1986.

9. Needlestick transmission of HTLV-III from a patient infected in Africa. Lancet 2:1376-1377, Dec. 15, 1984.

10. Oksenhendler, E. et al.: HIV infection with seroconversion after a superficial needlestick injury to the finger. N Engl J Med 315:582, Aug. 28, 1986.

11. Shouldice, E. E., and Martin, C. J.: Wound infections, surgical gloves and hands of operating personnel. Can Med Assoc J 81:636-640, Oct. 15, 1959.

12. Russel, T. R., Roque, F. E., and Miller, F. A.: A new method for detection of the leaky glove. Arch Surg 93:245-248, August 1966.

13. Denes, A. E., et al.: Hepatitis B infection in physicians. JAMA 239:210-21, Jan. 16, 1978.

14. Nardt, F. et al.: Hepatitis B virus infections among Danish surgeons. J Infect Dis 140:972-974, December 1979.

15. Hirsch, M. S. et al.: Risk of nosocomial infection with human T-cell lymphotropic virus III (HTLV-III). N Engl J Med 312:1-4, Jan. 3, 1985.

16. Weiss, S. N. et al.: HTLV-III infection among health care workers. Association with needle stick injuries. JAMA 254:2089-2093, Oct. 18, 1985.

17. Centers for Disease Control: Update: prospective evaluation of health care workers exposed via the parenteral or mucus-membrane route to blood or body fluids from patients with acquired immunodeficiency syndrome, United States. MMWR 34:101-103, Feb. 22, 1985.

18. Centers for Disease Control: Update: acquired immunodeficiency syndrome and human immunodeficiency virus among health-care workers. MMWR 37:229-234, 239, Apr. 22, 1988.

19. Centers for Disease Control: Update: human immunodeficiency virus infections in health care workers exposed to blood of infected patients. MMWR 36:285-289, May 22, 1987.

20. Centers for Disease Control: Summary: recommendations for preventing transmission of infection with human T-lymphotropic virus type III/lymphadenopathy-associated virus in the workplace. MMWR 34:681-685, 691-695, Nov. 15, 1985.

21. Centers for Disease Control: Recommendations for prevention of HIV transmission in health-care settings. MMWR 36:1S-13S, Aug. 21, 1987.

22. Gerberding, J. L.: Recommended infection-control policies for patients with human immunodeficiency virus infection. N Eng J Med 315:1562-1564, Dec. 11, 1986.

23. Conte, J. E.: Infection with human immunodeficiency virus in the hospital. Ann Intern Med 105:730-766, November 1986.

24. American Medical Association: Ethical issues involved in the growing AIDS crisis. Report of the Council on Ethical and Judicial Affairs, Nov. 12, 1987.

25. Gordin, F. et al.: Hospital workers' knowledge, behavior and attitudes toward AIDS. Communication 213. Program Abstracts, Second International Conference on AIDS, Paris, France, June 23, 1986.

26. Reed, P., Wise, T. N., and Mann, L. S.: Nurses' attitudes regarding acquired immunodeficiency syndrome (AIDS). Nurs Forum 21:153-156, April 1984.

27. Richardson, J. L., Lochner, T., McGuigan, K., and Levine, A. M.: Physician attitudes and experience regarding the care of patients with acquired immunodeficiency syndrome (AIDS) and related disorders (ARC). Med Care 25:625-685, July 1987.

28. Kelly, J. A. et al.: Stigmatization of AIDS patients by physicians. Am J Public Health 77:789-791, July 1987.

29. Centers for Disease Control: Recommendations for preventing transmission of infection with human T-lymphotropic virus type III/lymphadenopathy-associated virus during invasive procedures. MMWR 35:21-23, Jan. 17, 1986.

30. Institute of Medicine, National Academy of Sciences: Confronting AIDS. Directions for public health care and research. National Academy Press, Washington, DC, 1986, pp. 153-155.

31. Plumeri, P. A.: The refusal to treat: abandonment and AIDS. J Clin Gastroenterol 6:281-284, June 1984.

32. Current opinions of the Council on Ethical and Judicial Affairs of the American Medical Association, 1986. Chicago, IL, 1986, p. ix.

33. Charap, M. N., Levin, R. I., and Weinglass, J.: Physician choices in the treatment of angina pectoris. Am J Med 79:461-466, October 1985.

34. Sobal, J. et al.: Physicians' beliefs about the importance of 25 health promoting behaviors. Am J Public Health 75:1427-1428, December 1985.

35. Orleans, C. T., George, L. K., Noupt, J. L., and Brodie, H. K. H.: How primary care physicians treat psychiatric disorders: a national survey of family practitioners. Am J Psychiatry 142:52-57, January 1985.

11.3 Singer PA, Siegler M, Whitington PF, Lantos JD, Emond JC, Thistlethwaite JR, Broelsch CE (1989) Ethics of Liver Transplantation with Living Donors. N Engl J Med 321:620–2

620   THE NEW ENGLAND JOURNAL OF MEDICINE   Aug. 31, 1989

OCCASIONAL NOTES

ETHICS OF LIVER TRANSPLANTATION WITH LIVING DONORS

LIVER transplantation involving only a portion of a liver from a cadaveric donor is now performed in several major centers worldwide. We propose to transplant a liver lobe from a living donor — the parent of the recipient — to a noncritically ill infant with advanced liver disease. Although it is technically feasible, such transplantation of an organ from a living donor raises complex ethical issues involving the balance of risks and benefits, the selection of donor and recipient, and informed consent. This article describes the unique ethical aspects of liver transplantation with parents as living donors and describes our approach to these issues.

RESEARCH-ETHICS CONSULTATION

Research-ethics consultation[1] is the process in which the ethical issues raised by an innovative therapy are analyzed before a protocol is submitted to the institutional review board. This process has been an essential part of our liver-transplantation program in recent years. It begins with meetings between investigators and clinical ethicists to identify and address the key ethical aspects of a contemplated medical or surgical innovation. In the case of liver transplantation with living donors, our group of transplant physicians and clinical ethicists convened a yearlong series of seminars and discussions that were open to the entire university community. On the basis of these seminars, we drafted and circulated for comment a working paper on the ethics of liver transplantation with living donors. A revised version of that paper served as the basis of a proposal submitted to the institutional review board. We hope this publication will encourage discussion of this innovative therapy, preferably before its first use in this country. We here discuss the specific aspects of liver transplantation with living donors that we considered.

RISKS AND BENEFITS FOR RECIPIENTS AND DONORS

The main risk to the recipient relates to the implantation of a hepatic lobe obtained from a living donor, as compared with the risk of conventional, cadaveric whole-liver transplantation. Techniques for the transplantation of hepatic lobes have been developed in the course of reduced-size and split-liver transplantation. Reduced-size transplantation (the implanting of a lobe of a cadaveric liver into a recipient smaller than the donor) has had a survival rate of 80 percent, which is comparable to the survival rate with full-size liver transplantation.[2-5] Split-liver transplantation (the dividing of a larger liver from a cadaveric donor and the implanting of the lobes into two different recipients) has had a survival rate of 79 percent.[6] Like full-size transplants, transplanted liver lobes grow along with the child, and long-term graft failure has not been encountered.[5]

The main benefit to the recipient of transplantation from a living donor is a reduced risk of pretransplan-

tation mortality. At present, because of the shortage of donors, many infants, perhaps up to 50 percent nationwide, die awaiting transplantation.[5,7,8] Many of these children could be saved by allografts from living donors. Liver transplantation involving such donors may also offer improved survival after transplantation, as compared with cadaveric liver transplantation, because the donors and recipients will be haploidentical with respect to HLA antigens. In addition, the organ-damaging hemodynamic instability associated with the death of the donor is avoided, and the coordinated scheduling of operations in the donor and recipient holds ex vivo organ ischemia to a minimum.

The main risk to the donor is that of partial hepatectomy. Although some published reports describe a mortality rate from this operation that is as high as 11 percent,[9-11] no mortality has been reported from several centers where surgeons have considerable experience in performing partial hepatectomy.[12-15] At our institution, there have been no operative deaths or serious postoperative complications in 35 consecutive patients without cirrhosis who have undergone hepatic resection for tumors. Moreover, we have recently developed the living-donor operation in an animal model: eight of nine dogs provided a satisfactory liver graft, and all nine survived the procedure without complication (unpublished data). Because the liver regenerates fully, such a donation should not affect long-term hepatic function.[9,16]

The benefit to the donor is psychological. As a parent of the recipient, the prospective donor has a powerful motivation to participate. If transplantation succeeds, the donor has the extreme satisfaction of having saved the life of the child. Even if transplantation fails, the donor may take comfort in the knowledge of having done everything possible to save the child.

These considerations of risks and benefits are comparable to those in accepted procedures for transplantation with living donors, such as kidney or pancreas transplantation.[17-19] We believe that from the perspectives of both recipient and donor, the benefits outweigh the risks and that it is ethically appropriate to proceed with a trial of liver transplantation using a parent as a living donor.

SELECTION OF RECIPIENTS AND DONORS

Innovative transplantation procedures are often attempted first in the sickest patients, as a "desperate remedy."[20,21] By contrast, we propose to perform the initial transplantations in infants with advanced liver disease who are not critically ill but who will certainly require a liver transplant within about three months to survive. When transplantation is performed in a recipient who is not critically ill, the pressure on the donor is reduced because the need to make a decision under emergency circumstances is obviated. Also, time becomes available for a thorough medical and psychiatric evaluation of the donor, as well as for the two-step process of informed consent described below. Finally, since a living donor is placed at some risk, we believe that it is more appropriate ethically to select a recipient with a higher chance of survival. Infants who are not critically ill with advanced liver disease represent such recipients. Furthermore, they do not have the mortality and morbidity associated with waiting for a cadaveric liver. (Such infants often become critically ill before they can be considered for the scarce supply of small livers.) The infants are medically stable at the time of surgery. Under these criteria, approximately 50 percent of the children newly referred to our transplant program would be eligible for liver transplantation involving a living donor.

We propose that the donor should be the child's parent or, in rare cases, a mature sibling or grandparent. When the donor is genetically and emotionally related to the recipient, the intangible benefits of saving a life are most rewarding, and the risk–benefit ratio is most favorable. According to our proposal, the potential donor will be evaluated by the transplant team, an internist, and a psychiatrist with respect to the criteria for donation: compatible blood type, no history of liver disease, normal results of liver-function testing, appropriate size of left liver lobe on CT scanning, no vascular anomalies on hepatic arteriography, low operative risk, low risk of psychological decompensation, and informed consent. The final decision about donation will be made in conference between the liver-transplant team and the internist and the psychiatrist, and the discussion will focus on the donor's safety.

INFORMED CONSENT FOR RECIPIENT AND DONOR

Consent on behalf of the recipient will be obtained by the pediatric hepatologist on the transplant team. Because the recipient will be an infant, consent must be obtained from a proxy decision maker, usually a parent. The consent form conforms to a standard format, including a description of the nature and duration of the procedure and the risks, benefits, and alternatives. The consent form explicitly states, "The operation your child will have . . . has never been performed."

Two important elements affect the granting of consent on behalf of the recipient. First, the information about liver transplantation with the use of living donors is limited. Although uncertainty is a problem in consenting to any innovative therapy, our data from experiments in dogs and reduced-size and split-liver transplantation in humans allow us to estimate the survival of a recipient after transplantation from a living donor. Second, the parental decision maker may also serve as the donor of the hepatic graft. Although this situation may influence the decision maker's readiness to give consent, we believe that from the perspective of the recipient it validates the decision maker's good faith, because a proxy who is willing to accept some personal risk to benefit the recipient will also represent the recipient's best interests.

Consent for the operation in the donor will be obtained in two steps. The initial consent, obtained by the pediatric hepatologist and the hepatic surgeon on the transplant team, will focus on the evaluation needed for a person to become a living donor, as well as on the donor's operation itself. If the potential donor agrees, a complete medical evaluation will be performed by a consulting internist, and a complete psychiatric evaluation by a consulting psychiatrist. If the donor is considered medically and psychologically fit, a second consent will be obtained by the two transplantation physicians, as well as the consultant in internal medicine acting as a "consent advocate" for the donor.[22] The second consent will focus on the donor's operation and will review the published data on partial hepatectomy, local experience with the procedure, and the results in experiments with animals. The risk of dying is "estimated at close to zero," and that of a major postoperative complication at "less than 5 percent." After the second consent, there will be a mandatory two-week waiting period before transplantation, during which the donor may withdraw consent.

The donor's decision to give consent may be influenced by three factors. First, the donor may feel considerable internal pressure to donate, because he or she knows that otherwise the recipient may die.[23] Such pressure is unavoidable, and it is not unique to liver transplantation. The need to balance selfishness and altruism is a universal feature of family relationships. We do not think that it invalidates voluntary consent.

Second, family members or even health care workers may exert external pressure to donate.[24] Several elements of our protocol are designed to minimize such coercion, including psychiatric evaluation and counseling and the presence of a consent advocate for the donor who is not directly involved in the donor's operation.[25,26]

Third, pressures on potential donors may be exacerbated if the medical situation is urgent.[27] Our protocol minimizes such pressure by selecting recipients who are not critically ill and mandating a two-week waiting period during which donors can change their minds.

CONCLUSION

Moore has recently stressed the importance of "open display, public evaluation, and discussion" in the ethical conduct of therapeutic innovation.[21] We agree that public dialogue is beneficial in assessing controversial research protocols. Prospective research-ethics consultation,[1] central to our analysis of liver transplantation with living donors, provides the opportunity for such dialogue. Research-ethics consultation, and especially the ability and willingness of clinical investigators and clinical ethicists to analyze ethical issues in a collaborative fashion and anticipate ethical issues before protocols are submitted to an institutional review board, may represent an important step in clinical research.

PETER A. SINGER, M.D., MARK SIEGLER, M.D.,
PETER F. WHITINGTON, M.D.,
JOHN D. LANTOS, M.D., JEAN C. EMOND, M.D.,
J. RICHARD THISTLETHWAITE, M.D., PH.D.,
University of Chicago   AND CHRISTOPH E. BROELSCH,
Chicago, IL 60637   M.D., PH.D.

REFERENCES

1. Singer PA, Lantos JD, Whitington PF, Broelsch CE, Siegler M. Equipoise and the ethics of segmental liver transplantation. Clin Res 1988; 36:539-45.
2. Bismuth H, Houssin D. Reduced-sized orthotopic liver graft in hepatic transplantation in children. Surgery 1984; 95:367-70.
3. Broelsch CE, Emond JC, Thistlethwaite JR, et al. Liver transplantation, including the concept of reduced-size liver transplants in children. Ann Surg 1988; 208:410-20.
4. Broelsch CE, Emond JC, Thistlethwaite JR, Rouch DA, Whitington PF, Lichtor JL. Liver transplantation with reduced-size donor organs. Transplantation 1988; 45:519-24.
5. Emond JC, Whitington PF, Thistlethwaite JR, Alonso EM, Broelsch CE. Reduced-size orthotopic liver transplantation: use in the management of children with chronic liver disease. Hepatology (in press).
6. Alonso EM, Whitington PF, Broelsch CE, Emond JC, Thistlethwaite JR. "Split-liver" orthotopic liver transplantation (OLT). Pediatr Res 1989; 25:107A. abstract.
7. Malatack JJ, Schaid DJ, Urbach AH, et al. Choosing a pediatric recipient for orthotopic liver transplantation. J Pediatr 1987; 111:479-89.
8. Lilly JR, Hall RJ, Altman RP. Liver transplantation and Kasai operation in the first year of life: therapeutic dilemma in biliary atresia. J Pediatr 1987; 110:561-2.
9. McDermott WV Jr, Ottinger LW. Elective hepatic resection. Am J Surg 1966; 112:376-81.
10. Starzl TE, Koep LJ, Weil R III, Lilly JR, Putnam CW, Aldrete JA. Right trisegmentectomy for hepatic neoplasms. Surg Gynecol Obstet 1980; 150:208-14.
11. Adson MA. Diagnosis and surgical treatment of primary and secondary solid hepatic tumors in the adult. Surg Clin North Am 1981; 61:181-96.
12. Iwatsuki S, Shaw BW Jr, Starzl TE. Experience with 150 liver resections. Ann Surg 1983; 197:247-53.
13. Bismuth H, Houssin D, Michel F. Le risque opératoire des hépatectomies: expérience sur 154 hépatectomies: a propos de la communication de M.A. Rohner sur les hépatectomies, séance du 3 février 1982. Chirurgie 1983; 109:342-8.
14. Broelsch CE, Neuhaus P, Ringe B, Long W, Pichlmayr R. Hepatic resection in primary and secondary liver tumors. In: Axel-Girigi H, ed. Aspekte der klinischen Onkologie. Stuttgart: Gustav Fischer Verlag, 1984:483.
15. Nagao T, Inoue S, Mizuta T, Saito H, Kawano N, Morioka Y. One hundred hepatic resections: indications and operative results. Ann Surg 1985; 202:42-9.
16. Stone HH, Long WD, Smith RB III, Haynes CD. Physiologic considerations in major hepatic resections. Am J Surg 1969; 117:78-84.
17. Spital A. Living kidney donation: when is it justified? AKF Nephrol Lett 1988; 5:1-15.
18. Singer PA, Siegler M. Whose kidney is it anyway? Ethical considerations in living kidney donation. AKF Nephrol Lett 1988; 5:16-20.
19. Kendall DM, Sutherland DE, Goetz FC, Najarian JS. Metabolic effect of hemipancreatectomy in donors: preoperative prediction of postoperative oral glucose tolerance. Diabetes 1989; 38:Suppl 1:101-3.
20. Moore FD. Three ethical revolutions: ancient assumptions remodeled under pressure of transplantation. Tranplant Proc 1988; 20:Suppl 1:1061-7.
21. Idem. The desperate case: CARE (costs, applicability, research, ethics). JAMA 1989; 261:1483-4.
22. Levine RJ. Ethics and regulation of clinical research. 2nd ed. Baltimore: Urban & Schwarzenberg, 1986:130-4.
23. Simmons RG, Hickey K, Kjellstrand CM, Simmons RL. Family tension in the search for a kidney donor. JAMA 1971; 215:909-12.
24. Fox RC, Swazey JP. The courage to fail: a social view of organ transplants and dialysis. 2nd ed. Chicago: University of Chicago Press, 1978:20-7.
25. Gulledge AD, Buszta KC, Montague DK. Psychosocial aspects of renal transplantation. Urol Clin North Am 1983; 10:327-35.
26. House RM, Thompson TL II. Psychiatric aspects of organ transplantation. JAMA 1988; 260:535-9.
27. Grim PS, Singer PA, Gramelspacher GP, Feldman T, Childers RW, Siegler M. Informed consent in emergency research: prehospital thrombolytic therapy for acute myocardial infarction. JAMA 1989; 262:252-5.

11.4   Kodish E, Lantos JD, Stocking CB, Singer PA, Siegler M, Johnson FL (1991) Bone Marrow Transplantation for Sickle Cell Disease; A Study of Parents' Decisions. N Eng J Med 325:1349–53

SPECIAL ARTICLE

BONE MARROW TRANSPLANTATION FOR SICKLE CELL DISEASE

A Study of Parents' Decisions

Eric Kodish, M.D., John Lantos, M.D., Carol Stocking, Ph.D., Peter A. Singer, M.D., M.P.H.,
Mark Siegler, M.D., and F. Leonard Johnson, M.D.

Abstract *Background.* Bone marrow transplantation has been shown to cure sickle cell disease, but it carries a 15 percent mortality risk. To determine whether parents would accept this risk to cure their children of sickle cell disease, we interviewed parents of children with sickle cell disease who were being followed in a university hospital clinic.

Methods. We assessed parents' attitudes by using questions based on the standard reference-gamble paradigm. After we gave them descriptions of bone marrow transplantation and graft-versus-host disease (GVHD), the parents were presented with a series of hypothetical situations. In the first situation, bone marrow transplantation was described as offering certain (100 percent) survival with cure of sickle cell disease. In subsequent descriptions, the mortality rate associated with bone marrow transplantation was increased by 5 percent increments. The parents indicated the highest mortality risk at which they would consent to the procedure in order to cure their children.

Results. In order to obtain a cure for their children, 36 of 67 parents (54 percent) were willing to accept some risk of short-term mortality, 25 of 67 (37 percent) were willing to accept at least the 15 percent short-term mortality risk we estimate to be the current figure for bone marrow transplantation, and 8 of 67 (12 percent) were willing to accept a short-term mortality risk of 50 percent or more. Nine parents (13 percent) said they would accept both a mortality risk of 15 percent or more and an additional 15 percent risk of GVHD. The parents' decisions were not related to the clinical severity of their children's illness.

Conclusions. At current rates of mortality and morbidity with bone marrow transplantation, a substantial minority of the parents of children with sickle cell disease may consent to bone marrow transplantation for their children. Parental attitudes should be factored into decisions about whether to offer bone marrow transplantation to children with sickle cell disease. (N Engl J Med 1991;325: 1349-53.)

BONE marrow transplantation is the only therapy that has been reported to cure patients with sickle cell disease.[1-3] However, when performed for currently accepted indications, this procedure is associated with a 10 to 50 percent risk of mortality and substantial additional risk of morbidity due to graft-versus-host disease (GVHD).[4-8] The mortality and morbidity have been readily accepted when bone marrow transplantation is used for life-threatening diseases, such as leukemia, for which no better treatment is available. But is this treatment appropriate for diseases that are not immediately life-threatening, such as sickle cell disease?

Sickle cell disease has an extremely variable natural history. Although some children with the disease die in infancy[9] or have devastating complications such as strokes,[10] acute chest syndrome,[11] and recurrent vaso-occlusive pain crises, others have few medical complications or none. Recent data show that older patients with more frequent painful episodes have higher mortality rates.[12] Although actuarial data on the life expectancy of patients with sickle cell disease are lacking, hematology textbooks suggest that patients with this disease rarely survive beyond middle age.[13,14] Be-

cause of the unpredictable course of the disease and its tendency to cause chronic debilitation rather than death, the use of bone marrow transplantation for children with sickle cell disease raises difficult clinical and ethical dilemmas.

In July 1988, clinicians at the University of Chicago submitted a proposal to the institutional review board to offer bone marrow transplantation to carefully selected patients with sickle cell disease. The proposal generated a great deal of controversy over whether this treatment should be offered to any patients with sickle cell disease and, if so, what criteria should be used to select appropriate candidates.[15] The institutional review board decided to allow investigators to offer bone marrow transplantation to two groups of children: those who had already had a stroke and were therefore given monthly blood transfusions to lessen the risk of another stroke, and those with recurrent pain crises so severe that they had been hospitalized for narcotic analgesia during more than 60 percent of the past year. In approving this protocol, the institutional review board decided that, for these selected high-risk patients, the risk–benefit ratio for bone marrow transplantation matched that for conventional treatment; thus, the parents of these children might reasonably choose either course of treatment.

It was not known how many parents would accept the risk of early death from bone marrow transplantation in exchange for the prospect of a cure for their children and what factors might predict parents' willingness to consent to transplantation on behalf of their children. We therefore decided to study parents'

From the Department of Pediatrics and the Center for Clinical Medical Ethics, University of Chicago Pritzker School of Medicine, Chicago, and the Department of Medicine and Centre for Bioethics, University of Toronto, Toronto, Ont. Address reprint requests to Dr. Kodish at the Department of Pediatrics, University of Chicago, Box 97, 5841 S. Maryland Ave., Chicago, IL 60637.

The Center for Clinical Medical Ethics is supported by grants from the Henry J. Kaiser Family Foundation, the Andrew W. Mellon Foundation, and the Pew Charitable Trusts.

1350   THE NEW ENGLAND JOURNAL OF MEDICINE   Nov. 7, 1991

attitudes about acceptable risks entailed by treatment to cure their children of sickle cell disease. If parents disagreed with the institutional review board about the appropriate use of bone marrow transplantation for sickle cell disease, it would raise a fundamental question about the ethics of innovative therapy in pediatrics: Who should decide whether children should undergo innovative medical treatment with the potential for both great risk and great benefit?

METHODS

After obtaining informed consent for their participation in a study regarding a new treatment for sickle cell disease, we interviewed parents of children with sickle cell disease at the time of their visits to the pediatric hematology clinic at the University of Chicago. The subjects were selected at random from among the parents attending the clinic on each study day, regardless of the severity of the children's disease. No parent was allowed to participate more than once. Parents were told explicitly that their responses would remain confidential and that the interview would have no effect on their children's medical care.

We conducted a structured interview with each parent. After obtaining relevant information about the demographic characteristics of the family and the patient's medical history, we described the process of bone marrow transplantation. The information we gave parents about bone marrow transplantation was based on the informed-consent form approved by the institutional review board. The portions of the description that we read to the parents included the following:

One potential treatment for sickle cell disease is called bone marrow transplantation. This treatment has been used in the past for other diseases, but is not yet used for sickle cell disease. In the procedure strong medications are given to the patient to destroy his or her bone marrow. . . . If no problems occur, the entire procedure requires hospitalization for about one month. Although this treatment has very serious risks, if successful it would probably cure sickle cell disease. . . . The next set of questions involves trying to find out how much risk you would be willing for your child to accept for a bone marrow transplant to cure [him or her].

A board-certified pediatrician specializing in hematology and oncology, who is knowledgeable about both bone marrow transplantation and sickle cell disease, conducted the majority of the interviews and supervised the others. The parents were given several opportunities to ask questions. The interview did not proceed until the interviewer was certain that parents understood the information they had been given.

We assessed parents' decisions about acceptable risks of mortality and morbidity by using questions based on the standard reference-gamble paradigm.[16] The standard reference gamble and its variants are decision-analysis techniques that have been used in the past to elicit adults' preferences among treatments for lung cancer,[17] laryngeal cancer,[18] and prostate cancer.[19] The technique has not to our knowledge been used previously with parents' being asked to make decisions for their children.

The parents were asked whether they would consent to bone marrow transplantation for their children in various hypothetical situations. In the first situation, bone marrow transplantation was described as offering 100 percent survival (no risk of mortality from the transplantation) and certain cure of sickle cell disease. In subsequent descriptions, the mortality rate associated with bone marrow transplantation was gradually increased by 5 percent increments. Graphic representations of survival and mortality rates accompanied each question in order to facilitate clear understanding of the risks. In this way, each parent indicated the highest risk of mortality that he or she would accept in exchange for the prospect of cure for his or her child. The first situation in which the parent answered "no" was registered as the point of too much risk, and this section of the interview was concluded. For example, the fourth question was

accompanied by a pie chart showing 15 percent mortality and 85 percent survival; the text read as follows:

Suppose that for the transplant 85 percent lived and 15 percent died from the treatment. That is: 85 out of every 100 children lived and were cured of sickle cell disease, but 15 out of 100 died in the first 30 days after the treatment. If these were the risks, would you want [your child] to have this treatment?

We posed an additional question only to those parents who were willing to accept a risk of mortality of 15 percent or more. This question asked the parents to consider the additional risk of chronic morbidity due to GVHD. Our description of GVHD was based on the informed-consent form approved by the institutional review board for the protocol to offer transplantation to patients with sickle cell disease and read, in part:

After having a bone marrow transplantation, some patients develop a new problem called graft-versus-host disease. . . . Of those who survive [transplantation], most will be cured, but some will have graft-versus-host disease. Graft-versus-host disease is a chronic illness that some people who have had a bone marrow transplant develop. It can affect the lungs, liver, gastrointestinal tract, and skin. People with graft-versus-host disease can be very sick and die from it. . . . Less is known about graft-versus-host disease than sickle cell disease because it is a newer problem than sickle cell disease.

We then asked this group of parents if they would want bone marrow transplantation for their child if the risk of mortality were 15 percent, the risk of GVHD were 15 percent, and the chance for cure without GVHD were 70 percent. These percentages reflect the likely outcome of transplantation among such patients today and are based on data obtained from the experience with bone marrow transplantation in patients with thalassemia[8] and aplastic anemia.[20]

To analyze our data, we compared parents who accepted some risk associated with transplantation with those who did not by using the continuity-adjusted chi-square test for dichotomous variables and the Wilcoxon rank-sum test for ordinal variables. We then used a Wilcoxon analysis of the variable we called "too much risk" to look at factors that related to the degree of risk parents were willing to accept with transplantation. Finally, we performed a multivariate analysis with a linear regression model to examine the intercorrelation of associated variables. The study was approved by the institutional review board of the University of Chicago.

RESULTS

We interviewed 67 parents or guardians (we shall refer to both parents and guardians as "parents") of 67 children (35 girls and 32 boys) with sickle cell disease between October 1989 and April 1990. No parent whom we approached declined to participate. The children ranged from infancy to 20 years of age, with a mean age of 10 years. Seven (10 percent) of the children were 18 years old or older. Because our study was designed to assess parents' views, these young adults were not interviewed. All the children had homozygous disease. The parents ranged in age from 18 to 64 years, with a mean age of 34. They included 53 mothers, 3 fathers, 3 aunts, 4 grandmothers, 2 adult siblings, and 2 other guardians. Fifty-five of the 67 parents (82 percent) were currently unmarried.

Sixteen of 67 parents (24 percent) were unwilling to accept any risk of short-term mortality (death within 30 days) in order for their children to be cured of sickle cell disease. These parents said no to transplantation at the 100 percent survival–cure level (100 percent probability of cure and 0 percent short-term mortality). Another 15 parents (22 percent) were probably

Vol. 325   No. 19   BONE MARROW TRANSPLANTATION FOR SICKLE CELL DISEASE — KODISH ET AL.   1351

not willing to accept any risk. These 15 said yes to transplantation at the 100 percent survival–cure level but said no at the 95 percent level (95 percent probability of cure and 5 percent risk of short-term mortality). Thirty-six of the 67 parents (54 percent) were willing to accept some risk of short-term mortality for their children in exchange for a cure (Fig. 1). Twenty-five of the 67 parents (37 percent) were willing to accept a 15 percent or greater risk of short-term mortality, which we estimate to be the current risk for such a procedure. Eight parents (12 percent of our sample) were willing to accept a 50 percent or greater risk of short-term mortality due to transplantation in exchange for a cure for sickle cell disease.

We asked only the 25 parents who accepted a 15 percent or greater mortality risk about the additional risk of GVHD, to determine how a 15 percent risk of GVHD would modify their decision. Nine of the 25 (36 percent) were willing to accept both a short-term mortality risk of 15 percent and an additional 15 percent risk of GVHD. Thus, 9 of 67 parents (13 percent) said they would consent to bone marrow transplantation for their children given current estimates of the risk of morbidity and mortality, or worse conditions.

Parents who accepted some risk in exchange for a cure for their children were different in several ways from those who did not accept risk. Parents who had graduated from high school were significantly more likely to accept some risk in exchange for cure than those who were not high-school graduates (28 of 43 vs. 8 of 24, P = 0.012). Parents who were employed or in school were more likely to accept some risk than those who were not occupied outside the home (19 of 28 vs. 17 of 39, P = 0.05). Parents who had more than one child with sickle cell disease were more willing to risk mortality to obtain a cure (8 of 10 vs. 23 of 47, P = 0.07). Finally, parents were more willing to consent to bone marrow transplantation for girls than for boys (23 of 35 vs. 13 of 32, P = 0.04). Clinical factors such as the number of hospital admissions in the past year, history of stroke, admission to the intensive care unit, the frequency of pain medication, and the frequency of absence from school because of sickle cell disease were not significantly associated with parents' acceptance of risk.

Wilcoxon analysis to examine the degree of risk parents were willing to accept also demonstrated that having at least a high-school education was most strongly associated (P = 0.004) with the degree of risk accepted. Parents who had more than one child with sickle cell disease (P = 0.03), whose children were girls (P = 0.05), and who were employed or in school (P = 0.1) also accepted more risk to obtain a cure than did other parents. As before, the clinical severity of sickle cell disease did not correlate with the degree of risk parents were willing to accept in exchange for the cure of their children.

Finally, we used a linear regression model in which the degree of risk was the dependent variable and the

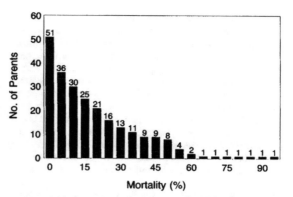

Figure 1. Number of Parents of Children with Sickle Cell Disease Who Said They Would Choose Bone Marrow Transplantation at Different Estimates of the Mortality Rate Associated with the Procedure.

There were 67 parents in the study. Sixteen said they would not consent to the procedure even if there was no risk of death associated with it. The numbers over the bars indicate how many parents said they would consent to the procedure at each risk level.

parent's education level, the sex of the child, the presence of other children with sickle cell disease in the family, the number of hospital admissions in the past year, the number of days of school missed, and previous admissions to the intensive care unit were the independent variables. When we used this model, the variable for female sex lost its statistical significance. Parental education and the presence of another child with sickle cell disease in the family remained significantly associated with a willingness to accept greater risk.

Discussion

Thirty-seven percent of the parents we interviewed were apparently willing to consent to bone marrow transplantation with a 15 percent or greater risk of short-term mortality for their children. Thirty-six percent of this group (13 percent of the entire cohort) said they would consent to transplantation if it entailed a 15 percent risk of chronic morbidity due to GVHD in addition to a 15 percent or greater risk of short-term mortality. Thus, at least 13 percent of parents might be expected to consent to bone marrow transplantation for sickle cell disease given current rates of morbidity and mortality. These data suggest that parents would weigh the risks and benefits of bone marrow transplantation for sickle cell disease in a different way from the members of our institutional review board. The results raise the question of whose judgment should prevail.

Before addressing this question, we should note four limitations of this study. First, the decisions made by the parents we interviewed were explicitly hypothetical, and therefore they may not accurately reflect the decisions that parents would make if their children were actually offered bone marrow transplantation.

Second, our cohort may be skewed toward parents of children with more severe disease because these are presumably the parents who bring their children to the hematology clinic more frequently. If more severe illness would predispose parents to consent to transplantation, this selection bias might lead us to overestimate the number of parents who would consent to the procedure.

Third, it is possible that some parents did not understand the standard-gamble questions, despite the pie charts and the simple question format used in the interview. Nevertheless, our presentation of the quantitative risks and benefits was probably as clear and understandable as that which parents would receive if they were actually offered the option of transplantation.

Finally, we may not have conveyed qualitative information about morbidity due to bone marrow transplantation graphically enough for parents to understand it fully. Previous studies have demonstrated that the language used to describe a procedure can dramatically affect the rate of consent.[21] We modeled our description of bone marrow transplantation and GVHD on the descriptions in the informed-consent form approved by the institutional review board, which parents would be given if their children were actually offered the option of transplantation. Specific details of the medications used and their potential complications were omitted, but the major organ-system complications were discussed, and the possibility that GVHD might be worse than sickle cell disease was stated. As with the quantitative information, our descriptions were comparable to what parents are told in real informed-consent situations. In all cases, the interviewer answered all questions from each parent.

Our data raise questions about decision making for children with sickle cell disease. At the outset of this study, we hypothesized that parents, like members of the institutional review board, would consider the severity of illness to be the most relevant factor in deciding whether to consent to bone marrow transplantation for their children, and we wondered what degree of severity parents would consider sufficient to justify the risks associated with transplantation. Unlike doctors, however, parents did not base their decisions on clinical factors indicating the severity of illness. Thus, parents may not think about risks and benefits the way doctors do.

Parents' decisions were related to certain social and demographic factors. Parents with more than one child with sickle cell disease tended to choose transplantation more often, and at higher risk levels, than those with only one affected child. This difference may reflect more intimate knowledge of the disease, or it may be an indication of the burdens of caring for children with sickle cell disease. The parents' education level was also strongly correlated with an acceptance of transplantation — a finding that is in sharp contrast to the results of a study that showed that parental education was inversely associated with willingness to allow children to participate in research.[22]

The differences between the parents' decisions and the criteria of the institutional review board raise a difficult question. Which set of factors is most appropriate in determining whether a child should be offered or allowed to undergo bone marrow transplantation to treat sickle cell disease? Do the medical indications used by the institutional review board protect children from well-intentioned, well-informed, but perhaps overzealous or desperate parents? Or do institutional review boards represent a paternalistic infringement on parents' right to make medical decisions for their children?

Institutional review boards were created to protect the rights and welfare of human subjects of research. Children are considered an especially vulnerable population, and research involving children is generally permissible only if it involves minimal risk (or none) to the child. Any research proposal that involved a 15 percent risk of death and a 15 percent risk of serious illness would almost surely be prohibited. If a treatment protocol is not research, however, then patients are not research subjects, and institutional review boards should not control the selection of patients. Instead, clinicians and parents must decide together whether the risks and burdens of treatment outweigh the benefits. Thus, a key question in deciding whether parents or an institutional review board should decide which children with sickle cell disease should be offered bone marrow transplantation is whether the procedure is considered clinical research or innovative therapy.

Research and the practice of medicine often overlap. Although it acknowledges that there will always be some ambiguity, the Declaration of Helsinki distinguishes between "medical research in which the aim is essentially diagnostic or therapeutic for a patient, and medical research, the essential object of which is purely scientific."[23] The declaration then states that "the doctor must be free to use a new diagnostic and therapeutic measure, if in his or her judgment it offers hope of saving life, reestablishing health, or alleviating suffering." Research, according to Levine, is an activity "designed to develop or contribute to generalizable knowledge."[24] The practice of medicine, by contrast, is an activity "designed solely to enhance the well-being of an individual patient or client."[24] According to these definitions, we suggest, bone marrow transplantation for sickle cell disease need not be considered research, and thus may not require approval from an institutional review board.

The regulations of the Department of Health and Human Services, which permit risky research involving children only if it "holds out the prospect of direct benefit for the individual subject,"[25] apply only to projects that have already been deemed to be research. The regulations do not address the issue of how to weigh the prospect of benefit to the patient against the goal of collecting generalizable knowledge in order to determine which innovations require approval from an institutional review board.

The primary motivation of the clinicians who wanted to offer bone marrow transplantation to children with sickle cell disease was to benefit the patient. Much is known about the use of bone marrow transplantation for other hemoglobinopathies.[8,26,27] Although some knowledge may be gained from offering transplantation to patients with sickle cell disease, we suggest that the use of transplantation for patients with sickle cell disease is not primarily a matter of research.

This is not to say that bone marrow transplantation should be offered to all patients with sickle cell disease. Clinicians who specialize in the procedure and in the care of patients with this disease must first decide whether they feel the procedure is medically indicated. The distinction between research and therapy has few implications for the doctor–patient relationship. Physicians must still judge the risks and benefits of various treatments and discuss the options realistically with patients and their parents.

Parents' views of the risks and benefits of bone marrow transplantation, and the factors they consider relevant in deciding whether to consent to the procedure for their children with sickle cell disease, challenge us to examine the reasons why such therapy should or should not be offered. In making clinical decisions, rigorous analysis of the risks and benefits of therapy should be combined with careful consideration of the values that underlie treatment decisions. Studies of the values that underlie parental choices might help clinicians to understand better the relation between clinical and moral factors in deciding how best to use innovative therapies.

We are indebted to Linda Drawhorn, R.N., Uma Subramanian, M.D., and Ruth Rudinsky, M.D., for their help with the enrollment of subjects, and to Aine Kresheck for assistance with the data collection.

REFERENCES

1. Johnson FL, Look AT, Gockerman J, Ruggiero MR, Dalla-Pozza L, Billings FT III. Bone-marrow transplantation in a patient with sickle-cell anemia. N Engl J Med 1984;311:780-3.
2. Vermylen C, Fernandez-Robles EF, Ninane J, Cornu G. Bone marrow transplantation in five children with sickle cell anaemia. Lancet 1988;1:1427-8.
3. Johnson FL. Bone marrow transplantation in the treatment of sickle cell anemia. Am J Pediatr Hematol Oncol 1985;7:254-7.
4. McGlave P. Bone marrow transplants in chronic myelogenous leukemia: an overview of determinants of survival. Semin Hematol 1990;27:Suppl 4:23-30.
5. Forman SJ, Blume KG. Allogeneic bone marrow transplantation for acute leukemia. Hematol Oncol Clin North Am 1990;4:517-33.
6. Durbin M. Bone marrow transplantation: economic, ethical, and social issues. Pediatrics 1988;82:774-83.
7. Locasciulli A, vant Veer L, Bacigalupo A, et al. Treatment with marrow transplantation or immunosuppression of childhood acquired severe aplastic anemia: a report from the EBMT SAA Working Party. Bone Marrow Transplant 1990;6:211-7.
8. Lucarelli G, Galimberti M, Polchi P, et al. Bone marrow transplantation in patients with thalassemia. N Engl J Med 1990;322:417-21.
9. Leikin SL, Gallagher D, Kinney TR, Sloane D, Klug P, Rida W. Mortality in children and adolescents with sickle cell disease. Pediatrics 1989;84:500-8.
10. Sarnaik SA, Lusher JM. Neurological complications of sickle cell anemia. Am J Pediatr Hematol Oncol 1982;4:386-94.
11. Sprinkle RH, Cole T, Smith S, Buchanan GR. Acute chest syndrome in children with sickle cell disease. Am J Pediatr Hematol Oncol 1986;8:105-10.
12. Platt OS, Thorington BD, Brambilla DJ, et al. Pain in sickle cell disease — rates and risk factors. N Engl J Med 1991;325:11-6.
13. Beutler E. The sickle cell diseases and related disorders. In: Williams WJ, Beutler E, Erslev AJ, Lichtman MA, eds. Hematology. 3rd ed. New York: McGraw-Hill, 1983:583-609.
14. Platt OS, Nathan DG. Sickle cell disease. In: Nathan DG, Oski FA, eds. Hematology of infancy and childhood. 3rd ed. Philadelphia: W.B. Saunders, 1987:655-98.
15. Kodish E, Lantos J, Siegler M, Kohrman A, Johnson FL. Bone marrow transplantation in sickle cell disease. Clin Res 1990;38:694-700.
16. Froberg DG, Kane RL. Methodology for measuring health-state preferences — II: scaling methods. J Clin Epidemiol 1989;42:459-71.
17. McNeil BJ, Weichselbaum R, Pauker SG. Fallacy of the five-year survival in lung cancer. N Engl J Med 1978;299:1397-401.
18. Idem. Speech and survival: tradeoffs between quality and quantity of life in laryngeal cancer. N Engl J Med 1981;305:982-7.
19. Singer PA, Tasch ES, Stocking C, Rubin S, Siegler M, Weichselbaum R. Sex or survival: tradeoffs between quality and quantity of life. J Clin Oncol 1991;9:328-34.
20. Storb R, Thomas ED, Buckner CD, et al. Marrow transplantation for aplastic anemia. Semin Hematol 1984;21:27-35.
21. Briggs NC, Piliavin JA, Lorentzen D, Becker GA. On willingness to be a bone marrow donor. Transfusion 1986;26:324-30.
22. Harth SC, Thong YH. Sociodemographic and motivational characteristics of parents who volunteer their children for clinical research: a controlled study. BMJ 1990;300:1372-5.
23. World Medical Association Declaration of Helsinki: recommendations guiding medical doctors in biomedical research involving human subjects. Presented at the 29th World Medical Assembly, Tokyo, Japan.
24. Basic concepts and definitions. In: Levine RJ. Ethics and regulation of clinical research. 2nd ed. New Haven, Conn.: Yale University Press, 1986:1-18.
25. Department of Health and Human Services. Additional protections for children involved as subjects in research. Fed Regist 1983;48:9814-20.
26. Galimberti M, Andreani M, Lucarelli G, et al. Patterns of graft rejection after bone marrow transplant in thalassemia. In: Buckner CD, Gale RP, Lucarelli G, eds. Advances and controversies in thalassemia therapy. Vol. 309 of Progress in clinical and biological research. New York: Alan R. Liss, 1989:223-9.
27. Or R, Naparstek E, Ciridalli G, et al. Bone marrow transplantation in beta-thalassemia major: the Israeli experience. Hemoglobin 1988;12:609-14.

11.5　Siegler M, Lantos JD (1992) Ethical Justification for Living Liver Donation. Camb Q Healthc Ethics 4:320–5

Reproduced with permission from Cambridge University Press.

Living Liver Donors: Bioethics

Commentary: Ethical Justification for Living Liver Donation
Mark Siegler and John D. Lantos

Introduction

In 1989, the distinguished Brazilian surgeon, Dr. Silvano Raia, performed the world's first liver transplantation using a liver segment graft obtained from a living donor, the mother of the 4-year-old recipient. In the accompanying paper by Professor Marco Segre, a second living donor operation is mentioned, one that apparently involved a 1-year-old recipient and an unrelated adult donor. Professor Segre, a member of the ethics committee of the University of São Paulo Medical College, describes the considerations that led the committee to approve these innovative and untested procedures. In describing the "reasons for the transplantation request," Professor Segre emphasizes issues of donor safety (see points 1, 3, 4, 5) and voluntary informed consent (see points 6, 7, 8) but hardly mentions potential recipient benefit (see point 2). The only justification for permitting living liver donors to assume any risk must relate to the potential benefits for recipients.

In the Discussion section of the paper, Professor Segre notes without further comment that "Clinically, the evaluation of risks and benefits presented by the surgical team was a favorable one." Presumably, Professor Segre is referring to donor risks and recipient benefits, but this point is not entirely clear. Nor does Segre present the basis for these conclusions. This omission is troubling.

Professor Segre then indicates the es-

Mark Siegler and John D. Lantos

sential basis for the committee's decision:

> The committee's favorable opinion on this request was based largely upon the principle of autonomy. . . . We strongly advocate the viewpoint of patient and donor autonomy as articulated in the North American bioethics literature. We believe that the individual who is considering donating organs has the controlling decision, and that the analysis by third parties of the reasons for donation is of secondary moral importance. Thus it is irrelevant whether the donation motivation arises from a wish to repay a potential organ recipient for something that was received, from financial interest, or from strong emotional links with a son, brother, or any other person.

The São Paulo committee's extreme and inappropriate reliance on donor autonomy is unsettling and may explain some of the following problems with their approval of the procedures. First, there is little mention of recipient need or potential benefit; second, they permitted an unrelated living donor to be used in a highly experimental and untested transplantation procedure; and finally, the committee authorized a procedure that on its face appears to contravene a provision of the Brazilian Federal Medical Ethics code which states that organ donation ". . . is only permitted in the case of double organs or tissues." We feel that Professor Segre and his colleagues may have misinterpreted the "North American bioethics literature" if they believe that voluntary consent constitutes adequate justification to perform any procedure. We will return to this point.

In a paper on organ transplantation and surgical innovation, Dr. Francis Moore noted that the ethical conduct of therapeutic innovation should involve ". . . open display, public evaluation,

and prior discussion."[1] Dr. Raia's group may have conducted prior discussions with the São Paulo ethics committee, but they performed their first living liver transplantation without ". . . open display [or] public discussion." By contrast, at the University of Chicago, we had been considering the use of living related donors to provide organ segments for infants and children since 1986. After extensive discussions were conducted within the University community and between the transplantation team and the Institutional Review Board, our group chose to announce our plans publicly in advance and to describe the ethical considerations of this innovative procedure before performing the first such operation. Three months before the Chicago team performed its first living donor liver transplantation, we published our ethical analysis and plans in the *New England Journal of Medicine* and invited public and professional response.[2]

At the University of Chicago, the first living donor liver transplantation was performed on 23 November 1989; the 20th case in the experimental series was completed on 12 February 1991; and the series was reported in the fall of 1991 in the *Annals of Surgery*.[3] Subsequently, the Chicago team has performed more than 25 additional living liver donor operations. The results from these 45 cases have been excellent; there have been no donor deaths, and graft survival in recipients has been greater than 80%.

Intensive private and public discussion of the plans of the Chicago team enabled us to identify and analyze the full range of ethical issues in the living donor procedure. Further, such discussion facilitated development of an experimental surgical protocol that constituted a useful prospective scientific experiment for a potentially valuable but also potentially dangerous surgical innovation. Unfortunately, in contrast to the Chicago approach, the São Paulo group proceeded without taking adequate account of Professor Moore's cautionary advice. As a result, they failed to recognize the full range of ethical issues associated with this new operation and failed also to develop an experimental protocol that could yield useable scientific results.

Is Autonomy the Whole Ethical Question?

The use of living organ donors remains controversial.[4-7] This is especially true for living liver transplantation, a new surgical procedure involving a nonpaired organ. Physicians who use living donors subject a healthy person to a procedure that entails some medical and surgical risk and that does not improve or maintain that person's health. The risk to the donor is justified only by the potential benefit to the recipient.

This dilemma is often mistakenly perceived as a problem of patient consent. However, Woodruff noted in 1964 that consent is not the crucial issue. Many competent adults freely consent to self-sacrificial actions for altruistic reasons. "The question is not whether the donor is right to offer to give up his kidney, but whether the doctor is right to allow him to do so."[8] Singer and Siegler echoed this conclusion and debunked the notion that individuals had a so-called "right" to donate organs in situations where surgeons were unwilling to accept such donations.[9]

Woodruff proposed that solutions to this dilemma would not be found in moral absolutes but in clinical judgments based on the probabilities of risks and benefits to both donor and recipient. This approach is still relevant. Most but not all transplant surgeons consider live donor transplants accept-able even though they involve some risk to a healthy donor. Prudent people might be allowed to consent to a small personal risk to give another person a great benefit but not to a great risk for a small benefit. In deciding whether to use a living donor, surgeons weigh the relative risks to the donor, which must be extremely low, against the potential benefits to the recipient.

Donor Risks

The donor requires a general anesthesia for a partial hepatectomy, and this is associated with risks. A partial hepatectomy can be quite risky in the face of underlying cirrhosis, and some surgeons have reported operative mortality rates as high as 11%.[10,11] In a number of series involving noncirrhotic patients, however, the operation has been performed with no or very low mortality.[12-15]

In our first experimental series involving 20 patients, living liver donors developed operative complications.[16] One patient required splenectomy as a result of an intraoperative laceration of the spleen. Two donors have required nonoperative management of bile leaks. No donor deaths have occurred. Long-term risks to the donor appear to be low. After partial hepatectomy, the liver regenerates,[17] so liver mass is expected to return to normal within 4–6 weeks, although this has not been studied in the living donor situation. Thus, although no long-term data on donors are currently available, there is reason to believe that donors will have normal hepatic function after partial liver donation.[18]

Recipient Benefits

There is no medical therapy for patients dying of end stage liver disease. The primary benefit to the recipient is the

Mark Siegler and John D. Lantos

availability of an organ for transplant at a time when the recipient is still medically suitable or appropriate for transplant. For a number of patients, especially infants and small children, the shortage of suitable cadaveric livers often leads to death or clinical deterioration while waiting for an organ. The use of reduced-size and split livers ameliorates the organ shortage for children, but the shortage remains.

Liver transplantation from living donors, rather than cadavers, may confer other benefits as well. The transplanted organs may be healthier because there would be decreased ischemic time between organ harvest and transplantation. In other organ transplant situations, organs from family members are less likely to be rejected, most likely as a result of better HLA matching. This may be true for livers as well.

It is hard to evaluate the efficacy of living liver donation because the procedure is so new. Our initial results are comparable or somewhat better than results after whole liver transplants from cadaver donors. If graft survival is comparable, and live donor transplants allow patients who would have died while waiting for an organ to survive, then many people will judge the recipient benefits to outweigh the small known and the unquantified unknown risks to the donor.

What about Informed Consent?

In most cases, donation is only acceptable if an autonomous patient consents to the procedure. Valid consent has three elements: the patient must have the cognitive capacity to make decisions, the patient must be given sufficient information to understand the medical situation, and the decision must be made without undue coercion.

As healthy individuals who are choosing to undergo potentially risky surgery,

living organ donors must meet the highest standards of decision-making capacity. We therefore disagree strongly with Segre's view that even doubts regarding the "donor's psychic fitness" may not be sufficient grounds to override the donor's right to donate. It is axiomatic that organ donors should have access to all relevant information about the risks of donation. Such information may not, however, be a key factor in donor decision making. Empirical studies show that most kidney donors make their decision to donate immediately after the subject of transplant is first mentioned to them, and no additional information has any effect on their decision.[19-21] Because potential donors appear unwilling or incapable of evaluating information about risks and benefits, physicians may recommend that donors undergo psychological or psychiatric evaluation to determine whether their decision is truly voluntary.[22,23]

Three Forms of Coercion: Altruism, Guilt, and Greed

Given high standards of decision-making capacity and adequate disclosure of information about donor risk, the potential for coercion becomes the key element of informed consent. Three possible components of donor coercion should be distinguished. The first is psychological or internal coercion created by the donor's own feelings of guilt because the patient may die without donor participation.[24] This negative or coercive psychological response may, of course, be balanced by positive emotional responses to donation, such as feelings of loyalty, responsibility, love, or duty toward a family member.

Psychological coercion may be unavoidable but may also be indistinguishable, in many cases, from laudable psychological motivations for donation. In any case, this sort of coercion is not

Living Liver Donors: Justification

unique to organ transplantation. The need to balance selfishness and altruism is a universal feature of an individual's relationship with his or her family. Because this is a universal element of human interaction, we do not think that it invalidates voluntary consent.

The second element of donor coercion is external. Pressure upon an unwilling donor to consent may come from family members or healthcare workers.[25] If family pressures appear to be unduly coercive and the donor seems conflicted about the decision to donate, psychiatric evaluation and counseling of both the potential donor and the family may be necessary.[26] Although controversial, physicians might also, with the consent of the patient, inform a family that the decision not to donate was based on medical criteria, such as tissue incompatibility, rather than lack of consent. This would offer the potential donor psychological protection from family pressures.

Pressure from the transplant team may be more difficult to avoid. Surgeons can avoid unintentionally coercing donors by highlighting the potential risks of donation and emphasizing that a decision not to donate would be understandable and acceptable. A "donor advocate," independent of the transplant team, may counsel the potential donor and help work through the tangle of conflicting emotions.[27]

A third form of coercion could come from financial incentives to donate. We strongly disagree with Segre when he says it is ". . . irrelevant whether the donation motivation arises . . . from financial interest. . . ." The legalization of organ selling would be coercive because it would create an irresistible financial incentive particularly for the poor, who would likely make decisions that they otherwise would not have made.[28] Further, the buying and selling of organs has been condemned by the World Health Organization.

Conclusion

In deciding whether the use of live donors is acceptable for any particular clinical situation, it is always necessary to weigh the potential benefits to the recipient against the risks to the donor. This crucial point is not adequately discussed in Professor Segre's paper. Physicians should set guidelines for when donation using living donors is acceptable. On this score, we strongly disagree with Segre's observation that ". . . it is irrelevant whether the donation motivation arises from a wish to repay a potential organ recipient for something that was received [or] from financial interest. . . ." Patient autonomy, although important, is not absolute. It is constrained by the traditional professional ethical obligation of physicians to do no harm. Guidelines for deciding when donation is acceptable and for selecting donors should reflect clinical data on outcomes, the normative values that prohibit donors from undergoing more than minimal risk, and procedural safeguards to prevent coercion. Surgical innovation, particularly when it involves living donors, should proceed according to Dr. Moore's recommendations for "open display, public evaluation and prior discussion." It should also proceed according to scientific norms that allow the experiment to be evaluated for its scientific merit. Unfortunately, this was not done in the two isolated cases described by Professor Segre.

Notes

1. Moore FD. Three ethical revolutions: ancient assumptions remodeled under pressure of transplantation. *Transplantation Proceedings* 1988;20(Suppl. 1):1061–7.
2. Singer PA, Siegler M, Lantos JD, *et al.* Ethics of liver transplantation with living donors. *New England Journal of Medicine* 1989;321: 620–2.
3. Broelsch CE, Whitington PF, Emond JC, *et al.* Liver transplantation in children from living

Mark Siegler and John D. Lantos

related donors: surgical techniques and results. *Annals of Surgery* 1991;214:428–39.

4. Kreir H. Why living related donors should not be used whenever possible. *Transplantation Proceedings* 1985;17:1510–4.

5. Sutherland DER. Living related donors should be used whenever possible. *Transplantation Proceedings* 1985;17:13–7.

6. Friedman EA, Najarian J, Starzl T, *et al.* Ethical aspects in renal transplantation. *Kidney International* 1983;23:S90–3.

7. Starzl TE. Living donors: con. *Transplantation Proceedings* 1987;19 (Part 1):174–5.

8. Woodruff MFA. Ethical problems in organ transplantation. *British Medical Journal* 1964; 1:1457–60.

9. Singer PA, Lowance D, Siegler M. Whose kidney is it anyway? Ethical considerations in living kidney donation. *American Kidney Foundation* 1988;5(1):16–20.

10. McDermott WV, Ottinger W. Elective hepatic resection. *American Journal of Surgery* 1966; 112:376–81.

11. Starzl TE, Weil R, Putnam CW. Right trisegmentectomy for hepatic neoplasms. *Surgery, Gynecology & Obstetrics* 1980;150:209–13.

12. Adson M. Diagnosis and surgical treatment of primary and secondary solid hepatic tumors in the adult. *Surgical Clinics of North America* 1981;61:181–92.

13. Iwatsuki S, Shaw BW, Starzl TE. Experience with 150 liver resections. *Annals of Surgery* 1983;197:247–53.

14. Bismuth H, Houssin D, Michel, F. Operative risks in hepatectomies. Experience with 154 hepatectomies. *Chirurgie* 1983;109:342–8.

15. Broelsch CE, Neuhaus P, Ringe B, *et al.* Hepatic resection in primary and secondary liver tumors. In: Axel-Girigi H, ed. *Aspekte der Klinischen Onkologie*. Stuttgart: Gustav Fischer Verlag, 1984:483.

16. Takeshi N, Inoue S, Mizuta T, *et al.* One hundred hepatic resections. *Annals of Surgery* 1985;202:42–9.

17. Nagasue N, Inokuchi K, Kanashima R. Release of lysosomal enzymes after partial hepatectomy: study of patients with and without cirrhosis of the liver. *Archives of Surgery* 1982;117:772–6.

18. Jansen PL, Chamuleau RA, van Leeuwen DJ, *et al.* Liver regeneration and restoration of liver function after partial hepatectomy in patients with liver tumors. *Scandinavian Journal of Gastroenterology* 1990;25:112–8.

19. Sadler HH, Davison L, Carroll C, *et al.* The living genetically unrelated kidney donor. *Seminars in Psychiatry* 1971;3:86–101.

20. Fellner CH. Selection of living kidney donors and the problem of informed consent. *Seminars in Psychiatry* 1971;3:79–85.

21. Fellner CH, Marshall JR. Twelve kidney donors. *Journal of the American Medical Association* 1968;206:2703–7.

22. Surman OS. Psychiatric aspects of organ transplantation. *American Journal of Psychiatry* 1989;146:972–82.

23. Singer PA, Siegler M, Lantos JD, *et al.* Liver transplantation using living donors: a clinical ethical analysis. *New England Journal of Medicine* 1989;321:620–1.

24. Simmons RG, Hickey K, Kjellstrand CM, et al. Family tension in the search for a kidney donor. *Journal of the American Medical Association* 1971;215:909–12.

25. Fox RC, Swazey JP. *The Courage to Fail.* 2nd ed. Chicago: The University of Chicago Press, 1978:20–7.

26. Gulledge AD, Buszta KC, Montague DK. Psychological aspects of renal transplantation. *Urologic Clinics of North America* 1983;10: 327–35.

27. House RM, Thompson TL. Psychiatric aspects of organ transplantation. *Journal of the American Medical Association* 1988;260:535–9.

28. Annas GJ. Life, liberty and the pursuit of organ sales. *Hastings Center Report* 1984 Feb.: 22–3.

11.6   Cronin D, Millis M, Siegler M (2001) Transplantation of Liver Grafts from Living Donors into Adults: Too Much, Too Soon. N Eng J Med 344:1633–7

Sounding Board

TRANSPLANTATION OF LIVER GRAFTS FROM LIVING DONORS INTO ADULTS — TOO MUCH, TOO SOON

SINCE 1995, many liver-transplantation programs in the United States,[1,2] Europe,[3] and Asia[4,5] have performed adult-to-adult transplantation of liver grafts from living donors. Since 1997, more than 30 U.S. transplantation programs have performed more than 400 of these procedures. Although six of these programs have performed only 1 procedure each, one program has performed more than 100. Twenty-three centers are planning to start such programs.[6,7] Liver transplantation in adults with the use of grafts from living donors may initially have been regarded as a technical extension of the procedure for transplanting liver grafts from living donors into children. However, we are unaware of any formal analyses of whether it is ethical to perform the operation, even if donors and recipients provide informed consent.

In this article, we examine the ethical aspects of liver transplantation in adults with the use of grafts from living donors by comparing the procedure with liver transplants in children with the use of grafts from living donors and by considering a number of potential concerns.[8,9] Although we acknowledge the benefits of the procedure for selected adults when it is performed by competent surgical teams, we believe that it has been disseminated too quickly, that more programs than are required currently perform the surgery or plan to start doing so in the near future, and that inadequate data are being collected on outcomes for both recipients and donors. As a result, regulatory oversight may be required to protect the interests of all parties.

TRANSPLANTATION OF GRAFTS FROM LIVING DONORS INTO CHILDREN

During the 1980s, the leading U.S. liver-transplantation centers reported mortality rates of 20 to 30 percent among children on their waiting lists for transplants.[10] The high rates were due primarily to the lack of grafts of an appropriate size for children. By the late 1980s, innovative surgical techniques, including the use of reduced-size and split-liver cadaveric grafts, had reduced the number of deaths among infants and children on waiting lists but had not eliminated them.[10]

A successful transplantation of a liver from a living donor was performed in Australia in 1989 by Strong and colleagues.[11] Subsequently, the liver-transplantation team at our institution, which had had success with innovative liver surgery, designed a formal clinical trial that was approved by the institutional review board. Before the trial began, the clinical and ethical aspects of the new operation were analyzed.[12]

Only after the favorable results of this clinical trial had been published[13] did several leading liver-transplantation programs in the United States,[14,15] Europe,[16] and Asia[17,18] begin transplanting liver grafts from living donors into carefully selected children. Substantial technical modifications[19-21] have improved the procedure, which is now usually effective and safe for both the recipient[21] and the donor.[22,23] More than 1500 such surgeries have been performed throughout the world. Only two donors have died,[24] although it is possible that there have been unreported deaths among donors.

The basic operation (a left lateral segmentectomy) has predictable, demonstrated risks and benefits. Complications have been reported in less than 10 percent of donors; most of these complications have involved the biliary system.[23] The rate of graft survival at one year has increased from 74 percent to 94 percent, and mortality before transplantation has decreased significantly.[21] Liver transplantation in children with the use of grafts from living donors has been performed only by the most experienced liver-surgery programs in the world.

TRANSPLANTATION OF GRAFTS FROM LIVING DONORS INTO ADULTS

The first liver transplantation in an adult with the use of a graft from a living donor was performed at the University of Chicago in 1991 as an emergency procedure.[25] In recent years, we have obtained approval from our institutional review board for a prospective case study that extends our pediatric program of transplantation with the use of grafts from living donors (a procedure we have performed approximately 150 times) to include adult donors and recipients. As of April 2001, we have evaluated additional donors and recipients but have not transplanted another liver graft from a living donor into an adult. Several centers have reported their experience with this operation in adults.[1-3,5,19,26,27] Many key aspects of liver transplantation in adults with the use of grafts from living donors remain unclear; the same is not true of the procedure performed in children. First, there is a lack of agreement on the technique that is most effective and that provides the greatest safety for donor and recipient. Second, indications for the surgery have not been clearly defined or standardized. Third, the procedure has been developed with variable standards for approval by institutional review boards. The rapid proliferation of programs that perform transplantation in adults with the use of grafts from living donors (most of those in the United States have performed fewer than 10 procedures each) is alarming for an innovative, nonstandardized operation that places two people, one of whom is healthy, at risk.

The New England Journal of Medicine

IS THERE A NEED FOR THE PROCEDURE IN ADULTS?

Subjecting a healthy donor to the risks of surgery can be justified only in clinical circumstances in which the potential recipient has a compelling need for a liver transplant from a living donor. According to current data obtained from the United Network for Organ Sharing, in 2000, a total of 10,887 patients in the United States were placed on a waiting list for a liver transplantation, 4934 liver transplantations were performed, and 853 of the patients placed on a waiting list that year died.[28] From 1998 to 1999, the number of liver transplantations performed in children with the use of grafts from living donors increased from 61 to 88, and the number of such procedures in adults increased from 25 to 131[28]; the total number of grafts from living donors increased further in 2000, to 355. Use of the procedure in adults has been justified by the disparity between the number of patients waiting for cadaveric organs and the number of organs that become available. Because of the disparity, the waiting period for a transplant can be long, and some patients die before an organ becomes available.

Whereas among children, use of liver transplants from living donors was justified by the significant effect of a prolonged waiting period,[10] waiting time alone does not appear to justify use of transplants from living donors in adults. Medical urgency and the severity of the underlying liver disease are better predictors of pretransplantation mortality than is the duration of the waiting period.[29] In fact, under the recently proposed Model for End-Stage Liver Disease system, organs would be allocated on the basis of the severity of a patient's liver disease, rather than on the basis of the time a patient has been on the waiting list.[30] Nonetheless, specific groups of adults may benefit from the availability of grafts from living donors, including patients with type A or O blood[31] and those with primary biliary cirrhosis,[32] small hepatocellular cancer,[33] or fulminant hepatic failure.[34]

RISKS AND BENEFITS FOR DONORS AND RECIPIENTS

Risks for Donors

The risks of liver donation are difficult to quantify. Procedures for evaluating donors are not uniform among transplantation programs. Some programs require a mesenteric angiogram[1-3,27] and liver biopsy,[1] whereas others do not.[5] There is also a lack of uniformity in the surgical technique used; some programs perform a right lobectomy,[1,5] removing approximately 60 percent of the hepatic mass, and others an extended right hepatectomy,[27] removing approximately 70 percent of the hepatic mass, including the middle hepatic vein. Different surgical teams perform each of these operations differently. The lack of standardization in the evaluation of donors and in the oper-

ative procedure, as well as variations in the experience and skill of surgical groups, makes it extremely difficult to assess the risks of complications and death to donors.

Morbidity attributable to surgical resection in donors of grafts for adult recipients has been reported to be as high as 50 percent, with complications including wound infection, injury to the nerves of the brachial plexus, and portal-vein thrombosis.[35] Furthermore, unlike a left lateral segmentectomy, a right lobectomy often results in postoperative hepatic insufficiency, although it has been reported to be reversible.[5] The rate and severity of complications are distinctly higher among donors of grafts for adults[35] than among donors of grafts for children.[23]

The most serious potential consequence of a right lobectomy or an extended right hepatectomy is death due to an intraoperative complication or postoperative liver failure. Although a right lobectomy performed in a healthy donor should carry a low risk of death, the mortality rate has not been clearly established. On the basis of discussions at professional meetings, as compared with reports in the literature, we are concerned that some centers may not be reporting deaths in a timely manner. In 1999, Strong stated that six persons had died as a result of liver donation[8] but did not specify whether the operations were performed to obtain grafts for children or adults.[36] We believe complications and deaths related to an innovative procedure — especially one involving living, healthy donors — should be reported in detail in a timely fashion in peer-reviewed journals and ideally to a registry.[36]

Benefits for Donors

For a donor, the benefit of donation is primarily psychological.[12] The outcome for the recipient notwithstanding, the donor usually has an elevated sense of self-esteem. A family member, spouse, or close friend may be strongly motivated to donate part of an organ, and such donors appear to benefit from knowing that they have done all they can to help, even if the recipient dies.

Risks for Recipients

The risks for the recipient can be divided into the risks associated with liver transplantation in general, such as hemorrhage, infection, primary nonfunctioning of the graft, and death, and those specific to the receipt of a right-lobe graft. For a right-lobe graft, the risks include those due to the cut surface, which include bile leaks and infections, and those due to the provision of insufficient hepatic mass.[37] Refinements in surgical techniques have reduced some of these risks.[38] Transplantation of grafts from living donors is associated with high rates of graft loss and death among recipients who are in poor condition before transplantation,[5] those with clinically significant portal hypertension at the time of surgery,[39] and those who receive a graft that is small for their body size.[40] The risks of graft loss and death are inversely related to the experience of the surgical team.[4]

Benefits for Recipients

To justify the use of a liver graft from a living donor, it is necessary to show that such a graft has a measurable, incremental benefit for the intended recipient, as compared with a full-size or split cadaveric graft. We are unaware of data demonstrating such a benefit. Although the survival advantage among children who receive liver grafts from living donors has been shown to be associated with the superior quality of the graft and the shorter period of ischemia before transplantation,[20] such studies have not been performed for liver transplantation in adults with the use of grafts from living donors.

Equipoise for Donors and Recipients

When standard therapy is compared with an innovative procedure, equipoise is required.[41] Equipoise is an initial balance between risks and benefits in the two study groups. In conventional clinical trials, the benefits and risks apply only to the patients in the study groups, but in trials of transplantation involving living donors, both the recipients and the donors have a stake in the outcome. The potential benefit for recipients varies according to their clinical status at the time of transplantation and their specific liver disease. For this operation, there is a double equipoise, which reflects a balance between potential benefits and risks for both the recipients and the donors. In certain situations, the use of a graft from a living donor cannot be justified ethically. For example, it would be unethical to transplant a graft from a living donor into a patient with end-stage liver disease and widely metastatic carcinoma who had severe multisystem organ failure and was in an intensive care unit, even if both the donor and the recipient were willing to proceed.

INFORMED CONSENT

The two informed-consent documents needed for an experimental surgical procedure involving a living donor and a recipient are related. The risks and benefits may be difficult to specify. Moreover, they are likely to vary among institutions according to the skill and experience of the team performing the surgery.

Because of the special circumstances of liver transplantation in adults with the use of grafts from living donors, informed consent should be obtained in three steps. First, the recipient should provide informed consent to the planned transplantation in general and to the additional risk of receiving a right-lobe graft from a living donor. Second, the donor should provide informed consent — this process must be as free from coercion as possible, and since the donor and the recipient usually know each other, the donor must be offered an opportunity to decline. Third, the recipient

should accept or decline the proposed gift from the donor. Both the recipient and the donor must be informed of the risks and benefits of transplanting a graft from a living donor and those of transplanting a graft from a cadaveric donor, as well as the risks and benefits of the lobectomy performed to obtain the graft from the donor. Ultimately, the potential recipient must have the right to decline a donation from a living donor.

In our view, the surgeon performing each operation must ultimately be responsible for obtaining informed consent. To protect both the recipient and the donor from the surgeon's enthusiasm for the procedure, which might be perceived as a conflict of interest, we recommend that a consultant in internal medicine who is uninvolved with the surgical team be designated as the "consent advocate" for both the donor and the recipient.

FIELD STRENGTH AND INSTITUTIONAL CLIMATE

The term "field strength" refers to the capacity of a surgical team to meet the technical demands of an innovative procedure.[9] Broelsch recently stated that a team planning to perform liver transplantation in adults with the use of grafts from living donors should have proven success, with validation of good outcomes, in performing transplantation with the use of reduced-size cadaveric grafts, transplantation of in situ and ex vivo split cadaveric grafts, transplantation in children, and complex biliary reconstructions and liver resections.[42] We agree. Although it is difficult to quantify the field strength of surgical teams, it is troubling that the performance of liver transplantation in adults with the use of grafts from living donors has not been restricted to high-volume transplantation centers that have track records in all facets of hepatobiliary and liver surgery. Centers that perform fewer than 20 transplantations involving cadaveric grafts per year have lower rates of survival among recipients than centers that perform 20 or more such procedures each year.[43] Brown recently reported that 22 of 54 programs responding to a survey had performed liver transplantation in adults with the use of grafts from living donors but that only 7 of these 22 programs had performed more than 10 such procedures.[7] We are concerned that many of the programs that currently perform liver transplantation in adults with the use of grafts from living donors or that plan to do so in the next year[7] may not have adequate field strength or the established record of success that is required to undertake this complex and dangerous operation.

Moore used the term "institutional climate" in discussing the motivation of a surgeon, surgical team, or institution to perform an innovative procedure.[9] Such a procedure can increase the prestige of individual surgeons and of the institution. For surgeons, the benefits may include scholarly publication, career advancement, increased status within the medical community, and monetary rewards. The possible benefits for the institution are greater market exposure and an increase in referrals — both for the particular procedure and for other services. We should consider whether the needs of patients or those of surgeons and institutions are the driving force behind programs of liver transplantation in adults with the use of grafts from living donors.

CONCLUSIONS

We recommend that all adults who are candidates for a liver graft from a living donor meet the criteria of the United Network for Organ Sharing for placement on the waiting list for a cadaveric graft[44] and that they be placed on the list. One reason for this recommendation is that patients who have graft loss (primary nonfunctioning of the graft or hepatic-artery thrombosis) within seven days after transplantation automatically qualify as a Status I candidate (one needing a transplant with the greatest urgency)[44] for a cadaveric liver graft. Patients who otherwise would not initially qualify for a cadaveric liver graft but who would qualify if a graft from a living donor failed should not place at a disadvantage those patients who do qualify and are awaiting a cadaveric graft.

The safety of both the donor and the recipient must be ensured through a process that balances the risks and benefits for each. This involves a three-step procedure for obtaining informed consent that provides protection for the donor–recipient pair and makes it clear that the recipient has the right to decline a donation from a living donor.

We believe it is unreasonable to expect that the surgeons and transplantation programs already performing liver transplantation in adults with the use of grafts from living donors, and those planning to do so, will regulate themselves. Surgical-specialty societies could have taken an earlier and more active role in self-regulation of the field by permitting only programs that met criteria such as those suggested by Broelsch[42] to perform the surgery. Realistically, however, specialty societies may not have enough clout to regulate the actions of surgeons and transplantation programs. In the absence of professional self-regulation, private health insurers and government agencies, such as the Health Care Financing Administration (HCFA), should provide oversight.

Private and public health insurance plans provide coverage for liver transplantation in adults with the use of grafts from living donors on a case-by-case basis. Insurers can be expected to collect data at least on short-term outcomes (i.e., survival rates among donors and recipients and costs), and they will eventually decide, retrospectively, which programs they will continue to cover. The transplantation community should work with insurance companies to identify centers of excellence by establishing a registry to which transplantation programs must report data on short- and long-term outcomes for donors and recipients.

HCFA has a list of criteria for determining whether a transplantation program is eligible for Medicare reimbursement. These criteria define minimally acceptable standards for the performance and outcomes of liver transplantation with the use of cadaveric grafts. Transplantation programs that are already accepted as Medicare providers should be required to apply for special certification to perform liver transplantation with grafts from living donors. Specialty societies should assist HCFA in establishing the minimal criteria for certification and the clinical indications for the procedure. We suspect that fewer than 15 high-volume programs in the United States with surgical expertise and field strength will initially meet the criteria for certification to perform liver transplantation in adults with the use of grafts from living donors.

We hesitate to propose changes in a tradition that has permitted the surgical community, through professional self-regulation, to be the sole arbiter in determining when an innovative surgical approach is introduced into practice. Unfortunately, in the case of this procedure, the surgical and transplantation communities in the United States have not established criteria for selecting donors and recipients or standards of surgical technique and have not required the certification of programs. This lack of self-regulation has resulted in the use by many liver-transplantation programs of liver grafts from living donors in adults. Therefore, we believe that this internal, professional control should be supplemented by an external mechanism for prospective regulation, which may include government intervention. Unless professional self-regulation for other innovative surgical procedures improves, government regulation may not be restricted to innovative liver transplantation.

DAVID C. CRONIN II, M.D., PH.D.
J. MICHAEL MILLIS, M.D.
MARK SIEGLER, M.D.
University of Chicago
Chicago, IL 60637

REFERENCES

1. Marcos A, Fisher RA, Ham JM, et al. Right lobe living donor liver transplantation. Transplantation 1999;68:798-803.
2. Wachs ME, Bak TE, Karrer FM, et al. Adult living donor liver transplantation using a right hepatic lobe. Transplantation 1998;66:1313-6.
3. Testa G, Malago M, Broelsch CE. Living-donor liver transplantation in adults. Langenbecks Arch Surg 1999;384:536-43.
4. Fan ST, Lo CM, Liu CL. Technical refinement in adult-to-adult living donor liver transplantation using right lobe graft. Ann Surg 2000;231:126-31.
5. Inomata Y, Uemoto S, Asonuma K, Egawa H. Right lobe graft in living donor liver transplantation. Transplantation 2000;69:258-64.
6. Marcos A. Live donor liver transplantation to adult recipients: the U.S. experience. Presented at the First Joint Annual Meeting of the American Society of Transplant Surgeons and the American Society of Transplantation, Chicago, May 13–17, 2000.
7. Brown R. Survey on current practice of LDLT in adults. Presented at the Workshop on Living Donor Liver Transplantation, Bethesda, Md., December 4–5, 2000.

SOUNDING BOARD

8. Strong RW. Whither living donor liver transplantation? Liver Transpl Surg 1999;5:536-8.

9. Moore FD. Three ethical revolutions: ancient assumptions remodeled under pressure of transplantation. Transplant Proc 1988;20:Suppl 1:1061-7.

10. Emond JC, Whitington PF, Thistlethwaite JR, Alonso EM, Broelsch CE. Reduced-size orthotopic liver transplantation: use in the management of children with chronic liver disease. Hepatology 1989;10:867-72.

11. Strong RW, Lynch SV, Ong TH, Matsunami H, Koido Y, Balderson GA. Successful liver transplantation from a living donor to her son. N Engl J Med 1990;322:1505-7.

12. Singer PA, Siegler M, Whitington PF, et al. Ethics of liver transplantation with living donors. N Engl J Med 1989;321:620-2.

13. Broelsch CE, Whitington PF, Emond JC, et al. Liver transplantation in children from living related donors: surgical techniques and results. Ann Surg 1991;214:428-37.

14. Amersi F, Farmer DG, Busuttil RW. Fifteen-year experience with adult and pediatric liver transplantation at the University of California, Los Angeles. In: Clinical transplants. Los Angeles: UCLA Tissue Typing Laboratory, 1998:255-61.

15. Emre S, Schwartz ME, Schneider B, et al. Living related liver transplantation for acute liver failure in children. Liver Transpl Surg 1999;5:161-5.

16. Rogiers X, Burdelski M, Broelsch CE. Liver transplantation from living donors. Br J Surg 1994;81:1251-3.

17. Tanaka K, Uemoto S, Tokunaga Y, et al. Surgical techniques and innovations in living related liver transplantation. Ann Surg 1993;217:82-91.

18. Fan ST, Lo CM, Chan KL, et al. Liver transplantation: perspective from Hong Kong. Hepatogastroenterology 1996;43:893-7.

19. Mori K, Nagata I, Yamagata S, et al. The introduction of microvascular surgery to hepatic artery reconstruction in living-donor liver transplantation — its surgical advantages compared with conventional procedures. Transplantation 1992;54:263-8.

20. Millis JM, Alonso EM, Piper JB, et al. Liver transplantation at the University of Chicago. In: Clinical transplants. Los Angeles: UCLA Tissue Typing Laboratory, 1995:187-97.

21. Millis JM, Cronin DC, Brady LM, et al. Primary living-donor liver transplantation at the University of Chicago: technical aspects of the first 104 recipients. Ann Surg 2000;232:104-11.

22. Yamaoka Y, Morimoto T, Inamot T, et al. Safety of the donor in living-related liver transplantation — an analysis of 100 parental donors. Transplantation 1995;59:224-6.

23. Grewal HP, Thistlethwaite JR Jr, Loss GE, et al. Complications in 100 living-liver donors. Ann Surg 1998;228:214-9.

24. Malago M, Rogiers S, Burdelski M, Broelsch CE. Living related liver transplantation: 36 cases at the University of Hamburg. Transplant Proc 1994;26:3620-1.

25. Piper JB, Whitington PF, Woodle ES, et al. Pediatric liver transplantation at the University of Chicago Hospitals. In: Clinical transplants. Los Angeles: UCLA Tissue Typing Laboratory, 1992:179-89.

26. Lo CM, Fan ST, Liu CL, et al. Extending the limit on the size of adult recipient in living donor liver transplantation using extended right lobe graft. Transplantation 1997;63:1524-8.

27. Lo CM, Fan ST, Liu CL, et al. Adult-to-adult living donor liver transplantation using extended right lobe grafts. Ann Surg 1997;226:261-9.

28. 2000 Annual report of the U.S. Scientific Registry for Transplantation Recipients and the Organ Procurement and Transplantation Network: transplant data: 1989-1999. Rockville, Md.: Department of Health and Human Services, 2000.

29. Freeman RB Jr, Edwards EB. Liver transplant waiting time does not correlate with waiting list mortality: implications for liver allocation policy. Liver Transpl 2000;6:543-52.

30. UNOS policy proposal for public comment. Richmond, Va.: United Network for Organ Sharing, March 29, 2001. (See http://www.unos.org/pdf/pubcomment_20010329.pdf.)

31. Everhart JE, Lombardero M, Detre KM, et al. Increased waiting time for liver transplantation results in higher mortality. Transplantation 1997;64:1300-6.

32. Kim WR, Wiesner RH, Therneau TM, et al. Optimal timing of liver transplantation for primary biliary cirrhosis. Hepatology 1998;28:33-8.

33. Llovet JM, Fuster J, Bruix J. Intention-to-treat analysis of surgical treatment for early hepatocellular carcinoma: resection versus transplantation. Hepatology 1999;30:1434-40.

34. Miwa S, Hashikura Y, Mita A, et al. Living-related liver transplantation for patients with fulminant and subfulminant hepatic failure. Hepatology 1999;30:1521-6.

35. Pomposelli JJ, Pomfret EA, Kamel IR, et al. Living donor adult liver transplantation (LDALT): donor evaluation, outcome and resource utilization. Transplantation 2000;69:S291. abstract.

36. Hirano I, Blei AT. Deaths after living related liver transplantation. Liver Transpl 2000;6:250.

37. Emond JC, Whitington PF, Thistlethwaite JR, et al. Transplantation of two patients with one liver: analysis of a preliminary experience with 'split-liver' grafting. Ann Surg 1990;212:14-22.

38. Goss JA, Yersiz H, Shackleton CR, et al. In situ splitting of the cadaveric liver for transplantation. Transplantation 1997;64:871-7.

39. Ben-Haim M, Emre S, Facciuto M, et al. Critical graft size in adult-to-adult living donor liver transplantation: the impact of the recipient's disease. Transplantation 2000;69:S290. abstract.

40. Kiuchi T, Kasahara M, Uryuhara K, et al. Impact of graft size mismatching on graft prognosis in liver transplantation from living donors. Transplantation 1999;67:321-7.

41. Freedman B. Equipoise and the ethics of clinical research. N Engl J Med 1987;317:141-5.

42. Broelsch C. Results with living donor liver transplants in Germany. Presented at the Workshop on Living Donor Liver Transplantation, Bethesda, Md., December 4–5, 2000.

43. Edwards EB, Roberts JP, McBride MA, Schulak JA, Hunsicker LG. The effect of the volume of procedures at transplantation centers on mortality after liver transplantation. N Engl J Med 1999;341:2049-53.

44. UNOS bylaws. Richmond, Va.: United Network for Organ Sharing, 1995-2001. (See http://www.unos.org/frame_Default.asp?Category=aboutbylawsTOC.)

11.7   Testa G, Angelos P, Crowley-Matoka M, Siegler M (2009) Elective Surgical Patients as Living Organ Donors: A Clinical and Ethical Innovation. Am J Transplant 9:2400–5

American Journal of Transplantation 2009; 9: 2400–2405
Wiley Periodicals Inc.

© 2009 The Authors
Journal compilation © 2009 The American Society of
Transplantation and the American Society of Transplant Surgeons

doi: 10.1111/j.1600-6143.2009.02773.x

Elective Surgical Patients as Living Organ Donors: A Clinical and Ethical Innovation

G. Testa[a,*], P. Angelos[b], M. Crowley-Matoka[c]
and M. Siegler[d]

[a] Department of Surgery, Director of Liver Transplantation
and Hepatobiliary Surgery, The University of Chicago,
Chicago, IL
[b] Department of Surgery, MacLean Center for Clinical
Medical Ethics, The University of Chicago, Chicago, IL
[c] University of Pittsburgh and Research Scientist, Center
for Health Equity Research and Promotion, Pittsburgh
Veterans Affairs Medical Center, Pittsburgh, PA
[d] Department of Medicine, MacLean Center for Clinical
Medical Ethics, The University of Chicago, Chicago, IL
*Corresponding author: Giuliano Testa,
gtesta@surgery.bsd.uchicago.edu

We propose a new model for living organ donation
that would invite elective laparoscopic cholecystectomy patients to become volunteer, unrelated living
kidney donors. Such donors would be surgical patients
first and living donors second, in contrast to the current system, which 'creates' a surgical patient by operating on a healthy individual. Elective surgery patients
have accepted the risks of anesthesia and surgery for
their own surgical needs but would face additional surgical risks when a donor nephrectomy is combined
with their cholecystectomy procedure. Because these
two procedures have never been performed together,
the precise level of additional risk entailed in such a
combined approach is unknown and will require further study. However, considering the large number of
elective cholecystectomies performed each year in the
United States, if as few as 5% of elective cholecystectomy patients agreed to also serve as living kidney donors, the number of living kidney donors would
increase substantially. If this proposal is accepted by
a minority of patients and surgeons, and proves safe
and effective in a protocol study, it could be applied to
other elective abdominal surgery procedures and used
to obtain other abdominal donor organs (e.g. liver and
intestinal segments) for transplantation.

Key words: Clinical ethics, living donor kidney transplantation, surgery kidney donation

Received 04 March 2009, revised 14 May 2009 and accepted for publication 07 June 2009

Introduction

We propose a new model for living organ donation that
would invite elective laparoscopic cholecystectomy patients to become volunteer, unrelated living kidney donors.
In our approach, the donor would be a surgical patient first
and a living donor second, in contrast to the current system, which 'creates' a surgical patient by operating on an
otherwise healthy individual. Elective cholecystectomy patients have accepted the risks of general anesthesia and
abdominal surgery for their own needs but would face
additional surgical risks if a donor nephrectomy is combined with the elective cholecystectomy. Because these
two procedures have never been performed together, the
precise level of additional risk entailed in such a combined approach—as compared to either cholecystectomy
alone or donor nephrectomy alone—is not known. Given
the large volume of elective cholecystectomies performed
each year in the United States, it would require only 3–5%
of patients agreeing to serve as living kidney donors under
this model to increase substantially the current supply of
kidneys for transplantation (1,2). Based on the existing literature on stranger donation, such a modest level of potential
acceptance does not seem unrealistic (3–5). Moreover, if
our proposal is accepted by even a minority of patients,
surgeons and payers, and if it proves safe and effective in
a protocol study, it could encourage applying this approach
to other elective abdominal surgery procedures and even
to obtaining other abdominal donor organs (e.g. segments
of liver and intestine).

This paper provides a brief background on the long-
standing ethical objections to living donation and the current organ shortage in the United States. We then examine
the key clinical and ethical issues raised by our proposal to
use elective surgical patients as living donors. Finally, we
describe our plan for moving this model from the conceptual stage, through a period of rigorous analysis, to
eventual implementation in an institutional review board
(IRB)-approved experimental trial.

Background

In the United States, kidney transplantation using living
donors currently relies almost entirely upon using healthy
individuals who are related biologically or emotionally to
someone who needs a kidney transplant. The only reason

these healthy individuals face the harm, risks and discomforts of surgery and general anesthesia is because they have agreed to be organ donors. Beginning with the first living kidney donor in 1954, critics as well as supporters of living donation have raised concerns about whether it is ethical for surgeons to subject donors to harm and risk by operating on them not for their own good but in order to benefit another person in need of kidney transplantation (6,7). As Dr. Frances Moore, under whose leadership, living donor kidney transplantation was first performed successfully, wrote: '[Living donor] tissue transplantation is a unique field of surgery. It flaunts the ancient principles upon which medical and surgical care are based: do no harm and help the patient to help himself. The welfare of a healthy person, heretofore never sacrificed in human medicine, is now jeopardized when tissue is obtained from the healthy donor' (8). Despite such concerns, however, living kidney donation has grown substantially and in 2008 provided more than 35% of kidneys transplanted in the United States (9). The main reason for the increased use of living kidney donors is the worsening shortage of kidneys, which is reflected by the current waiting list of more than 70 000 people with an additional 30 000 new patients being added annually in 2006, 2007 and 2008 (9).

Many approaches have been tried to increase the supply of *deceased* donor kidneys, but existing data suggest that even maximizing the use of deceased donors is unlikely to solve the organ shortage (10). As a result, efforts to address the supply–demand gap in abdominal organs for transplantation increasingly have turned in the United States to *living* donors (11–14). Recently, much attention has been directed to developing programs using paired kidney exchanges, nondirected living donors and marginal living donors (15–20). Thus far, the impact of these initiatives is limited. Moreover, in the face of apparently stagnant donation rates, there have been increased calls for ethically controversial proposals to provide compensation for organ donation, although the impact of commercialization on increasing the number of available organs for transplantation is unknown (21–24).

The Proposed Model: Critical Issues

In this section, we examine the arguments for and against the proposed approach to using elective cholecystectomy patients as living kidney donors by exploring three key areas: technical feasibility, practical issues and ethical issues.

Technical feasibility
The individual techniques and risks for cholecystectomy and nephrectomy are well-established and each has been performed separately many times (25,26). In terms of technical feasibility, it would be possible for a general surgeon working with a transplant surgeon to perform the two operations sequentially. This could be done using the same anterior abdominal laparoscopic approach and two additional operative ports. Although generally it has been more common to remove the left kidney in living donation, several recent reports suggest there is no difference in donor and recipient outcome when the right kidney is taken (27–29).

Anticipated increased risks for the combined procedure over the cholecystectomy procedure alone would include longer anesthesia time, larger incision, increased length of hospital stay, the operative risks of the nephrectomy and the loss of the donated kidney. In the literature, the average time for a donor nephrectomy varies between 160 and 200 min from incision to bandage application (29,30). We estimate that combining the cholecystectomy and nephrectomy would add about 2 h to the laparoscopic cholecystectomy. The patient will be told that the incision will be about 7 cm in length, which is between 4 and 5 cm longer than is needed for the extraction of the gallbladder. Most kidney donors stay in hospital less than 72 h, but this is about 24–48 h longer than the stay for cholecystectomy patient, some of whom are discharged on the day of surgery (31,32). The greatest risk of the donor nephrectomy is bleeding, especially from the renal artery, and this is regarded as the number one cause of death after kidney donation, with an incidence of 0.02% (25). Finally, the loss of a kidney is also a risk incurred by donation, but this controversial issue has been studied since living donor kidney transplantation started more than 50 years ago, and most believe that the loss of a kidney does not increase donor morbidity and mortality (33).

To our knowledge, no one has reported performing a cholecystectomy and a right nephrectomy as part of a single planned laparoscopic surgical procedure. For this reason, the precise level of additional risk entailed in *combining* the two procedures for the first time is not known, making this a form of innovative or experimental surgery. As such, we believe that initial implementation of this model should occur only under an IRB-approved protocol as part of a trial clinical series. At all times the cholecystectomy (performed by the general surgeon) would remain the primary and prioritized procedure, and the nephrectomy (performed by the transplant surgeon) would proceed only in the absence of any surgical problems with the gallbladder removal and with the general surgeon's permission.

Practical issues
We envision a number of potential practical barriers to the feasibility of implementing this approach to living donation. First and foremost, it is not known whether unrelated elective cholecystectomy patients would ever consider serving as altruistic living kidney donors. This proposal could founder because of a lack of patients willing to take an increased risk in order to donate to strangers. However, existing programs, in nondirected living organ and bone marrow donation for example, suggest that there are *some* altruistic individuals willing to assume some level of personal

Testa et al.

risk for a stranger (3–5). Indeed, a recent survey reported 24% of people declared themselves willing to freely donate a kidney to a stranger in need, and an additional 21% said that they would probably would do so (3). While such numbers are likely to reflect a social desirability bias and be unrealistically high as an indication of actual *behavior*, they do indicate generally positive *attitudes* toward the concept of altruistic kidney donation among a significant proportion of the population.

Second, even if some potential donors would consent, would surgeons agree to participate? General surgeons may be extremely reluctant to let their patients undergo an experimental 'combined' donor nephrectomy and cholecystectomy with increased and currently unknown risks. For their part, would transplant surgeons, some of whom continue to harbor serious concerns about living organ donation, agree to obtain and use kidneys for transplant using this innovative approach? While such critical questions will only be answered fully upon completion of our proposed protocol study, informal discussions with surgical colleagues at our own institution and others suggest that at least some general and transplant surgeons would be willing to participate in this form of living donation. Moreover, the history of willingness to initiate other innovative surgical procedures in an attempt to alleviate the organ shortage (e.g. living liver donation and living lung donation) further suggests that at least some surgeons would find the potential contribution to the organ supply a reasonable justification for exploring and possibly participating in this new approach.

Third, would hospital administrators and payers support and facilitate this form of living organ donation? More specifically, who would pay for this surgical 'experiment', the company that insured the patient for the gallbladder operation or the organ recipient's insurer who generally pays the cost of living donor organ procurement? Although existing systems for covering the costs of living organ donation under the insurance of the organ recipient provide some guideposts, clearly the financial and insurance issues entailed in this new model of living donation are complex and will require additional study.

Lastly, how should kidneys obtained using this approach be allocated? An independent allocation authority or a cooperation system between Organ Procurement Organizations and Transplant Centers have been proposed for the allocation of kidneys currently obtained from altruistic donors (17,34). Under this new model, either system for the distribution of organs could be considered and studied as long as the criteria followed for the allocation are the same across the nation.

Ethical issues
Finally, our proposed model raises several ethical questions, centered around three key issues: 1) the level of risk entailed in this form of living organ donation; 2) the potential vulnerability to coercion of patients in need of surgery; and 3) the informed consent process proposed for this approach.

Donor risk: Minimizing the risk to altruistic organ donors is an ethical imperative. Exactly how to conceptualize the risk of living donation under this new proposed model is a complex issue. When a healthy individual who otherwise does not require abdominal surgery agrees to serve as a living kidney donor, he or she assumes the full panoply of risks and surgical discomfort that are associated with abdominal surgery, general anesthesia and the donor nephrectomy. Of course, the risk to each individual surgical patient who also agrees to be a donor is undoubtedly increased by combining the kidney donation procedure with the planned and needed elective cholecystectomy. But in the unusual situation where a patient needs elective surgery *and* also expresses a desire to be an altruistic living kidney donor, we believe it should be studied whether it is less risky to perform the two procedures sequentially with a single anesthesia, rather than subjecting the patient/donor to two separate surgery and anesthesia procedures. This study is warranted because many of the morbidity and mortality risks of serving as a traditional living kidney donor are the risks of undergoing abdominal surgery and general anesthesia (including adverse reactions to medications and anesthesia, as well as postoperative bleeding, infection and pulmonary emboli) and because elective surgery patients have already consented to accept these risks *for their own benefit* as part of their elective surgical procedure.

It is possible that the overall risks for a healthy person who accepts abdominal surgery solely to serve as a volunteer donor would be greater than the *incremental* surgical and postoperative risks faced by an already-scheduled surgical patient who agrees to also have a donor nephrectomy as part of the same procedure. It is this potentially favorable though still unproved risk profile that might offer one ethical justification for moving forward with an IRB-approved protocol series to study the comparative risks.

Patient vulnerability: Of particular concern is the possibility that elective cholecystectomy patients may be especially vulnerable to being coerced into serving as unrelated kidney donors because they have gallbladder disease that requires surgery and may thus feel beholden to and dependent upon their general surgeon. That is, patients might agree to donation because they fear that their surgeon will not treat them as well or will be disappointed with them if they do not agree to serve as a living kidney donor. Such psychological vulnerability is of serious ethical concern. Accordingly, in the section below on informed consent, we outline a planned process designed to scrupulously protect patients and to respond to their potential concerns that refusing to donate could damage relations with their surgeon or compromise their surgical care in any way.

It is not clear, however, that the potential vulnerability to coercion of *unrelated* potential living donors in our model is necessarily greater than the coercion living *related* donors often report feeling when they are invited to serve as donors for a loved one (35,36). Indeed, it may prove easier to minimize coercion for unrelated patients—with a well-designed informed consent process—than for traditional living related donors, who often face both subtle and overt coercion based on family dynamics. Some have suggested that living related donors should be permitted to take higher risks than unrelated donors because of the possibility that they derive a greater degree of psychological benefit for donating than do unrelated donors (37). We disagree and believe the ethical imperative in living donation rests on minimizing the risks assumed by both related and unrelated living donors.

Informed consent: Because of the experimental nature of using surgical patients as living organ donors, special attention must be paid to assuring the highest level of informed consent from patients. We propose initially to approach the general surgeon for permission to have a donor advocate team, independent from the transplant team, contact that surgeon's elective patient. If the surgeon agrees, the donor advocate team will provide information to the patient about this experimental living kidney donor operation and leave written material with the potential donor, who will be asked to contact the donor team if he/she is interested in further discussion. Only if the potential donor takes the initiative to recontact the donor advocate team, would a first-stage consent then be negotiated to permit potential donors to undergo further evaluation to determine if they would qualify as a kidney donor. If patients pass this initial evaluation, they would be given a cooling-off period of 2 weeks, after which, the patient could sign the consent and the general surgeon would be informed that the patient has consented to donate a kidney. In cases where the donation does not go forward, the general surgeon would not know whether the patient was rejected for donation on medical grounds or had declined to donate. This almost complete separation between the general surgeon who will perform the cholecystectomy and the donation evaluation and consent process will substantially minimize the potential vulnerability of the donor.

Discussion

Efforts to increase the organ supply

In the 55 years since the first successful living donor kidney transplant, living kidney donors have become increasingly important, especially in the United States, for meeting the transplantation needs of patients with end-stage renal disease. Our proposal to approach elective abdominal surgery patients is a major change in the way potential living kidney donors would be identified and invited to become altruistic living unrelated donors. This new approach to living donation relies upon the high volume of elective abdominal surgery procedures in the United States as an opportunity to possibly increase the supply of donor organs. Moreover, only low levels of acceptance among elective surgical patients would be required to substantially increase the organ supply. Concerted efforts to increase the supply of donor kidneys over the past two decades have had limited success. We believe the potential of using elective surgical patients as living donors merits further exploration.

Efforts to decrease overall donor risk

Our proposal to invite elective surgical patients to serve as kidney donors also aims to explore whether it is possible to decrease the overall risk for the population of potential living kidney donors. The individual risk faced by a cholecystectomy patient who agrees to donate a kidney during the same operative procedure will be increased compared to the risk of cholecystectomy alone or a donor nephrectomy alone. However, if a sufficient number of living donor kidneys were obtained through this new approach, it might no longer be necessary to subject as many healthy persons to surgery solely for the purpose of serving as living kidney donor. In a protocol trial of this approach, we intend to test whether the incremental risk to the cholecystectomy patient is greater or less than the entire risk profile for the traditional living kidney donor. Many recent proposals to increase the supply of living donors, such as the use of expanded criteria living donors and efforts to develop a commercial system for buying and selling organs, are likely to further increase donor risk, because these approaches depend upon donors who are more medically and/or socioeconomically vulnerable (18–24). Moreover, while our focus in this paper has been on the potential risk to *donors*, it is possible that expanded criteria living donors and commercial sellers may also increase the risk to organ *recipients*, by decreasing the quality of organs available for transplantation (38). Compared to such alternatives, our proposal, may offer a more effective and ethically sound approach to living organ donation.

Next steps in advancing a new model for living organ donation

We believe it is essential to compare the risks of current standard approaches to living donation with our new model to use surgical patients as living donors. Accordingly, we propose to move this model forward from the conceptual stage through a period of focused analysis and evaluation to implementation in an IRB-approved protocol trial. To this end, we are first initiating rigorous qualitative and quantitative research to explore whether the proposed model has any realistic feasibility for the key stakeholders who would be most directly involved with this procedure, including elective cholecystectomy patients, general surgeons and transplant surgeons. In conjunction with these data collection efforts, we also have initiated an analysis of the clinical and ethical issues posed by this concept through a series of planned presentations and publications designed to invite public and professional examination, discussion

Testa et al.

and criticism. Following a model developed at our center for initiating surgical innovation in an ethical way (39), this public analysis and evaluation process—in combination with our research findings—will be used to develop an IRB protocol for implementing this experimental surgical model. Finally, we plan to conduct an IRB-approved trial series involving elective cholecystectomy patients as living kidney donors. Results from this trial will be analyzed and published in order to assess whether there is evidence of safety and effectiveness to warrant continuing the experimental study of this procedure and to justify moving toward its more widespread and routine use.

Conclusion

If our proposal to obtain kidneys for transplantation from surgical patients who need and have consented to an elective laparoscopic cholecystectomy proves technically feasible, acceptable to patients, surgeons and payers and ethically sound, then the procedure may achieve some of the following results:

1. This model could contribute to reducing the US shortage of kidneys for transplantation even if as few as 3–5% patients undergoing elective abdominal agreed to serve as altruistic living kidney donors.
2. This approach might reduce the risk of living kidney donation, not for individual donors, but for the population of living kidney donors because overall fewer patients would require general anesthesia and abdominal surgery solely to recover donor kidneys for transplantation.
3. Our proposal could obviate the need to embark on a dangerous social experiment to develop a market system in the United States and elsewhere for buying and selling human organs.

Contributions and Conflict of Interest Statement

We declare that we each participated in the conceptualization, writing and revision of this manuscript and that we have each seen and approved the final version. We declare that we have no conflict of interest.

References

1. Csikesz N, Ricciardi R, Tseng JF, Shah SA. Current status of surgical management of acute cholecystitis in the United States. World J Surg 2008; 32: 2230–2236.
2. Centers for Disease Control and Prevention. National health statistics report. 2008; 5: 1–20.
3. Spital A. Public attitudes toward kidney donation by friends and altruistic strangers in the United States. Transplantation 2001; 71: 1061–1064.
4. Mark PJ, Baker K, Aguayo C, Sorenson JB. Experience with an organ procurement organization-based non-directed living kidney donor programme. Clin Transpl 2006; 20: 427–437.
5. Crowley-Matoka M, Switzer G. Nondirected living donation: A preliminary survey of current trends and practices. Transplantation 2005; 79: 515–519.
6. Starzl T. Living donors: Con. Transplant Proc 1987; 19: 174–176.
7. Truog RD. The ethics of organ donation by living donors. New Eng J Med 2005; 353: 444–446.
8. Moore FD. Transplant: The Give and Take of Tissue Transplantation. New York: Simon and Schuster, 1964: 313.
9. United Network for Organ Sharing Web Site. Organ procurement and transplantation network data. Available at: http://www.unos.org. Accessed January 26, 2009.
10. Sheehy E, Conrad SL, Brigham LE et al. Estimating the number of potential organ donors in the United States. N Engl J Med 2003; 349: 667–674.
11. Pomfret EA. Solving the organ shortage crisis: The 7th annual American Society of Transplant Surgeons' state-of-the-art winter symposium. Am J Transplant 2008; 8: 745–752.
12. Shah SA, Levy GA, Greig PD et al. Reduced mortality with right-lobe living donor compared to deceased-donor liver transplantation. Am J Transplant 2007; 7: 998–1002.
13. Kato T, Tzakis A. Living donor intestinal transplantation should it be used more frequently? Pediatr Transplant 2006; 10: 140–141.
14. Tan M, Kandaswamy R, Sutherland DE, Gruessner R. Laparoscopic donor distal pancreatectomy for living donor pancreas and pancreas-kidney transplantation. Am J Transplant 2005; 5: 1966–1970.
15. Segev DL, Gentry SE, Warren DS et al. Kidney paired donation and optimizing the use of live donor organs. JAMA 2005; 293: 1883–1890.
16. Jacobs CL, Roman D, Garvey C, Kahn J, Matas AJ. Twenty-two nondirected kidney donors: An update on a single center's experience. Am J Transplant 2004; 4: 1110–1116.
17. Gilbert JC, Brigham L, Batty DS Jr, Veatch RM. The nondirected living donor program: A model for cooperative donation, recovery and allocation of living donor kidneys. Am J Transplant 2005; 5: 167–174.
18. Matas AJ. Transplantation using marginal living donors. Am J Kidney Dis 2006; 47: 353–355.
19. Karpinski M, Knoll G, Cohn A, Yang R, Garg A, Storsley L. The impact of accepting living kidney donors with mild hypertension or proteinuria on transplantation rates. Am J Kidney Dis 2006; 47: 317–323.
20. Woodle ES, Khatib ME. The marginal donor. In: Gruessner RWG, Bendetti E, eds. Living Donor Organ Transplantation, New York: McGraw-Hill, 2007: 154–158.
21. Epstein RA. Thinking the unthinkable: Organ sales. In: Barnet S, Bedau H, eds. Current Issues and Enduring Questions: A Guide to Critical Thinking and Argument, with Readings. MA: Bedford, St. Martins, 2005: 102–105.
22. Matas A. The case for kidney sales: Rationale, objections and concerns. Am J Transplant 2004; 4: 2007–2017.
23. Becker GS, Elias JJ. Introducing incentives in the market for live and cadaveric organ donations. J Econ Perspec 2007; 21: 3–24.
24. Meckler L. Kidney shortage inspires a radical idea: Organ sales. Wall Street Journal, November 14, 2007.
25. Matas AJ, Bartlett ST, Leichtman AB, Delmonico FL. Morbidity and mortality after kidney donation, 1999–2001: Survey of United States transplant centers. Am J Transplant 2003; 3: 830–834.
26. Deziel DJ, Millikan KW, Economou SG, Doolas A, Ko ST, Airan MC. Complications of laparoscopic cholecystctomy: A national survey

of 4292 hospitals and an analysis of 77604 cases. Am J Surg 1993; 165: 9–14.

27. Buell JF, Hanaway MJ, Potter SR et al. Surgical technique in right laparoscopic donor nephrectomy. J Am Coll Surg 2002; 95: 131–137.

28. Posselt AM, Mohanty H, Kang SM et al. Laparoscopic right donor nephrectomy: A large single center experience. Transplantation 2004; 78: 1665–1669.

29. Dols LFC, Kok NFM, Alwayn IPJ, Khe Tran TC, Weimar W, IJzermans JNM. Laparoscopic donor nephrectomy: A plea for the right-sided approach. Transplantation 2009; 87: 745–750.

30. Jacobs SC, Cho E, Foster C, Liao P, Bartlett ST. Laparoscopic donor nephrectomy: The university of maryland 6-year experience. J Urol 2004; 171: 47–51.

31. Kenlemans Y, Eshnis J, de Haes H, de Wilt LT, Gouma DJ. Laparoscopic cholecystectomy: Day-care versus clinical observation. Ann Surg 1998; 228: 734–740.

32. Victorozon M, Tolonen P, Vuorialho T. Day-care laparoscopic cholecystectomy: Treatment of choice for selected patients? Surg Endos 2007; 21: 70–73.

33. Barry Y, Parker T, Kaplan B, Glassock R. Primum non nocere: Is chronic kidney disease staging appropriate in living kidney transplant donor? Am J Transplant 2009; 9: 657–660.

34. Weimar W, Zuidema W, Klerk M, Haase-Kromceijk B, IJzermans. Altruistic kidney donation. Lancet 2006; 368: 987.

35. Simmons RG, Simmons RL, Marine SK. Gift of Life: The Effect of Organ Transplantation on Individual, Family and Societal Dynamics. New Brunswick: Transaction Books.

36. Biller-Andorno N. Gender imbalance in living organ donation. Med, Health Care Philos 2002; 5: 199–203.

37. Ross LF, Glannon W, Josephson MA, Thistlethwaite JR. Should all living donors be treated equally? Transplantation 2002; 74: 418–421.

38. Goyal M, Mehta RL, Schneiderman LJ, Sehgal AF. Economic and health consequences of selling a kidney in India. JAMA 2002; 288: 1589–1593.

39. Singer PA, Siegler M, Lantos JD et al. Ethics of liver transplantation with living donors. N Engl J Med 1989; 321: 620–622.

Appendix: Photos

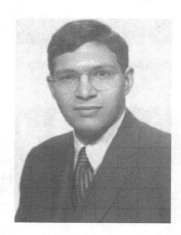

Photo 1 Dr. Siegler's University of Chicago Medical School graduation picture, 1967

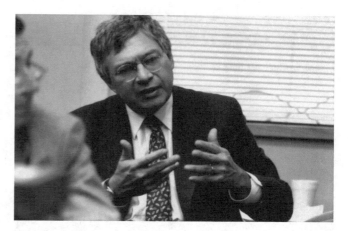

Photo 3 Drs. Ronald Miller and Mark Siegler, c. 1989

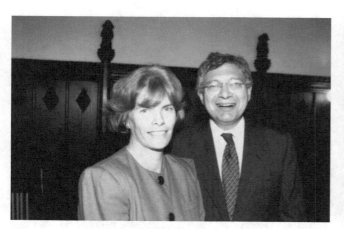

Photo 2 Anna Hollinger Siegler and Dr. Mark Siegler, c. 1975

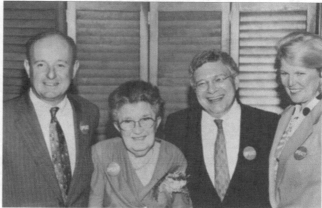

Photo 4 Dr. Siegler, Dorothy J. MacLean (Founder of the MacLean Center), Barry MacLean, and Mary Ann MacLean, c. 1989

© Springer International Publishing AG 2017
L.W. Roberts, M. Siegler (eds.), *Clinical Medical Ethics*, DOI 10.1007/978-3-319-53875-4

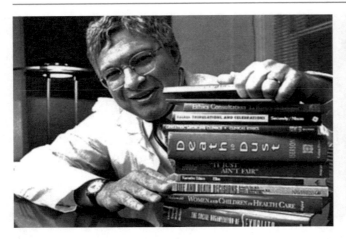

Photo 5 Clinical ethics by the book. Dr. Siegler, c. 1990

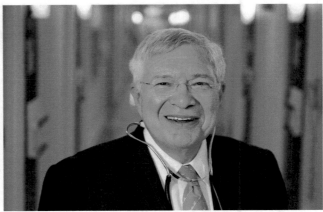

Photo 8 Dr. Siegler in the general medicine clinic, c. 2010

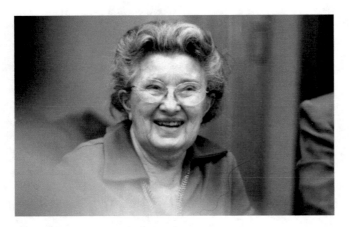

Photo 6 Dorothy Jean MacLean, MacLean Center Founder, c. 1991

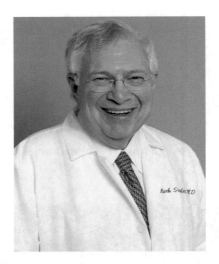

Photo 9 Dr. Siegler on rounds, c. 2010

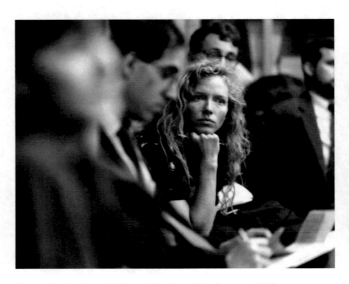

Photo 7 Dr. Laura Roberts, MacLean Conference, 1992

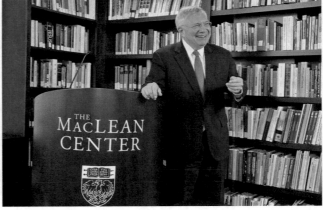

Photo 10 Dr. Siegler lecturing in the Clinical Ethics Fellowship, c. 2013

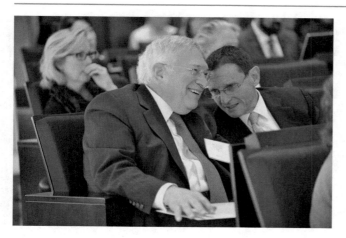

Photo 11 Dr. Mark Siegler and Dean Kenneth Polonsky, MacLean Conference, 2014

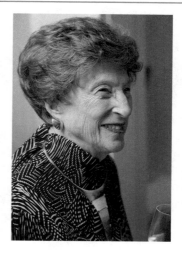

Photo 14 Carolyn Bucksbaum, founder of the Bucksbaum Institute for Clinical Excellence, c. 2015

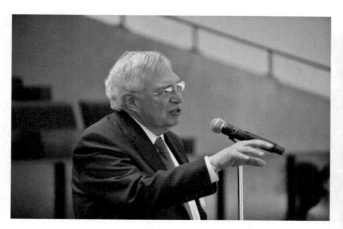

Photo 12 Dr. Siegler, MacLean Conference, 2014

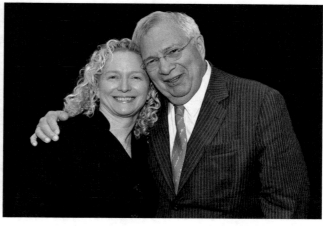

Photo 15 Drs. Laura Roberts and Mark Siegler, MacLean Conference, 2015

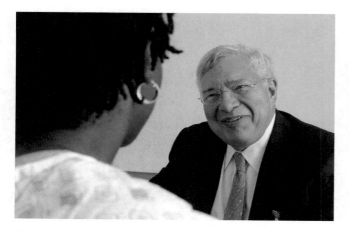

Photo 13 Dr. Siegler taking a patient's history, c. 2014

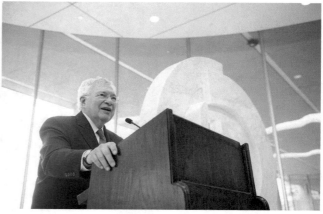

Photo 16 Dr. Siegler speaking at the dedication of the monumental marble sculpture *Caring*, commissioned by the Bucksbaum Institute for Clinical Excellence and created by Virginio Ferrari, 2015

Index